HANDBOOK OF LEARNING DISABILITIES

Also Available

Handbook on the Science of Early Literacy
Edited by Sonia Q. Cabell, Susan B. Neuman,
and Nicole Pattón Terry

Handbook of LEARNING DISABILITIES

THIRD EDITION

edited by
Cynthia M. Okolo
Nicole Patton Terry
Laurie E. Cutting

Foreword by Karen R. Harris,
H. Lee Swanson, and Steve Graham

THE GUILFORD PRESS
New York London

A Division of Guilford Publications, Inc.
www.guilford.com

Printed in the United States of America

This book is printed on acid-free paper.

For product and safety concerns within the EU, please contact *GPSR@taylorandfrancis.com,* Taylor & Francis Verlag GmbH, Kaufingerstraße 24, 80331 München, Germany.

Last digit is print number: 9 8 7 6 5 4 3 2 1

Library of Congress Cataloging-in-Publication Data is available from the publisher

ISBN 978-1-4625-5906-0 (paperback)
ISBN 978-1-4625-5907-7 (cloth)

About the Editors

Cynthia M. Okolo, PhD, is Professor Emeritus of Counseling, Educational Psychology, and Special Education at Michigan State University. Her research focuses on technology and literacy for students with mild disabilities, universal design for learning, and history instruction for students with learning challenges. Dr. Okolo is a former special education teacher, and her scholarship is rooted in applied issues related to instruction in inclusive classrooms. She has played a leadership role in numerous state, regional, and national boards and organizations; has directed undergraduate, master's, and doctoral programs; and has been a frequent contributor to the scholarly literature as an author and editor. Dr. Okolo is a recipient of the Lifetime Achievement Award from the Council for Exceptional Children.

Nicole Patton Terry, PhD, is the Olive and Manuel Bordas Professor of Education in the School of Teacher Education and Director of the Florida Center for Reading Research (FCRR) at Florida State University. She is the founding director of The Urban Child Study Center at Georgia State University and The Village at FCRR, two research entities where researchers collaborate with school and community partners to promote student success. Dr. Patton Terry's work focuses on young learners who are vulnerable to experiencing difficulty with language and literacy achievement in school, in particular, African American children, children growing up in poverty, and children with disabilities. A former special education teacher, she currently serves as president of the Society for the Scientific Study of Reading and is a Fellow of the American Speech–Language–Hearing Association and the American Educational Research Association.

Laurie E. Cutting, PhD, is the Patricia and Rodes Hart Professor of Neuroscience in the Departments of Special Education, Psychology and Human Development,

Radiology, Pediatrics, and Electrical and Computer Engineering at Vanderbilt University. She is also Associate Director of the Vanderbilt Kennedy Center, a member of the Vanderbilt Brain Institute, and training faculty for Vanderbilt's Neuroscience PhD program, and was the recipient of the 2017–2018 Joe B. Wyatt Distinguished University Professorship. Dr. Cutting recently completed a 2-year assignment as Associate Provost in the Office of the Vice Provost for Research and Innovation. Her work focuses on brain–behavior relations in children and adolescents, with a particular emphasis on academic and cognitive development.

Contributors

Heba Z. Abdelnaby, PhD, Department of Special Education, College of Education and Human Development, University of Missouri, Columbia, Missouri

Suzanne M. Adlof, PhD, Department of Communication Sciences and Disorders, University of South Carolina, Columbia, South Carolina

Stephanie Al Otaiba, PhD, Annette Caldwell Simmons School of Education and Human Development, Southern Methodist University, Dallas, Texas

Tim T. Andress, PhD, Department of Special Education and Communication Disorders, University of Nebraska, Omaha, Omaha, Nebraska

Alfredo J. Artiles, PhD, Department of Education, Stanford Graduate School of Education, Stanford University, Stanford, California

Marcia A. Barnes, PhD, Department of Special Education, Peabody College of Education and Human Development, Vanderbilt University, Nashville, Tennessee

Amber E. Benedict, PhD, Mary Lou Fulton College for Teaching and Learning Innovation, Arizona State University, Tempe, Arizona

Mary T. Brownell, PhD, Collaboration for Effective Educator Development, Accountability, and Reform Center, University of Florida, Gainesville, Florida

Matthew K. Burns, PhD, Department of Special Education, University of Florida, Gainesville, Florida

Philip Capin, PhD, Department of Education, Graduate School of Education, Harvard University, Cambridge, Massachusetts

Nathan H. Clemens, EdD, Department of Special Education, The University of Texas at Austin, Austin, Texas

Donald L. Compton, PhD, Florida Center for Reading Research, Florida State University, Tallahassee, Florida

Bryan G. Cook, PhD, Department of Special Education, School of Education and Human Development, University of Virginia, Charlottesville, Virginia

Michael D. Coyne, PhD, Department of Special Education, Neag School of Education, University of Connecticut, Storrs, Connecticut

Laurie E. Cutting, PhD, Departments of Special Education, Psychology, and Human Development, Vanderbilt University, Nashville, Tennessee

Susan De La Paz, PhD, Department of Special Education, College of Education, University of Maryland, College Park, College Park, Maryland

McKinzie D. Duesenberg-Marshall, PhD, Thrive Child Psychology, Bloomington, Illinois

Ashley A. Edwards, PhD, Florida Center for Reading Research, Florida State University, Tallahassee, Florida

Daniel Espinas, PhD, Department of Special Education, George Mason University, Fairfax, Virginia

Emily A. Farris, PhD, Meadows Center for Preventing Educational Risk, The University of Texas at Austin, Austin, Texas

Amy L. Ferrell, PhD, Department of Special Education, School of Education and Human Development, University of Colorado Denver, Denver, Colorado

Laura L. Feuerborn, PhD, School of Education, University of Washington Tacoma, Tacoma, Washington

Jesse I. Fleming, PhD, Department of Special Education, Mary Lou Fulton College for Teaching and Learning Innovation, Arizona State University, Tempe, Arizona

Jack M. Fletcher, PhD, Department of Psychology, Texas Institute for Measurement, Evaluation, and Statistics (TIMES), University of Houston, Houston, Texas

Sally K. Fluhler, PhD, Department of Special Education, The University of Texas at Austin, Austin, Texas

Douglas Fuchs, PhD, Department of Psychology and Human Development, Vanderbilt University, Nashville, Tennessee

Lynn S. Fuchs, PhD (deceased), Department of Psychology and Human Development, Vanderbilt University, Nashville, Tennessee

Allison Gruner Gandhi, EdD, American Institutes for Research (AIR), Arlington, Virginia

Kelly-Ann Gesuelli, PhD, Institute for Educational Initiatives, University of Notre Dame, Notre Dame, Indiana

Steve Goodman, PhD, Center on Positive Behavioral Interventions and Supports, Arlington, Virginia

Steve Graham, PhD, Division of Leadership and Innovation, Mary Lou Fulton College for Teacher Training and Learning Innovation, Arizona State University, Tempe, Arizona

Barbara A. Gueldner, PhD, private practice, Steamboat Springs, Colorado

Nuria Gutiérrez, PhD, Florida Center for Reading Research, Florida State University, Tallahassee, Florida

Emily M. Harriott, BS, Department of Educational Neuroscience, Peabody College of Education and Human Development, Vanderbilt University, Nashville, Tennessee

Karen R. Harris, EdD, Mary Lou Fulton College for Teacher Training and Learning Innovation, Arizona State University, Tempe, Arizona

Nancy C. Jordan, EdD, Department of Education, University of Delaware, Newark, Delaware

Rachel L. Juergensen, PhD, Department of Special Education, Delaware State University, Dover, Delaware

Jennifer E. Kong, PhD, Department of Special Education, Attallah College of Educational Studies, Chapman University, Irvine, California

Kathleen Lynne Lane, PhD, Department of Special Education, University of Kansas, Lawrence, Kansas

Melinda M. Leko, PhD, Collaboration for Effective Educator Development, Accountability, and Reform Center, University of Florida, Gainesville, Florida

Erica S. Lembke, PhD, Department of Special Education, University of Missouri, Columbia, Missouri

Alexa Levison, MA, Karuna House, LLC, Perrysburg, Ohio

Susan M. Loftus-Rattan, PhD, Acadience Learning, Eugene, Oregon

Nancy C. Marencin, PhD, Department of Communication Sciences and Disorders, University of South Florida, Tampa, Florida

Jeremy Miciak, PhD, Department of Psychology, Texas Institute for Measurement, Evaluation, and Statistics (TIMES), University of Houston, Houston, Texas

Anna E. Middleton, PhD, Luke Waites Center for Dyslexia and Learning Disorders at Scottish Rite for Children, Dallas, Texas

Dana Miller-Cotto, PhD, School of Education, University of California, Berkeley, Berkeley, California

Timothy N. Odegard, PhD, Department of Psychology, Middle Tennessee State University, Murfreesboro, Tennessee

Josue Otarola, PhD, Department of Counseling, Higher Education, and Special Education, College of Education, University of Maryland, College Park, College Park, Maryland

Peng Peng, PhD, Department of Special Education, College of Education, The University of Texas at Austin, Austin, Texas

Stephen A. Petrill, PhD, Department of Psychology, The Ohio State University, Columbus, Ohio

Valeria M. Rigobon, PhD, Australian Centre for the Advancement of Literacy, Australian Catholic University, Sydney, Australia

Sheryl Rimrodt-Frierson, PhD, Luke Waites Center for Dyslexia and Learning Disorders at Scottish Rite for Children, Dallas, Texas

Monica E. Romero, PhD, Educational Psychology Department, The University of Texas at Austin, Austin, Texas

William Romine, PhD, Department of Biology, Wright State University, Dayton, Ohio

Dayna Russell Freudenthal, PhD, Department of Education, Mount Saint Joseph University, Cincinnati, Ohio

Ashley M. Adams Sanabria, PhD, Department of Speech, Language, and Hearing Sciences, San Diego State University, San Diego, California

Katherine Sargent, PhD, Department of Special Education, Indiana University South Bend, South Bend, Indiana

Pamela M. Seethaler, PhD, Department of Psychology and Human Development, Vanderbilt University, Nashville, Tennessee

Sarah W. Siegal, PhD, School of Education, University of California, Irvine, Irvine, California

Brandi Simonsen, PhD, Department of Special Education, Neag School of Education, University of Connecticut, Storrs, Connecticut

Cassandra M. Smith, PhD, Department of Special Education, College of Education and Human Development, University of Missouri, Columbia, Missouri

Laura M. Steacy, PhD, Florida Center for Reading Research, Florida State University, Tallahassee, Florida

H. Lee Swanson, PhD, Department of Educational Psychology, College of Education, University of New Mexico, Albuquerque, New Mexico

William J. Therrien, PhD, Department of Special Education, School of Education and Human Development, University of Virginia, Charlottesville, Virginia

Ashli D. Tyre, EdD, Department of School Psychology, Seattle University, Seattle, Washington

Delinda van Garderen, PhD, Department of Special Education, College of Education and Human Development, University of Missouri, Columbia, Missouri

Rebecca M. Vasile, BS, Florida Center for Reading Research, Florida State University, Tallahassee, Florida

Sharon Vaughn, PhD, The Meadows Center for Preventing Educational Risk, The University of Texas at Austin, Austin, Texas

Lesly Wade-Woolley, PhD, Educational Psychology Department, University of Alberta, Edmonton, Alberta, Canada

Hoi Ting Wan, MEd, Department of School Psychology, University of Missouri, Columbia, Missouri

Jeanne Wanzek, PhD, Department of Special Education, Peabody College, Vanderbilt University, Nashville, Tennessee

Julie A. Washington, PhD, Department of Language Science, School of Education, University of California, Irvine, Irvine, California

Erik G. Willcutt, PhD, Department of Psychology and Neuroscience, University of Colorado Boulder, Boulder, Colorado

Daniel R. Wissinger, PhD, Department of Education, Indiana University of Pennsylvania, Indiana, Pennsylvania

Vivian C. Wong, PhD, Department of Research, Statistics, and Evaluation, School of Education and Human Development, University of Virginia, Charlottesville, Virginia

Mai W. Zaru, PhD, Department of Education, Annette Caldwell Simmons School of Education and Human Development, Southern Methodist University, Dallas, Texas

Foreword

As Torgesen (1991, pp. 30–31) stated,

> *The field of learning disabilities is presently a strong and vital force within the larger special and regular education communities. Its services, which are mandated by law, are offered to vast numbers of children with a variety of very difficult and unusual educational problems. Professionals in the field have organized themselves into strong associations that provide adequate means for communication about research and professional issues. Research in the area is growing and becoming more diverse, and many new research initiatives are being supported by governmental agencies . . . [However,] science is raising fundamental questions about the nature of learning disabilities, and educational politics are challenging current methods of service delivery. One of the most serious challenges . . . as many acknowledge, arises from the likely overutilization of the LD label to provide services to a wide variety of children for whom special services are not otherwise available . . . Educational politics and scientific concerns have become very complex and we have many thorny questions facing us. The only firm prediction I can offer is that the coming decade should prove very interesting indeed.*

Wong (1991) quoted two leading scholars in the field of learning disabilities (LD):

> *In our quest to provide effective, appropriate services to students who have learning disabilities, we must preserve and strengthen the framework established to protect the rights of students who were once denied access to a free, appropriate public education . . . The challenge is development and reliable implementation of effective, research-based interventions within the structure of each model [of service delivery]. As Meyen (1990, p. 13) commented:*
>
>> *If instruction that is appropriate to the needs of learners who have exceptionalities is the purpose of special education, then the profession must discipline itself to invest in developing interventions that make a difference in how students learn. (Kauffman & Trent, 1991, pp. 477–478)*

As we began to think about and plan this Foreword for the third edition of the *Handbook of Learning Disabilities*, we reviewed articles and texts about the history of our field as well as the first two volumes of the *Handbook of Learning Disabilities*. The roots of our field go back to the 1800s and research on the effects of brain injury on language, reading, spelling, behavior, and more; definitions of and research on "dyslexia," a term that appeared in 1884; and early and ongoing fights for social justice (e.g., Hallahan & Mock, 2003; Hallahan et al., 2013; Johnson & Myklebust, 1967; Morgan, 1896; Pelka, 2012). Use of the term *LD* evolved over time and first appeared in print in 1962 (Hallahan & Mock, 2003).

Torgesen (1991) accurately predicted that the decade following 1991 would prove "very interesting indeed," as has each decade that followed. The quote above highlights many of the challenges facing the field of LD early on. Many of these same challenges continue today, although we have come a long way in each of these areas. Kauffman and Trent (1991) identified the crucial challenge of developing effective and evidence-based interventions for students with LD. This is also an area where the field has made impressive strides, although more remains to be done.

So much was happening in the field of LD that a handbook was needed to help bring together advancements being made across multiple areas. We agreed to edit the first *Handbook of Learning Disabilities* in 2001 with The Guilford Press, which came out in 2003, and the second edition of the *Handbook of Learning Disabilities,* published in 2013. The first and second editions were organized across areas that reflect the epigraphs above: Foundations and Current Perspectives, Causes and Behavioral Manifestations, Effective Instruction and Formation of Instruction Models (Domain-Specific Instruction/Intervention Research and General Instructional Models in the second edition), and Methodology (Measurement and Methodology in the second edition). By 2020, it was time for new editors to undertake the third volume of the *Handbook of Learning Disabilities*.

We were delighted and excited when this powerful team of researchers and scholars in LD, Drs. Cynthia M. Okolo, Nicole Patton Terry, and Laurie E. Cutting, agreed to develop and edit the current third edition of the *Handbook of Learning Disabilities*. Each a leader in the field of LD, they have carefully crafted one of the most valuable resources we have in understanding the challenges and progress being made in the field of LD today. They have gathered a team of impressive scholars for the chapters in this book. The third edition is divided into three parts: Causes, Correlates, and Manifestations of Learning Disabilities; Instructional Interventions; and Future Directions in Learning Disabilities. The current chapter authors address many of the areas of research and practice included in the first two editions of the *Handbook*, but also expand the scope of the *Handbook*, making this third edition a must-read.

The development and publication of any handbook is a significant challenge, one that these editors and authors have met. Strong handbooks also require collaboration with a representative or Senior Editor for the publisher. This person must be organized, highly knowledgeable in the field, able to provide feedback and support, and truly care about the book being developed. Chris Jennison, Senior

Education Editor for The Guilford Press during the development of the first edition of the *Handbook of Learning Disabilities,* was outstanding in this role. Rochelle Serwator, Senior Editor in Special Education at The Guilford Press, worked with us and the current editorial team with grace and dedication on the second and third editions.

The third edition of the *Handbook of Learning Disabilities* is a critical and outstanding contribution to our field and all who are deeply committed to individuals with LD. Our appreciation and thanks go out to all who have made this happen.

Karen R. Harris, PhD
Regents Professor Emeritus
Mary Lou Fulton College
for Teaching and Learning Innovation
Arizona State University

H. Lee Swanson, PhD
Research Professor
Department of Educational Psychology
University of New Mexico

Steve Graham, PhD
Regents Professor and the Warner Professor
in the Division of Leadership and Innovation
at Mary Lou Fulton College for Teaching
and Learning Innovation
Arizona State University

REFERENCES

Hallahan, D. P., & Mock, D. R. (2003). A brief history of the field of learning disabilities. In L. Swanson, K. R. Harris, & S. Graham (Eds.), *Handbook of learning disabilities* (pp. 16–29). Guilford Press.

Hallahan, D. P., Pullen, P., & Ward, D. (2013). A brief history of the field of learning disabilities. In L. Swanson, K. R. Harris, & S. Graham (Eds.), *Handbook of learning disabilities* (2nd ed., pp. 405–438). Guilford Press.

Johnson, D. J. & Myklebust, H. R. (1967). *LD: Educational principles and practices.* Grune & Stratton.

Kauffman, J. M., & Trent, S. C. (1991). Issues in service delivery for students with learning disabilities. In B. Y. L. Wong (Ed.), *Learning about learning disabilities* (pp. 477–478). Academic Press.

Morgan, W. P. (1896). A case of congenital word blindness. *British Medical Journal, 2,* 1378.

Pelka, F. (2012). *What we have done: An oral history of the disability rights movement.* University of Massachusetts Press.

Torgesen, J. K. (1991). Learning disabilities: Historical and conceptual issues. In B. Y. L. Wong (Ed.), *Learning about learning disabilities* (pp. 30–31). Academic Press.

Wong, B. Y. L. (Ed.). (1991). *Learning about learning disabilities.* Academic Press.

Preface

We were delighted to accept an offer to coedit the third *Handbook of Learning Disabilities*. As you might expect, we also experienced some trepidation, as we are following in the footsteps of H. Lee Swanson, Karen R. Harris, and Steve Graham, coeditors of the first and second editions. We are extremely grateful for the contributions that these researchers have and continue to make to our field. And we are thankful for their generous assistance with this edition.

Since the publication of the second edition, we have seen major upheavals in social, economic, and political institutions and practices. Technology has evolved in ways we could not have predicted, ushering in developments that can have a positive impact on all of society, as well as introducing serious concerns about the future of human agency. Global concern for climate change has led to international cooperation and scientific advancements. The Black Lives Matter movement drew attention to diversity, equity, and inclusion, and the #MeToo movement brought international attention to sexual harassment and abuse. The worldwide pandemic brought the world to a stop, requiring educators, students, and families to pivot to technology-based remote education. All of these developments, and many more, have had an impact on education and services for students with learning disabilities (LD).

Over these years, the fields of special education and related disciplines have both matured and expanded. The reader will find continuities as well as fascinating new developments in this edition of the *Handbook*. As was the tradition in the first two editions, we have invited renowned scholars to write about topics best aligned with their expertise. Authors were asked to situate their own research programs in the larger context of knowledge, developments, and practices in the field of LD. The result is a third edition comprised of 25 chapters that cover, arguably, the most important contemporary issues in our community of scholars and practitioners. Evident in many of the chapters is the evolution of topics with a long history in the field, including diagnosis, cognitive processes, effective instructional practices, and assessment and progress monitoring. As the reader will see, the systematic nature of the authors' research programs is impressive. One can trace the development of increasingly nuanced and sophisticated scholarship and refined approaches to intervention, all aimed at better understanding and improving outcomes for individuals with LD.

New lines of research also are represented in the *Handbook*. Advances in neuroimaging, gene sequencing, big data, and artificial intelligence approaches have led to breakthroughs in studies of the brain and cognitive processes, research regarding risk factors for disability, and new approaches to knowledge production and synthesis—among other topics.

This edition of the *Handbook* is divided into three parts, which we discuss in turn below. We did not differentiate domain-specific instructional practices from general instructional models, as our predecessors did. Most chapters about instructional interventions in this edition discussed both domain-specific (e.g., mathematics word problem solving) and general instructional models (e.g., self-regulated strategy development). Nor did we attempt to assemble a set of chapters about methods and methodology, as these topics are woven throughout most of the chapters in the context of specific research questions and the approaches used to investigate them.

In Part I, Causes, Correlates, and Manifestations of Learning Disabilities, ten chapters address the diagnosis and characteristics of learning disabilities. In Part II, Instructional Interventions, eight chapters focus on research about teaching and learning in literacy, mathematics, and content area subjects. These chapters also offer detailed explanations of research-based instructional interventions. Finally, Part III, Future Directions in Learning Disabilities, is comprised of seven chapters that offer insights into emerging and future trends such as dyslexia law, teacher education, and crowdsourcing research.

In conclusion, we cannot begin to do justice to the theoretical and empirical richness of these chapters. We encourage the reader to take a deep dive into the wealth of information contained in each. Research and practice will continue to evolve, despite the challenges and changes that have beset education and society. We are curious about what the next edition of the *Handbook of Learning Disabilities* might have to say.

Contents

PART I

CAUSES, CORRELATES, AND MANIFESTATIONS OF LEARNING DISABILITIES

This part provides in-depth coverage of diagnosis and characteristics of learning disorders. In Chapter 1, Miciak and Fletcher examine current research and practices related to classification and diagnosis. The authors review controversies surrounding the construct of LD and explicate the challenges inherent in its classification, identification, and definition. The use of, support for, and reliability and validity of a variety of identification frameworks are discussed. These include aptitude–achievement discrepancy, patterns of cognitive strengths and weaknesses, and instructional response. The chapter concludes with the presentation of the Texas Center for Learning Disabilities' treatment-oriented, "hybrid" approach to the identification of LD, which characterizes LD as an instructional problem that meets three criteria: (1) evidence for low achievement, (2) evidence of inadequate instructional response, and (3) evidence to rule out exclusionary factors contraindicative of LD. The authors acknowledge that challenges to reliable identification of LD will not be solved by a hybrid approach but contend that reducing focus on eligibility and foregrounding instructional planning is likely to reduce the harms of LD identification.

In Chapter 2, Compton, Steacy, Rigobon, Edwards, Gutiérrez, Marencin, and Vasile discuss the processes that early readers undergo to develop high-quality orthographic representations upon which fluent word reading is based. The authors provide a detailed explanation of orthographic learning and the essential role it plays in skilled reading, as well as the sources of knowledge needed to support an orthographic lexicon. The key roles of precision and redundancy in orthographic learning, as well as the regularity of an orthography and the symmetry between one's native language and English, are discussed in detail. Throughout the chapter, the authors discuss orthographic learning challenges faced by English learners (ELs), speakers of nonmainstream American English, and students with dyslexia. The authors conclude the chapter with recommendations for helping these learners develop high-quality orthographic representations through systematic attention to the relations between orthography, phonology, and semantics.

In Chapter 3, Jordan, Miller-Cotto, and Gesuelli address mathematics learning difficulties among elementary school learners. Reporting that alarmingly few students with disabilities score proficient on national assessments, the authors present data showing how mathematics difficulties disadvantage students' future educational and employment opportunities as well as their everyday lives. The authors document how mathematical knowledge, concepts, and procedures are supported by three domain-general cognitive processes: the central executive system, the visual–spatial system, and the language system. The authors discuss each of these in turn and explicate the processes within each system and how difficulties in each impact mathematical proficiency.

Following a detailed discussion of arithmetic and word problem skills among students who struggle with mathematics, the authors describe screening procedures to identify students at risk for mathematics learning difficulties and document the importance of early intervention. They describe their empirically validated Fraction Sense Intervention, which embodies evidence-based principles of effective mathematics instruction. The authors commend the growth of rigorous research about mathematics but note the need for additional studies with learners in middle grades and above, as well as further investigation of the value of integrating general cognitive training into mathematics interventions.

Although there is considerable variability in reports, social–emotional challenges may affect between one-third and three-quarters of students with LD. In Chapter 4, Feuerborn, Gueldner, and Tyre first describe the impact of social–emotional competence on overall health, relationships, employment, and other outcomes throughout the lifespan. Research shows that social–emotional skills can be taught, spurring the growth of school-based social–emotional learning (SEL) programs. With roots in diverse fields, including education, psychology, and neuroscience, the authors note that there are many different frameworks, approaches, and terms for SEL. They base their chapter on the framework developed by CASEL (Collaborative for Academic, Social, and Emotional Learning), which is inclusive of knowledge, skills, attitudes, identities, emotions, empathy, goal setting, relationships, responsibility, and caring. The framework gives explicit attention to equity, social justice, and inclusion and addresses values and skills in both collectivist and individualistic societies. The authors discuss how LD can affect social–emotional competence and note that further investigation of relationships among different types of LD (e.g., reading, math, and comorbid attention-deficit/hyperactivity disorder [ADHD]) might be useful in clarifying the degree to which these students experience social–emotional challenges.

The authors review research about both strengths and weaknesses among students with LD in five key areas: self-awareness, self-management, social awareness, relationship skills, and responsible decision making. They detail SEL approaches and programs that have been evaluated in school-based programs for students with disabilities and then set SEL efforts in the larger context of school climate, relationships, and partnerships. The chapter concludes with a detailed discussion of SEL assessment, specifically within the multi-tiered system of support (MTSS) framework, and a plea for a better understanding of SEL-related needs, attributes, and strengths for students with LD.

In Chapter 5, "Cognitive Processes, Neuroscience, and Learning Disabilities," Harriott and Cutting examine the cognitive and neurobiological foundations of reading and math disabilities, highlighting their impact on individuals and society. Reading disabilities, particularly dyslexia and Specific Reading Comprehension Disorder (S-RCD), involve distinct deficits in word recognition and text comprehension. The Simple View of Reading (SVR) model explains reading as the product of decoding and language comprehension, with neurobiological research identifying key brain regions such as the left occipitotemporal, temporoparietal, and inferior frontal regions. Individuals with dyslexia show reduced activation in these areas, while those with S-RCD exhibit deficits in language and memory-related brain functions. The chapter underscores the long-term consequences of reading difficulties, including academic failure, mental health challenges, and societal costs, and introduces a new neurobiological model of reading that captures word-, sentence-, and discourse-level processing, as well as executive functions (EFs).

The authors then review the neurobiological correlates of math disabilities, which involve deficits in numerical cognition, working memory, and executive function. They review the triple code model, which identifies three key components of math processing: numerical representation, visuospatial skills, and verbal processing. Neuroimaging studies highlight the role of the intraparietal sulci, prefrontal cortex, and inferior temporal cortex in math cognition, with individuals with math disabilities displaying functional abnormalities in these regions. The authors also explore the frequent comorbidity between reading and math disabilities, suggesting shared cognitive and neurobiological mechanisms. The chapter closes with a call for further research to refine diagnostic criteria, improve early intervention strategies, and develop targeted educational support for affected individuals.

In Chapter 6, "Genetics, Learning Abilities, and Disabilities," Petrill and Levison discuss the considerable advancement in genetic studies of LD and other learning and behavioral challenges over the past two decades. This literature is complex, but the authors do not assume extensive prior knowledge of the reader and provide an overview of genetic models with an accompanying table of definitions. They then present two approaches to genetic studies of LD: behavioral genetics and molecular. Describing the relevant methods that characterize each of these approaches, they review studies that have been conducted using them. The first category, behavioral genetics, relies on the relatedness of family members to estimate the degree to which underlying genetic characteristics account for observable characteristics (e.g., reading disability, LD, and

ADHD). Molecular genetics, made feasible after the human genome was fully sequenced in 2003, can directly examine the impact of DNA differences.

The many studies reviewed by the authors present considerable evidence of the substantial heritability of reading disability and LD while also showing the influences of biological and environmental mediators. The authors conclude with a look toward future directions, such as the development of ways to identify risk sooner, the design of environments that ameliorate those risks, and better differentiation of instruction to remediate or prevent reading and learning disabilities. They also describe the many challenges that remain before research can reliably and appropriately be translated into practice.

In Chapter 7, "Executive Functions and Learning Disabilities," Barnes and Peng review bodies of research and note that studies of EFs have burgeoned across the last three decades and are now dispersed across a range of disciplines, including special education. The authors provide a review of the history of EFs, a discussion of conceptual and measurement models, and a review of research about the role of EFs in academic performance for students with LD. The authors review meta-analyses of the relations between EFs and reading and theoretical models and individual studies of EFs and written expression.

The authors explicate the considerable variability across the literature in definitions of EFs and the number and nature of EF subcomponents. This variability poses significant challenges to synthesizing theory and research. Additionally, the authors note that EF deficits are associated with many different learning and behavioral disorders and are not limited to LD, raising empirical questions about the value of EFs in LD diagnosis while still highlighting their potential importance in the design of interventions.

In Chapter 8, "Memory Difficulties in Children with Specific Learning Disabilities," Swanson and Kong review meta-analyses of research that link LD in reading and other areas to working memory (WM) and short-term memory (STM). Research findings consistently show deficits in both WM and STM among students with reading, math, and both reading and mathematics disabilities. They note that fMRI studies support their conclusions and highlight that some of the regions of the brain that have an overlapping role in reading and mathematics are also involved in the executive processing component of WM.

The authors then present their research about the characteristics of three working memory components in students with LD: visual–spatial sketchpad, phonological loop, and central executive (Baddeley, 2012; Baddeley & Logie, 1999). Briefly, this body of research shows that students with math and reading disabilities have deficits in the phonological loop related to accurate and fluent access to speech codes in STM and in the executive system related to monitoring the processing and storage while concurrently suppressing irrelevant information. However, individuals with reading and mathematics disabilities in these studies do not have deficits in all aspects of the phonological loop or the executive system. In fact, they demonstrate intact abilities related to spontaneous speech and oral language comprehension (related to the processing of the phonological loop) and do not show deficits in planning (a function of the executive system).

The authors conclude the chapter by highlighting two foci of their current research. The first set is an investigation of English language learners (ELLs) exploring whether the role of memory processes involved in reading and second language acquisition is limited to the phonological domain and whether the similarities in cognitive processes underlie difficulties in second language acquisition and monolingual students' reading and math disabilities. The second area of investigation explores the identification and design of interventions for children with WM difficulties. The authors conclude with a review of challenges, limitations, and contradictions in bodies of research about WM and lay out questions for future research to resolve.

In Chapter 9, "Language Development, Developmental Language Disorder, and Reading Disabilities," Adlof and Wade-Woolley address developmental language disorder (DLD), which is characterized by difficulties in producing and understanding spoken language. Children with DLD usually display weakness across multiple aspects of language, including phonology, morphology, syntax, vocabulary, and discourse. The authors cite studies that report 7–9% of 5-year-olds have DLD but are underidentified for speech and language services. Early identification and intervention are important, as the authors report that DLD is likely to have a stronger negative impact when unidentified after 5 years of age. Furthermore, research shows that, for many students, oral language impairments are particularly disadvantageous as text becomes more complex in the upper elementary grades.

Illustrating the characteristics and impact of DLD, the authors provide three case studies of children who have participated in their past studies. In presenting an interpretation of each case, they illustrate the variability in profiles of students with DLD and the different intervention approaches that fit each profile. Unresolved issues in the education of students with DLD include minimal awareness, lack of appropriate screening, the delay between the time students appear to be at risk until the time they meet criteria for services, disproportionalities in identification and intervention, and limited knowledge and resources for the identification of learners who speak languages and dialects other than general American English.

In Chapter 10, "Learning Disabilities and Comorbidity: Prevalence, Etiology, and Implications," Willcutt provides a nuanced examination of LDs in reading, mathematics, and writing, with a focus on their comorbidity with ADHD and other psychological disorders. This comorbidity presents a complex challenge, affecting the interpretation of research, the efficacy of treatments, and the degree of functional impairment experienced by individuals. Drawing from extensive data from the Colorado Learning Disabilities Research Center (CLDRC) and the International Longitudinal Twin Study of Early Reading and Attention (ILTSERD), the author offers in-depth cross-sectional and longitudinal analyses, revealing the profound and enduring impact of comorbid LDs on both academic performance and nonacademic domains of life, such as social relationships and work performance.

The chapter further explores the etiology of these comorbidities, proposing that they may arise from shared genetic and environmental influences, which manifest as cognitive processing weaknesses that are common to RD, MD, and ADHD. Contrary to previous models that posited a single cognitive deficit underlying each disorder, contemporary research suggests that multiple neurocognitive deficits contribute to the development of LDs, requiring a multifaceted approach to diagnosis and intervention. The author emphasizes the importance of comprehensive clinical assessments that screen for a wide range of academic difficulties and associated psychopathologies to ensure that all comorbid conditions are identified and addressed. The author also highlights the need for interventions that are responsive to the presence of comorbid conditions and ongoing research to better understand the early risk factors that may predispose individuals to develop comorbid LDs, the specific cognitive weaknesses that underlie these disorders, and how these factors influence long-term outcomes.

CHAPTER 1

Classification and Definition of Learning Disabilities

A Hybrid Approach to Identification

Jeremy Miciak and Jack M. Fletcher

This chapter addresses the classification, definition, and related identification processes for learning disabilities (LD). It begins with an overview of classification research, which provides a framework for understanding and comparing the reliability, validity, and utility of different conceptual frameworks for LD, which is the primary focus of this chapter. Questions underlying the classification and definition of LD have important implications in research and practice. In practice, identification with LD is one of the most common mechanisms by which children receive specialized instruction and services in the United States and internationally. Thus, the reliability and validity of the diagnostic methods employed to identify individual students with LD address important questions of fairness and access. Within educational and psychological research, students with LD represent a frequent subgroup for study with overarching questions about the neurobiological and educational characteristics of students with LD, as well as questions about effective methods to reliably identify and treat students with LD. Careful scrutiny of the assumptions underlying different conceptual frameworks of LD, as well as the criteria by which individuals are identified with LD within a specific research study, is necessary to evaluate the external validity, or generalizability, of its findings.

LD in Context

The construct of LD has long been controversial, with active debate regarding the best ways to treat and identify LDs and extending to questions about the basic scientific validity of the construct (Elliott & Grigorenko, 2014; Fletcher & Miciak,

2017; Schneider & Kaufman, 2017). Despite these controversies, the conceptual basis and definition remain largely consistent: LD represents "unexpected" underachievement in one or more academic domains (Fletcher et al., 2019). That students with LD experience underachievement in the academic domains of reading, writing, or mathematics is uncontroversial; academic difficulties represent a necessary (but not sufficient) inclusion criteria for any conception of LD.

The question of what makes observed underachievement "unexpected" is fraught with controversy. This controversy is frequently framed as disagreement about the most reliable and valid methods to identify individual students with LD, but often extends to foundational disagreements about the nature of LD, which we review in this chapter. For much of the past 50 years, LD has represented underachievement that is unexpected due to higher intellectual or cognitive capacity (Mercer & Hallahan, 2002). Throughout this chapter, we refer to this approach and more modern instantiations as cognitive discrepancy frameworks for LD. We contrast this with an instructional framework for LD, an approach that has taken increased prominence in research and practice on LD—although not without controversies of its own (Fuchs et al., 2010; Hale et al., 2010). Within an instructional framework, underachievement is unexpected because it occurs despite the provision of generally effective instruction (Fletcher et al., 2019). All approaches to LD identification presume the absence of other conditions that might negatively impact academic achievement, such as sensory disorders, intellectual disabilities, and other pervasive disorders of development, behavioral disorders, or environmental factors, such as limited educational opportunity, poverty, or minority language status, commonly referred to as *exclusionary criteria*.

Seeds of the conceptual controversies around LD can be traced to the historical origins of the construct (Mercer & Hallahan, 2002). Historically, much of the early advocacy and legislation addressing LDs emerged during the civil rights era, as part of a worldwide disability rights movement. Early advocates obtained significant victories for children with diverse learning differences, including children with moderate to pervasive difficulties such as intellectual disabilities and sensory disorders, as well as more specific learning difficulties such as LD and speech and language impairments. In the United States, the most important of these victories was adoption of Public Law 94-142, The Education for All Handicapped Children Act (later renamed the Individuals with Disabilities Education Act). Since adoption, this law and its reauthorizations have mandated outreach and services and provided legal protections for millions of vulnerable children. Further, it has solidified the notion of LD in public consciousness as a real disorder with a significant impact on education and public health (Grigorenko et al., 2020). However, it must also be acknowledged that the situation of LD in a legal and civil rights framework has at times served to complicate or obscure fundamental characteristics of the disorder, further fomenting controversies. For example, individual identification as a gateway to service has placed undue emphasis on identification processes and encouraged categorical conceptions of LD as an intrinsic, qualitative difference among learners that is immutable. In fact, our best evidence indicates that LD is none of these things. Additionally, the prominence of legislation and statute in shaping conceptions of LD has often served to conflate the legal construct of LD with its underlying scientific construct. Although legislators are well within their rights to put forth whatever definition of LD they wish, scientists must rely on empirical observation to demonstrate the reliability, validity, and utility of their classification, definition, and operational definition. In the section that follows, we describe several features of LD that often stand in contrast to public (and occasionally scientific) understanding of the disorder. Additionally, we identify key areas of disagreement about the nature of LD, which we trace to conceptual disagreements about the hypothetical classification itself. We then propose a framework by which to evaluate these disagreements based on different conceptions of LD.

Challenges for Classification, Definition, and Identification

A classification is a framework by which we partition a larger group of entities into a smaller, more homogeneous subgroup based on similarities and dissimilarities on some identified set of attributes. Classifications represent hypotheses about the organization of observed phenomena, which can be evaluated based on the extent to which observed phenomena conform to the proposed classification hypothesis. Although often conflated, classifications are distinct from definitions, which represent a clear statement of what attributes the classification includes and excludes. A definition is derived from a classification hypothesis. Both classifications and definitions are abstractions. To evaluate these abstractions, we must put forth an operational definition, which explicitly states the measurable attributes that mark boundaries for a disorder. That operational definition can be utilized for identification or diagnosis, the process by which individuals (or groups of individuals) are placed in subgroups demonstrating the disorder (LD) or not (not LD). For example, our operational definition might state that to be identified with LD, a student must demonstrate a 1.5 standard deviation discrepancy between their measured full-scale IQ and a measure of their current academic functioning, in addition to excluding other potential causes of low achievement (e.g., lack of educational opportunity, second language acquisition, and other exclusionary criteria). This operational definition provides sufficient detail that individuals (or groups of individuals) can be identified as demonstrating or not demonstrating the disorder, which is fundamentally a categorical decision based on the criteria that leads to the formation of groups with and without the presumed attributes of LD.

The Attributes of LD Are Continuous

Although the decision about the presence of LD is categorical and related to resource allocation or group comparisons used in research, the attributes on which this categorical decision is based are continuous (and often correlated) with no clear demarcation that would mark disordered versus not disordered. For example, reading and math represent the two most common academic domains in which an individual might be identified with LD. Population studies of achievement in these domains show a continuous, uninterrupted distribution of skills when individuals with acquired brain injuries and intellectual disabilities are excluded (Jorm et al., 1986; Shaywitz et al., 1992). IQ and other cognitive processes are attributes that are commonly employed in cognitive discrepancy models for LD identification and also demonstrate continuous, largely normal distributions (McGrew & Wendling, 2010). Even attributes that are more complex to operationalize and measure, such as intervention response, appear to be continuous with individual differences in intervention response indicative of differences of degree, not kind (Fletcher et al., 2011; Vellutino et al., 2006). Because the underlying attributes upon which we identify LD are continuous with no clear threshold to mark the disability, the cut points we may apply to operationally define an attribute of LD are somewhat arbitrary. Generally, these cut points are based on studies that predict important educational outcomes, but it must be acknowledged that such predictions are done in aggregate and are imperfect at the individual level.

The Attributes of LD Are Imperfectly Measured

One reason that these predictive studies are imperfect is that the attributes underlying LD are latent constructs, unobservable except as indicated by imperfect tests. The fields of psychology and education are replete with latent constructs because these fields attempt to understand unobservable processes, such as thinking and feeling. For example, a child's reading skill is unobservable independently of the tasks that we impose and measure to evaluate their understanding of the meaning of texts or their accuracy in identifying words during the reading task. Importantly, these tasks are not perfectly reliable, and the resulting score will contain some unknown amount of error around the individual's "true score." This error can result from reliability challenges such as examiner error, as well as differences in the individual's performance on different occasions (Francis et al., 2005). However, even here reality is somewhat more complex than a confidence interval might suggest, as no assessment task will perfectly overlap with the latent construct of interest. This assertion is obvious when considering broad notions such as intelligence, but extends even to more sharply defined constructs such as reading, math, or writing.

Reliability Is a Universal Challenge

Because the attributes of LD are measured by imperfect tests and are continuously distributed in the population, any attempt to impose a rigid categorical structure (LD vs. not LD) based on strict cut points on psychometric data will lead to unreliability at the individual level. Due to differences in cut points, formulae applied, measurement occasion, or test employed, individual identification decisions will shift. This fact is well established across methods and approaches to identification, including aptitude–achievement discrepancies (Francis et al., 2005; Macmann & Barnett, 1985), methods based on instructional response (Barth et al., 2008; Hendricks & Fuchs, 2020), and methods based on identifying a pattern of cognitive processing strengths and weaknesses (Miciak et al., 2015, 2018; Taylor et al., 2017). Even seemingly straightforward methods that employ a low achievement criterion demonstrate fluctuation in individual identification decisions over time (Francis et al., 2005). Although this situation is often seen as a problem because different districts will identify different students as LD, it is important to recognize that this situation is an inherent problem because of measurement error and the use of different identification procedures—even when the districts are using the same method and the same tests for identification.

Types of Classifications

Categorical Classifications

Categorical and dimensional classifications differ in the distribution of the underlying attributes that mark the classification (Brown & Barlow, 2005; Widiger, 1992). Categorical classifications are marked primarily by the presence or absence of binary attributes. Examples of categorical classifications are common in medicine, including viral infections, cancers, or conditions such as pregnancy. In these conditions, the disease or disorder is marked by the presence (or sometimes absence) of a particular attribute (e.g., the presence of a tumor) or constellation of attributes. Medical models built on categorical classifications have had persistent influence on conceptions of LD (Grigorenko et al., 2020), as both practitioners and scientists have adopted identification and treatment protocols that rely on a binary decision-making framework. Categorical classifications rely upon clear qualitative differences among entities: *differences of kind*. Traditional conceptions of LD often hypothesize a categorical classification, though this hypothesis is frequently implicit. For example, approaches to LD identification that rely on differentiating among "garden-variety struggling learners" and students with LD represent a hypothesis that qualitative differences exist among struggling learners (Kavale, 2005; Mather & Gregg, 2006). Proponents of this conception hold that students with LD and students with academic difficulties not indicative of LD differ in educationally meaningful ways; these hypothesized differences may be found in their psychoeducational characteristics, educational prognoses, or response to specific educational interventions. These hypothesized differences should be investigated to determine the extent to which reality conforms to the resultant predictions—an evaluative framework we describe below.

Dimensional Classifications

In contrast with categorical classifications, dimensional classifications are based upon attributes that are continuously distributed and typically do not include a clear demarcation that would mark "disordered" versus "nondisordered" (Ellis, 1984). Although we most commonly use categorical language even for classifications of this nature, medicine, psychology, and education feature a large number of conditions based on dimensional classifications. In medicine, obesity is an easily understood example: obesity is generally defined as occurring when an individual's body mass index is 30 or greater. However, there is very little difference in the underlying health attributes of an individual with a body mass index of 29 and another with 31. The difference is one of degree, and the cut point that marks obesity is somewhat arbitrary. Hypertension is a second informative example for understanding a dimensional conception of LD. Thresholds for type I and type II hypertension are somewhat arbitrary, and individuals whose scores tend to cluster on either side of these thresholds will demonstrate similar health outcomes. Diagnosis with hypertension is further complicated by the fact that blood pressure varies not only across but within individuals. Dependent upon circumstances, one's blood pressure may vary considerably even within the same day. Thus, to diagnose hypertension, a physician will typically work with the patient to take repeated measures of their blood pressure. Diagnosis is based on repeated measures and an emerging pattern (Flack & Adekola, 2020).

The attributes of LD are similar. Individuals who receive standard scores of 84 and 85 on a standardized measure of math calculations will perform very similarly in computation tasks, and their expected outcomes in math are likely similar when we control for instruction. Further, it is likely that if we administer a different test of math calculations, or even the same test of math calculations on a different day, their individual scores will vary. In this circumstance, applying a strict cut point of 85 or below may result in different individual decisions on different days. As a result, identification processes for LD should rely on multiple data sources (Fletcher & Miciak, n.d.).

Evaluating Conceptual Frameworks for LD

It is well understood that there is no gold standard for LD identification against which arguments for validity, reliability, and utility can be evaluated (Fletcher et al., 2019). Different conceptual frameworks must be evaluated to determine the extent to which observed reality conforms to their hypotheses. This process can be done in isolation, or different frameworks can be evaluated simultaneously to compare their accordance with reality. This process is called *classification research* and is a hallmark of the scientific process (Morris & Fletcher, 1988). It stands in contrast to circular approaches that forestall inquiry by appealing to proposed definitions, an approach that asserts "*LD must be this because it is defined as that.*" In fact, such assertions are logical fallacies, examples of tautological thinking in which an assertion is claimed to be true by virtue of its definition. Scientific thinking requires that we collect data and evaluate assertions. These assertions can be evaluated through consideration of multiple factors.

Different conceptual frameworks for LD should be directly evaluated in empirical research. Evidence for different conceptual frameworks may take many forms, including cross-sectional studies that investigate: (1) the characteristics of students at risk for and not at risk for learning disabilities (e.g., Cho et al., 2015); (2) associations between hypothesized attributes of individuals with LD (e.g., Johnson et al., 2010); (3) intervention outcomes for students with different learning profiles (e.g., Stuebing et al., 2015); and (4) the reliability of the approach when applied with empirical data (e.g., Hendricks & Fuchs, 2020; MacMann et al., 1989). Studies such as this can provide indirect evidence for a particular conception of LD—an argument for its validity (Kane, 2013).

Most important are studies that directly apply a proposed operational definition and compare the resulting groups on other meaningful attributes (Morris & Fletcher, 1988). For example, a researcher who wishes to investigate the reliability and validity of a cognitive discrepancy approach to LD could conduct a study in which a large group of struggling learners is identified as either demonstrating an IQ achievement discrepancy or not and then compare the resulting groups on external, educationally meaningful factors. These factors are considered external because they represent dimensions or data that were not utilized in group formation. There are numerous educationally meaningful external dimensions on which performance can be compared, including behavior, cognition, long-term academic outcomes, response to specific interventions, and even neurobiological indicators such as brain structure and function. The extent to which groups resulting from our proposed criteria differ in these educationally meaningful dimensions serves as strong evidence for the validity of the classification.

Proposed classifications, definitions, and their operational definitions should also be evaluated for the reliability of individual decisions. As described above, all strictly psychometric methods for the identification of LD will demonstrate limited reliability at the individual level. This is because all psychometric test data are imperfect. Scores will fluctuate based on task demands, testing occasion, and factors such as examiner error. However, not all identification methods are impacted similarly; thus, an important consideration for classification research in LD is how reliably the identification methods can be employed. For example, complex methods that rely on multiple intra-individual comparisons of test data may demonstrate unique reliability challenges.

Finally, proposed classification frameworks and their resulting identification methods should be evaluated for their utility. Here, we define utility broadly as an indicator of the extent to which a proposed classification and its methods improve psychoeducational outcomes for individuals who interact with its implementation. Importantly, this forces consideration not just of individuals who are ultimately identified as LD, but also of individuals who are potentially LD, but found ineligible. The utility of a classification framework for LD might be based on its potential to improve instruction for individuals who interact with its process by collecting educationally relevant data or implementing a rigorous intervention framework. All of these factors might contribute to the asserted utility of a classification framework.

Cognitive Discrepancy Methods

Aptitude–Achievement Discrepancy

Overview

Aptitude–achievement discrepancy approaches to LD have featured prominently in LD research and practice for over 50 years (Mercer & Hallahan, 2002). This approach holds that observed academic underachievement is "unexpected" because the individual demonstrates higher aptitude presumably associated with the capacity to achieve at higher levels. This approach requires the identification of a discrepancy between an individual's ability (typically indexed by their full-scale IQ or a listening comprehension score) and their current academic achievement (typically indexed on a standardized measure of academic achievement). Thus, the fundamental classification hypothesis for these approaches holds that LD (as marked by low achievement and an aptitude–achievement discrepancy) can be differentiated from expected low achievement (when low achievement is commensurate with measured aptitude). Due to the long history of this approach, its challenges in reliability, validity, and utility are well documented.

Reliability of Aptitude–Achievement Discrepancies

The identification of an aptitude–achievement discrepancy most frequently relies on documentation of a difference score of some specified magnitude between an individual's full-scale IQ and their current academic achievement. The psychometric challenges associated with this strict formulaic approach are many. First, any approach that relies on applying strict cut points to imperfect test data will demonstrate poor reliability at the individual level (Francis et al., 2005). Further, a difference score is derived from scores on two imperfect tests, each of which contains some unknown amount of error around an individual's true score. The confidence interval for a difference score is typically broader than that for a single test (Bereiter, 1967; Rogosa, 1995). The correlation between tests of IQ and academic achievement also affects the magnitude of the difference score and impacts identification reliability (Macmann & Barnett, 1985). Because a simple difference score relies on individual performance on multiple tests, the pattern of scores will be influenced by regression to the mean. Thus, individuals who demonstrate extreme scores on either aptitude or achievement are more likely to be identified as LD; in practice, individuals with higher aptitude are likely to be overidentified, while those individuals scoring lower on aptitude measures are less likely to be identified as LD.

In a series of influential studies investigating the reliability of aptitude–achievement discrepancy approaches, Macmann et al. (1985, 1989) highlighted the impact to reliability of three factors: (1) the diminished reliability of the difference score; (2) variability in performance due to test selection; and (3) variability due to the application of different cut scores or different approaches to identifying a discrepancy. Across simulations manipulating differences on each of these three factors, agreement for individual LD identification decisions was quite low, with very few scenarios demonstrating agreement on more than 50% of LD decisions. In a subsequent study to parse the source(s) of this observed low agreement, Macmann et al. (1989) observed that moderate to good agreement could be obtained across different methods to calculate a significant aptitude–achievement discrepancy. Agreement using the kappa index (*k*), where perfect agreement is 1.0, ranged from .57–.86. However, the use of different tests of achievement with different normative bases in the same academic domain had a significant, deleterious effect on agreement, with observed drops in *k* indicating only poor to fair agreement (range: .19–.47).

Validity and Utility of Aptitude–Achievement Discrepancies

For decades, aptitude–achievement discrepancy approaches have been criticized as lacking both validity and utility—criticisms that raise fundamental questions about fairness and resource allocation. The imbalance of evidence against these approaches makes a lengthy recitation unnecessary in this chapter; few within the special education research community argue for the validity and utility of these approaches today. This accumulated evidence is best summarized in two seminal meta-analyses (Hoskyn & Swanson, 2000; Stuebing et al., 2002) that informed the influential Learning Disabilities Summit in 2001 and the 2004 reauthorization of the Individuals with Disabilities Education Act, which removed the requirement to identify an aptitude–achievement discrepancy as part of the LD identification process from U.S. federal law. Both meta-analyses compared the psychoeducational profiles of struggling learners who demonstrated an IQ–achievement discrepancy and struggling learners who did not demonstrate a discrepancy between their IQ and observed low achievement. Results were generally consistent: neither meta-analysis found educationally meaningful differences between these groups. In Stuebing et al. (2002), which explicitly excluded outcomes used to define the groups, the resultant groups of struggling readers were comparable in behavior and achievement. The small differences observed in cognition were largely attributable to differences introduced by selection criteria. These meta-analytic results are supported by studies of prognosis, which fail to demonstrate long-term differences in outcomes between the two groups (Shaywitz et al., 1999). Neurobiological comparisons of struggling learners have not identified reliable differences in brain activation patterns of struggling learners who vary in IQ (Simos et al., 2014; Tanaka et al., 2011). There is one imaging study of a small sample (Hancock et al., 2016) and behavior genetic studies (Wadsworth et al., 2010) that show small differences in relation to IQ), but the bulk of the evidence is null.

The largely null evidence for educationally meaningful differences between groups of students with and without an IQ–achievement discrepancy in the domains of behavior, achievement, and cognition highlights the limited utility of assessing IQ as part of the LD identification process. In reading, the most common academic domain for LD, struggling learners with and without an IQ–achievement discrepancy do not differ in their reading skill and development at any age (Francis et al., 1996). Additionally, individuals with and without an IQ–achievement discrepancy demonstrate substantively similar responses to intensive academic interventions (Stuebing et al., 2009; Vellutino et al., 2000). In their meta-analytic review, Stuebing et al. (2002) found that IQ explained very small amounts of unique variance in intervention response when compared to direct measures of baseline academic skills. These results suggest that routine measurement of IQ as part of the LD identification process is unlikely to generate data useful for treatment planning. IQ tests should be used if there is a question about an intellectual disability (see Fletcher et al., 2019).

Patterns of Cognitive Processing Strengths and Weaknesses

Overview

In recent years, there have been increasing calls for a new cognitive discrepancy approach that requires documentation of an intra-individual pattern of cognitive processing strengths and weaknesses as an inclusionary criterion for the identification of LD. In the sections that follow, we refer to these approaches as *PSW methods*, which we intend as an umbrella term to refer to modern instantiations of the cognitive discrepancy approach. These methods are also frequently referred to as *Third Way methods*, a reference to their place as an alternative to aptitude–achievement discrepancy approaches and approaches that utilize instructional response. PSW methods hold that LD is marked by intra-individual variability as indexed by an academic weakness in the presence of unrelated cognitive processing strength(s) and a cognitive processing weakness(es) that holds potential to explain the observed academic weakness. These strengths and weaknesses are variably defined, including normative and relative strengths and weaknesses depending upon the method considered. Multiple methods have been proposed to operationally define these PSW methods, including: (1) the concordance/discordance method (C/DM; Hale & Fiorello, 2017); (2) the dual discrepancy/consistency method (DDCM), which we have previously referred to as the cross-battery assessment method (Flanagan et al., 2018); (3) the discrepancy/consistency method (D/CM; Naglieri, 1999); and (4) the core selective evaluation process (C-SEP; Schultz & Stevens, 2015). These methods differ in multiple important ways, including their use of relative or normative comparisons, what tests are required to be administered, and how exclusionary factors are considered.

Despite the recent origins of this approach to LD identification, proponents of PSW methods make strong evidentiary claims. This is best illustrated in a white paper issued by the Learning Disabilities Association of America that claimed to summarize an expert consensus on evidence-based practices for the identification and treatment of LD (Hale et al., 2010). This paper concluded that PSW methods "make the most empirical and theoretical sense" (Hale et al., p. 283). However, the white paper was controversial, and a response issued by The Consortium for Evidence-Based Early Intervention Practices (2010) criticized both its conclusions and methods. Of particular note, the response to the white paper highlighted the paucity of direct empirical research on PSW methods, a gap acknowledged in subsequent evidentiary reviews (McGill & Busse, 2017; Schneider & Kaufman, 2018) and highlighted below.

Reliability of PSW Methods

Despite differences in their operational definition, PSW methods require identification of three factors: (1) an academic weakness; (2) a cognitive processing weakness; and (3) a cognitive processing strength. All PSW methods also recommend the application of clinical judgment, the incorporation of multiple data, and consideration of exclusionary conditions. However, these recommendations are unlikely to overcome the considerable reliability challenges these complex methods introduce, as evidenced by both empirical studies of the methods and data simulations evaluating their technical adequacy.

In a series of studies, our group at the Texas Center for Learning Disabilities has highlighted these challenges for proposed PSW methods. Although empirical studies focus on the C/DM and DDCM methods, the poor reliability we observe is likely to generalize to all PSW methods that rely on complex comparisons of imperfect test data in multiple domains. In one of the first studies investigating the reliability of PSW methods, Stuebing et al. (2012) simulated latent datasets across a broad range of plausible parameters. Within these latent datasets, latent LD status was identified across multiple scenarios informed by the assumptions of three prominent PSW methods: C/DM, DDCM, and DC/M. Then, observed data were generated at different levels of test reliability to examine whether LD identification decisions at the observed level were in agreement with latent LD status.

Across the three methods, a clear pattern emerged. All three identified very few individuals as LD at the latent level (1–2% across most parameterizations). This low base rate resulted in generally high agreement for "not LD" identification decisions, as evidenced by very high specificity and negative predictive value estimates. However, moderate to low sensitivity and very low positive predictive values were observed, indicating that none of the three methods performed adequately at positively identifying individuals with LD.

Similar results were reported by Kranzler et al. (2016) using normative data from the Woodcock Johnson III (Woodcock et al., 2001). Similar to Stuebing et al. (2012), Kranzler et al. (2016) found a low base rate of LD, meaning that agreement was generally high for "not LD" identification decisions, but poor agreement was observed for positive LD identification decisions. As these methods are premised on identifying specific patterns of cognitive performance to tailor academic interventions. This means an unacceptably high number of students would receive inappropriate interventions.

In subsequent work, we sought to parse the sources of disagreement for PSW methods. For example, in two studies (Miciak et al., 2014; Miciak et al., 2016), we examined whether the LD identification decisions emerging from two proposed PSW methods agree. In both studies, we identified a sample of students who had not responded to an intensive intervention, following recommendations for implementation of PSW methods (Hale et al., 2010). We then applied criteria for the C/DM (Hale & Fiorello, 2004) and the DDCM (Flanagan et al., 2018). Even within a sample demonstrating substantial educational risk, both approaches identified a low percentage of individuals as LD (range: 24–66%). Further, agreement for LD identification decisions across the two approaches was poor, with most scenarios not exceeding chance agreement (kappa range: -.10–.31). These studies suggest that different operational definitions of PSW methods are not interchangeable; therefore, evidence for validity must be accrued separately.

Following the approach of Macmann and Barnett (1985) described above, we next investigated the effect of test selection on agreement for LD identification decisions within the C/DM (Hale & Fiorello, 2004). Second-grade students who had demonstrated inadequate response to an intensive intervention were assessed, and C/DM criteria were applied with two assessment batteries that were theoretically equivalent but differed only in the achievement test utilized for applying the C/DM criteria. Across the two batteries, agreement was poor (.29), particularly when considering the domain of achievement in which the child was identified as LD.

In a related data simulation, Taylor et al. (2017) found that differences in test selection resulted in low positive agreement across a wide range of test reliabilities and intercorrelations between measures. Agreement for positive LD identification demonstrated a strong linear relationship with test reliability, an illustration of the deleterious effects of measurement error. Further, the effects of measurement error are not likely to be overcome via the use of multiple measures within the C/DM. To illustrate, we simulated latent LD status following procedures utilized by Stuebing et al. (Miciak et al., 2018). We then determined agreement for LD identification decisions at the observed level for (1) a single indicator; (2) two indicators as part of a test–retest confirmation model; and (3) a mean score of two indicators. Similar to previous simulations, we found high specificity and negative predictive value, but low sensitivity and positive predictive value when utilizing a single observed indicator in each academic and cognitive domain. When we evaluated whether agreement improved for decisions based on multiple indicators, we observed small, inconsistent improvements in "not LD" decisions for the test–retest procedure and small improvements in agreement (mean improvement = 2.0%, range = .3–2.8%) when using mean scores for two indicators. In order to achieve these small improvements in agreement, the test battery had to be doubled for every individual assessed.

Validity and Utility of PSW Methods

Despite the increasing use of PSW methods in practice (Maki & Adams, 2019), there is very little empirical research investigating the validity and utility of PSW methods. Recent reviews of the evidence for these methods highlight these significant gaps in evidence (McGill & Busse, 2017; Schneider & Kaufman, 2017). In one of the first empirical investigations of the external validity of PSW classifications (Miciak et al., 2014), we compared academic profiles of struggling learners who met CDM or DDCM criteria for LD and participants who did not meet these criteria. For this comparison, the critical differences were the presence or absence of an intra-individual pattern of strengths and weaknesses. Across reading measures, these comparisons did not yield differential patterns of performance, as would be expected if the presence of a pattern of strengths and weaknesses resulted in meaningful differences in academic performance.

In a subsequent large-scale study, we investigated whether PSW status was associated with differential intervention response within a sample of struggling readers in fourth grade (Miciak et al., 2016). We hypothesized that if the presence or absence of a pattern of cognitive processing strengths and weaknesses is educationally meaningful, we would observe consistent measurable differences in how participants would respond to an intensive intervention in reading. Prior to the intervention, we identified groups of participants who met PSW criteria for LD in reading based on procedures for the C/DM and DDCM. Multiple comparisons of posttest performance for students who met PSW criteria with those who did not were largely null, with small, inconsistent effect sizes. These results suggest that students with reading difficulties with and without an intra-individual pattern of strengths and weaknesses demonstrate similar educational prognoses (Miciak et al., 2016).

Additionally, the assertions by many PSW proponents that an assessment of cognitive processes is necessary to individually tailor interventions should be weighed against the resounding lack of evidence for the effectiveness of cognitively tailored interventions. Recent literature reviews and meta-analyses conclude that the evidence for aptitude by treatment interactions and cognitively tailored interventions is preliminary at best and does not support widespread adoption (Burns et al., 2016; Kearns & Fuchs, 2013). Moreover, the evidence that cognitive assessments contribute value-added information to identification or predictive information for intervention response is limited, except in the case of young children with little exposure to instruction. One potential reason that such evidence has been slow to emerge may be the well-documented challenges associated with cognitive profile analysis (McGill et al., 2018). Cognitively tailored interventions require interpreting variance in subtest scores on cognitive tests. However, in a series of studies, Canivez and colleagues have demonstrated that most modern intelligence tests are unidimensional and cannot be interpreted reliably as multidimensional (Canivez et al., 2017, 2019, 2020). Further, recent analyses demonstrate that within-person subscore reliability estimates are poor, including for students identified with LD (Styck et al., 2019). Such studies call into question the clinical utility of subscores on cognitive assessments.

Instructional Methods

Instructional Response

Overview

The reauthorization of the Individuals with Disabilities Education Act in 2004 (U.S. Department of Education) allowed U.S. states and districts to utilize an approach that relies on response to intervention as an inclusionary criterion for

LD identification. This shift in federal policy resulted in confusion, in large part due to the conflation of the term *response to intervention* as an individual indicator for LD identification with a response-to-intervention service delivery framework (e.g., Reynolds & Shaywitz, 2009). To avoid this confusion, we use the term *instructional response* to describe data that inform LD identification and the term *multi-tier systems of support* (MTSS) to describe a service delivery framework that includes universal screening, interventions of increasing intensity, and ongoing progress monitoring (Fletcher & Vaughn, 2009; Fuchs et al., 2008). Data on individual instructional responses are most efficiently collected within an MTSS framework but can also be collected in other contexts. Additionally, data about instructional response is required as part of any LD identification process to document sufficient educational opportunity. For LD identification methods that rely on documentation of inadequate instructional response, these data are considered inclusionary, indicative of an attribute that individuals must demonstrate. In contrast, cognitive discrepancy methods consider instructional response as an exclusionary criterion, data that can be used to rule out inadequate instructional opportunity.

There is additional confusion about the assessment process within LD identification methods that rely on instructional response. For example, some have criticized instructional response methods for not ruling out exclusionary factors contraindicative of LD (e.g., Hale et al., 2010). However, under IDEA statutes, eligibility can never be established based on a single criterion or data point. Instead, all children evaluated for LD must undergo a comprehensive assessment, regardless of the specific LD identification approach employed. This comprehensive evaluation must (1) use a variety of fair, technically sound assessment tools and strategies; (2) be sufficiently comprehensive to assess all areas of suspected disability and identify all special education and service needs; and (3) include data that directly assist in identifying the child's intervention needs. Thus, documentation of inadequate instructional response is never sufficient for LD identification. Instead, data documenting inadequate instructional response can inform a comprehensive assessment process for the identification of LD. In the sections that follow, we describe studies on the reliability, validity, and utility of inadequate instructional response as a criterion for group formation while acknowledging that these data are not sufficient for LD identification.

Reliability of Methods Based on Instructional Response

The application of a rigid cut point to differentiate adequate from inadequate instructional response will demonstrate unreliability at the individual level, regardless of the specific indicator of instructional response employed (Fletcher et al., 2018). This includes final-status indicators that assess post-intervention achievement, growth indicators that calculate a rate of improvement during the intervention period, and dual-discrepancy approaches that combine final status and growth. This fluctuation in instructional response status is an inherent artifact of measurement error and the dimensional nature of the underlying construct described above. Evaluation of the reliability of instructional response methods is further complicated by the lack of agreement on how instructional response should be measured. Some proponents of instructional response methods argue that curriculum-based measures of instructional response are sufficient (Koveleski et al., 2013), while others have argued that standardized, norm-referenced assessments administered following intervention provide a more defensible indicator if used in conjunction with curriculum-based measures (Fletcher & Miciak, n.d.).

The challenges to reliability highlighted above are well documented in empirical research. Studies of this type apply target criteria and compare resulting groups to evaluate how consistent the identification decisions are across differences in measures, measurement occasion, and the specific cut points or criteria employed. Variations along any of these dimensions will result in changes in individual responder status (Barth et al., 2008; Waesche et al., 2011; Burns et al., 2010; Hendricks & Fuchs, 2020). The use of different criteria for differentiating adequate from inadequate instructional response is particularly impactful. For example, Waesche et al. (2011) compared groups resulting from three potential indicators of instructional response: (1) a final-status indicator following intervention; (2) a growth indicator across the intervention period; and (3) a dual-discrepancy approach that combined final status and growth. Agreement between these indicators was highly variable and affected by the indicator employed, as well as the cut point to dichotomize responder status. However, across all comparisons, agreement was generally poor to moderate, highlighting the psychometric limitations of instructional response methods.

Further, there is evidence that the application of different response criteria results in groups that differ in their psychoeducational characteristics (Frijters et al., 2013; Wanzek et al., 2016). In one recent study, Hendricks and Fuchs (2020) illustrated that differences in response criteria and measures are associated with individual differences in achievement and cognition within the resulting groups. Across variation in criteria (final status vs. growth) and measures, agreement varied from chance levels of agreement to moderate agreement, replicating results from previous studies (e.g., Barth et al., 2008; Burns et al., 2010). Additionally, there were systematic differences in how individual differences predicted response status based on method employed. For example, participants with higher pre-intervention scores in reading were more likely to be identified as adequate responders when final-status indicators were employed. Conversely, participants with lower achievement prior to intervention were more likely to be identified as an adequate responder when growth indicators were employed.

Even when the same method for determining instructional response is employed, there will be variation in responder status due to differences in measure and cut point (Barth et al., 2008; Waesche et al., 2011). Fletcher et al. (2011) investigated how test selection impacted agreement. Using empirical data, they observed poor to fair agreement across pairs of measures that could be used to identify inadequate intervention response (k range: .14–.48). In a subsequent data simulation to parse the sources of this disagreement, they found diminished agreement due to five potential sources: (1) imperfect correlations between measures (k = .72–.77); (2) imperfect reliability of the measures (k = .72–.78); (3) both imperfect correlations and reliability (k = .62–.68); (4) differences in the normative sample of the measures (k = .39); and (5) sampling error inherent to small samples (k = .39). These sources of diminished agreement are not unique to instructional response methods, but instead reflect universal challenges to methods that employ imperfect psychometric data. Particular attention should be paid to the influence of differences in the normative samples, given the common practice of using tests from different assessment batteries that are normed on different samples.

Validity and Utility Methods Based on Instructional Response

As we have highlighted throughout this chapter, the challenges to individual identification with LD are universal; individual decisions should be based on converging data. Yet, these challenges to individual identification do not preclude an evaluation of validity and utility, which occurs at the group level. Across indicators of instructional response, resulting groups of adequate and inadequate responders can be compared using external dimensions. If instructional response status results in groups that differ in educationally meaningful ways, the underlying classification accrues validity (Morris & Fletcher, 1988). It is through studies of this type that we observe significant differences in external validity when comparing methods based on instructional response with cognitive discrepancy approaches. There is a growing body of evidence in support of the assertion that differences in instructional response (both dimensional differences and categorical differences) are meaningful; groups differentiated by responder status demonstrate different academic, behavioral, and cognitive characteristics (Al Otaiba & Fuchs, 2002; Nelson et al., 2003). Additionally, neurobiological research finds measurable differences in the brain activation patterns of adequate and inadequate responders following intensive interventions in reading (Molfese et al., 2013; Rezaie et al., 2011).

Our research group has conducted a series of non-overlapping studies comparing the academic and cognitive characteristics of participants demonstrating adequate versus inadequate response to a standardized intervention (Cho et al., 2015; Fletcher et al., 2011; Miciak et al., 2014). In each of these studies, students at risk for reading disabilities received an intensive, long-term intervention. Following intervention, participants were empirically classified as inadequate or adequate responders based on performance on final-status indicators of reading. Across a broad range of cognitive and academic assessments, we observed clear differentiation on measures not utilized for group formation, such as cognitive performance. However, these differences parallel differences in level of achievement. We interpret these differences as evidence for a continuum of severity hypothesis (Vellutino et al., 2006), in which observed differences in cognition parallel differences in reading proficiency, as would be expected for correlated domains within a dimensional disorder.

A Hybrid Approach for LD Identification

Our research group at the Texas Center for Learning Disabilities has long advocated for a treatment-oriented, hybrid approach for the identification of LD (Fletcher & Miciak, n.d.). We describe this as a hybrid approach because it utilizes multiple data to provide evidence for three criteria for LD identification. Based on consensus recommendations of the Learning Disability Summit (Bradley et al., 2002), these criteria include: (1) evidence for low achievement; (2) evidence of inadequate instructional response; and (3) evidence to rule out exclusionary factors contraindicative of LD. We consider this approach treatment-oriented for two reasons. First, much of the data should be generated within an MTSS that emphasizes early intervention for all students at risk for academic difficulties. Second, the hybrid approach limits assessment to domains that guide intervention design; we do not recommend routine assessment of cognitive processes because these data do not inform intervention design. It generally eschews concepts of etiology and prognosis. The orientation of this approach toward treatment planning informs the entire assessment process, differentiating it from traditional assessment processes focused on identifying the right kid. Limiting the assessment burden incurred as part of a comprehensive assessment for LD identification conserves resources and shifts its emphasis toward intervention planning.

In the United States, federal statutes require that the comprehensive assessment process document evidence of low achievement, adequate instructional opportunity, and a consideration of exclusionary clauses regardless of the specific approach to LD identification a state or district chooses to employ. Although it is not strictly necessary to implement an MTSS to collect these data, these data are routinely collected as part of a well-implemented MTSS. Thus, MTSS is an efficient framework to facilitate the LD identification process. However, the goal of MTSS is never LD identification, but improved outcomes for all students. Thus, the hybrid approach for which we advocate is dynamic, treatment-oriented, and preventative.

Regardless of the specific method employed to identify LD, there are multiple steps that an assessment team can take to increase confidence in any resulting decision. First, the use of multiple data points provides stronger evidence for ruling in or out hypothesized attributes. The use of multiple indicators meets statutory requirements and increases the likelihood of identifying all academic deficits in need of remediation. Second, assessment teams should avoid the use of fixed cut points and consider confidence intervals in their decision making. Confidence intervals reflect the degree of uncertainty associated with a test score and provide a range of possible values. Diagnostic decisions in other disability categories have moved toward incorporation of confidence intervals and clinical judgment; teams identifying LD should do the same. Additionally, the treatment orientation that we have described as guiding our hybrid approach can be adopted across any LD identification process. Assessment teams should strongly consider intervention planning and error toward providing necessary academic interventions. Finally, in recognition of the inherent challenges related to identifying LD, we suggest that all decision making be located within a recursive framework that allows for decisions to be revisited and errors corrected.

As the field of LD research and practice moves toward the future, we encourage the incorporation of (multi) dimensional and probabilistic conceptions of LD (Wagner et al., 2019). Practitioners should utilize psychometrically sound achievement data to provide timely interventions of appropriate intensity. These interventions should be systematic and explicit and address all of the individual child's instructional needs, regardless of special education eligibility status or label. Future research can assist with this process, as our understanding of individual differences in development and learning improves from neurological, genetic, cognitive, and instructional perspectives (Grigorenko, 2020). Such research can assist by identifying multivariate risk indicators that inform the early identification of individuals with higher probabilities to develop academic difficulties and LD (Catts & Petscher, 2022; Wagner et al., 2019) with an eye toward early intervention.

Conclusions

In this chapter, we reviewed issues related to the classification, definition, and identification of LD. We described a shift in understanding about the nature of LD, away from categorical conceptions of the disorder focused on identifying qualitative differences between individuals with academic difficulties and toward a dimensional understanding that de-emphasizes strict cut points and prioritizes convergent data, particularly data collected in the context of instruction. This shift has implications for how researchers and practitioners identify LD, as well as how we might prioritize evidence for the validity and utility of proposed methods. The numerous psychometric challenges to reliable LD identification are unlikely to be fully ameliorated. However, a reduced focus on issues of eligibility combined with increased attention to treatment planning can serve to reduce the harm resulting from these challenges. Within this conception, LD is best understood as an instructional problem; our response must be oriented toward improved instruction.

REFERENCES

Al Otaiba, S., & Fuchs, D. (2002). Characteristics of children who are unresponsive to early literacy intervention: A review of the literature. *Remedial and Special Education, 23*(5), 300–316.

Bandalos, D. L., & Leite, W. (2013). The use of Monte Carlo studies in structural equation modeling research. In G. R. Hancock & R. O. Mueller (Eds.), *Structural equation modeling: A second course* (2nd ed., pp. 625–666). Information Age Publishing.

Barth, A. E., Stuebing, K. K., Anthony, J. L., Denton, C. A., Mathes, P. G., Fletcher, J. M., & Francis, D. J. (2008). Agreement among response to intervention criteria for identifying responder status. *Learning and Individual Differences, 18*, 296–307.

Bereiter, C. (1967). Some persisting dilemmas in the measurement of change. In C. W. Harris (Ed.), *Problems in the measurement of change* (pp. 3–20). University of Wisconsin Press.

Bradley, R., Danielson, L., & Hallahan, D. P. (2002). *Identification of learning disabilities: Research to practice.* Routledge.

Brown, T. A., & Barlow, D. H. (2005). Dimensional versus categorical classification of mental disorders in the fifth edition of the *Diagnostic and Statistical Manual of Mental Disorders* and beyond: Comment on the special section. *Journal of Abnormal Psychology, 114*(4), 551.

Burns, M. K., Peterson-Brown, S., Haegele, K., Rodriguez, M., Schmitt, B., & VanDerHeyden, A. M. (2016). Meta-analysis of academic interventions derived from neuropsychological data. *School Psychology Quarterly, 31*, 28–42.

Burns, M. K., Scholin, S. E., Kosciolek, S., & Livingston, J. (2010). Reliability of decision-making frameworks for response to intervention for reading. *Journal of Psychoeducational Assessment, 28*(2), 102–114.

Canivez, G. L., McGill, R. J., Dombrowski, S. C., Watkins, M. W., Pritchard, A. E., & Jacobson, L. A. (2020). Construct validity of the WISC-V in clinical cases: Exploratory and confirmatory factor analyses of the 10 primary subtests. *Assessment, 27*(2), 274–296.

Canivez, G. L., Watkins, M. W., Good, R., James, K., & James, T. (2017). Construct validity of the WISC–IVUK with a referred Irish sample: Wechsler and CHC model comparisons with 15 subtests. *British Journal of Educational Psychology, 87*(3), 383–407.

Canivez, G. L., Watkins, M. W., & McGill, R. J. (2019). Construct validity of the Wechsler Intelligence Scale For Children–Fifth U.K. Edition: Exploratory and confirmatory factor analyses of the 16 primary and secondary subtests. *British Journal of Educational Psychology, 89*(2), 195–224.

Catts, H. W., & Petscher, Y. (2022, May/June). A cumulative risk and resilience model of dyslexia. *Journal of Learning Disabilities, 55*(3), 171–184. [Epub ahead of print]

Cho, E., Roberts, G. J., Capin, P., Roberts, G., Miciak, J., & Vaughn, S. (2015). Cognitive attributes, attention, and self-efficacy of adequate and inadequate responders in a fourth grade reading intervention. *Learning Disabilities Research & Practice, 30*(4), 159–170.

Consortium for Evidence-Based Early Intervention Practices. (2010). *A response to the Learning Disabilities Association of America (LDA) white paper on specific learning disabilities (SLD) identification. www.isbe.net/Documents/LDA_SLD_white_paper_response.pdf.*

Elliott, J. G., & Grigorenko, E. L. (2014). *The dyslexia debate* (No. 14). Cambridge University Press.

Ellis, A. W. (1984). The cognitive neuropsychology of developmental (and acquired) dyslexia: A critical survey. *Cognitive Neuropsychology, 2*, 169–205.

Flack, J. M., & Adekola, B. (2020). Blood pressure and the new ACC/AHA hypertension guidelines. *Trends in Cardiovascular Medicine, 30*(3), 160–164.

Flanagan, D. P., Alfonso, V. C., Sy, M. C., Mascolo, J. T., McDonough, E. M., & Ortiz, S. O. (2018). Dual discrepancy/consistency operational definition of SLD: Integrating multiple data sources and multiple data-gathering methods. *Essentials of Specific Learning Disability Identification*, 329–430.

Fletcher, J. M., Lyon, G. R., Fuchs, L. S., & Barnes, M. A. (2018). *Learning disabilities: From identification to intervention.* Guilford Press.

Fletcher, J. M., & Miciak, J. (2017). Comprehensive cognitive assessments are not necessary for the identification and treatment of learning disabilities. *Archives of Clinical Neuropsychology, 32*(1), 2–7.

Fletcher, J. M., & Miciak, J. (n.d.). *The identification of specific learning disabilities: A summary of research on best practices. https://texasldcenter.org/files/resources/SLD-Manual_Final.pdf.*

Fletcher, J. M., Stuebing, K. K., Barth, A. E., Denton, C. A., Cirino, P. T., Francis, D. J., & Vaughn, S. (2011). Cognitive correlates of inadequate response to intervention. *School Psychology Review, 40*, 2–22.

Fletcher, J. M., & Vaughn, S. (2009). Response to intervention: Preventing and remediating academic difficulties. *Child Development Perspectives, 3*(1), 30–37.

Francis, D. J., Fletcher, J. M., Stuebing, K. K., Lyon, G. R., Shaywitz, B. A., & Shaywitz, S. E. (2005). Psychometric approaches to the identification of learning disabilities: IQ and achievement scores are not sufficient. *Journal of Learning Disabilities, 38*, 98–110.

Francis, D. J., Shaywitz, S. E., Stuebing, K. K., Shaywitz, B. A., & Fletcher, J. M. (1996). Developmental lag versus deficit models of reading disability: A longitudinal, individual growth curves analysis. *Journal of Educational Psychology, 88*(1), 3.

Frijters, J. C., Lovett, M. W., Sevcik, R. A., & Morris, R. D. (2013). Four methods of identifying change in the context of a multiple component reading intervention for struggling middle school readers. *Reading and Writing, 26*(4), 539–563.

Fuchs, D., Fuchs, L. S., & Stecker, P. M. (2010). The "blurring" of special education in a new continuum of general education placements and services. *Exceptional Children, 76*(3), 301–323.

Fuchs, L. S., Fuchs, D., & Zumeta, R. O. (2008). Response to intervention. *Educating Individuals with Disabilities: IDEIA 2004 and Beyond*, 115.

Grigorenko, E. L., Compton, D. L., Fuchs, L. S., Wagner, R. K., Willcutt, E. G., & Fletcher, J. M. (2020). Understanding, educating, and supporting children with specific learning disabilities: 50 years of science and practice. *American Psychologist, 75*(1), 37.

Hale, J., Alfonso, V., Berninger, V., Bracken, B., Christo, C., Clark, E., & Yalof, J. (2010). Critical issues in response-to-intervention, comprehensive evaluation, and specific learning disabilities identification and intervention: An expert white paper consensus. *Learning Disability Quarterly, 33*(3), 223–236.

Hale, J. B., & Fiorello, C. A. (2004). *School neuropsychology: A practitioner's handbook.* Guilford Press.

Hancock, R., Gabrieli, J. D. E., & Hoeft, F. (2016). Shared temporoparietal dysfunction in dyslexia and typical readers with discrepantly high IQ. *Trends in Neuroscience and Education, 5*(4), 173–177.

Hendricks, E. L., & Fuchs, D. (2020). Are individual differences in response to intervention influenced by the methods and measures used to define response? Implications for identifying children with learning disabilities. *Journal of Learning Disabilities, 53*(6), 428–443.

Hoskyn, M., & Swanson, H. L. (2000). Cognitive processing of low achievers and children with reading disabilities: A selective meta-analytic review of the published literature. *The School Psychology Review, 29*, 102–119.

Johnson, E. S., Humphrey, M., Mellard, D. F., Woods, K., & Swanson, H. L. (2010). Cognitive processing deficits and students with specific learning disabilities: A selective meta-analysis of the literature. *Learning Disability Quarterly, 33*(1), 3–18.

Jorm, A. F., share, D. L., Matthews, M., & Matthews, R. (1986). Cognitive factors at school entry predictive of specific reading retardation and general reading backwardness: A research note. *Journal of Child Psychology, 27*, 45–54.

Kane, M. (2013). The argument-based approach to validation. *School Psychology Review, 42*(4), 448–457.

Kavale, K. A. (2005). Identifying specific learning disability: Is responsiveness to intervention the answer? *Journal of Learning Disabilities, 38*(6), 553–562.

Kearns, D. M., & Fuchs, D. (2013). Does cognitively focused instruction improve the academic performance of low-achieving students? *Exceptional Children, 79*, 263–290.

Kovaleski, J. F., VanDerHeyden, A. M., & Shapiro, E. S. (2013). *The RTI approach to evaluating learning disabilities.* Guilford Press.

Kranzler, J. H., Floyd, R. G., Benson, N., Zaboski, B., & Thibodaux, L. (2016). Classification agreement analysis of Cross-Battery Assessment in the identification of specific learning disorders in children and youth. *International Journal of School & Educational Psychology, 4*, 124–136.

Macmann, G. M., & Barnett, D. W. (1985). Discrepancy score analysis: A computer simulation of classification stability. *Journal of Psychoeducational Assessment, 4*, 363–375.

Macmann, G. M., Barnett, D. W., Lombard, T. J., Belton-Kocher, E., & Sharpe, M. N. (1989). On the actuarial classification of children: Fundamental studies of classification agreement. *Journal of Special Education, 23*(2) 127–149.

Maki, K. E., & Adams, S. R. (2019). A current landscape of specific learning disability identification: Training, practices, and implications. *Psychology in the Schools, 56*(1), 18–31.

Mather, N., & Gregg, N. (2006). Specific learning disabilities: Clarifying, not eliminating, a construct. *Professional Psychology: Reseearch and Practice, 37*, 99–106.

McGill, R. J., & Busse, R. T. (2017). When theory trumps science: A critique of the PSW model for SLD identification. *Contemporary School Psychology, 21*(1), 10–18.

McGill, R. J., Dombrowski, S. C., & Canivez, G. L. (2018). Cognitive profile analysis in school psychology: History, issues, and continued concerns. *Journal of School Psychology, 71*, 108–121.

McGrew, K. S., & Wendling, B. J. (2010). Cattell–Horn–Carroll cognitive-achievement relations: What we have learned from the past 20 years of research. *Psychology in the Schools, 47*(7), 651–675.

Mercer, C., & Hallahan, D. (2002). Learning disabilities: Historical perspectives. *Identification of Learning Disabilities: Research to Practice*, 1–65.

Miciak, J., Fletcher, J. M., Stuebing, K. K., Vaughn, S., & Tolar, T. D. (2014). Patterns of cognitive strengths and weaknesses: Identification rates, agreement, and validity for learning disabilities identification. *School Psychology Quarterly, 29*(1), 21.

Miciak, J., Stuebing, K. K., Vaughn, S., Roberts, G., Barth, A. E., & Fletcher, J. M. (2014). Cognitive attributes of adequate and inadequate responders to reading intervention in middle school. *School Psychology Review, 43*(4), 407–427.

Miciak, J., Taylor, W. P., Denton, C. A., & Fletcher, J. M. (2015). The effect of achievement test selection on identification of learning disabilities within a patterns of strengths and weaknesses framework. *School Psychology Quarterly, 30*(3), 321.

Miciak, J., Taylor, W. P., Stuebing, K. K., & Fletcher, J. M. (2018). Simulation of LD identification accuracy using a pattern of processing strengths and weaknesses method with multiple measures. *Journal of Psychoeducational Assessment, 36*(1), 21–33.

Miciak, J., Williams, J. L., Taylor, W. P., Cirino, P. T., Fletcher, J. M., & Vaughn, S. (2016). Do processing patterns of strengths and weaknesses predict differential treatment response? *Journal of Educational Psychology, 108*(6), 898.

Molfese, P. J., Fletcher, J. M., & Denton, C. A. (2013). Adequate versus inadequate response to reading intervention: An event-related potentials assessment. *Developmental Neuropsychology, 38*(8), 534–549.

Morris, R. D., & Fletcher, J. M. (1988). Classification in neuropsychology: A theoretical framework and research paradigm. *Journal of Clinical and Experimental Neuropsychology, 10*, 640–658.

Naglieri, J. A. (1999). *Essentials of CAS Assessment.* John Wiley & Sons.

Nelson, J., Benner, G. J., & Gonzalez, J. (2003). Learner characteristics that influence the treatment effectiveness of early literacy interventions: A meta-analytic review. *Learning Disabilities Research & Practice, 18*(4), 255–267.

Paxton, P., Curran, P. J., Bollen, K. A., Kirby, J., & Chen, F. (2001). Monte Carlo experiments: Design and implementation. *Structural Equation Modeling, 8*, 287–312.

Reynolds, C. R., & Shaywitz, S. E. (2009). Response to intervention: Prevention and remediation, perhaps. Diagnosis, no. *Child Development Perspectives, 3*(1), 44–47.

Rezaie, R., Simos, P. G., Fletcher, J. M., Cirino, P. T., Vaughn, S., & Papanicolaou, A. C. (2011). Temporo-parietal brain activity as a longitudinal predictor of response to educational interventions among middle school struggling readers. *Journal of the International Neuropsychological Society, 17*(5), 875–885.

Rogosa, D. (1995). Myths and methods: "Myths about longitudinal research" plus supplemental questions. *The Analysis of Change, 3*, 66.

Schneider, W. J., & Kaufman, A. S. (2017). Let's not do away with comprehensive cognitive assessments just yet. *Archives of Clinical Neuropsychology, 32*(1), 8–20.

Schultz, E. K., & Stephens, T. L. (2015). Core-selective evaluation process: An efficient & comprehensive approach to identify students with SLD using the WJ IV. *Dialog: Journal of the Texas Educational Diagnosticians Association, 44*(2).

Shaywitz, S. E., Escobar, M. D., Shaywitz, B. A., Fletcher, J. M., & Makuch, R. (1992). Evidence that dyslexia may represent the lower tail of a normal distribution of reading ability. *New England Journal of Medicine, 326*, 145–150.

Simos, P. G., Fletcher, J. M., Rezaie, R., & Papanicolaou, A. C. (2014). Does IQ affect the functional brain network involved in pseudoword reading in students with reading disability? A magnetoencephalography study. *Frontiers in Human Neuroscience, 7*, 932.

Stuebing, K. K., Barth, A. E., Molfese, P. J., Weiss, B., & Fletcher, J. M. (2009). IQ is not strongly related to response to reading instruction: A meta-analytic interpretation. *Exceptional Children, 76*(1), 31–51.

Stuebing, K. K., Barth, A. E., Trahan, L. H., Reddy, R. R., Miciak, J., & Fletcher, J. M. (2015). Are child cognitive characteristics strong predictors of responses to intervention? A meta-analysis. *Review of Educational Research, 85*(3), 395–429.

Stuebing, K. K., Fletcher, J. M., Branum-Martin, L., Francis, D. J., & VanDerHeyden, A. (2012). Evaluation of the technical adequacy of three methods for identifying specific learning disabilities based on cognitive discrepancies. *School Psychology Review, 41*(1), 3–22.

Stuebing, K. K., Fletcher, J. M., LeDoux, J. M., Lyon, G. R., Shaywitz, S. E., & Shaywitz, B. A. (2002). Validity of IQ-discrepancy classifications of reading disabilities: A meta-analysis. *American Educational Research Journal, 39*(2), 469–518.

Styck, K. M., Beaujean, A. A., & Watkins, M. W. (2019). Profile reliability of cognitive ability subscores in a referred sample. *Archives of Scientific Psychology, 7*(1), 119.

Tanaka, H., Black, J. M., Hulme, C., Stanley, L. M., Kesler, S. R., Whitfield-Gabrieli, S., Reiss, A. L., Gabrieli, J. D., & Hoeft, F. (2011). The brain basis of the phonological deficit in dyslexia is independent of IQ. *Psychological Science, 22*(11), 1442–1451.

Taylor, W. P., Miciak, J., Fletcher, J. M., & Francis, D. J. (2017). Cognitive discrepancy models for specific learning disabilities identification: Simulations of psychometric limitations. *Psychological Assessment, 29*(4), 446.

Vellutino, F. R., Scanlon, D. M., & Lyon, R. G. (2000). Differentiating between difficult-to-remediate and readily remediated poor readers: More evidence against the IQ-achievement discrepancy definition of reading disability. *Journal of Learning Disabilities, 33*(3), 223–238.

Vellutino, F. R., Scanlon, D. M., Small, S., & Fanuele, D. P. (2006). Response to intervention as a vehicle for distinguishing between children with and without reading disabilities: Evidence for the role of kindergarten and first-grade interventions. *Journal of Learning Disabilities, 39*(2), 157–169.

Wadsworth, S., Olson, R., & DeFries, J. (2010). Differential genetic etiology of reading difficulties as a function of IQ: An update. *Behavior Genetics, 40*, 751–758.

Waesche, J. S. B., Schatschneider, C., Maner, J. K., Ahmed, Y., & Wagner, R. K. (2011). Examining agreement and longitudinal stability among traditional and response-to-intervention-based definitions of reading disability using the affected-status agreement statistic. *Journal of Learning Disabilities, 44*(3), 296.

Wagner, R. K., Edwards, A. A., Malkowski, A., Schatschneider, C., Joyner, R. E., Wood, S., & Zirps, F. A. (2019). Combining old and new for better understanding and predicting dyslexia. *New Directions for Child and Adolescent Development, 2019*(165), 11–23.

Wanzek, J., Petscher, Y., Al Otaiba, S., Kent, S. C., Schatschneider, C., Haynes, M., Rivas,

B. K., & Jones, F. G. (2016). Examining the average and local effects of a standardized treatment for fourth graders with reading difficulties. *Journal of Research on Educational Effectiveness, 9*(Suppl.), 45–66.

Widiger, T. A. (1992). Categorical versus dimensional classification: Implications from and for research. *Journal of Personality Disorders, 6*(4), 287–300.

Woodcock, R. W., McGrew, K. S., & Mather, N. (2001). *Woodcock–Johnson III NU Complete.* Riverside.

CHAPTER 2

Representational Quality in Children with Dyslexia

Issues of Precision and Redundancy That Affect Long-Term Word Reading and Decoding Development

Donald L. Compton, Laura M. Steacy, Valeria M. Rigobon, Ashley A. Edwards, Nuria Gutiérrez, Nancy C. Marencin, and Rebecca M. Vasile

Automatic and effortless word recognition is a hallmark of skilled reading (see Stanovich, 1991). During the earliest stages of reading development, children are tasked with establishing and storing high-quality orthographic representations that allow automatic word reading. Fully specified orthographic representations are "deterministic" (Perfetti, 1991) and impenetrable to factors such as knowledge and expectation (Perfetti, 2007; Perfetti & Hart, 2002; Stanovich, 1991); thus, permitting an orthographic input to sufficiently and uniquely identify the word to be read (see Castles et al., 2018). This, in turn, activates phonological, syntactic, and semantic information to be used by the reader to form faithful representations of text (see Foorman et al., 2016; Kintsch & Rawson, 2005; Snow, 2002). Our group has spent years studying variability in the quality of orthographic representations in children, the cognitive and experiential determinants of individual differences in these representations, and the possible reasons why children with dyslexia experience difficulties forming high-quality representations. This work has been heavily influenced by Perfetti's (1991, 1992) early writings on the formation of orthographic representations, leading to the lexical quality hypothesis (Perfetti & Hart, 2002), as well as the architecture and mechanistic explanations provided by computational models of word reading, specifically the triangle model (Harm, McCandliss, & Seidenberg, 2003; Harm & Seidenberg, 1999, 2004; Seidenberg, 2005; Seidenberg & McClelland, 1989). Here, we review work, both our own and that of others, that has influenced how we currently think about the formation of orthographic representations in children with dyslexia and those from linguistically diverse backgrounds who are at risk for developing dyslexia. Specifically, we consider how the lexical principles of *precision* and *redundancy* (see Perfetti,

1992) help explain word reading and decoding behavior of children with dyslexia and those who are at risk for developing dyslexia.

To accomplish our goal, we first review key tenets of symptomology and etiology related to developmental dyslexia; provide an overview of a developmental word reading model (orthographic learning) that guides our work; offer a summary of the knowledge sources supporting the development of the orthographic lexicon; and, finally, introduce Perfetti's concepts of redundancy and precision that affect the quality of representations in developing readers. We then present results from two studies that suggest the importance of considering issues of precision and redundancy in the formation of high-quality orthographic representations that affect word reading development in children with dyslexia and those from linguistically diverse backgrounds. We conclude by providing some general comments on how intervention programs that promote the development of skills and knowledge that support the formation of precise and redundant orthographic representations may be particularly effective for at-risk readers.

Developmental Dyslexia

Dyslexia is a developmental word reading and spelling disorder affecting anywhere from 6% to 17% of school-age children with variability in prevalence estimates depending largely on the severity of the cut point adopted for diagnosis (Fletcher et al., 2018). While definitions vary (see Fletcher, 2009), the vast majority contain a common set of key elements, including (1) dyslexia is neurobiological in origin; (2) the dominant characteristics or symptoms are persistent and severe difficulties in the development of accurate and/or fluent word recognition, decoding, and spelling skills; and (3) the neurocognitive influences are multifactorial, primarily involving phonological processing deficits as well as weaknesses in other oral language skills and processing speed (Pennington, 2009; Peterson & Pennington, 2015). Developmentally, phonological processing deficits—impaired representation of, or access to, the abstract units of spoken language—have been implicated as the principal source of reading difficulties in dyslexic children by disrupting the ability to establish various levels of spelling-to-sound correspondence knowledge (Brady & Schankweiler, 1991; Bruck, 1992; Juel, Griffith, & Gough, 1986; Shankweiler et al., 1999; Stanovich & Siegel, 1994; Torgesen, 2000; Vellutino et al., 1996). This knowledge underlies accurate and fluent word recognition development through the process of phonological decoding (see Vellutino et al., 2004), supporting self-teaching (Share, 1995) and/or orthographic learning (see Castles & Nation, 2006; Nation & Castles, 2017). As such, deficits in individuals with dyslexia are more likely to be observed when the phonological demands of the word reading task are greater (e.g., decoding of pronounceable nonwords), giving rise to the well-documented nonword reading deficit in children with developmental dyslexia (e.g., Harm & Seidenberg, 1999; Metsala et al., 1998; Rack et al., 1992). Here, we explore how phonological processing difficulties and associated difficulties developing orthography-to-phonology (O→P) knowledge result in orthographic representations low in redundancy and precision that affect word reading and decoding development across time among children with dyslexia and children from linguistically diverse backgrounds who are at risk of dyslexia. To help anchor our discussion of orthographic representation development and the role of precision and redundancy in the formation of high-quality orthographic representations in children with dyslexia, we first present a model of item-level word reading development known as *orthographic learning.*

Orthographic Learning: Mechanism for Word Reading Development

Orthographic learning (see Nation & Castles, 2017; Perfetti, 1992) explains the transition from novice to skilled word reading through the continuous addition of high-quality and fully specified word-specific representations to the orthographic lexicon. Orthographic learning is an item-based acquisition process that relies heavily on the application of phonological decoding skills to novel printed words via self-teaching (see Share, 1995, 2011), which results in the formation of stable item-specific orthographic representations. Studies of early reading development have reported that relatively few successful exposures to a word are required for the acquisition of word-specific representations in typically developing readers (e.g., Brooks, 1977; Ehri & Saltmarsh, 1995; Reitsma, 1983), implying that word-specific representations form relatively rapidly as children develop reading skills. Furthermore, item-based acquisition theories acknowledge that, at any point in time, a child may be reading some words slowly and with great effort, while other words are read automatically (Castles & Nation, 2006; Share, 1995). This item-level variation likely depends on individual differences in variables like the frequency and richness of reading (Cunningham & Stanovich, 1998), phonological decoding skill (de Jong et al., 2009; Nation & Castles, 2017), and semantic knowledge (Ouellette & Fraser, 2009; Perfetti & Stafura, 2014).

Quasiregular orthographies, such as English, contain substantial ambiguities between orthography and phonology, which place added demands on developing readers (see Seymour et al., 2003) and an increased level of complexity to the process of orthographic learning. At the level of the item (e.g., the specific word to be learned), there are word features and child characteristics that either promote or inhibit orthographic learning. For developing readers, attempting to decode an unfamiliar letter string can result in either full or partial decoding (see Castles & Nation, 2006; Elbro et al., 2012; Keenan & Betjemann, 2008; Tunmer & Chapman, 2012; Venezky, 1999). Full decoding occurs when a reader has sufficient phonological decoding skills to sound out words containing regular (or decodable) relationships between orthography and phonology. Partial decoding, on the other hand, occurs when the reader does not have sufficient phonological decoding skills to sound out the word or the word is irregular and cannot be pronounced correctly by applying common decoding rules (e.g., *was*, *have*, *come*, *said*, *shoe*, *wasp*, *stomach*, and *soup*) (Wang et al., 2013). During full or partial decoding, the role of the reader is to match the assembled phonology from phonological decoding with the lexical phonological representation of the word (see Share, 2008; Venezky, 1999). Thus, the decodability of a word depends on both the decoding knowledge of the child (e.g., Steacy et al., 2020) and the relative regularity of the orthographic-to-phonological (O→P) relationships of the word (Seidenberg et al., 1984). Further, the availability of top-down support, either through activation of the stored phonological form (e.g., Duff & Hulme, 2012; Wang et al., 2013) or meaning (Ouellette & Fraser, 2009), help a child to determine the exact pronunciation of a novel letter string based on a partial decoding attempt. This suggests lexical support in orthographic learning under conditions of decoding ambiguity (see Wang et al., 2012, 2013). As such, orthographic learning is relevant to the learning of all words with differences in a child's ability to acquire a reliable orthographic representation being influenced by a combination of child- (e.g. phonological awareness, phonological decoding skill, and availability of semantic and phonological forms) and word-characteristics (e.g., the word's regularity, orthographic complexity, and frequency) and the overall number of word exposures the child experiences (see Cunningham & Stanovich, 1998; Reitsma, 1983). Our work suggests that there are substantial individual differences in developing readers' ability to form high-quality orthographic representations (Compton, 2002; Edwards et al., in press; Gilbert et al., 2011; Kearns et al., 2016; Siegelman et al., in press; Steacy & Compton, 2019; Steacy et al., 2017, 2019a, 2019b, 2021a, 2021b); we have concentrated our efforts on identifying significant cognitive and experiential predictors that help explain why some children have difficulty forming and storing high-quality representations available for reading and spelling. To fully understand our perspective on representation quality as it relates to children with dyslexia, we present a more detailed explanation of the lexical knowledge sources that support the critical development of high-quality orthographic representations.

Evolution of the Knowledge Sources Supporting Development of the Orthographic Lexicon

A typically developing reader's orthographic lexicon contains approximately 10,000 word-specific representations (excluding inflectional forms) by eighth grade (Ehri, 2005; Harris & Jacobson, 1982). This requires a lexical system that can quickly establish and reliably retrieve word-specific spellings that activate pronunciation, meaning, and syntax. The orthographic lexicon comprises four major components (i.e., knowledge sources): word-specific representations, orthographic units, phonological units, and sublexical O→P connections (see Compton et al., 2014; Perfetti et al., 2005). As children learn to read, the orthographic lexicon changes in two important ways (Compton, 2002; Ehri, 2014; Perfetti, 1992). First, there is a continuous increase in the absolute number of orthographically addressable entries, referred to as word-specific representations. Word-specific representations are considered less dependent on phonological processes because they have been supplanted by specific connections linking spelling directly to pronunciation (Harm & Seidenberg, 2004; Perfetti, 1992; Share, 1995).

The second change in the orthographic lexicon associated with reading development is an increase in the overall quantity and quality of sublexical O→P connections (Perfetti, 1992). Sublexical connections between orthographic and phonological codes exist at multiple levels: for instance, individual letter-phonemes, letter cluster-phonemes, letter cluster-rimes, letter cluster-syllables, and letter cluster-morphemes (see Berninger, 1994; Ziegler & Goswami, 2005). Early O→P connections are initially based on simple one-to-one correspondences that are relatively insensitive to orthographic context (see Share, 1995). With reading experience O→P connections evolve to represent abstract context-dependent O→P relationships (see Steacy et al., 2019a; Treiman et al., 2003; Treiman et al., 2006) that are "*implicit, very numerous, and very fast*" (Gough et al., 1992, p. 38). We maintain that disruptions in the formation of both basic and sophisticated sublexical O→P knowledge in children with dyslexia result in orthographic representations that are of low quality, lacking redundant and precise O→P connections, and, ultimately, compromise the development of context-dependent decoding rules. To better understand the relationship between disruptions in the phonological system in children with dyslexia and the associated paucity of complex O→P connections, we draw upon Perfetti's (1991, 1992) concepts of precision and redundancy as they apply to the development of high-quality orthographic representations.

The Role of Precision and Redundancy in the Formation of High-Quality Representations

Increases in word reading skill not only bring about the addition of more word-specific entries but also produce important changes in the representations. Changes in representational quality at the item-level drive the formation of complex O→P connections by increasing the number of sophisticated context-sensitive connections. As Perfetti puts it, "the more powerful the context-sensitive decoding rules (or analogic capabilities), the more entries the learner can acquire. And the more entries, the more powerful the decoding rules" (1992, pp. 161–162). Additionally, the application of increasingly sophisticated O→P connections during decoding refines stored phonological representations and improves overall quality of representations (see Ehri, 2020). From Perfetti's perspective, there are two principles that characterize the development of high-quality lexical representations: *precision* and *redundancy*. The precision principle is that fully specified representations are superior to partially specified ones. Precise representations are determinant with respect to the input features that will trigger it, meaning that a given letter string will be sufficient to fully activate spelling, exact pronunciation, meaning, and part of speech. In contrast, variable or less precise representations (i.e., memory for specific letters and their positions within a word is incomplete or inaccurate) are often "fuzzy" in terms of eliciting spelling and activating an exact phonological pronunciation, as well as lacking specificity in meaning. From Perfetti's perspective, lexical representations evolve toward completeness and specification through the process of becoming more precise. We further enumerate on the process by suggesting that high-quality representations can only form in the presence of a precise phonological representation along with the requisite O→P knowledge to allow successful phonological decoding. To support "amalgamation" between the orthographic and phonological representations (see Ehri, 2020) that is the hallmark of a precise and high-quality orthographic representation, we and other colleagues (e.g., Elbro & de Jong, 2017) suggest that a decoded form of the word must be formed and likely stored as part of a word's lexical representation. The decoded form of a word is viewed as a stepping stone between the orthographic representation of a word and its standard pronunciation. Elbro and de Jong stress that beginning readers must learn to associate the novel sound pattern, what we refer to as the *decoded form*, with an existing pronunciation in the phonological lexicon, a process that requires some degree of phonological flexibility. As Elbro and de Jong put it, "readers learn spelling pronunciations [decoded form] as alternative (variant) phonological representations in addition to the familiar spoken ones that are already stored in their mental lexicon. So, for example, a reader who comes across the printed word answer may form a phonological representation *answer* that contains a "w" sound in addition to the already familiar representation *anser*" (p. 177). There is strong evidence that creating the decoded form influences phonological representations of the words in the reader's mental lexicon (e.g., Morais & Kolinsky, 2005; Nation & Hulme, 2011; Ranbom & Connine, 2011), leading Elbro and de Jong to suggest that decoded forms are learned just like any other variant of a spoken language—both on an item basis and by means of patterns that emerge from the relationships between spelling pronunciations and standard pronunciations. All of this suggests that precise lexical representations for reading and spelling consist of knowledge of the orthographic pattern, the phonological representation of the word, and the decoded form of the word. It is important to note that the stored phonological representation of a word can vary significantly across individuals, whereas the decoded form should be much more invariant. As such, children with phonological processing difficulties (e.g., children with dyslexia) often store less precise phonological representations and also fail to develop the essential O→P knowledge to allow successful phonological decoding. The lack of precise phonological representations presents fundamental issues that limit the formation of high-quality orthographic representations through the formation of decoded forms of the word. We illustrate how the principle of precision affects children's ability to complete what is known as "phonological cleanup" during decoding and how this likely affects overall word reading development in children with dyslexia and perhaps those from linguistically diverse backgrounds.

The second principle of qualitative changes in a representation is that of redundancy. Just as representations become more fully specified, they also increase in their inclusion of redundant information sources. The main source of redundancy results from O→P connections at various levels or grain sizes (see Ziegler & Goswami, 2005). As we noted above, O→P connections exist at multiple levels (e.g., individual letter-phonemes, letter cluster-phonemes, letter cluster-rimes, letter cluster-syllables, and letter cluster-morphemes), and this overlap between connections at various levels results in O→P redundancy and helps push precision (e.g., letters in the word *drinking* represented at the individual phoneme level, /dr/ as a two-consonant cluster, /ink/ and /ing/ as different cluster-rimes, and /ing/ as a morpheme, too). With reading development, initially incomplete and oversimplified, representations become sophisticated context-dependent connections (Steacy et al., 2019; Treiman et al., 2003, 2006). The redundancy advantage is important in reading both for bootstrapping the identification of unfamiliar words and for the rapid automatic recognition of familiar words. We demonstrate the importance of redundancy by illustrating the consequence of children with dyslexia relying on a single O→P connection at the whole word level, which leads to what we have termed *lexical asymmetry*. We extend the idea of redundancy to help account for poor word reading development in at-risk bilingual children and children who speak dialects.

Redundancy Principle: Lexical Asymmetry and Word Reading in Developmental Dyslexia

As mentioned previously, deficits in phonemic awareness skill limit the growth of important sublexical O→P associations in children with dyslexia (see Brady & Schankweiler, 1991; Harm & Seidenberg, 2004; Torgesen, 2000; Vellutino et al., 1996). As a result, children with dyslexia exhibit a general tendency to process only partial information about words and further rely on sources of information other than sublexical O→P associations that are considerably less efficient to facilitate word recognition (see Harm et al., 2003; Stanovich, 1988). This is consistent with the view that children with dyslexia may be overreliant on a global processing strategy that results in insufficient attention to individual letters or groupings of letters (Ehri & Saltmarsh, 1995; Frith, 1985; Siegel et al., 1995) and the corresponding phonological representations. The result is that children with dyslexia tend to add word-specific representations to the lexicon without associated growth in sublexical O→P associations (i.e., the behavioral equivalent of overfitting). These representations lack redundancy and, therefore, are also considered less precise.

From a grain-size perspective (see Ziegler & Goswami, 2005), attention to the coarser whole word-phonological grain prevents the development of finer O→P associations that support the development and expansion of important context-dependent sublexical O→P associations (see also Harm et al., 2003; Steacy et al., 2019). We (Compton, 2002; Compton et al., 2014; Steacy et al., 2021b) have conceptualized this as *asymmetric* development of the lexical system in which children with dyslexia add word-specific representations (i.e., whole word-phonological) to their orthographic lexicons without the corresponding development of sublexical associations (i.e., fine-grained O→P associations) seen in typically developing readers. The asymmetry explanation is consistent with the behavioral observation of the nonword reading deficit in children with developmental dyslexia (e.g., Metsala et al., 1998; Metsala, 1999; Rack et al., 1992).

Our data is consistent with the hypothesized time course of nonword and word reading development associated with asymmetric lexical development in children with dyslexia. Namely, initially weak phonological representations lead to a global processing strategy in word learning, resulting in a lack of redundant O→P associations, which, in turn, leads to asymmetric development of the lexical system in children with dyslexia such that word-specific representations are added to the orthographic lexicon without the corresponding development of sublexical O→P associations that allow the decoding of nonwords. In a recent developmental study (see Steacy et al., 2021b), we modeled parallel growth of word reading and nonword reading factor scores across the entire distribution of reading skills (N = 588 children) using a growth curve of factors approach, focusing specifically on those children with low levels of initial reading skill in first grade (i.e., children at risk for developing dyslexia). Vector plots (see ***https://qmi-fcrr.shinyapps.io/vector_plot*** for a demonstration) were used to visualize the co-development between individual word reading–nonword reading factor trajectories across grades 1–4 as a function of initial word reading and nonword reading skill in first grade. This was the first study to model, and display visually, the relations between word reading and nonword reading growth trajectories in a large sample of developing readers, thus allowing the asymmetry hypotheses of dyslexia to be appraised.

Vectors are quantities that have both direction and magnitude; allowing visualization of the direction and magnitude of simultaneous growth in two sets of constructs. In our case, the vector plot for estimated word reading and nonword reading co-development displays estimated word reading scores on the x-axis and estimated nonword reading scores on the y-axis. Each arrow represents the word reading–nonword reading vector for an individual child. The arrows provide several key pieces of information for interpreting co-development. First, the base of the arrow indicates the estimated initial status of a child's word reading and nonword reading (i.e., spring of first grade). Second, the head of an arrow represents the final estimated factor scores on both the word reading and nonword reading assessments. Third, the length of an arrow describes the amount of growth in both word reading and nonword reading during grades 1–4. Finally, the angle of the arrow characterizes co-development. Arrows pointed closer to 0° reflect individual growth that is dominant for the measured domain on the x-axis (i.e., word reading), whereas arrows pointed closer to 45° represent relatively equal co-development in both word reading and nonword reading domains (Petscher et al., 2016). Thus, each vector plot represents initial word reading and nonword reading performance in first grade, final word reading and nonword reading performance in fourth grade, the magnitude of growth in word reading and nonword reading across grades 1–4, and the relative co-development of word reading and nonword reading growth between grades 1–4.

Vector visualization indicated that children with low initial word reading and nonword reading skills tend to exhibit relatively flat word reading–nonword reading co-development (i.e., word reading growth without concomitant nonword reading growth), again supporting the well-documented nonword reading deficit in children with developmental dyslexia (see Rack et al., 1992). Additionally, results indicate that while word reading and nonword reading growth factors are highly related in the sample, the relation between word reading and nonword reading trajectories changes in a nonlinear fashion as a function of initial word reading and nonword reading skills. Specifically, the angle of word reading–nonword reading vectors moves from nearly 45° in children with average and high initial word reading skill to much more horizontal in children with low initial word reading. Flat vectors indicate word reading growth without concomitant growth in nonword reading. In addition, children with low initial word reading skills also had lower phonological awareness skills compared to children with average and high initial word reading skills. From a lexical asymmetry standpoint, Ehri and Saltmarsh (1995) have hypothesized that children with dyslexia lack sufficient "grapho-phonic" knowledge to fully analyze matches between orthographic and phonological units in order to store high-quality representations that include complete sublexical O→P associations. This is consistent with the view that phonological processing deficits in children with dyslexia lead to a processing strategy that affords insufficient attention to sublexical O→P relations and representations that lack redundancy across O→P connections of different grain sizes. It is important to emphasize that the lexical asymmetry hypothesis views this dependence on more global orthographic structure in dyslexia not as a strategy, but rather as a consequence of how O→P mappings are learned. Results suggest that phonological processing problems in children with dyslexia result in the inability to form redundant O→P mappings, decreasing the ability to establish decoded forms of words and thus affecting the overall quality of orthographic representations, which significantly decreases the process of orthographic learning.

From the standpoint of children from linguistically diverse backgrounds, the possibility that word-specific representations are formed without adequate redundancy between subword O→P associations is quite plausible, but for very different reasons than children with dyslexia. In the case of English learners (ELs) in the United States, the evidence that points to a distinct lag in word reading skills, even among ELs with high listening comprehension (Vaughn et al., 2009) and oral language skills, is suggestive of a struggle with forming connections from phonological representations to orthographic representations at the beginning of English acquisition (Mancilla-Martinez & Lesaux, 2010; Nakamoto et al., 2007). Particularly for ELs who are acquiring oral language skills in a home language that is more orthographically transparent than English, such as Spanish, there is no necessity to form O→P connections beyond the simple one-to-one correspondences that are insensitive to orthographic context when beginning to read in the home language. Therefore, a lack of attention to larger grain sizes of O→P connections in the home language can contribute to some ELs' difficulty in establishing sublexical connections at multiple levels that are crucial for developing word-specific representations in English. While typically developing ELs may catch up in word-level reading skills with peers who learned English as a first language (O'Connor et al., 2019), it is important to acknowledge that in the context of English acquisition in the United States, the impact of this initial difficulty with forming redundant sublexical O→P connections can be seen in persistently slower vocabulary growth and lags in reading comprehension (Kieffer, 2008).

Rather than an initial lack of sensitivity to grain sizes beyond simple one-to-one correspondences, students who speak Nonmainstream American English

(NMAE), including any dialect of English with phonological and morphosyntactic features that deviate from Mainstream American English (MAE), are tasked with navigating even more irregularities in sublexical O→P associations than other MAE-speaking peers who are beginning to read in English (Brown et al., 2015). For example, children who speak African American English (AAE, a systematic, rule-governed dialect of American English) learn to pronounce words with reduced final consonant clusters (e.g., "depen" for "depend"). When these children begin to internalize this rule of the spoken language they hear at home and in their community, they are already forming precise and high-quality representations for the phonological units in words that they have in their oral vocabulary but are doing so in a way that does not include information about the letter(s) that the child does not pronounce (final /d/ in "depend"). Therefore, a child who speaks AAE at home may struggle to decode "depend" in text, even after explicitly learning the most frequent MAE pronunciations of each grapheme in the word, and subsequently fail to realize that the decoded form of "depend" is semantically identical to their stored representation of "depen" after the first decoding attempt. Such differences between dialects and complicated encounters with increasingly more irregular words in English text (i.e., higher inconsistency between spelling and pronunciation and lower decodability) can impact phonological development of children who speak NMAE as they learn how to read and write in MAE at school (Thomas-Tate et al., 2006), contributing to fewer successful decoding attempts and slower establishment of redundant sublexical O→P associations at different grain sizes. Without forming those redundant associations in early reading experiences or obtaining a clear understanding of how to be flexible with words' pronunciations between mainstream and non-mainstream English dialects when introduced to MAE in school, a beginning reader will likely continue to struggle with the conflict between their phonological representations of words in the two different dialects and ultimately fall behind in building new orthographic representations for both unknown words and known words in their oral vocabulary that are encountered in text.

In sum, we hypothesize that the developmental consequence of lexical asymmetry is a significant reduction of successful self-teaching opportunities in children with dyslexia and, by analogy, at-risk children from linguistically diverse backgrounds because of limited sublexical O→P connections necessary for phonological decoding and thus the ability to establish decoded forms of words. We now turn to the principle of precision by examining the relationship between the process of phonological cleanup and word reading skill in developing readers.

Precision Principle: The Role of Phonological Cleanup in Word Reading Development

While phonological decoding skill is certainly necessary to support orthographic learning, it is not sufficient to guarantee the formation of a particular word-specific representation (see Nation & Castles, 2017; Share, 2008). As mentioned previously, for developing readers, attempting to decode an unfamiliar letter string can result in either full or partial decoding (see Castles & Nation, 2006; Elbro et al., 2012; Keenan & Betjemann, 2008; Tunmer & Chapman, 2012; Venezky, 1999), in which the role of the reader is to match the assembled decoded form of the letter string with the stored phonological form of the word (see Share, 2008; Venezky, 1999). Thus, the probability that a child will correctly decode an unfamiliar letter string depends on the decoding knowledge of the reader, the relative regularity of the orthographic-to-phonological (O→P) relationships of the word, and the ability of the reader to bridge any differences between the decoded form and the correct phonological form stored in memory.

The "distance" between the decoded form and correct phonological form affects the probability that a developing reader will successfully make the match (see Edwards et al., in press), as does the precision of the child's stored phonological representation. Certainly, the task of disambiguating the decoded form to identify the stored phonological form of the word places primary demands on the phonological system in what can be thought of as a cleanup process. Connectionist models of reading (see Harm & Seidenberg, 1999, 2004; Harm et al., 2003; Rueckl et al., 2019) contain a set of phonological cleanup units that contribute to decoding by cleaning up noisy or incomplete phonological representations resulting from orthographic input. This allows hidden units from the orthographic component of the model to provide the phonological system with somewhat incomplete input, akin to the decoded form that a child might produce, which captures the regularities in the mapping from orthography to phonology.

The distributed nature of connectionist models allows phonological cleanup units to be influenced by phonological, orthographic, and semantic components of the model, thus providing various sources of information to bear on the problem of disambiguating a mismatch between the decoded and phonological forms, particularly ones that result from orthographic to phonological mapping. With more training, the phonological cleanup units within the model become attuned to corpus orthography-to-phonology relations, which allows the cleanup units to efficiently disambiguate ever more complicated and noisy inputs. This suggests that the overall precision of stored phonological representations significantly aids in the cleanup process. Connectionist modeling studies have shown that disruptions to the phonological cleanup units result in network performance that degrades performance and mimics that of children with moderate to severe phonological dyslexia, that is, severely impaired nonword reading and moderately impaired exception word reading (see Harm & Seidenberg, 2004; Steacy et al., 2021b). In an unimpaired model, the phonological system contributes to decoding by cleaning up noisy or incomplete phonological representations that result from generating the decoded form of a word. However, in the impaired phonological system, more work must be done by the hidden units because the phonological system is less able to repair degraded or incomplete phonological representations that result from the decoding process, in part because the stored form of the phonological representation is less precise. Furthermore, the lack of precise phonological representations limits the influence of subword O→P information available to the cleanup units and inhibits the normal functions of the cleanup units to disambiguate noisy or incomplete phonological representations. From a computational standpoint, impaired phonological cleanup units impair the formation of precise and redundant orthographic representations, which further limits the ability of the cleanup units to draw upon distributed O→P relations within the system to help clean up and disambiguate a noisy input.

In our behavioral work, we have used the set for variability (SfV) task as a proxy for the mechanisms involved in the phonological cleanup process. The SfV task is a purely oral language task (see Tunmer & Chapman, 1998) requiring an individual to disambiguate the mismatch between the decoded form of an irregular word (provided orally by the assessor) and its actual lexical pronunciation (produced by the child). In the task, children are asked to identify the correct pronunciation of spoken English words that are "mispronounced" by the assessor based on regular decoding rules (e.g., /brikfəst/ for /brɛkfəst/; /wæsp/ for /wɒsp/). We have recently reported a correlation of .79 between SfV and word reading skill (with the effects of age removed) in a sample of 489 children in grades 2–5 (see Steacy et al., submitted). In addition, we used regression analyses to demonstrate the strength of the SfV–word reading relationship in the presence of other important word reading-related predictors (i.e., phonological awareness, rapid automatized naming, vocabulary, and attention). Results indicate that SfV explained an additional 16.5% of unique variance in word reading, whereas phonological awareness only predicted 1.2% of unique variance in word reading above all other predictors. We used quantile regression to explore whether the strength of the association between SfV and word reading varies as a function of word reading ability and found that the magnitude of the association between SfV and word reading differed across quantiles. The strength of the association between SfV and word reading was higher at the lower end of word reading (see Figure 2.1). Results suggest that in children with dyslexia, the SfV task may represent a true measure of phonological cleanup by stressing the phonological system without the availability of other types of representations (spellings and decoded forms) and, therefore, represents a "purer" index of phonological processing as it relates to word reading. We interpret these results as evidence that precise phonological representations are likely necessary for the phonological cleanup process that undergirds successful orthographic learning.

While phonological processing difficulties hamper the phonological cleanup system in children with dyslexia by limiting the formation of precise representations, the mechanisms that affect the phonological cleanup process in at-risk children from linguistically diverse backgrounds appear more experiential. Lack of well-established semantic and phonological representations in ELs may stem from having generally fewer opportunities to consolidate whole-word semantic representations and subword O→P associations compared to their peers who are learning Mainstream American English (MAE) as their first language with family members who also speak it at home. For example, ELs who more often speak with non-fluent English-speaking family members at home are likely participating in fewer English conversations that are enriched with reliable pronunciations of

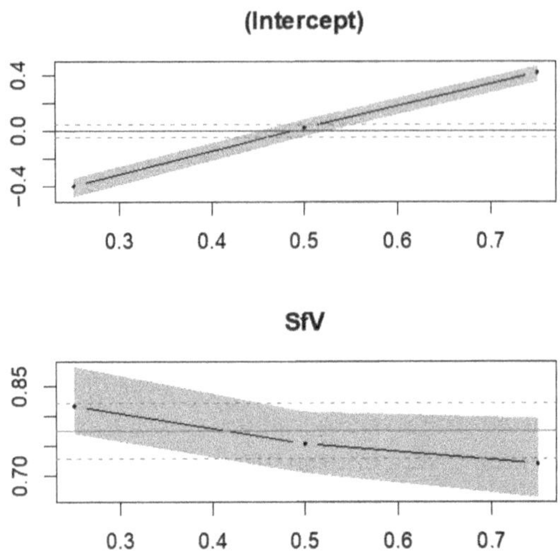

FIGURE 2.1. Coefficient values at each of the three quantiles (.25, .50, and .75) are represented by a black dot, with the surrounding gray area representing the confidence interval. The solid line represents the coefficient that would be observed in OLS regression when conditioned at the mean, with the dashed lines representing the upper and lower bounds of the confidence interval of that estimate.

English words and a diverse vocabulary that a child can use as reliable knowledge sources for building precise phonological representations. So when a partial orthographic representation (i.e., decoded form) results from an EL's attempt to decode an unfamiliar letter string with limited O→P sublexical connections, the lack of existing high-quality phonological or semantic representations of the word does not leave the EL child with other helpful sources of information about the word to disambiguate the orthographic input (Goldenberg, 2020). Additionally, prior reading experience in more orthographically transparent languages than English would not require an EL to store more than one fully specified representation of the word or develop some form of a phonological cleanup system given that the consistency of spelling to sound mappings would result in the decoded and actual word pronunciations being the same or nearly identical for the majority of words in that transparent language. Therefore, a phonological cleanup system may not be necessary for an EL to rely on until being tasked with reading written words in English.

Rather than experiencing a lack of opportunities for forming precise phonological associations, students who speak Nonmainstream American English (NMAE) dialects of English already form precise phonological representations of words in their oral vocabulary in both their NMAE dialect and MAE. Findings from Terry and Scarborough (2011) suggest that a child's usage of NMAE in settings where MAE is necessary (e.g., reading) may indicate a lack of "metalinguistic insights that underlie contextually appropriate flexibility of language usage and an appreciation of the phonological structure of words" (p. 112). In other words, a dialect speaker attempting to decode an unfamiliar word can struggle with connecting its decoded form to either of the individual's stored pronunciations, particularly if reading instruction has not included explicit training to think flexibly about the different phonemes that can be represented by a single grapheme in English (i.e., linguistic awareness of complex phonological structure within English words). The lack of linguistic awareness among NMAE speakers who struggle with word reading skills can account for why some NMAE speakers do not benefit from a phonological cleanup system when deciding which of their stored phonological representations most closely maps onto the printed spelling of the unfamiliar word encountered in text. Similarly, to how ELs' lack of sensitivity to different grain-size O→P connections can limit their formation of redundant sublexical connections, NMAE speakers' lack of sensitivity to variation in language structure between dialects can limit the usefulness of cleanup units in the context of partial/incomplete decoding attempts.

Results from our work (Edwards et al., in press; Steacy et al., submitted) suggest that the ability of the reader to bridge differences between the decoded form and the correct phonological form stored in memory (i.e., phonological cleanup) is a critical aspect of forming high-quality orthographic representations in developing readers. Furthermore, the distance between the decoded form and phonological form affects the probability that a developing reader will successfully make the match, as does the precision of the child's stored phonological representation. We present these results as evidence that precise phonological representations are necessary for the phonological cleanup process that undergirds successful orthographic learning and, further, that a lack of the decoded form or greater distance between decoded and already stored phonological forms in at-risk readers makes the cleanup process more difficult. We conclude by exploring how the principles of precision and redundancy may play an important role in how we consider instruction/intervention for children at risk for poor word reading outcomes.

The Potential Role of Precision and Redundancy in Interventions for At-Risk Learners

The goal of early word reading instruction/intervention for children at risk of developing poor reading outcomes is to provide pedagogical experiences that promote a progression of skill development that supports word reading and decoding skills. From our perspective, this means instructional procedures that support symmetrical development of word-specific representations and advanced sublexical O→P connections by systematically supporting relations between orthography, phonology, and semantics. Our vision of effective instruction for at-risk children promotes advanced decoding and word identification skill development in a way that promotes symmetrical growth of the two orthographic lexicon systems, as described by Perfetti (1991, 1992). Furthermore, we argue this approach has the potential to promote "typical" learning mechanisms in children who struggle to learn to read. While it is important to note that the etiology of word reading difficulties in children with dyslexia may differ from those of at-risk children from linguistically diverse backgrounds, it appears that the basic components needed to support word reading and decoding skill development in these groups are similar, with the relative emphasis of different components perhaps differing across groups. With this in mind, it makes sense to consider how intervention programs might productively promote the formation of precise and redundant representations that are the foundation of high-quality orthographic entries.

Considering the development of precision first, we believe that encouraging precise phonological representations that can be connected to semantics and various grain sizes of the orthography is critical. We consider that one of the most plausible levels for influencing precision during orthographic learning is to support the formation of the decoded form of words during children's encounters with unfamiliar letter strings. This can be done both during oral language practice (presenting the decoded form while children are decoding and spelling) and during decoding to support accurate formation of the decoded form. We argue that providing opportunities to create an accurate decoded form of a word, which is connected to the child's actual phonological and semantic representations for that word, will increase the precision of that word's orthographic representation in at-risk learners. An example of how this might work is provided by Boyer and Ehri (2011), who conducted a phonemic awareness experiment to determine whether teaching children to analyze articulatory gestures in words would better secure spellings to pronunciations in memory and hence improve their word reading. It was reasoned by the researchers that if articulation is central to the phonemic representation of words in memory, then enhancing children's sensitivity to the articulatory properties of phonemes should strengthen the grapheme–phoneme connections that are formed to remember how to read words. We further posit that teaching articulatory properties of phonemes in words significantly increases the precision of the phonological representation, allows for easier connection to be made between orthography and phonology, and increases the probability that an accurate decoded form will be established. Results from the study indicate that the articulation group learned to read the words more easily than the other active contrast group (letter-sound learning without articulation). Boyer and Ehri suggest that articulation training improved children's access to the motoric gestures configuring the phonemic representations of words in memory. As a result, during sight word learning trials, letters in the words became more securely attached to these motoric phonemic constituents to support word reading. Other studies have also shown the role of articulation influences children's sight word learning (Laing & Hulme, 1999; Rack et al., 1994). We posit that teaching articulatory properties of phonemes in words significantly increases the precision of the phonological representation and allows for easier connections to be made between orthography and phonology. We wonder whether providing children with accurate auditory input of phonological representations, while also encouraging accurate, and perhaps exaggerated, oral repetitions of the word's decoded form, may also promote the formation of precise phonological representations in the absence of overt articulatory training. The evidence thus far suggests that activities that promote precision of phonological representations have the potential to aid the formation of word-specific representations and advanced sublexical O→P connections and improve the word reading development of children at risk for poor outcomes.

We now turn to the importance of instruction supporting the development of redundant O→P connections in promoting symmetrical development of word-specific representations and advanced sublexical O→P connections. Lovett et al. (2000) tested the efficacy of a combination of a synthetic decoding program and strategy-based word reading approach (focused on teaching O→P connections of varying grain sizes) on the reading outcomes of children with dyslexia. Results suggested that combining the synthetic decoding program and strategy-based word reading approach proved superior to either approach on nonword reading, letter-sound and keyword knowledge, and three other word identification measures. Generalization of nonword decoding to real word identification was achieved with a combination of effective remedial components. We interpret the results as supporting the importance of providing at-risk children with opportunities to develop redundant O→P connections that support the development of advanced decoding skills and, more importantly, high-quality orthographic representations.

Importantly, while it is critical to provide ELs and dialect speakers with practices that have already been deemed effective for foundational skill development in phonemic awareness, decoding, oral reading fluency, and vocabulary acquisition (August, 2018), the needs of linguistically diverse students must also be met with tailored approaches to support the development of word-specific representations and advanced sublexical O→P connections. For ELs who already have some phonological and vocabulary skills in another language, recommendations for academic language instruction (see August et al., 2014; Carlo et al., 2004) can extend beyond prioritizing vocabulary recognition and comprehension to provide several opportunities for students to practice articulating correct word pronunciations (i.e., building more precise phonological representations), mapping those pronunciations onto correct spellings, via formation of the decoded form, with more spelling and writing practice (i.e., strengthening orthographic representations), and using the words in oral and written activities to build a stronger network of links between the phonological, orthographic, and semantic representations of a new word. Particularly for ELs with more orthographically transparent home language exposure, we speculate that learning to decode words that have high spelling-sound inconsistency can be facilitated with special attention to cognates (i.e., words that share similar spelling, meaning, and sometimes pronunciation across languages) that allow for capitalizing on shared language features and focusing on sublexical O→P connections at different grain sizes in English.

For children who speak an NMAE dialect, findings from Brown et al. (2015) reinforce the notion of the ambiguity in reading a word that is pronounced differently between a child's home dialect and MAE being lessened by drawing explicit distinctions between the pronunciations early on in reading development. Combined with repeated exposures to carefully selected vocabulary words that support academic language development (similar to the approach described above with ELs), reading instruction for these students could be more effective by providing instruction that supports accurate formation of the decoded form of a word that is explicitly linked to the child's store phonological representation. It is important to note that this approach is not intended to change the child's stored phonological representations but instead to add the decoded form to that representation to aid in the formation of precise and redundant relations between orthography and the child's stored phonological representation. There is ample evidence to support that AAE speakers can store precise phonological representations in AAE and MAE (Terry & Scarborough, 2011), but we still lack knowledge on best practices for bridging more distant non-MAE representations to decoded forms of irregular words and their MAE pronunciations. The key here is that instead of dismissing a non-MAE or accented word pronunciation as incorrect or completely detached from the MAE pronunciation of a word, reading instruction with linguistically diverse students can reframe foundational reading activities to prioritize *flexibility* with word pronunciations in English while acknowledging the connections that can be made from vocabulary in another home language (in the case of ELs) or precise phonological representations (in the case of NMAE speakers) to the establishment of high-quality orthographic representations. Just as we propose that students with dyslexia may benefit from intervention targeted at forming high-quality word-specific representations based on precise phonological representations and redundant O→P connections, students from linguistically diverse backgrounds may benefit from a set of strategies that are tailored to bridging existing representations to new word representations that foster fluent word reading.

Conclusions

In this chapter, we have made the case for considering Perfetti's lexical principles of precision and redundancy as they relate to the formation of high-quality orthographic representations. Specifically, we consider how these principles help explain the formation of high-quality orthographic representations and how this may help us to better understand the word reading and decoding behaviors of children with dyslexia and those who are at risk for developing poor word reading outcomes due to navigating the challenges of being raised in linguistically diverse backgrounds and educated in MAE classrooms. We present evidence from two studies to suggest that children at risk for poor word reading outcomes fail to form precise and redundant orthographic representations. We further suggest that helping children to form and store precise and redundant decoded forms of words may be one way to improve the formation of high-quality representations in at-risk words. Certainly, more work in this area is warranted as we continue to explore ways to support early word reading development in at-risk children.

ACKNOWLEDGMENTS

This research was supported in part by Grant P20HD091013 from the Eunice Kennedy Shriver National Institute of Child Health and Human Development (NICHD). Statements do not reflect the position or policy of these agencies, and no official endorsement by them should be inferred.

REFERENCES

August, D. (2018). Educating English language learners: A review of the latest research. *American Educator, 42*(3), 4.

August, D., Branum-Martin, L., Cárdenas-Hagan, E., Francis, D. J., Powell, J., Moore, S., & Haynes, E. F. (2014). Helping ELLs meet the Common Core State Standards for literacy in science: The impact of an instructional intervention focused on academic language. *Journal of Research on Educational Effectiveness, 7*(1), 54–82.

Berninger, V. W. (1994). *The varieties of orthographic knowledge I: Theoretical and developmental issues.* Kluwer Academic Press.

Boyer, N., & Ehri, L. C. (2011). Contribution of phonemic segmentation instruction with letters and articulation pictures to word reading and spelling in beginners. *Scientific Studies of Reading, 15*(5), 440–470.

Brady, S. A., & Shankweiler, D. P. (Eds.). (1991). *Phonological processes in literacy: A tribute to Isabelle Y. Liberman.* Erlbaum.

Brooks, L. (1977). Visual pattern in fluent word identification. In A. S. Reber & D. L. Scarborough (Eds.), *Towards a psychology of reading* (pp. 95–110). Erlbaum.

Brown, M. C., Sibley, D. E., Washington, J. A., Rogers, T. T., Edwards, J. R., MacDonald, M. C., & Seidenberg, M. S. (2015). Impact of dialect use on a basic component of learning to read. *Frontiers in Psychology, 6*, 196.

Bruck, M. (1992). Persistence of dyslexics' phonological awareness deficits. *Developmental Psychology, 28*, 874–886.

Carlo, M. S., August, D., McLaughlin, B., Snow, C. E., Dressler, C., Lippman, D. N., & White, C. E. (2004). Closing the gap: Addressing the vocabulary needs of English-language learners in bilingual and mainstream classrooms. *Reading Research Quarterly, 39*(2), 188–215.

Castles, A., & Nation, K. (2006). How does orthographic learning happen? In S. Andrews (Ed.), *From inkmarks to ideas: Current issues in lexical processing* (pp. 151–179). Psychology Press.

Castles, A., Rastle, K., & Nation, K. (2018). Ending the reading wars: Reading acquisition from novice to expert. *Psychological Science in the Public Interest, 19*(1), 5–51.

Compton, D. L. (2002). The relationship between phonological processing, orthographic processing, and lexical development in reading-disabled children. *Journal of Special Education, 35*, 201–210.

Compton, D. L., Miller, A. C., Elleman, A. M., & Steacy, L. M. (2014). Have we forsaken reading theory in the name of "quick fix" interventions for children with reading disability? *Scientific Studies of Reading, 18*(1), 55–73.

Cunningham, A. E., & Stanovich, K. E. (1998). What reading does for the mind. *American Educator, 22*, 8–17.

de Jong, P. F., Bitter, D. J., Van Setten, M., & Marinus, E. (2009). Does phonological recoding occur during silent reading, and is it necessary for orthographic learning? *Journal of Experimental Child Psychology, 104*(3), 267–282.

Duff, F. J., & Hulme, C. (2012). The role of children's phonological and semantic knowledge in learning to read words. *Scientific Studies of Reading, 16*(6), 504–525.

Edwards, A., Steacy, L. M., Seigelman, N., Rigobon, V. M., Kearns, V. M., Rueckl, J. R., & Compton, D. L. (in press). Unpacking the unique relationship between set for variability and word reading development: Examining word- and child-level predictors of performance. *Journal of Educational Psychology.*

Ehri, L. C. (2005). Learning to read words: Theory, findings, and issues. *Scientific Studies of Reading, 9*, 167–188.

Ehri, L. C. (2014). Orthographic mapping in the acquisition of sight word reading, spelling memory, and vocabulary learning. *Scientific Studies of Reading, 18*(1), 5–21.

Ehri, L. C. (2020). The science of learning to read words: A case for systematic phonics instruction. *Reading Research Quarterly, 55*, S45–S60.

Ehri, L. C., & Saltmarsh, J. (1995). Beginning readers outperform older disabled readers in learning to read words by sight. *Reading and Writing, 7*, 295–326.

Elbro, C., & de Jong, P. F. (2017). Orthographic learning is verbal learning. In K. Cain, D. L. Compton, & R. Parilla (Eds.), *Theories of reading development* (pp. 169–189). John Benjamins.

Elbro, C., de Jong, P. F., Houter, D., & Nielsen, A. M. (2012). From spelling pronunciation to lexical access: A second step in word decoding? *Scientific Studies of Reading, 16*(4), 341–359.

Fletcher, J. M. (2009). Dyslexia: The evolution of a scientific concept. *Journal of the International Neuropsychological Society, 15*, 501–508.

Fletcher, J. M., Lyon, G. R., Fuchs, L. S., & Barnes, M. A. (2018). *Learning disabilities: From identification to intervention*. Guilford Press.

Foorman, B., Beyler, N., Borradaile, K., Coyne, M., Denton, C. A., Dimino, J., & Wissel, S. (2016). *Foundational skills to support reading for understanding in kindergarten through 3rd grade. Educator's practice guide*. NCEE 2016-4008. What Works Clearinghouse.

Frith, U. (1985). Beneath the surface of developmental dyslexia. In K. Patterson, J. Marshall, & M. Coltheart (Eds.), *Surface dyslexia* (pp. 301–330). Erlbaum.

Gilbert, J. K., Compton, D. L., & Kearns, D. K (2011). Word and person effects on decoding accuracy: A new look at an old question. *Journal of Educational Psychology, 103*, 489–507.

Goldenberg, C. (2020). Reading wars, reading science, and English learners. *Reading Research Quarterly, 55*, S131–S144.

Gough, P. B., Juel, C., & Griffith, P. L. (1992). Reading, spelling, and the orthographic cipher. In P. B. Gough, L. C. Ehri, & R. Treiman (Eds.), *Reading acquisition* (pp. 35–48). Erlbaum.

Harm, M. W., McCandliss, B. D., & Seidenberg, M. S. (2003). Modeling the successes and failures of interventions for disabled readers. *Scientific Studies of Reading, 7*(2), 155–182.

Harm, M. W., & Seidenberg, M. S. (1999). Phonology, reading acquisition, and dyslexia: Insights from connectionist models. *Psychological Review, 106*, 491–528.

Harm, M. W., & Seidenberg, M. S. (2004). Computing the meanings of words in reading: Cooperative division of labor between visual and phonological processes. *Psychological Review, 111*(3), 662–720.

Harris, A., & Jacobson, M. (1982). *Basic reading vocabulary*. Macmillan.

Juel, C., Griffith, P. L., & Gough, P. B. (1986). Acquisition of literacy: A longitudinal study of children in first and second grade. *Journal of Educational Psychology, 78*(4), 243.

Kearns, D. K, Steacy, L. M., Compton, D. L., Gilbert, J. K., Goodwin, A. P., Cho, E., Lindstrom, E. R., & Collins, A. A. (2016). Modeling polymorphemic word recognition: Exploring differences among children with early-emerging and late-emerging word reading difficulty. *Journal of Learning Disabilities, 49*, 368–394.

Keenan, J. M., & Betjemann, R. S. (2008). Comprehension of single words: The role of semantics in word identification and reading disability. In E. Grigorenko (Ed.), *Single-word reading: Behavioral and biological perspectives* (pp. 191–209). Erlbaum.

Kieffer, M. J. (2008). Catching up or falling behind? Initial English proficiency, concentrated poverty, and the reading growth of language minority learners in the United States. *Journal of Educational Psychology, 100*(4), 851.

Kintsch, W., & Rawson, K. A. (2005). Rereading effects depend on time of test. *Journal of Educational Psychology, 97*(1), 70–80.

Laing, E., & Hulme, C. (1999). Phonological and semantic processes influence beginning readers' ability to learn to read words. *Journal of Experimental Child Psychology, 73*(3), 183–207.

Lovett, M. W., Lacerenza, L., Borden, S. L., Frijters, J. C., Steinbach, K. A., & De Palma, M. (2000). Components of effective remediation for developmental reading disabilities: Combining phonological and strategy-based instruction to improve outcomes. *Journal of Educational Psychology, 92*(2), 263.

Mancilla-Martinez, J., & Lesaux, N. K. (2010). Predictors of reading comprehension for struggling readers: The case of Spanish-speaking language minority learners. *Journal of Educational Psychology, 102*(3), 701.

Metsala, J. L. (1999). The development of phonemic awareness in reading-disabled children. *Applied Psycholinguistics, 20*(1), 149–158.

Metsala, J. L., Stanovich, K. E., & Brown, G. D. (1998). Regularity effects and the phonological deficit model of reading disabilities: A meta-analytic review. *Journal of Educational Psychology, 90*(2), 279.

Morais, J., & Kolinsky, R. (2005). Literacy and cognitive change. In M. Snowling & C. Hulme (Eds.), *The science of reading: A handbook* (pp. 188–203). Blackwell.

Nakamoto, J., Lindsey, K. A., & Manis, F. R. (2007). A longitudinal analysis of English language learners' word decoding and reading comprehension. *Reading and Writing, 20*(7), 691–719.

Nation, K., & Castles, A. (2017). Putting the learning in orthographic learning. In K. Cain, D. Compton, & R. Parrila (Eds.), *Theories of reading development* (pp. 147–168). John Benjamins.

Nation, K., & Hulme, C. (2011). Learning to read changes children's phonological skills: Evidence from a latent variable longitudinal study of reading and nonword repetition. *Developmental Science, 14*(4), 649–659.

O'Connor, M., Geva, E., & Koh, P. W. (2019). Examining reading comprehension profiles of grade 5 monolinguals and English language learners through the lexical quality hypothesis lens. *Journal of Learning Disabilities, 52*(3), 232–246.

Ouellette, G., & Fraser, J. R. (2009). What exactly is a yait anyway: The role of semantics in orthographic learning. *Journal of Experimental Child Psychology, 104*, 239–251.

Pennington, B. F. (2009). *Diagnosing learning disorders: A neuropsychological framework* (2nd ed.). Guilford Press.

Perfetti, C. A. (1991). Representations and awareness in the acquisition of reading competence. In L. Rieben & C. A. Perfetti (Eds.), *Learning to read: Basic research and its implications* (pp. 33–44). Erlbaum.

Perfetti, C. A. (1992). The representation problems in reading acquisition. In P. B. Gough, L. C. Ehri, & R. Treiman (Eds.), *Reading acquisition* (pp. 145–174). Erlbaum.

Perfetti, C. (2007). Reading ability: Lexical quality to comprehension. *Scientific Studies of Reading, 11*(4), 357–383.

Perfetti, C. A., & Hart, L. (2002). The lexical quality hypothesis. *Precursors of Functional Literacy, 11*, 67–86.

Perfetti, C. A., Landi, N., & Oakhill, J. (2005). The acquisition of reading comprehension skill. In M. J. Snowling & C. Hulme (Eds.), *The science of reading: A handbook* (pp. 227–247). Blackwell.

Perfetti, C. A., & Stafura, J. (2014). Word knowledge in a theory of reading comprehension. *Scientific Studies of Reading, 18*(1), 22–37.

Peterson, R. L., & Pennington, B. F. (2015). Developmental dyslexia. *Annual Review of Clinical Psychology, 11*, 283–307.

Petscher, Y., Quinn, J. M., & Wagner, R. K. (2016). Modeling the co-development of correlated processes with longitudinal and cross-construct effects. *Developmental Psychology, 52*(11), 1690.

Rack, J., Hulme, C., Snowling, M., & Wightman, J. (1994). The role of phonology in young children learning to read words: The direct-mapping hypothesis. *Journal of Experimental Child Psychology, 57*(1), 42–71.

Rack, J. P., Snowling, M. J., & Olson, R. K. (1992). The nonword reading deficit in developmental dyslexia: A review. *Reading Research Quarterly, 27*(1), 29–53.

Ranbom, L. J., & Connine, C. M. (2011). Silent letters are activated in spoken word recognition. *Language and Cognitive Processes, 26*(2), 236–261.

Reitsma, P. (1983). Printed word learning in beginning readers. *Journal of Experimental Child Psychology, 36*(2), 321–339.

Rueckl, J. G., Zevin, J. D., & Wolf, H. (2019). Using computational techniques to model and better understand developmental word-reading disorders (i.e., dyslexia). In J. A. Washington, D. L. Compton, & P. McCardle, (Eds.), *Dyslexia: Revisiting etiology, diagnosis, treatment, and policy* (pp. 57–70). Brookes Publishing Co.

Seidenberg, M. S. (2005). Connectionist models of word reading. *Current Directions in Psychological Science, 14*, 238–242.

Seidenberg, M. S., & McClelland, J. L. (1989). A distributed, developmental model of word recognition and naming. *Psychological Review, 96*, 523.

Seidenberg, M. S., Waters, G. S., Barnes, M. A., & Tanenhaus, M. K. (1984). When does irregular spelling or pronunciation influence word recognition? *Journal of Verbal Learning & Verbal Behavior, 23*(3), 383–404.

Seymour, P. H. K., Aro, M., & Erskine, J. M. (2003). Foundation literacy acquisition in European orthographies. *British Journal of Psychology, 94*(Pt. 2), 143–174.

Shankweiler, D., Lundquist, E., Katz, L., Stuebing, K. K., Fletcher, J. M., Brady, S., & Shaywitz, B. A. (1999). Comprehension and decoding: Patterns of association in children with reading difficulties. *Scientific Studies of Reading, 3*(1), 69–94.

Share, D. L. (1995). Phonological recoding and self-teaching: Sine qua non of reading acquisition. *Cognition, 55*, 151–218.

Share, D. L. (2008). Orthographic learning, phonological recoding, and self-teaching. *Advances in Child Development and Behavior, 36*, 31–82.

Share, D. L. (2011). On the role of phonology in reading acquisition: The self-teaching hypothesis. In S. A. Brady, D. Braze, & C. A. Fowler (Eds.), *Explaining individual differences in reading: Theory and evidence* (pp. 45–68). Psychology Press.

Siegel, L. S. (1989). IQ is irrelevant to the definition of learning disabilities. *Journal of Learning Disabilities, 22*(8), 469–478.

Siegel, L. S., Share, D., & Geva, E. (1995). Evidence for superior orthographic skills in dyslexics. *Psychological Science, 6*(4), 250–254.

Siegelman, N., Rueckl, J. G., Steacy, L. M., Frost, S. J., van den Bunt, M., Zevin, J. D., Seidenberg, M. S., Pugh, K. R., Compton, D. L., & Morris, R. D. (in press). Individual differences in learning the regularities between orthography, phonology, and semantics predict early reading skills. *Journal of Memory and Language, 114*, 104–145.

Snow, C. E. (2002). *Reading for understanding: Toward a research and development program in reading comprehension.* RAND

Stanovich, K. E. (1991). Word recognition: Changing perspectives. In P. D. Pearson, R. Barr, M. L. Kamil, & P. Mosenthal (Eds.), *Handbook of reading research* (Vol. II, pp. 418–452). Erlbaum.

Stanovich, K. E. (1988). Explaining the differences between the dyslexic and the garden-variety poor reader: The phonological-core variable-difference model. *Journal of Learning Disabilities, 21*, 590–604.

Stanovich, K. E., & Siegel, L. S. (1994). Phenotypic performance profile of children with reading disabilities: A regression-based test of the phonological-core variable difference model. *Journal of Educational Psychology, 86*(1), 24–53.

Steacy, L. M., & Compton, D. L. (2019). Examining the role of imageability and regularity in word reading accuracy and learning efficiency among first and second graders at-risk for reading disabilities. *Journal of Experimental and Child Psychology, 178*, 226–250.

Steacy, L. M., Compton, D. L., Petscher, Y., Elliott, J. D., Smith, K., Rueckl, J., Sawi, O. Frost, S., & Pugh K. (2019a). Development and prediction of context-dependent vowel pronunciation in elementary readers. *Scientific Studies of Reading, 23*, 49–63.

Steacy, L. M., Edwards, A. A., Himelhoch, A., Rigobon, V. M., Gutierrez, N., Marencin, N. C., Siegelman, N., Himelhoch, C., Rueckl, J., & Compton, D. L. (submitted). Set for variability dominates phonological awareness as a predictor of word reading: Potential implications for early identification and treatment of dyslexia. *Reading Research Quarterly.*

Steacy, L. M., Elleman, A. M., & Compton D. L. (2017). Opening the "black box" of learning to read: Inductive learning mechanisms supporting word-learning development with a focus on interventions for children who struggle to read. In K. Cain, D. L. Compton, & R. K. Parilla (Eds.), *Theories of reading development*, (pp. 99–121). John Benjamins Publishing.

Steacy, L. M., Fuchs, D., Gilbert, J. K., Kearns, D. M., Elleman, A. M., & Edwards, A. A. (2020). Sight word acquisition in first grade students at risk for reading disabilities: An item-level exploration of the number of exposures required for mastery. *Annals of Dyslexia, 70*(2), 259–274.

Steacy, L. M., Kearns, D. N, Gilbert, J. K., Compton, D. L., Cho, E., Lindstrom, E. R., & Collins, A. A. (2017). Exploring individual differences in irregular word recognition among children with early-emerging and late-emerging word reading difficulty. *Journal of Educational Psychology, 109*, 51–69.

Steacy, L. M., Petscher, Y., Elliott, J. D., Smith, K., Rigobon, V. M., Abes, D., Edwards, A. A., Himelhoch, A., Rueckl, J. G., & Compton, D. L. (2021a). The effect of facilitative vs. inhibitory word training corpora on word reading accuracy growth in children with dyslexia. *Learning Disability Quarterly, 44*(3), 158–169.

Steacy, L. M., Petscher, Y., Rueckl, J. R., Edwards A., & Compton, D. L. (2021b). Modeling and visualizing the co-development of word and nonword reading in children from first through fourth grade: Informing developmental trajectories of children with dyslexia. *Child Development, 92*(3), e252–e269.

Steacy, L. M., Wade-Woolley, L., Rueckl, J. G., Pugh, K. R., Elliott, J. D., & Compton, D. L. (2019b). The role of set for variability in irregular word reading: Word- and child-predictors in typically developing readers and students at-risk for reading disabilities. *Scientific Studies of Reading, 23*, 523–532.

Terry, N. P., & Scarborough, H. S. (2011). The phonological hypothesis as a valuable framework for studying the relation of dialect variation to early reading skills. In S. Brady, D. Braze, & C. Fowler (Eds), *Explaining individual differences in reading: Theory and evidence* (pp. 97–117). Taylor & Francis.

Thomas-Tate, S. R., Washington, J. A., Craig, H. K., & Packard, M. E. W. (2006). Performance of African American preschool and kindergarten students on the Expressive Vocabulary Test. *Language, Speech, and Hearing Services in Schools, 37*, 143–149.

Torgesen, J. K. (2000). Individual differences in response to early interventions in reading: The lingering problem of treatment resisters. *Learning Disabilities Research & Practice, 15*(1), 55–64.

Treiman, R., Kessler, B., & Bick, S. (2003). Influence of consonantal context on the pronunciation of vowels: A comparison of human readers and computational models. *Cognition, 88*(1), 49–78.

Treiman, R., Kessler, B., Zevin, J. D., Bick, S., & Davis, M. (2006). Influence of consonantal context on the reading of vowels: Evidence from children. *Journal of Experimental Child Psychology, 93*(1), 1–24.

Tunmer, W. E., & Chapman, J. W. (1998). Language prediction skill, phonological recoding ability and beginning reading. In C. Hulme & R. M. Joshi (Eds.), *Reading and spelling: Development and disorder* (pp. 33–67). Erlbaum.

Tunmer, W. E., & Chapman, J. W. (2012). Does set for variability mediate the influence of vocabulary knowledge on the development of word recognition skills? *Scientific Studies of Reading, 16*, 122–140.

Vaughn, S., Martinez, L. R., Linan-Thompson, S., Reutebuch, C. K., Carlson, C. D., & Francis, D. J. (2009). Enhancing social studies vocabulary and comprehension for seventh-grade English language learners: Findings from two experimental studies. *Journal of Research on Educational Effectiveness, 2*(4), 297–324.

Vellutino, F. R., Fletcher, J. M., Snowling, M. J., & Scanlon, D. M. (2004). Specific reading disability (dyslexia): What have we learned in the past four decades? *Journal of Child Psychology and Psychiatry, 45*(1), 2–40.

Vellutino, F. R., Scanlon, D. M., Sipay, E. R., Small, S. G., Pratt, A., Chen, R., & Denckla, M. B. (1996). Cognitive profiles of difficult-to-remediate and readily remediated poor readers: Early intervention as a vehicle for distinguishing between cognitive and experiential deficits as basic causes of specific reading disability. *Journal of Educational Psychology, 88*(4), 601.

Venezky, R. L. (1999). *The American way of spelling: The structure and origins of American English orthography.* Guilford Press.

Wang, H.-C., Castles, A., & Nickels, L. (2012). Word regularity affects orthographic learning. *The Quarterly Journal of Experimental Psychology, 65*, 856–864.

Wang, H., Nickels, L., Nation, K., & Castles, A. (2013). Predictors of orthographic learning of regular and irregular words. *Scientific Studies of Reading, 17*(5), 369–384.

Ziegler, J. C., & Goswami, U. (2005). Reading acquisition, developmental dyslexia, and skilled reading across languages: A psycholinguistic grain size theory. *Psychological Bulletin, 131*(1), 3.

CHAPTER 3

Mathematics Learning Difficulties

Nancy C. Jordan, Dana Miller-Cotto, and Kelly-Ann Gesuelli

Far too many students fail to develop math proficiency, despite years of education. According to the most recent U.S. Nation's Report Card (National Assessment of Educational Progress, 2019), just 24% of 12th graders demonstrated math proficiency (vs. 37% in reading). Among students with diagnosed disabilities, only 7% demonstrated math proficiency; this number has remained virtually unchanged since 2005. Moreover, students who performed in the lowest percentile groups (i.e., 10th and 25th percentiles) appeared to be losing ground, compared to the lowest-performing students in previous years. Math failure has serious long-term consequences for an individual's well-being and society. According to the Program for International Student Assessment Young Adult Follow-up Study (PISA YAFS) (Mamedova et al., 2021), students who are not proficient in math at age 15 are much less likely than their proficient peers to pursue advantageous educational outcomes (e.g., attending college) by age 19; about 17% of these students did not yet have a high school diploma versus only 5% of math-proficient students. Increasingly, well-paying jobs require advanced math capabilities (Rittle-Johnson & Jordan, 2016). In addition to limiting educational and associated workforce opportunities, math difficulties negatively affect an individual's daily life skills, such as making sound financial and healthcare decisions (Knuth et al., 2016).

In the present chapter, we focus on elementary school-age children with or at risk for developing mathematics learning difficulties (MLD). Although students struggle in math for many reasons, including inadequate teaching, a growing body of research points to the influence of domain-specific numerical cognitive knowledge and domain-general cognitive competencies in supporting mathematical learning (e.g., Kauffman et al., 2013). We address the potential impact of deficiencies in one or more of these areas on math achievement. Concurrently, a growing body of research has shown that risk for MLD can be identified early (e.g., Gersten et al., 2005) and that it is possible to improve achievement levels for elementary school students with MLD through targeted intervention (Fuchs et al., 2021). As such, we also address essential features of early screening for MLD along with principles of effective math intervention programs in the elementary grades. Fuchs et al. (this volume) address intervention for students with mathematics learning disabilities in further detail.

Defining MLD

Although math learning difficulties have been defined differently in the research literature, they typically are determined by performance at least one standard deviation below the mean—or at or below the 25th percentile—on norm-referenced diagnostic tests, such as the *Key Math* (Connolly, 2007) or the *Test of Early Mathematics Abilities* (TEMA) (Ginsburg & Baroody, 2003). Math learning disabilities or *dyscalculia* (Van Luit, 2019) may be further differentiated within the MLD category with a more stringent criterion of performing at or below the 10th percentile (about two standard deviations below the mean), despite normal intelligence. These more severe forms of MLD are extremely persistent: kindergartners who perform below the 10th percentile in math have a 70% chance of scoring below the 10th percentile at the end of elementary school (Morgan et al., 2009). MLD also might be identified when a student fails to meet proficiency on criterion-referenced tests based on national benchmarks, such as the U.S. Common Core State Standards (CCSS) (Common Core State Standards Initiative, 2010) or in one or more math content areas (e.g., fractions). Clinically, many of these children do not respond to typical classroom math instruction and require intensive help in small group or one-to-one tutorial settings (Clarke et al., 2015).

Conceptual and Procedural Mathematical Knowledge

Knowledge of mathematical concepts and procedures applies to all mathematical content areas (Geary, 2004), including those involving whole and rational numbers. Procedural mathematics knowledge in elementary school is most relevant to learning arithmetic operations with integers and rational numbers (Hecht & Vagi, 2012; Siegler et al., 2013). For example, students may learn a counting on from the first number procedure for adding two integers or a cross-multiplication procedure to compare the size of two fractions. Conceptual mathematics knowledge involves understanding the properties of all numbers, such as linear relations between numbers and knowing why one fraction is bigger than another one (Hiebert & Lefevre, 1986). Both concepts and procedures are important for mathematical learning and typically support each other (Rittle-Johnson, 2017). Students with MLD may struggle with one or both types of knowledge, within or between math content areas. For example, students who struggle with whole-number concepts are almost certain to struggle with fraction concepts. Some children may memorize the procedure for multiplying fractions easily but do not understand why multiplying two fractions can lead to a smaller number (e.g., $\frac{1}{2} \times \frac{1}{2} = \frac{1}{4}$). Relatedly, automatic retrieval of procedural information facilitates mathematical learning. Many children with MLD, for example, can apply counting procedures to solve arithmetic combinations but do not shift to automatic retrieval, despite intensive practice (e.g., Geary, 2011). Consequently, problem solving for students with MLD is slow, laborious, and error-prone.

Number-Specific Cognitive Competencies

To provide context for discussing numerical competencies and their relation to MLD, it is important to consider numerical development as an integrated, continuous process that centers on the number line (Siegler & Lortie-Forgues, 2014; Siegler et al., 2011). Typically, researchers, as well as educators, have viewed numerical development as being segmented into whole numbers and fractions or rational numbers, with the former learned somewhat naturally and the latter with greater difficulty (e.g., Geary, 2004; Gelman & Williams, 1998). However, all real numbers (i.e., integers and rational numbers) are integrated by having specific magnitudes that can be represented as spatial positions on a number line (Siegler & Lortie-Forgues, 2014).

Numbers and their magnitudes appear in three forms, referred to as the triple code model of numerical processing (Dehaene, 1992; Landerl, 2019): analog magnitude (e.g., four dots on the page; four dots are more than two dots), number words presented orally (e.g., "four"; "four" is more than "two"), and written number symbols or Arabic numerals (e.g., 4 > 2). Although the time frame for learning these three interrelated numerical formats varies, young children first acquire *nonsymbolic* magnitude representations and then link these understandings to small oral numbers and written symbols through everyday experiences (e.g., seeing numerals on board games) (Siegler, 2009). Young children by around 3 years of age can subitize or immediately apprehend cardinal values of small quantities (i.e., five or less) without counting. Gradually, children acquire accurate representations of larger whole numbers through conventional counting. For example, when enumerating sets of any size, children count each object once (one-to-one correspondence) in a stable order and recognize that the last number in the count sequence always indicates how many items are in the set (cardinality principle) (Gelman & Gallistel, 1978). By kindergarten and first grade, many children form a mental number line and can see that numbers are represented linearly, with the next number in the count sequence always exactly one more than the previous one ($N + 1$ principle) (Baroody et al., 2006). They understand, for example, that 6 is 1 more than 5 or 1 less than 7, which allows them to engage in simple number operations. Eventually, children learn place value (one, tens, hundreds, etc.) and how to operate with larger numbers. Place value in multidigit written numbers can be confusing to many children since the same numeral can have a different meaning depending on its position (e.g., 27 vs. 702) (Landerl, 2019).

Throughout schooling, children also come to see that there are other numbers between whole numbers (fractions) and that an infinite set of whole and rational numbers can be represented on the number line. However, a deeper understanding of numbers is required for learning fractions. Children must see that properties of whole numbers do not always apply to fractions and decimals (Siegler & Lortie-Forgues, 2014). For example, the magnitude of a fraction is determined by the relation between the numerator and the denominator and not the absolute value of either number (e.g., ¼ is smaller than ½). For decimal notation, .05 is larger than .005, even though the latter has more numerals. All these ideas are critical for engaging in more advanced math, such as algebra (e.g., Booth et al., 2014).

Numerical Processing and MLD

Many children with MLD (including developmental dyscalculia) display core deficits in numerical processing (Butterworth & Laurillard, 2010; Dehaene, 1997; Rousselle & Noël, 2007; Skagerlund & Träff, 2016; Träff et al., 2017). Research on *nonsymbolic* numerical discrimination skills in children with MLD reveals inconsistent findings. Some studies show MLD students possess lower approximate number system (ANS) acuity on dot array tasks that require them to indicate which of two sets has more dots compared to their typically developing (TD) peers (e.g., Mazzocco et al., 2011; Piazza et al., 2010). However, a longitudinal study by Desoete, Ceulemans, De Weerdt, and Pieters (2012) found students with MLD displayed both nonsymbolic and symbolic skill deficits in kindergarten, but only symbolic deficits when reassessed in second grade. Research further indicates that task congruency and other perceptual cues impact MLD students' nonsymbolic magnitude comparison skills, with children performing worse on incongruent trials (e.g., inverse relation between surface area and magnitude) than congruent ones (Bugden & Ansari, 2016; Mejias et al., 2012; Mussolin et al., 2010). These findings suggest that lower ANS performance in students with MLD may reflect non-numerical weaknesses related to the executive system, such as visual–spatial working memory and inhibition of irrelevant non-numerical information—rather, deficits in numerical discrimination. (See also discussion in domain-general processes and MLD.)

Research has more consistently identified symbolic numerical processing as a key area of weakness among MLD students (e.g., Cañizares et al., 2012; Iuculano et al., 2008; Morsanyi et al., 2018; Mussolin et al., 2010; Wong et al., 2017). These skills are also shown to be more negatively impacted in students with MLD compared to those for nonsymbolic processing (e.g., Mejias et al., 2012). Students with MLD demonstrate poorer accuracy than TD peers on various symbolic magnitude comparison tasks involving Arabic numerals and number words (e.g., Geary Hoard et al., 2008; Mejias et al., 2012; Morsanyi et al., 2018; Skagerlund & Träff, 2016). Children with MLD also display greater distance effects in their symbolic magnitude processing, as evidenced by increased reaction times when comparing numbers that are closer in distance (e.g., 2 vs. 3), suggesting the presence of a less precisely developed mental number line (Mussolin et al., 2010). According to eye-tracking data, children with MLD exhibit more unidentifiable visual fixation patterns when processing multidigit symbolic numbers and more erratic visual scanning strategies when attempting to estimate numerical magnitudes on the number line than TD students (van Viersen Slot et al., 2013). Taken together, studies illustrate that children with MLD struggle to access and represent magnitudes from symbolic stimuli, which can subsequently impede their ability to discriminate and manipulate such quantities through addition and subtraction. These weaknesses in numerical processing skills negatively impact students' future mathematics performance related to both procedural and concept knowledge (Desoete et al., 2012; Jordan et al., 2009).

General Cognitive Competencies

Domain-general cognitive competencies support number knowledge as well as mathematical concepts and procedures. Three systems guide these competencies: the central executive system, the visual–spatial system, and the language system (e.g., Geary, 2004). Weaknesses in each of these systems are associated with MLD and thus can inform teaching approaches and interventions.

Central Executive System

Executive function (EF) refers to an interrelated set of cognitive processes, which includes ignoring distractions and inhibiting inappropriate responses (inhibitory control), holding and manipulating information in memory (working memory), and shifting between tasks (cognitive flexibility) (e.g., Best et al., 2011). Children with MLD frequently demonstrate poor performance in one or more areas of EF (e.g., Fuchs et al., 2014).

Inhibitory Control

Many children with MLD show broad deficits in inhibition (e.g., Geary et al., 2007). Some theories have been asserted as to why this might be the case. Bull and Lee (2014) argue that inhibitory control plays a role in math performance by suppressing inappropriate calculation strategies, such as using addition when subtraction is more appropriate or subtracting the larger number from the smaller one on multidigit written calculations regardless of its position. Thinking about numerical magnitudes relies on inhibitory control as well; when working with whole numbers, students learn that large numbers mean greater magnitude, but with fractions, this is not always the case (e.g., Braithwaite & Siegler, 2018). Research on whole-number-line estimation suggests that core deficits in inhibition underlie difficulties in understanding numerical magnitude in children with MLD (Geary et al., 2008; Szucs et al., 2013), as well as in some TD children (e.g., Bos et al., 2014). For example, when children estimate the magnitude of fractions on the number line, they need to consider the size of the line and estimate the fractions accordingly. Children with MLD often place ½ in the middle of the number line, regardless of whether the line is from 0 to 1 or 0 to 2 (Rodrigues et al., 2016).

Working Memory

The correlation between working memory and mathematics performance varies in size across samples of TD children, children with MLD, and children with MLD and co-occurring developmental disorders (e.g., ADHD, neurodevelopmental disorders, and reading difficulties). Indeed, associations between mathematics and working memory are larger for children with several comorbidities (e.g., Barnes & Raghubar, 2017). Further, relative to other EF skills, working memory ability contributes unique variance to arithmetic skills (Peng et al., 2016; Swanson & Alloway, 2012), and children with poor counting and memory for single digits also tend to have underlying working memory deficits (e.g., Allen & Giofrè, 2021; Siegel & Ryan, 1989).

Studies have shown that there are individual differences in severity of working memory deficits among students with MLD, which may affect their response to instructional approaches. In one intervention designed to improve fraction knowledge (e.g., Fuchs et al., 2014), fourth graders with MLD were randomly assigned to a fluency practice condition where students completed strategic speeded activities to build fraction fluency or a conceptual condition where students explained their reasoning about fractions using manipulatives. Findings showed that students with MLD with weak working memory benefited most from supplementary conceptual work, whereas supplemental fluency practice better supported MLD students with relatively stronger working memory. These findings are likely attributable to the speeded activities involved in the fluency practices, which build automaticity in retrieving information; this placed a heavier demand on working memory and thus would disadvantage students with poorer working memory. Conceptual practice likely benefited children with poor working memory because this condition focused on helping students build representations of fractions and knowledge of how fractions differ.

So why might working memory and mathematics performance be so highly correlated? One possibility is that concurrent and longitudinal relations between working memory and math tasks reflect a problem of retrieval from long-term memory for students with poor working memory rather than (or in addition to) a filtering issue or a problem of the lesser ability to temporarily holding information in mind (Ericsson & Kintsch, 1995; Jones & Macken, 2015). Young children with MLD may need to rely more on working memory to execute calculation strategies because their fact knowledge is not well automatized. However, as knowledge accumulates and aspects of math knowledge become more integrated, working memory may become less important (Zhang et al., 2021). This theory is consistent with the finding that a key diagnostic indicator for children diagnosed with MLD is a developmental delay in the retrieval of math facts (e.g., Geary et al., 2012). For example, Geary et al. (2012) compared the fact retrieval skill across four groups of primary grade students: TD children, moderate MLD children (performing between the 10th and 25th percentile on a math achievement test) with mild fact retrieval deficits, moderate MLD children with severe fact retrieval deficits, and children with severe MLD (performing at or below the 10th percentile on a math achievement test) and severe fact retrieval deficits. Relative to the other groups, children with severe fact retrieval deficits, regardless of level of MLD, showed difficulty inhibiting irrelevant information while retrieving addition facts. That is, their errors suggested counting string intrusions (e.g., on the problem 6 + 3 giving an answer of 7 or 4). The authors propose that lack of inhibitory control explains these mistakes. Children with better inhibitory control skills may suppress prior counting knowledge to prevent interference. Thus, inhibitory control may partially explain deficits in mathematical skills as well as in working memory (Laski & Dulaney, 2015).

Cognitive Flexibility

Cognitive flexibility has also been associated with mathematics performance (McClelland et al., 2013). Some work has demonstrated a unique contribution of cognitive flexibility, relative to other components of EF and intelligence, in fourth- and sixth-grade students (Magalhaes et al., 2020). Our own work has indicated that while working memory is strongly related to math performance in kindergarten and first grade, as children age, this association decreases, whereas the association between cognitive flexibility and mathematics performance increases with age (Zhang et al., 2021). Early on, children may not have the prior knowledge to facilitate math performance and thus must rely on working memory to solve math calculations. As math knowledge increases, cognitive flexibility may assist in switching between specific strategies and goals for problem solving. Children with MLD tend to demonstrate poor cognitive flexibility (e.g., Morgan et al., 2017, on a card sorting task), especially in later grades. However, of the three components of EFs, cognitive flexibility is least investigated among researchers, requiring more work to elucidate the role of cognitive flexibility in MLD.

Visual–Spatial System

The visual–spatial system helps children think about numbers and their relations in space, which relies in part on spatial reasoning (Gunderson et al., 2012). Spatial reasoning involves awareness of space itself, representation of spatial information in the mind and externally through graphical representations, and interpreting spatial information (Resnick et al., 2019). The relation between spatial reasoning and math skills appears to maintain throughout development and even increase with grade level as math becomes more complex (e.g., Lowrie et al., 2018). Visuospatial attention uniquely predicts fraction arithmetic performance, over and above working memory and intelligence (e.g., Geary et al., 2021). Further, it has been shown that spatial tasks involving mental rotation, visual–spatial working memory, and visual–motor integration predict math performance in elementary grades (Mix et al., 2016). Spatial reasoning also supports children's numerical magnitude understanding, a core area of concern in many children with MLD. For example, it has been documented that number line estimation at age six mediates the relationship between children's spatial visualization at age five and math performance at age eight, suggesting that spatial visualization may be foundational to forming an accurate linear number representation (e.g., Gunderson et al., 2012). Nonsymbolic proportional reasoning about continuous quantities, another area of spatial thinking, relates to understanding multiplicative relations between equivalent fractions (e.g., a mixture of 3 parts of juice to 6 parts of water will taste the same as a solution of 6 parts of juice to 12 parts of water) (Boyer & Levine, 2012). This type of proportional reasoning is uniquely associated with fraction skill development in later elementary school (Ye et al., 2016).

Although there appears to be a clear connection between elements of spatial reasoning and mathematics, studies examining children with MLD have produced equivocal findings (Resnick et al., 2019). That is, some studies have shown children with MLD do not differ from their TD counterparts on measures of spatial reasoning skills (Mazzocco & Thompson, 2005; Szucs et al., 2013). A study comparing visual and spatial reasoning demonstrated that poor problem solvers demonstrated deficits in spatial reasoning (e.g., location of objects in space) but not general visual (e.g., knowledge of shapes and colors) or phonological abilities (e.g., Passolunghi & Mammarella, 2010). However, children with MLD do consistently appear to have relative weaknesses in visual–spatial working memory compared to TD children (e.g., Geary, 2004; Keeler & Swanson, 2001; Passolunghi & Siegel, 2001), an area that is also associated with the executive system.

Language System

Language is crucial for comprehending terms relevant to learning mathematics (e.g., "equal," "plus," "minus," "numerator," and "denominator") and for solving applied word problems (Seethaler et al., 2011). Not surprisingly, facility with language predicts early mathematical success (e.g., Purpura & Reid, 2016). In a meta-analysis, Peng and colleagues (2016) found a moderate relationship ($r = .42$) between language and mathematics performance across 344 studies. Language also helps explain early disparities in mathematics performance (e.g., Elliot & Bachman, 2018; King & Purpura, 2021). Many children with MLD exhibit poorer language skills than their peers. One study found that children with MLD significantly underperformed on measures of vocabulary, morphology, and syntax relative to their TD peers (e.g., Chow et al., 2021).

Reading and math difficulties often co-occur, with studies showing up to 66% of children with MLD also demonstrating reading difficulties (e.g., Prediger et al., 2019). Language helps children interpret both symbolic and nonsymbolic representations, as well as graphic representations in word problems (Prediger et al., 2019). Children who demonstrate reading difficulties often struggle with word problems; this is especially true for English language learners (e.g., Martiniello, 2008). Thus, for these children, it is not a math learning disability per se but rather a language difference that is preventing them from success in mathematics. To address this issue, Driver and Powell (2017) developed a schema-based intervention approach to improve word problem-solving performance for English language learners who also demonstrated math difficulties. The intervention explicitly highlighted the grammatical structure of word problems to help students identify types of word problems and learn how to solve each type accordingly. Students were exposed to similar word problem structures, which guided them to create schemas (i.e., hierarchically organized cognitive structures in the form of chunks stored in long-term memory) for similar word problems to promote transfer to novel contexts. Results from this randomized controlled study indicated that this direct type of instruction, with a focus on using grammatical structures to identify problem types and associated strategies, benefited children with math difficulties who were also English language learners, with a large effect size.

Difficulties in Math Content Areas

Arithmetic and MLD

Accurate representation and manipulation of numerosities is critical for carrying out basic arithmetic calculations (Ansari, 2008). Children initially learn to add and subtract by combining and separating quantities (see Butterworth, 2005, for a review). Nonverbal arithmetic tasks require the child to form a mental model of each numerical magnitude, compare their relation, and then manipulate them to produce an exact answer (e.g., Gilmore et al., 2010; Huttenlocher et al., 1994). Verbal arithmetic skills require the ability to access magnitudes from number words or Arabic numerals and simultaneously process the relation between numbers (e.g., Lyons & Beilock, 2011; Yu et al., 2016).

Arithmetic difficulties are common among students with MLD, particularly related to fact fluency (Butterworth et al., 2011; Mazzocco & Räsänen, 2013). Fact fluency, or quick recognition and retrieval of number combinations from long-term memory (e.g., Baroody et al., 2014; Zaunmüller et al., 2009), serves as a critical factor in the development of more complex calculation skills and students' overall mathematics success (National Mathematics Advisory Panel [NMAP], 2008). Arithmetic strategy development for addition and subtraction occurs in overlapping waves (Siegler, 1996), beginning with more time-consuming physical manipulations and counting strategies, such as joining/separating sets of objects, finger counting, and verbal counting (e.g., Bailey et al., 2012; Carpenter & Moser, 1984). Young children typically start with *count all* strategies, where they count both addends, followed using *min* (i.e., counting on from larger addend) and *max* (i.e., counting on from the smaller addend) procedures (Groen & Parkman, 1972; Siegler & Shrager, 1984). As associations between number combinations and solutions are formed on individual combinations, students' use of physical manipulation and counting procedures is replaced with memory-based fact retrieval and decomposition strategies ($4 + 4 = 8$, so $4 + 5 = 9$) (e.g., Bailey et al., 2012).

Slow retrieval of arithmetic combinations is a signature characteristic of many students with MLD (Geary et al., 2012; Jordan et al., 2003; Jordan & Montani,1997). Students with MLD recall fewer arithmetic facts, display longer retrieval response times (e.g., Andersson, 2010; Geary, 2011; Lambert & Moeller, 2019), make more counting errors, and employ more immature strategies (i.e., persistent use of finger and verbal counting and infrequent and delayed use of decomposition) than TD students (Geary et al., 2012). Neuropsychological studies also show that MLD students display increased brain activity in subregions of the parietal cortex related to numerical processing (e.g., Ashkenazi et al., 2012; Berteletti et al., 2014) while performing simple addition problems. Researchers interpret this increased activation as an indicator of MLD students' use of more effortful and time-consuming counting strategies compared to their TD peers. Additionally, working memory deficits among children with MLD (e.g., Andersson & Östergren, 2012) impede students' ability to represent, store, and manipulate numeric information, resulting in their greater reliance on counting strategies than automatized fact retrieval (see Menon, 2016, for a review).

Given the prevalence of number combination difficulties among children with MLD, it is not surprising that they also struggle with more complex calculation skills. Studies show primary school students with MLD display lower accuracy and make more errors on multidigit addition and subtraction (Andersson, 2010; Lambert & Moeller, 2019; Nelson & Powell, 2018; Raghubar et al., 2009) than those without MLD. Common errors include basic miscalculations, using the wrong operation, misapplication of commutative properties to subtraction (i.e., subtracting smaller from larger numbers), and failure to regroup. This latter error suggests difficulties in the understanding of place-value structures (e.g., Andersson, 2010; Lambert & Moeller, 2019; Nelson & Powell, 2018). Moreover, MLD students' performance on place value and arithmetic fluency tasks contribute unique variance in their multidigit calculation skills (Andersson, 2010). MLD students' multidigit calculation difficulties thus appear to be impacted by both underlying conceptual (e.g., place value) and procedural (e.g., fact fluency) arithmetic deficits.

Fraction arithmetic poses additional challenges for children with MLD, who may already have tenuous whole-number arithmetic skills. Symbolic processing with whole numbers provides a basis for thinking about fractions and their magnitudes (Jordan et al., 2019). Because children with MLD have poorly established numerical skills as well as deficits in inhibitory processing, they often have trouble suppressing the whole-number bias that properties of whole numbers are true for all numbers in general (e.g., multiplication of two fractions may yield a product smaller than either multiplicand; Jordan et al., 2017; Siegler et al., 2011). Errors of students with MLD are characterized by adding or subtracting across denominators or misapplying the procedure for fraction addition to fraction multiplication, that is, failing to change the denominator instead of multiplying across both denominators (Newton et al., 2014; Siegler & Pyke, 2013). Many students with MLD show little improvement in their fraction arithmetic skills through sixth grade when these skills are typically taught (Common Core State Standards Initiative, 2010; Hansen et al., 2015).

Word Problem Solving and MLD

Word problems pose challenges for students with MLD who already have difficulties with arithmetic and fluency. Word problem solving requires the ability to identify pertinent information and numbers from text, select the correct operation, and translate text information into an equation (e.g., Fuchs et al., 2008). These steps result in increased cognitive demands and can exacerbate working memory, language, and arithmetic difficulties commonly demonstrated by students with MLD (e.g., Anderson & Östergren, 2012; Cowan & Powell, 2014). Studies demonstrate that students with MLD are less accurate and make slower growth in their word problem-solving skills than both TD students and those with reading difficulties (RD) (e.g., Andersson, 2008, 2010; Kingsdorf & Krawec, 2014; Träff & Passolunghi, 2015). For example, Andersson (2010) showed third and fourth graders with MLD were initially less accurate in their arithmetic word problem solving than TD and RD groups and demonstrated smaller accuracy gains through sixth grade, thus widening the performance gaps between groups. Moreover, the demonstration of higher word problem-solving performance among RD students indicates that MLD students' difficulties are not solely due to their reading and comprehension skills but those unique to mathematics.

Analysis of MLD students' word problem errors indicates that they experience similar, yet unique, difficulties compared to those for symbolic arithmetic. Like symbolic multidigit arithmetic, MLD students demonstrate miscalculations and use of incorrect operations when solving arithmetic word problems (Kindgsdorf & Krawec, 2014). However, students also demonstrate difficulties generating accurate representations (e.g., visuals, diagrams, or general schemas), paraphrasing and integrating important information, and developing a solution plan (Andersson, 2008; Kingsdorf & Krawec, 2014; Krawec, 2014), reflecting the increased complexity involved in arithmetic word problem solving. Regression analyses demonstrate that MLD students' word problem performance is only partially explained by their poor calculation skills (Andersson, 2010). Together, these findings emphasize that MLD students' word problem-solving difficulties are affected by calculation weaknesses and the unique presentation of arithmetic problems within word problem formats.

Screening

Early screening measures that identify students who will have difficulties learning math are essential for providing instructional support and intervention (Van Luit, 2019). Screeners for young children focus on numerical competencies, including the three core elements of number knowledge: number (e.g., counting and cardinality), number relations (comparisons of the magnitudes of numbers), and number operations (simple addition and subtraction concepts). Core number knowledge supports formal learning of mathematical concepts and procedures in elementary school. For example, it is difficult to learn addition and subtraction facts by rote memory without a good sense of numerical magnitude (Jordan et al., 2003). Even geometry, measurement, and data analysis involve applications of number knowledge, such as knowing the number of angles in a triangle or interpreting a linear representation on a graph (National Research Council, 2009).

Research studies have demonstrated the usefulness of screening measures for teachers to document kindergarten and first-grade students' number competencies. Chard et al. (2005) found four number areas in early kindergarten that predict performance on a standardized mathematics achievement test at the end of the year: oral counting, number identification, quantity comparison (e.g., name the larger of two numerals), and finding a missing number in a sequence (e.g., 4, __, 6). Multiple screeners have been developed that begin in kindergarten and use fast 1- to 3-minute assessments—most notably *Assessing Student Proficiency in Early Number Sense* (*ASPENS*) (Clarke et al., 2011), *AimsWeb Plus* (Pearson, 2017), and *Acadience Math* (Wheeler et al., 2019). Quick screening methods allow universal screening of large numbers of students to sort out those who may be at risk for MLD. Timed 1- to 3-minute screeners, while fast to administer, should be interpreted cautiously, however. These measures may penalize young children who have not yet automatized skills and encourage teachers to focus their instruction on rote learning of facts and procedures.

The *Screener for Early Number Sense* (*SENS*) (Jordan et al., in press), in contrast, is a more comprehensive screener that provides opportunities to examine problem-solving strategies. For example, the *SENS* provides items specifically in number, number relations, and number operations at three grade levels: PreK, kindergarten, and first grade. Level of representation (i.e., nonsymbolic vs. symbolic) is explicitly varied. Thus, at each grade, teachers can see if a kindergartner can add and subtract on nonsymbolic tasks with concrete referents but not on symbolic tasks, such as word problems and number combinations. Established *SENS* cutoff points for risk have high diagnostic accuracy, discriminating between a child at risk for later MLD and a child not at risk for later MLD in 90% of cases for PreK, 76% of cases for kindergarten, and 86% of cases for first grade (Beliakoff, 2021).

Later in elementary school, children can be screened for their knowledge of rational numbers, among other skills. For example, Rodrigues et al. (2020) found that a screener that measured fraction number line estimation accuracy, general fraction concepts, and fraction arithmetic accurately identified fourth graders who are at risk for failing to meet math benchmarks on a statewide math achievement test at the end of fourth, fifth, and sixth grades, respectively. Cutoff points for risk discriminated between a student at risk for failing to meet benchmarks and a child not at risk for failing to reach benchmarks over 80% of the time in each of the three grade levels. Overall, screeners on core components of the mathematics curriculum—such as whole-number knowledge and fractions—accurately predict later achievement and can be used to identify children who might benefit from intervention.

Intervention

Research showing predictive relations between domain-general and number-specific competencies, as well as the diagnostic accuracy of early screening, has coincided with and spurred interventions that have successfully increased achievement levels in elementary school students with MLD. In the past, far more research had been devoted to literacy interventions than math interventions (Gersten et al., 2005), but this situation has changed, given international interest in STEM achievement. In 2021, the What Works Clearinghouse (WWC) of the U.S. Department of Education assembled a panel to review and synthesize the growing body of methodologically rigorous experimental and quasi-experimental studies that evaluated math interventions for assisting struggling students in the elementary grades. The resulting practice guide (Fuchs et al., 2021) made six recommendations for math interventions:

1. Systematic Instruction: Provide systematic instruction during intervention to develop student understanding of mathematical ideas.
2. Mathematical Language: Teach clear and concise mathematical language and support students' use of the language to help students effectively communicate their understanding of mathematical concepts.
3. Representations: Use a well-chosen set of concrete and semi-concrete representations to support students' learning of mathematical concepts and procedures.
4. Number Lines: Use the number line to facilitate the learning of mathematical concepts and procedures, build understanding of grade-level material, and prepare students for advanced mathematics.
5. Word Problems: Provide deliberate instruction on word problems to deepen students' mathematical understanding and support their capacity to apply mathematical ideas.
6. Timed Activities: Regularly include timed activities as one way to build fluency in mathematics. (p. 3)

Relatedly, our team has developed a successful fraction sense intervention (FSI) for students with MLD (Dyson et al., 2018; Barbieri et al., 2020; Jordan et al., 2024) that meets WWC standards (Fuchs et al., 2021). Because the FSI is a prototype of an intervention that explicitly incorporates the practice guide's recommendation, we show how it aligns with the six practice guide recommendations. First, *systematic instruction* is the cornerstone of the FSI. According to Fuchs et al. (2021), systematic instruction includes multiple evidence-informed practices to promote learning more generally. In the FSI, all fraction concepts (e.g., equivalency and multiplicative reasoning) and procedures (e.g., fraction arithmetic) are presented *incrementally*, starting with fractions involving familiar denominators of two and four, which students can more easily understand. New denominators are introduced one at a time in lessons, following a logical progression (i.e., halves, fourths, eighths, and, later, thirds, sixths, and twelfths). *Visual and verbal supports* (e.g., diagrams and verbal explanations) are intentionally provided together to reduce the student's cognitive demands. *Information from previous learned content is integrated and reviewed in subsequent lessons.* For example, students might learn how to add with simple common denominators in one lesson but continue to practice this skill in subsequent lessons with uncommon denominators. *Different types of problems are presented side by side to help students discriminate among problem types* (e.g., fraction addition where students do not add across denominators versus multiplication of fractions where they multiply across, such as ¾ + ¾ and ¾ × ¾). Students are given *immediate feedback to address progress and misunderstandings*. For example, children might be reminded to think about whether the error of ½ + ½ = 2/4 makes sense conceptually, given that it is equivalent to ½.

Throughout all FSI lessons, clear and precise *mathematical language* is taught (Karp et al., 2014), such as using the term "simplifying" rather than "reducing" fractions; using the words "numerator" and "denominator" when discussing the different parts of the fractions (e.g., unit fractions always have 1 in the numerator, and the denominator signifies the number of equal size parts in the whole); and saying one fourth of the area or the length rather than one out of four to describe one fourth. Precise mathematical language helps students explain their reasoning about problems. Gesturing is used to provide context and meaning to the words (e.g., Brooks & Goldin-Meadow, 2016). For example, a sweeping hand gesture is used to help students see the magnitude of a particular unit fraction, such as 0 to ¼, along a number line (Dyson et al., 2018).

FSI activities incorporate familiar *representations* of fractions, such as fraction bars, set models, and rulers, to strengthen understanding and promote flexibility and transfer. For example, to support learning of fraction concepts and procedures, students are given a metal sheet with fraction bar magnets, which show three wholes and the corresponding number of halves or fourths. Students use these fraction bars to solve problems involving halves and fourths. They also use the fraction bars to measure and mark miles and half miles in a 3-mile racecourse.

The majority of FSI activities center on the *number line*. Number lines vary in difficulty and type of representation. Number line racecourses provide a physical model for partitioning into fractional parts and finding equivalent fractions for a given distance. Number lines may range from 0 to 1 to 0 to 5 to help students think about fractions that may be greater than one. Number lines also help students see relations between integer and fraction magnitudes and visually represent relationships between fractions of different or equivalent magnitudes (Gersten et al., 2017).

Deliberate attention is given to *word problems* to support fraction concepts and procedures that are introduced in each FSI lesson. When learning about fraction arithmetic, for example, students talk about word problems that look similar but have different actions (e.g., "Adrian walked 2 miles on Monday and ¾ mile on Tuesday. How far did Adrian walk altogether?" versus "Adrian walked ¾ mile each day for 2 days. How far did Adrian walk altogether?"). They learn to represent the problems on a number line to make explicit the different actions represented in each problem.

Finally, *timed activities* are used to help students retrieve multiplication facts that are relevant for finding equivalent fractions for addition and subtraction. Student are also asked to quickly indicate which of two fractions is larger (e.g., ¼ or 6/8). However, they are encouraged to use a more appropriate strategy in real time if an incorrect response is given. For example, if a student says more parts make 6/8 larger than ¼, the instructor will show the child a more efficient benchmarking strategy that can be accessed when solving equivalency problems (e.g., "These fractions have different denominators, so we can't simply compare number of portions. We know that ¼ is closer to 0 and ⁶⁄₈ is closer to 1. Therefore, ⁶⁄₈ is larger than ¼.").

Conclusions

Math learning difficulties are a serious educational concern. Although students with MLD are heterogeneous in nature, many show core weaknesses in numerical processing that affect their understanding, accuracy, and fluency with math concepts and procedures. Math learning and learning difficulties are also associated with basic weaknesses in EF, spatial reasoning, and language, and some studies suggest causal connections. Importantly, children at risk for MLD can be reliably identified in early childhood with valid number screeners. Such screening informs early intervention practices, which pave the way for later math success. Rigorous intervention research has led to informed recommendations for helping elementary school children with MLD achieve success in math. However, additional work is needed to ensure positive long-term outcomes as students progress beyond the elementary and early middle school years. For example, students with MLD who make gains through intensive support should be followed into later grades to document whether these gains hold and lead to better outcomes in more advanced topics, such as algebra. Moreover, additional randomized controlled studies are needed to determine the best way to integrate training in general cognitive processes (e.g., EFs) into math interventions for students with MLD at different grade levels.

REFERENCES

Allen, K., & Giofrè, D. (2021). A distinction between working memory components as unique predictors of mathematical components in 7–8 year old children. *Educational Psychology, 41*(6), 678–694.

Andersson, U. (2008). Mathematical competencies in children with different types of learning difficulties. *Journal of Educational Psychology, 100*(1), 48–66.

Andersson, U. (2010). Skill development in different components of arithmetic and basic cognitive functions: Findings from a 3-year longitudinal study of children with different types of learning difficulties. *Journal of Educational Psychology, 102*(1), 115–134.

Andersson, U., & Östergren, R. (2012). Number magnitude processing and basic cognitive functions in children with mathematical learning disabilities. *Learning and Individual Differences, 22*(6), 701–714.

Ansari, D. (2008). Effects of development and enculturation on number representation in the brain. *Nature Reviews Neuroscience, 9*(4), 278–291.

Ashkenazi, S., Rosenberg-Lee, M., Tenison, C., & Menon, V. (2012). Weak task-related modulation and stimulus representations during arithmetic problem solving in children with developmental dyscalculia. *Developmental Cognitive Neuroscience, 2*(Suppl. 1), S152–S166.

Bailey, D. H., Littlefield, A., & Geary, D. C. (2012). The codevelopment of skill at and preference for use of retrieval-based processes for solving addition problems: Individual and sex differences from first to sixth grades. *Journal of Experimental Child Psychology, 113*(1), 78–92.

Barbieri, C. A., Rodrigues, J., Dyson, N., & Jordan, N. C. (2020). Improving fraction understanding in sixth graders with mathematics difficulties: Effects of a number line approach combined with cognitive learning strategies. *Journal of Educational Psychology, 112*(3), 628.

Barnes, M. A., & Raghubar, K. P. (2017). Neurodevelopmental disorders as model systems for understanding typical and atypical mathematical development. In D. C. Geary, D. B. Berch, R. Ochsendorf, & K. M. Koepke (Eds.), *Acquisition of complex arithmetic skills and higher-order mathematics concepts* (pp. 67–97). Academic Press.

Baroody, A. J., Lai, M.-L., & Mix, K. S. (2006). The development of young children's early number and operation sense and its implications for early childhood education. In B. Spodek & O. Saracho (Eds.), *Handbook of research on the education of young children* (pp. 187–221). Lawrence Erlbaum Associates.

Baroody, A. J., Purpura, D. J., Eiland, M. D., & Reid, E. E. (2014). Fostering first graders' fluency with basic subtraction and larger addition combinations via computer-assisted instruction. *Cognition and Instruction, 32*(2), 159–197.

Beliakoff, A. (2021). *Predicting mathematics difficulties with an early number sense screener.* University of Delaware, ProQuest Dissertation Publishing.

Berteletti, I., Prado, J., & Booth, J. R. (2014). Children with mathematical learning disability fail in recruiting verbal and numerical brain regions when solving simple multiplication problems. *Cortex, 57*, 143–155.

Best, J. R., Miller, P. H., & Naglieri, J. A. (2011). Relations between executive function and academic achievement from ages 5 to 17 in a large, representative national sample. *Learning and Individual Differences, 21*(4), 327–336.

Booth, J. L., Newton, K. J., & Twiss-Garrity, L. K. (2014). The impact of fraction magnitude knowledge on algebra performance and learning. *Journal of Experimental Child Psychology, 118*(1), 110–118.

Bos, I. F. V. D., Kolkman, M. E., Kroesbergen, E. H., & Leseman, P. P. (2014). Explaining variability: Numerical representations in 4- to 8-year-old children. *Journal of Cognition and Development, 15*(2), 325–344.

Boyer, T. W., & Levine, S. C. (2012). Child proportional scaling: Is $1/3 = 1/6 = 3/9 = 4/12$? *Journal of Experimental Child Psychology, 111*(3), 516–533.

Braithwaite, D. W., & Siegler, R. S. (2018). Developmental changes in the whole number bias. *Developmental Science, 21*(2), e12541.

Brooks, N., & Goldin-Meadow, S. (2016). Moving to learn: How guiding the hands can set the stage for learning. *Cognitive Science, 40*(7), 1831–1849.

Bugden, S., & Ansari, D. (2016). Probing the nature of deficits in the "Approximate Number System" in children with persistent developmental dyscalculia. *Developmental Science, 19*(5), 817–833.

Bull, R., & Lee, K. (2014). Executive functioning and mathematics achievement. *Child Development Perspectives, 8*(1), 36–41.

Butterworth, B. (2005). The development of arithmetical abilities. *Journal of Child Psychology and Psychiatry and Allied Disciplines, 46*(1), 3–18.

Butterworth, B., & Laurillard, D. (2010). Low numeracy and dyscalculia: Identification and intervention. *ZDM—International Journal on Mathematics Education, 42*(6), 527–539.

Butterworth, B., Varma, S., & Laurillard, D. (2011). Dyscalculia: From brain to education. *Science, 332*(6033), 1049–1053.

Cañizares, D. C., Crespo, V. R., & Alemañy, E. G. (2012). Symbolic and non-symbolic number processing in children with developmental dyslexia. *The Spanish Journal of Psychology, 15*(3), 952–966.

Carpenter, T. P., & Moser, J. M. (1984). The acquisition of addition and subtraction concepts in grades one through three published by: National Council of Teachers of Mathematics. *Journal for Research in Mathematics Education, 15*(3), 179–202.

Chard, D. J., Clarke, B., Baker, S., Otterstedt, J., Braun, D., & Katz, R. (2005). Using measures of number sense to screen for difficulties in mathematics: Preliminary findings. *Assessment for Effective Intervention, 30*(2), 3–14.

Chow, J. C., Majeika, C. E., & Sheaffer, A. W. (2021). Language skills of children with and without mathematics difficulty. *Journal of Speech, Language, and Hearing Research, 64*(9), 1–7.

Clarke, B., Doabler, C. T., Nelson, N. J., & Shanley, C. (2015). Effective instructional strategies for kindergarten and first-grade students at risk in mathematics. *Intervention in School and Clinic, 50*(5), 257–265.

Common Core State Standards Initiative. (2010). *Common Core State Standards for mathematics.* National Governors Association Center for Best Practices and the Council of Chief State School Officers.

Connolly, A. J. (2007). *KeyMath-3 Diagnostic Assessment.* Pearson Assessments.

Cowan, R., & Powell, D. (2014). The contributions of domain-general and numerical factors to third-grade arithmetic skills and mathematical learning disability. *Journal of Educational Psychology, 106*(1), 214–229.

Dehaene, S. (1992). Varieties of numerical abilities. *Cognition, 44*(1–2), 1–42.

Dehaene, S. (1997). *The number sense: How the mind creates mathematics.* Oxford University Press.

Desoete, A., Ceulemans, A., De Weerdt, F., & Pieters, S. (2012). Can we predict mathematical learning disabilities from symbolic and non-symbolic comparison tasks in kindergarten? Findings from a longitudinal study. *British Journal of Educational Psychology, 82*(1), 64–81.

Driver, M. K., & Powell, S. R. (2017). Culturally and linguistically responsive schema intervention: Improving word problem solving for English language learners with mathematics difficulty. *Learning Disability Quarterly, 40*(1), 41–53.

Dyson, N., Rodrigues, J., Barbieri, C, Rinne, L., & Jordan, N. C. (2018). A fraction sense intervention for students with or at risk for mathematics difficulties. *Remedial and Special Education, 41*(4), 1–11.

Elliott, L., & Bachman, H. J. (2018). SES disparities in early math abilities: The contributions of parents' math cognitions, practices to support math, and math talk. *Developmental Review, 49*, 1–15.

Ericsson, K. A., & Kintsch, W. (1995). Long-term working memory. *Psychological Review, 102*(2), 211.

Fuchs, L. S., Fuchs, D., Stuebing, K., Fletcher, J. M., Hamlett, C. L., & Lambert, W. (2008). Problem solving and computational skill: Are they shared or distinct aspects of mathematical cognition? *Journal of Educational Psychology, 100*(1), 30–47.

Fuchs, L. S., Newman-Gonchar, R., Schumacher, R., Dougherty, B., Bucka, N., Karp, K. S., et al. (2021). *Assisting students struggling with mathematics: Intervention in the elementary grades* (WWC 2021006). National Center for Education Evaluation and Regional Assistance (NCEE), Institute of Education Sciences, U.S. Department of Education. *http://whatworks.ed.gov*

Fuchs, L. S., Schumacher, R. F., Sterba, S. K., Long, J., Namkung, J., Malone, A., et al. (2014). Does working memory moderate the effects of fraction intervention? An aptitude–treatment interaction. *Journal of Educational Psychology, 106*(2), 499.

Fuchs, L. S., Seethaler, P. M., Sterba, S. K., Craddock, C., Fuchs, D., Compton, D. L., et al. (2021). Closing the word-problem achievement gap in first grade: Schema-based word-problem intervention with embedded language comprehension instruction. *Journal of Educational Psychology, 113*(1), 86–103.

Geary, D. C. (2004). Mathematics and learning disabilities. *Journal of Learning Disabilities, 37*(1), 4–15.

Geary, D. C. (2011). Cognitive predictors of achievement growth in mathematics: Cognitive predictors of achievement growth in mathematics. *Developmental Psychology, 47*(6), 1539–1552.

Geary, D. C., Hoard, M. K., & Bailey, D. H. (2012). Fact retrieval deficits in low achieving children and children with mathematical learning disability. *Journal of Learning Disabilities, 45*(4), 291–307.

Geary, D. C., Hoard, M. K., Byrd-Craven, J., Nugent, L., & Numtee, C. (2007). Cognitive mechanisms underlying achievement deficits in children with mathematical learning disability. *Child Development, 78*(4), 1343–1359.

Geary, D. C., Hoard, M. K., Nugent, L., & Bailey, D. H. (2012). Mathematical cognition deficits in children with learning disabilities and persistent low achievement: A five-year prospective study. *Journal of Educational Psychology, 104*(1), 206.

Geary, D. C., Hoard, M. K., Nugent, L., & Byrd-Craven, J. (2008). Development of number line representations in children with mathematical learning disability. *Developmental Neuropsychology, 33*(3), 277–299.

Geary, D. C., Hoard, M. K., Nugent, L., & Scofield, J. E. (2021). In-class attention, spatial ability, and mathematics anxiety predict across-grade gains in adolescents' mathematics achievement. *Journal of Educational Psychology, 113*(4), 754.

Gelman, R., & Gallistel, C. R. (1978). *The child's understanding of number.* Harvard University Press.

Gelman, R., & Williams, E. M. (1998). Enabling constraints for cognitive development and learning: Domain specificity and epigenesis. In W. Damon (Ed.), *Handbook of child psychology: Vol. 2. Cognition, perception, and language* (pp. 575–630). Wiley.

Gersten, R., Jordan, N. C., & Flojo, J. R. (2005). Early identification and intervention for students with mathematics difficulties. *Journal of Learning Disabilities, 38*(4), 293–304.

Gersten, R., Schumacher, R. F., & Jordan, N. C. (2017). Life on the number line: Routes to understanding fraction magnitude for students with difficulties learning mathematics. *Journal of Learning Disabilities, 50*(6), 655–657.

Gilmore, C. K., McCarthy, S. E., & Spelke, E. S. (2010). Non-symbolic arithmetic abilities and mathematics achievement in the first year of formal schooling. *Cognition, 115*(3), 394–406.

Ginsburg, H. P., & Baroody, A. J. (2003). *TEMA-3: Test of Early Mathematics Ability–Third Edition.* PRO-ED.

Groen, G. J., & Parkman, J. M. (1972). A chronometric analysis of simple addition. *Psychological Review, 79*, 329–343.

Gunderson, E. A., Ramirez, G., Beilock, S. L., & Levine, S. C. (2012). The relation between spatial skill and early number knowledge: The role of the linear number line. *Developmental Psychology, 48*(5), 1229.

Hansen, N., Jordan, N. C., Fernandez, E., Siegler, R. S., Fuchs, L. S., Gersten, R., & Micklos, D. A. (2015). Predictors of fraction knowledge in sixth grade. *Cognitive Development, 35*, 34–49.

Hecht, S. A., & Vagi, K. J. (2012). Patterns of strengths and weaknesses in children's knowledge about fractions. *Journal of Experimental Child Psychology, 111*(2), 212–229.

Hiebert, J., & Lefevre, P. (1986). Conceptual and procedural knowledge in mathematics: An introductory analysis. In J. Hiebert (Ed.), *Conceptual and procedural knowledge: The case of mathematics* (pp. 1–27). Erlbaum.

Huttenlocher, J., Jordan, N. C., & Levine, S. C. (1994). A mental model for early arithmetic. *Journal of Experimental Psychology: General, 123*(3), 284–296.

Iuculano, T., Tang, J., Hall, C. W. B., & Butterworth, B. (2008). Core information processing deficits in developmental dyscalculia and low numeracy. *Developmental Science, 11*(5), 669–680.

Jones, G., & Macken, B. (2015). Questioning short-term memory and its measurement: Why digit span measures long-term associative learning. *Cognition, 144*, 1–13.

Jordan, N. C., Dyson, N., Guba, T., Botello, M., Suchanec-Cooper, H., & May, H. (2024). Exploring the impact of a fraction sense intervention in authentic school environments: An initial investigation. *Journal of Experimental Child Psychology, 244*, 105954.

Jordan, N. C., Hanich, L. B., & Kaplan, D. (2003). Arithmetic fact mastery in young children: A longitudinal investigation. *Journal of Experimental Child Psychology, 85*, 103–119.

Jordan, N. C., Kaplan, D., Ramineni, C., & Locuniak, M. N. (2009). Early math matters: Kindergarten number sense and later mathematics outcomes. *Developmental Psychology, 45*, 850–867.

Jordan, N. C., Klein, A., & Huang, C. (in press). *Screener for early number sense.* Hammill Institute.

Jordan, N. C., & Montani, T. O. (1997). Cognitive arithmetic and problem solving: A comparison of children with specific and general mathematics difficulties. *Journal of Learning Disabilities, 30*(6), 634–684.

Jordan, N. C., Rinne, L., & Hansen, N. (2019). Mathematics learning difficulties in the United States: Current issues in screening and intervention. In A. Fritz-Stratman, V. G. Haase, & P. Rasanen (Eds.), *International handbook of mathematics learning difficulties* (pp. 183–199). Springer International AG.

Jordan, N. C., Rodrigues, J., Hansen, N., & Resnick, I. (2017). Fraction development in children: Importance of building numerical magnitude understanding. In D. C. Geary, D. B. Berch, R. Ochsendorf, & K. M. Koepke (Eds.), *Acquisition of complex arithmetic skills and higher-order mathematics concepts* (pp. 125–140). Academic Press.

Karp, K. S., Bush, S. B., & Dougherty, B. J. (2014). 13 rules that expire. *Teaching Children Mathematics, 21*(1), 18–25.

Kauffman, L., Mazzocco, M. M., Dowker, A., von Aster, M., Gobel, S., Grabner, R. H., et al. (2013). Dyscalculia from a developmental and differential perspective. *Frontiers in Developmental Psychology, 4.*

Keeler, M. L., & Swanson, H. L. (2001). Does strategy knowledge influence working memory in children with mathematical disabilities? *Journal of Learning Disabilities, 34*(5), 418–434.

King, Y. A., & Purpura, D. J. (2021). Direct numeracy activities and early math skills: Math language as a mediator. *Early Childhood Research Quarterly, 54*, 252–259.

Kingsdorf, S., & Krawec, J. (2014). Error analysis of mathematical word problem solving across students with and without learning disabilities. *Learning Disabilities Research & Practice, 29*(2), 66–74.

Knuth, E., Stephens, A., Blanton, M., & Gardiner, A. (2016). Build an early foundation for algebra success. *Phi Delta Kappan, 97*(6), 65–68.

Krawec, J. L. (2014). Problem representation and mathematical problem solving of students of varying math ability. *Journal of Learning Disabilities, 47*(2), 103–115.

Lambert, K., & Moeller, K. (2019). Place-value computation in children with mathematics difficulties. *Journal of Experimental Child Psychology, 178*, 214–225.

Landerl, K. (2019). Neurocognitive perspective on numerical development. In A. Fritz-Stratman, V. G. Haase, & P. Rasanen (Eds.), *International handbook of mathematics learning difficulties* (pp. 9–24). Springer International AG.

Laski, E. V., & Dulaney, A. (2015). When prior knowledge interferes, inhibitory control matters for learning: The case of numerical magnitude representations. *Journal of Educational Psychology, 107*(4), 1035.

Lowrie, T., Logan, T., Harris, D., & Hegarty, M. (2018). The impact of an intervention program on students' spatial reasoning: Student engagement through mathematics-enhanced learning activities. *Cognitive Research: Principles and Implications, 3*(1), 1–10.

Lyons, I. M., & Beilock, S. L. (2011). Numerical ordering ability mediates the relation between number-sense and arithmetic competence. *Cognition, 121*(2), 256–261.

Magalhães, S., Carneiro, L., Limpo, T., & Filipe, M. (2020). Executive functions predict literacy and mathematics achievements: The unique contribution of cognitive flexibility in grades 2, 4, and 6. *Child Neuropsychology, 26*(7), 934–952.

Mamedova, S., Stephens, M., Liao, Y., Sennett, J., & Sirma, P. (2021). *2012–2016 Program for International Student Assessment Young Adult Follow-up Study (PISA YAFS): How reading and mathematics performance at age 15 relate to literacy and numeracy skills and education, workforce, and life outcomes at age 19* (NCES 2021-029). U.S. Department of Education, National Center for Education Statistics. *https://nces.ed.gov/pubs2021/2021029.pdf*

Martiniello, M. (2008). Language and the performance of English-language learners in math word problems. *Harvard Educational Review, 78*(2), 333–368.

Mazzocco, M. M., Feigenson, L., & Halberda, J. (2011). Impaired acuity of the approximate number system underlies mathematical learning disability (dyscalculia). *Child Development, 82*(4), 1224–1237.

Mazzocco, M. M., & Räsänen, P. (2013). Contributions of longitudinal studies to evolving definitions and knowledge of developmental dyscalculia. *Trends in Neuroscience and Education, 2*(2), 65–73.

Mazzocco, M. M., & Thompson, R. E. (2005). Kindergarten predictors of math learning disability. *Learning Disabilities Research & Practice, 20*(3), 142–155.

McClelland, M. M., Acock, A. C., Piccinin, A., Rhea, S. A., & Stallings, M. C. (2013). Relations between preschool attention span-persistence and age 25 educational outcomes. *Early Childhood Research Quarterly, 28*(2), 314–324.

Mejias, S., Mussolin, C., Rousselle, L., Grégoire, J., & Nol, M. P. (2012). Numerical and nonnumerical estimation in children with and without mathematical learning disabilities. *Child Neuropsychology, 18*(6), 550–575.

Menon, V. (2016). Working memory in children's math learning and its disruption in dyscalculia. *Current Opinion in Behavioral Sciences, 10*, 125–132.

Mix, K. S., Levine, S. C., Cheng, Y. L., Young, C., Hambrick, D. Z., Ping, R., & Konstantopoulos, S. (2016). Separate but correlated: The latent structure of space and mathematics across development. *Journal of Experimental Psychology: General, 145*(9), 1206.

Morgan, P., Farkas, G., & Wu, Q. (2009). Five-year growth trajectories of kindergarten children with learning difficulties in mathematics. *Journal of Learning Disabilities, 42*, 306–321.

Morgan, P. L., Li, H., Farkas, G., Cook, M., Pun, W. H., & Hillemeier, M. M. (2017). Executive functioning deficits increase kindergarten children's risk for reading and mathematics difficulties in first grade. *Contemporary Educational Psychology, 50*, 23–32.

Morsanyi, K., van Bers, B. M. C. W., O'Connor, P. A., & McCormack, T. (2018). Developmental dyscalculia is characterized by order processing deficits: Evidence from numerical and non-numerical ordering tasks. *Developmental Neuropsychology, 43*(7), 595–621.

Mussolin, C., Mejias, S., & Noël, M. P. (2010). Symbolic and nonsymbolic number comparison in children with and without dyscalculia. *Cognition, 115*(1), 10–25.

National Assessment of Educational Progress (2019). *The nation's report card.* U.S. Department of Education, National Center for Education Statistics. *www.nationsreportcard.gov*

National Mathematics Advisory Panel (NMAP) (2008). *Foundations for success: The final report of the National Mathematics Advisory Panel.* U.S. Department of Education.

National Research Council. (2009). *Mathematics learning in early childhood: Paths toward excellence and equity.* National Academies Press.

Nelson, G., & Powell, S. R. (2018). Computation error analysis: Students with mathematics difficulty compared to typically achieving students. *Assessment for Effective Intervention, 43*(3), 144–156.

Newton, K. J., Willard, C., & Teufel, C. (2014). An examination of the ways that students with learning disabilities solve fraction computation problems. *The Elementary School Journal, 115*(1), 1–21.

Passolunghi, M. C., & Mammarella, I. C. (2010). Spatial and visual working memory ability in children with difficulties in arithmetic word problem solving. *European Journal of Cognitive Psychology, 22*(6), 944–963.

Passolunghi, M. C., & Siegel, L. S. (2001). Short-term memory, working memory, and inhibitory control in children with difficulties in arithmetic problem solving. *Journal of Experimental Child Psychology, 80*(1), 44–57.

Pearson. (2017). *AimsWeb Plus.*

Piazza, M., Facoetti, A., Trussardi, A. N., Berteletti, I., Conte, S., Lucangeli, D., et al. (2010). Developmental trajectory of number acuity reveals a severe impairment in developmental dyscalculia. *Cognition, 116*(1), 33–41.

Peng, P., Namkung, J., Barnes, M., & Sun, C. (2016). A meta-analysis of mathematics and working memory: Moderating effects of working memory domain, type of mathematics skill, and sample characteristics. *Journal of Educational Psychology, 108*(4), 455.

Prediger, S., Erath, K., & Opitz, E. M. (2019). The language dimension of mathematical difficulties. In A. Fritz-Stratman, V. G. Haase, & P. Rasanen (Eds.), *International handbook of mathematical learning difficulties* (pp. 437–455). Springer.

Purpura, D. J., & Reid, E. E. (2016). Mathematics and language: Individual and group differences in mathematical language skills in young children. *Early Childhood Research Quarterly, 36*, 259–268.

Raghubar, K., Cirino, P., Barnes, M., Ewing-Cobbs, L., Fletcher, J., & Fuchs, L. (2009). Errors in multi-digit arithmetic and behavioral inattention in children with math difficulties. *Journal of Learning Disabilities, 42*(4), 356–371.

Resnick, I., Newcombe, N. S., & Jordan, N. C. (2019). The relation between spatial reasoning and mathematical achievement in children with mathematical learning difficulties. In A. Fritz-Stratman, V. G. Haase, & P. Rasanen (Eds.), *International handbook of mathematical learning difficulties* (pp. 423–435). Springer.

Rittle-Johnson, B. (2017). Developing mathematics knowledge. *Child Development Perspectives, 11*(3), 184–190.

Rittle-Johnson, B., & Jordan, N. C. (2016). *Synthesis of IES-funded research on mathematics: 2002–2013* (NCER 2016–2003). National Center for Education Research.

Rodrigues, J., Dyson, N., Hansen, N., & Jordan, N. C. (2016). Preparing for algebra by building fraction sense. *Teaching Exceptional Children, 49*(2).

Rodrigues, J., Hansen, N., & Jordan, N. C. (2020). Identifying fraction measures as screeners of mathematics risk status. *Journal of Learning Disabilities, 52*(6), 480–497.

Rousselle, L., & Noël, M. P. (2007). Basic numerical skills in children with mathematics learning disabilities: A comparison of symbolic vs non-symbolic number magnitude processing. *Cognition, 102*(3), 361–395.

Seethaler, P. M., Fuchs, L. S., Star, J. R., & Bryant, J. (2011). The cognitive predictors of computational skill with whole versus rational numbers: An exploratory study. *Learning and Individual Differences, 21*(5), 536–542.

Siegel, L. S., & Ryan, E. B. (1989). The development of working memory in normally achieving and subtypes of learning disabled children. *Child Development, 60*(4), 973–980.

Siegler, R. S. (1996). *Emerging minds: The process of change in children's thinking.* Oxford University Press.

Siegler, R. S. (2009). Improving the numerical understanding of children from low-income families. *Child Development Perspectives, 3*(2), 118–124.

Siegler, R. S., Fazio, L. K., Bailey, D. H., & Zhou, X. (2013). Fractions: The new frontier for theories of numerical development. *Trends in Cognitive Sciences, 17*(1), 13–19.

Siegler, R. S., & Lortie-Forgues, H. (2014). An integrative theory of numerical development. *Child Development Perspectives, 8*(3), 144–150.

Siegler, R. S., & Pyke, A. A. (2013). Developmental and individual differences in understanding of fractions. *Developmental Psychology, 49*(10), 1994.

Siegler, R. S., & Shrager, J. (1984). Strategy choice in addition and subtraction: How do children know what to do? In C. Sophian (Ed.), *Origins of cognitive skills* (pp. 229–293). Erlbaum.

Siegler, R. S., Thompson, C. A., & Schneider, M. (2011). An integrated theory of whole number and fractions development. *Cognitive Psychology, 62*(4), 273–296.

Skagerlund, K., & Träff, U. (2016). Number processing and heterogeneity of developmental dyscalculia: Subtypes with different cognitive profiles and deficits. *Journal of Learning Disabilities, 49*(1), 36–50.

Swanson, H. L., & Alloway, T. P. (2012). Working memory, learning, and academic achievement. In *APA educational psychology handbook, Vol 1: Theories, constructs, and critical issues.* (pp. 327–366). American Psychological Association.

Szucs, D., Devine, A., Soltesz, F., Nobes, A., & Gabriel, F. (2013). Developmental dyscalculia is related to visuo-spatial memory and inhibition impairment. *Cortex, 49*(10), 2674–2688.

Träff, U., Olsson, L., Östergren, R., & Skagerlund, K. (2017). Heterogeneity of developmental dyscalculia: Cases with different deficit profiles. *Frontiers in Psychology, 7,* 1–15.

Träff, U., & Passolunghi, M. C. (2015). Mathematical skills in children with dyslexia. *Learning and Individual Differences, 40*, 108–114.

Van Luit, J. E. H. (2019). Diagnostics of dyscalculia. In A. Fritz-Stratman, V. G. Haase, & P. Rasanen (Eds.), *International handbook of mathematics learning difficulties* (pp. 654–667). Springer International AG.

van Viersen, S., Slot, E. M., Kroesbergen, E. H., van't Noordende, J. E., & Leseman, P. P. M. (2013). The added value of eye-tracking in diagnosing dyscalculia: A case study. *Frontiers in Psychology, 4*, 679.

Wheeler, C. E., Lembke, E. S., Richards-Tutor, C., Wallin, J., Good, R. H., Dewey, E. N., & Warnock, A. N. (2019). *Acadience Math. Assessment Manual.* Pearson.

Wong, T. T. Y., Ho, C. S. H., & Tang, J. (2017). Defective number sense or impaired access? Differential impairments in different subgroups of children with mathematics difficulties. *Journal of Learning Disabilities, 50*(1), 49–61.

Ye, A., Resnick, I., Hansen, N., Rodrigues, J., Rinne, L., & Jordan, N. C. (2016). Pathways to fraction learning: Numerical abilities mediate the relation between early cognitive competencies and later fraction knowledge. *Journal of Experimental Child Psychology, 152*, 242–263.

Yu, X., Liu, J., Li, D., Liu, H., Cui, J., & Zhou, X. (2016). Dynamic mental number line in simple arithmetic. *Psychological Research, 80*(3), 410–421.

Zaunmüller, L., Domahs, F., Dressel, K., Lonnemann, J., Klein, E., Ischebeck, A., & Willmes, K. (2009). Rehabilitation of arithmetic fact retrieval via extensive practice: A combined fMRI and behavioral case-study. *Neuropsychological Rehabilitation, 19*(3), 422–443.

Zhang, H., Miller-Cotto, D., & Jordan, N. C. (2021, February). *Exploring co-development of executive functions and math achievement using cross-lagged panel model with fixed effects.* Presentation at Annual Conference, Mathematical Cognition and Learning Society (MCLS), Virtual meeting.

CHAPTER 4

Social and Emotional Learning and Learning Disabilities

Laura L. Feuerborn, Barbara A. Gueldner, and Ashli D. Tyre

At the time of this writing, the social and emotional needs of our youth are dire. Rates of mental health problems among children and adolescents have been on the rise for over a decade, with suicide rates and attempts reported to be at an all-time high in 2019 (Curtin & Heron, 2019) and markedly increasing since the COVID-19 pandemic (Yard et al., 2021). Recently, leading mental health and healthcare organizations declared a state of emergency for child and adolescent mental health (American Academy of Pediatrics, 2021). One preliminary analysis of data suggests children and adolescents accessed emergency healthcare at higher rates between 2020 and 2022 compared to 2019 for serious behavioral health concerns such as self-harm, drug poisoning, substance use, eating disorders, and other mental health concerns (Radhakrishnan et al., 2022). Before the pandemic, many youths did not have access to and/or did not receive sufficient mental health care (Whitney & Peterson, 2019), and although the social and emotional-related effects of the pandemic are yet to be fully realized, it is already exacerbating existing service gaps and inequities, creating a critical need for school-based supports that are effective and well-coordinated (Chadi et al., 2022).

Social and emotional competence is linked to physical health, emotional well-being, educational attainment, healthy relationships, and employment (Durlak et al., 2011; Jones & Doolittle, 2017) and can be more predictive of life outcomes than IQ (Zins, 2004). The skills associated with social and emotional competence are malleable and teachable and yield increased academic, behavioral, and mental health outcomes across demographics and populations (Mahoney et al., 2019). Social and emotional learning (SEL) emphasizes a school-based approach to promote social and emotional competence and equitable learning environments where all can thrive with resilience in the face of life challenges. In addition to programs and strategies, SEL includes multiple points of ecological support for students and educators across layers of prevention or tiers.

Considering the needs of students with exceptionalities, the importance of SEL is underscored. Most students with an IDEA-classified disability are identified with an LD (33%; National Center for Education Statistics, 2021), and over four decades of research has clearly demonstrated that those with an LD are at an increased risk for social and emotional challenges. If these needs remain unaddressed, students may experience psychological distress, poor mental health, school dropout, and employment problems (American Psychiatric Association, 2013).

Social and Emotional Learning Frameworks and School-Based Applications

The field of SEL is predicated on diverse theories and disciplines, including the fields of psychology, neuroscience, and education; as a result, there are numerous organizing frameworks and approaches using different terms for SEL competencies, such as 21st-century skills, noncognitive skills, and character education (Jones & Doolittle, 2017). Herein, we use the SEL framework from the Collaborative for Academic, Social, and Emotional Learning (CASEL) to organize this content because it is commonly applied in schools and discussed in the literature. CASEL, a prominent research, policy, and practice-based organization, defines SEL as the process through which youth and adults acquire and apply the knowledge, skills, and attitudes to develop healthy identities, manage emotions, achieve personal and collective goals, have empathy for others, establish and maintain supportive relationships, and make responsible and caring decisions (CASEL, 2020).

The CASEL framework is applied across school, home, and community settings and incorporates five broad SEL competencies with both intrapersonal and interpersonal knowledge and skills (CASEL, 2020). Recently, the framework and competencies were recast to include a more explicit emphasis on social justice, equity, and inclusion, along with a more balanced emphasis on values and skills prominent in collectivist societies (e.g., cooperation) as compared to skills and values emphasized in individualistic societies (Jagers et al., 2018). The following competencies and indicators are but a brief overview; more complete definitions can be found at *https://casel.org/fundamentals-of-sel/what-is-the-casel-framework*.

- *Self-awareness:* identify and integrate various dimensions of personal identity (e.g., cultural, racial, and gender); sense of purpose; understand strengths and limitations; understand emotional and physiological experiences, thought processes, values, and biases.

- *Self-management:* regulate strong emotions and impulses; tolerate discomfort; sustain attention; manage stress; motivate oneself; perception of agency, courage, and ability to attain goals.

- *Social awareness:* empathy, compassion, and understanding; appreciate sociocultural norms and the perspectives of others from diverse backgrounds and contexts.

• *Relationship skills:* building healthy connections with others from diverse backgrounds; communication skills; cooperation; conflict management; intercultural competence; leadership; seek and offer help as appropriate.

• *Responsible decision making:* make decisions considering ethics, safety, and the potential outcomes on self and others; personal and societal problem-solving skills, including curiosity, receptivity to others' perspectives, innovation, and reasoning.

SEL Applied in Schools

The uptake and application of SEL have blossomed in recent years, with more than 70% of elementary principals surveyed reportedly implementing or planning to implement SEL in their buildings (Atwell & Bridgeland, 2019). At the time of this writing, 18 states have adopted SEL standards and benchmarks, with 21 states including guidance on the implementation of SEL (Yoder et al., 2020). Most SEL-related efforts in schools are programs with instructional activities to target specific skills as well as program-independent activities and strategies (Gueldner et al., 2020). Immediate and sustained outcomes of SEL programming include improved academic performance, social and emotional knowledge and skills, attitudes toward self and others, and prosocial behavior and reduced emotional and behavioral symptoms (e.g., Corcoran et al., 2018; Durlak et al., 2011; Taylor et al., 2017).

The diversity of existing SEL frameworks notwithstanding, common themes include systemic planning and implementation (Durlak, 2015; Mahoney et al., 2019) and the importance of contextual and cultural fit (Durlak, 2015). A systemic approach to SEL includes assessing needs and resources, identifying SEL priorities, supporting SEL for adults in the building, establishing internal capacity (e.g., professional development) and infrastructure (e.g., climate, policy), involving stakeholders (e.g., staff, students, community agencies, and families), creating schoolwide leadership teams with clear roles and responsibilities, and developing a long-term plan for implementation and evaluation. The implementation of SEL can be guided by a school team designated specifically for SEL or by an MTSS team designated to include SEL and positive discipline practices. Key implementation and evaluation activities include ongoing coaching, reflection, and support for implementers; monitoring implementation; assessing school and student outcomes; and establishing a continuous cycle for refinement and improvement that involves staff, students, and families. The CASEL school and district resource center contains more detailed guidance on this topic of systemic SEL (*https://schoolguide.casel.org*).

Research on the Social and Emotional Needs of Students with LD

Decades of research findings corroborate the co-existence of LD with SEL challenges (Bryan et al., 2004; Elias, 2004; Nelson & Harwood, 2011). Findings that document the social and emotional challenges experienced by individuals with LD are consistent across lifespan, location, informant (teachers, peers, parents, and self), research methodology, and time (Bryan et al., 2004). Estimations of the prevalence of social and emotional problems range from 38% to 75% of all youth with LD (Baum et al., 1988; Kavale & Forness, 1996). When Kavale and Forness (1996) completed a meta-analytic study analyzing 152 studies and found that 75% of youth with LD experienced social problems, they asserted that social challenges were integral to the experiences of students with LD. Since then, research has corroborated the interrelationship between LD and social–emotional learning needs (Al-Yagon, 2016; Cavioni et al., 2017).

The relationship between LDs and SEL needs is complex. Youth with LD may experience biological differences in social, emotional, and cognitive development and may also experience academic failure, special education exclusion, classroom isolation, and even discrimination within school and community settings (Darrow, 2014). These circumstances can limit opportunities for skill building, creating a social–emotional learning opportunity gap (Beyer, 2017). Developmental trajectories, life experiences, and opportunities to learn social and emotional skills may be fundamentally different for youth with and without LD. Although the issue of underrepresentation and overrepresentation is debated (e.g., Morgan et al., 2016), research has shown that the population of students identified with LD includes a misrepresentation of students who are male, Black, Latinx, linguistically diverse, and economically marginalized (Shifrer et al., 2011). When we consider the intersectionality of student identities, including race, culture, sexuality, and gender, numerous ecological considerations arise. Youth with LD from marginalized populations often experience additional systemic and environmental limitations on their opportunities for SEL that must be considered in understanding their strengths and needs (Beyer, 2017).

Considerations for LD Subtypes

Much of the research examining the SEL needs of youth with LD has not adequately distinguished between subtypes of LD (Fletcher et al., 2019). Many students with LDs have underlying language difficulties that characterize their disability (Grigorenko et al., 2019), and there is evidence that language difficulties are interconnected with social challenges (Elias, 2004; Peterson et al., 2013). Research has shown that 25–50% of those with reading LD meet diagnostic criteria for ADHD (Pennington, 2009), anxiety, and depressive disorders (Cederlof et al., 2017). Yet, comorbidity with conduct disorder appears to be largely restricted to those with both reading LD and ADHD (Willcutt et al., 2007). Studies seldom investigate the social and emotional needs of youth with math LDs, but available findings suggest higher risk for comorbidity with ADHD, anxiety, and depression (Willcutt et al., 2013). Youth with nonverbal LD are also more likely to experience challenges with social aspects of communication (Elias, 2004), including understanding nonverbal emotion cues (Fisher et al., 2022).

Social and Emotional Strengths and Needs in Students with LD

Prior research exploring the social and emotional competence of students with LD has focused on identifying their deficits through an examination of mean group differences between those with and without an LD diagnosis, as well as those with other diagnoses, such as ADHD and emotional behavioral disability (EBD). However, not all students with LD struggle with social and emotional competencies. Of those who do struggle, we must also attend to their strengths, assets, and sources of resilience as a leverage point for intervention programming and support in the educational setting (Carnazzo et al., 2019; Elias, 2004). It is important to understand the unique experiences, strengths, and identities of an individual student with LD while also seeking to understand their disability, its unique manifestations, and any associated challenges they experience with SEL. For example, positive parent, teacher, and peer relationships act as protective factors that mediate many of the social and emotional challenges experienced by students with LD (Al-Yagon, 2016), suggesting supportive positive relationships as a strength-based factor. In the section that follows, we review research findings on youth with LD in the five SEL competency areas.

Self-Awareness

Students with LD are more likely than students without LD to experience challenges with self-awareness, including self-efficacy, academic self-concept, and growth mindset (Bryan et al., 2004). They may experience challenges with recognizing their own feelings and may have a limited emotional labeling vocabulary beyond basic terms, such as happy, sad, and mad (Cavioni et al., 2017; Elias, 2004). They are more likely to make attributional errors as to the causes of their own successes and failures, especially when they also experience low self-esteem (Carnazzo et al., 2019). For example, after performing poorly on a test, a student with LD may attribute the cause to their ability rather than their lack of preparation in advance of the exam. Their experiences with academic failure may negatively impact their self-efficacy and cause them to avoid academic work that requires skill and effort, especially in the presence of peers (Cavioni et al., 2017; Nelson & Harwood, 2011). For example, a student with LD may act out when asked to read aloud in the presence of peers to avoid embarrassment.

Self-Management

Students with LD can have difficulty managing their emotions and behavior to achieve their goals as compared to students without LD. They may have difficulty managing strong emotions, both positive and negative (Carnazzo et al., 2019), which can interfere with learning (Elias, 2004). In the classroom, this may be evidenced as difficulty attending to instructions or social cues while experiencing excitement for a favored activity. Dysregulation, particularly with strong negative emotions (e.g., anger, anxiety, and depression), interferes with behavioral responses in social situations and may result in rejection by peers (Bryan et al., 2004).

Social Awareness

Students with LD have been found to experience challenges in social information processing, such as recognizing social norms and the emotions and perspectives of others (Bauminger et al., 2005; Elias, 2004). A student with LD might have difficulty understanding complex emotional situations in others, such as someone experiencing feelings of love and disdain simultaneously (Bauminger et al., 2005). They are also more likely to make attributional errors when interpreting the intent of others in social situations (Cavioni et al., 2017), such as attributing negative intent in an otherwise typical playground interaction.

Relationship Skills

Students with LD may experience social and behavioral challenges that negatively impact their interactions with peers and overall relationships. They may have trouble initiating and sustaining positive social interactions (Elias, 2004). They are likely to perform more poorly across measures of social communication skills, which is likely related to associated language deficits (Bryan et al., 2004; Henry & Reed, 1995). Research utilizing sociometric ratings by peers suggests students with LD are more likely to display aggression and disruptive behavior, and as a result, youth with LD can experience peer rejection (Cavioni et al., 2017; Elias, 2004).

Responsible Decision Making

Students with LD may experience challenges with decision making in social contexts. For example, research has shown that students with LD are more likely to generate ineffective solutions to hypothetical social dilemmas when compared to peers without an LD diagnosis who have low academic achievement (Cavioni et al., 2017).

Effective SEL Support for Students with LD

It is clear that many students with LD are at risk of or are experiencing social and emotional challenges, and that social and emotional skills are interconnected with academic functioning; thus, attending to students' areas of strengths and challenges is critical. The adoption of effective and meaningful SEL practices may be particularly relevant. Yet, the research on universal implementation of SEL with students with LD (and coordinating this approach with other interventions often used in special education) is complex and incomplete (Wiley & Siperstein, 2015). For example, most students with high-incidence disabilities such as LD receive instruction in general education classrooms and likely receive universally delivered, program-based SEL instruction (Wiley & Siperstein, 2015). However, most SEL programming has not been intentionally designed for students with disabilities and may not allow for the specificity that is required to address their needs (Wiley & Siperstein, 2015). Furthermore, compared to the research that has evaluated universal interventions with general populations, which may or may not include students with disabilities, less attention has been paid to the effects of universal SEL with students identified with IDEA-defined disabilities (Daley & McCarthy, 2020) and SLD in particular (Cavioni et al., 2017; Wiley & Siperstein, 2015). This gap makes it difficult to understand how students with LD are responding to universally delivered SEL programs. Universally and selected implementation of SEL and other interventions used in special education may improve areas such as social and emotional skills, attitudes toward school, symptoms associated with anxiety and depression, and academic difficulties (Clarke et al., 2015; Daley & McCarthy, 2020; Weare & Nind, 2011). To this end, Tier 1 SEL instruction can be helpful for students with LD from both an effectiveness and inclusiveness perspective (Cavioni et al., 2017), and integrating such practices with Tier 2 or Tier 3 level interventions may be essential (Buckley & Madhavi, 2018; Wiley & Siperstein, 2015). Herein, we review SEL and SEL-complementary approaches to support students with LD and/or students who are at risk for or who have developed social and emotional challenges.

Theoretical Bases and a Tiered Approach to SEL

Approaches to SEL in students with LD and other high-incidence disabilities often have a basis in social learning theory, cognitive-behavioral theory, problem solving, behaviorism, and explicit instruction (Whitcomb & Feuerborn, 2020; Wiley & Superstein, 2015). SEL programming at a universal level, and related social–emotional interventions often implemented in Tiers 2 and 3, can vary in terms of content, intensity, and the ability to tailor materials, instruction, and behavioral supports in response to students' needs and preferences. Universally designed and implemented SEL programs often use lesson-based materials (e.g., a curriculum), activities (e.g., circle time), and strategies to teach/learn/practice a specific skill in one or more competency areas. Such programs can be used at Tier 2 and 3 but would need to be increasingly individualized according to students' needs (e.g., content modifications; applying instructional strategies known to be effective with students with disabilities; and more opportunities for skills practice and generalization). Other activities may include the inclusion of social and emotional competency-focused IEP goals; small group instruction; individual counseling; and coordinating programs and strategies with teachers, parents, mental health providers, and community partners (Buckley & Madhavi, 2018; Gueldner et al., 2020). Perhaps key to SEL programming for students with LD is an interest in whether a coordinated and integrated approach between interventions delivered at Tier 1 and Tier 2 and 3 would improve outcomes for students (Espelage et al., 2015; Wiley & Superstein, 2015), decrease stigma associated with social–emotional challenges

(Cavioni, 2017), and increase opportunities to engage in prosocial interactions (Bryan et al., 2004).

SEL Approaches and Programs

Some SEL programs that are implemented in universal settings have been evaluated with students with disabilities, including LD. For example, *Second Step: Student Success Through Prevention (SS-SSTP)* is a lesson-based program that teaches students SEL skills, such as emotion regulation, effective communication, and social problem solving, including helping others who are being bullied, and includes direct and active forms of instruction (e.g., role-plays) (Committee for Children, 2008). An evaluation of 123 middle school students with IDEA-identified disabilities (47% of whom identified as having an SLD) indicated that after participating in the program over 3 years, students were significantly more interested in taking prosocial and helpful action in the context of bullying incidents and experienced improvements in their grades compared to those students who did not receive the program (Espelage et al., 2016). Furthermore, incidents of these students engaging in bullying behaviors significantly decreased over 3 years (Espelage et al., 2015). *Promoting Alternative Thinking Strategies* (PATHS) is another lesson-based program for preschool through grade 6 that focuses on emotional, social, and behavioral awareness and regulation and self-esteem (Kusché & Greenberg, 1994). A modified version emphasizing self-control was used with elementary students receiving special education services, 40% of whom were identified with LD. Results indicated student improvements in identifying emotions, behaviors, internalizing problems (e.g., depression), and problem solving (Kam et al., 2004).

Mindfulness-based approaches have garnered interest in recent years for use with all students. In one study with a small group of high school students with LD, students participated in a mindfulness meditation strategy for 5–10 minutes, 5 days per week, and over the course of 5 weeks. Results indicated significant decreases in anxiety and problem behaviors and increases in social skills and academic performance (Beauchamin et al., 2008). Another study also applied mindfulness-based practices with 15 male elementary school students with LD over the course of 10 weeks, leading to significant reductions in impulsive behaviors compared to students in the control condition (Alqarni & Hammad, 2021). Student engagement in the activities was improved through physical practices (e.g., walking and tasting food), games, student reflection and sharing, reinforcement, and tailoring instruction based on students' moods and attention.

Social Skills

Social skills training (SST) is a widely known intervention for students with high-incidence disabilities, including LD, and students with difficulties not necessarily identified with a disability (Maag, 2005). "Social skills" is a broad category that includes qualities found in CASEL's 5 Competency Areas framework (e.g., making and sustaining friendships; positive school functioning; understanding social norms and expectations; and responding prosocially).

In contrast to SEL programming, which draws from a large theoretical basis and focuses on universally implemented approaches to skill building, SST is influenced largely by behavioral theory and is typically implemented at a Tier 2 or 3 level to improve skill deficits (Gresham, 2010; Wiley & Siperstein, 2015). SST often involves focused assessment to clarify whether there are skills acquisition and/or performance difficulties (Gresham, 2010). Furthermore, functional assessment and replacement behavior training are recommended to design precise and meaningful interventions that can be more effective (Maag, 2005). SST instruction is typically focused on teaching, practicing, maintaining, and generalizing prosocial social skills (Cook et al., 2008) and does so through direct instruction, active forms of learning such as students practicing through role-playing and behavioral reinforcement techniques that can support engagement (Maag, 2005). These instructional methods can also be found in other SEL interventions but are more individualized in Tiers 2 and 3.

Research on the effectiveness of SST with students with social skills difficulties and LD varies (Gresham et al., 2006; Walker & Barry, 2018) and remains limited (Wiley & Siperstein, 2015). Forness and Kavale (1996) found that SST with an average implementation time of 30 hours produced small benefits for these students in terms of overall social skills, with the largest and statistically significant improvement found in self-reported social status compared to students without LD. Forness and Kavale (1996) speculated, and Gresham et al. (2006) concluded, that more time-intense SST may provide more benefits for students with LD who have difficulty acquiring social skills (e.g., 60 hours vs. 30 hours). Limitations to SST research include assorted components applied in various interventions diminish our ability to identify the components required to produce effectiveness, imprecise construct measurement, limited use of single-subject designs to evaluate effects, not measuring implementation fidelity (Forness & Kavale, 1996), and limited fidelity of implementation, skills generalization to other contexts, and matching students' needs and preferences to interventions (Gresham, 2010; Maag, 2005).

SEL Strategies

Several SEL and SEL-complementary strategies have been suggested for students with LD. Strategies are either included in pre-packaged programs or used independently (Walker & Barry, 2018). Table 4.1 highlights SEL strategies that have been recommended for students with LD, as well as instructional strategies that are indicated for both students with LD and a general population. Additional research would be helpful to precisely match SEL and/or general instructional strategies to SEL instruction with students with LD. Until more is known, we recommend that educators choose and apply such strategies in a thoughtful manner, taking into consideration students' needs and preferences, and existing and emerging research, to increase the likelihood of goodness-of-fit and effectiveness.

TABLE 4.1. SEL and Instructional Strategies

Strategy (reference)	Purpose of strategy	Example in use
Choice of topics, methods for investigation, and reporting (student-centered) (Elias, 2004)	Improve critical thinking skills, motivation, and effort when students are given choices.	Students choose a topic, ways in which they can find information, and media to use for reporting on this information.
Collaborative strategic reading (see Moore et al., 2020, for a review)	Apply collaborative learning skills in language arts to promote reading, comprehension, engagement, social skills, and self-regulation.	Students work together in groups on a project that is chunked. Every student works on each part, and they discuss, problem-solve, and offer feedback within their group.
Computer/software-assisted learning (Elias, 2004)	Use a complementary technology to learn SEL skills.	Use software that supports a variety of SEL skills.
Emotion vocabulary word list (Elias, 2004; Feuerborn & Tyre, 2009)	Improve emotion vocabulary identification in self and others.	Student- and teacher-created vocabulary lists that grow in complexity over time.
Feelings thermometer (Elias, 2004)	Learn how emotions normally change over time in intensity. Teachers validate students' emotions and normalize them to decrease confusion and stigma regarding emotional experiences.	Using a thermometer, or other indicator, as a visual aid for individual or group to illustrate change in and intensity of emotions over time.
Identify physical sensations and cues associated with emotions in self and others (Feuerborn & Tyre, 2009; Carrizales-Engelmann et al., 2016)	Connect physical experiences and external cues with emotions, thoughts, and behaviors to improve awareness and regulation.	Students identify physical sensations experienced with particular emotions. Students also identify physical cues or body language in others that can help one understand how someone else is feeling.
Mindset instruction (Garwood & Ampuja, 2019)	Strategies that encourage growth mindset to improve students' ability to look at challenges as opportunities, reduce stereotype threat, and improve achievement and social and emotional competence.	Psychoeducation regarding mindset, praise, and modeling growth mindset through verbalization to self and others.

Modeling coping strategies (teacher) (Feuerborn & Tyre, 2009; Jones et al., 2013)	Behavioral modeling is one way we learn. Students can learn healthy SEL strategies through observation of teacher behaviors.	Teacher models how they might use a coping strategy, such as positive "self-talk" during instruction or "in the moment."
Rehearsal of skills (Kazdin, 2008)	Practice skills through engaging activities.	Role-playing examples and non-examples of skills.
Reminders to use skills, precorrection, and reinforce use of skills (Feuerborn & Tyre, 2009)	Learn how to use, practice skills in other settings to promote generalization and maintain skills over time.	Remind student to take breaths when worried, model breathing strategy before implementing skills, and praise student's effort to implement skill.
Replacement behavior training (Maag, 2005)	Functional behavioral assessment is used to precisely identify students' needs and preferences. Focus of intervention is for the student to learn and use a helpful behavior that serves the same function as the identified unhelpful behavior.	Assessment suggests student avoids written work to cope with anxiety associated with diminished performance. Intervention teaches student diaphragmatic breathing to calm parasympathetic nervous system and agreeing to work for 10 minutes, after which student rates emotional intensity on feelings thermometer.
Self-advocacy skills (Buckley & Madhavi, 2018; Woods et al., 2013).	Increase understanding of disability and civil rights, participate in educational planning, and identify strengths.	Use of the Self-Directed IEP (e.g., Woods et al., 2013). Role-playing; *WhyTry® Curriculum*; narrative counseling (for review, see Hatch et al., 2009).
Self-reflection using video and guided questions (Moore et al., 2020)	Improve student engagement in learning skills and collaborative work. Provides more precise information on desired and actual behaviors being performed. Improves work quality.	Student views videos of behaviors that are considered to be skillful, along with the student's current behavior as demonstrated individually or in the context of group work.
Strengths and preferences (Beckmann & Minnaert, 2018; Elias, 2004)	Focus on strengths and preferences in contrast to focusing solely on areas of difficulty. Extends student identity to connect student to others, improve self-concept, and increase time spent in areas of challenge.	Student-teacher–identified strengths and preferences. Students join group with similar strengths/interests. Students as experts to highlight these skills with peers. For students identified with giftedness and LD, educator awareness that sometimes student strengths can "mask" disabilities (Beckmann & Minnaert, 2018, p. 15).

Note. Strategies are listed alphabetically.

Ecological Considerations: Climate, Relationships, and Partnerships

SEL utilizes a developmental and ecological framework to guide SEL implementation using a planful, thoughtful, supportive, and interactive approach (CASEL, 2020; Durlak, 2015; Gueldner et al., 2020). This section provides a highly condensed summary of a few ecological and alterable areas to consider: school climate, relationships, and partnerships.

School Climate

School climate has been conceptualized as the way in which people experience the school ecology and includes safety, support, relationships, and collaboration amongst educators and partners (National School Climate Council, 2007). For students with disabilities, climate and "social, emotional, and school-related adjustment" have been correlated (Murray & Greenberg, 2001, p. 37), which is encouraging when students are doing well but concerning when students are struggling. A study with elementary through high school students with a range of IDEA-identified disabilities found a positive association between their perceptions of school climate and achievement (Sanders et al., 2018). Yet, these students experienced differences in achievement compared with peers without a disability, suggesting the importance of school climate for students with disabilities.

Relationships

Relationships are essential to children's social, emotional, and academic development, and the teacher–student relationship plays a very important role (Bergin & Bergin, 2009). Some students with LD have reported more loneliness and less acceptance by their teachers compared to peers not identified with a disability (Al-Yagon & Mikulincer, 2004). One study found that students with LD relied on teacher feedback when reflecting upon their own academic performance (Bear & Minke, 1996), and this finding identifies one way a teacher's behavior (e.g., feedback) can be internalized by students. Positive teacher and peer relationships can also improve school climate (see review in Doll et al., 2014), especially for students with LD (Cavioni et al., 2017; Murray & Pianta, 2007).

For all students, teacher behaviors and classroom- and school-oriented practices that have been found to support students include helpful and attuned responsiveness to student cues; providing a sense of warmth, comfort, trust, and respect; having high expectations and low conflict in the relationship; appropriate use of humor; valuing relationships and student voice; teacher–student check-ins; scheduling that allows for more time spent between teachers and students; structured and safe classrooms (Bergin & Bergin, 2009; Doll et al., 2014; Murray & Pianta, 2007); and emotion coaching practices (Gus et al., 2015). Trauma-sensitive practices may also play an essential role in facilitating safe and supportive relationships and environments, particularly when these are led by educators (see Jennings [2018] for a comprehensive review). Some SEL programs may include relationship-building strategies (Albright & Weissberg, 2010); therefore, choosing an SEL program could include reviewing materials to identify such content. The *Students, Teachers, and Relationship Support (STARS)* program is an example of a classroom-based program that prioritizes time spent in positive teacher–student interactions and managing behavioral concerns (Pianta & Hamre, 2001).

Partnerships

Partnerships among families, schools, and community agencies are associated with myriad positive student outcomes (Albright & Weissberg, 2010; Smith et al., 2020). For students with LD, facilitating collaborative and equitable partnerships between schools and families is essential, given the extra complexities involved in educational decision making (Cavendish & Connor, 2018). Some SEL programs have partnership practices embedded in their design. For example, *Caring School Community* includes guidance on forming school teams with educators and parents (Battistich, 2008). Other activities may support SEL-oriented school–home partnerships, such as bidirectional and responsive communication, schools supporting parents as educators at home, and including parents in school-based programming and decisions (Albright & Weissberg, 2010). Students with LD may also need family–school–community partnerships to coordinate multiple points of support, such as mental health services (Buckley & Madhavi, 2018). Essential to these relationships is respect for all, excellent communication, understanding diverse practices (Weist et al., 2012), inclusionary practices that value family voice, and recognizing our personal biases that can interfere with effective partnerships (Albright & Weissberg, 2010).

Responsive and Thoughtful Implementation

Implementing SEL has many components and requires a thoughtful and coordinated approach. This section highlights five areas that may be especially helpful for students with LD.

Integrating SEL into Academics

Academic learning periods and everyday moments are common times to engage in SEL lessons and practice skills (e.g., reflecting on emotions experienced, decisions made by literary or historical figures, and using a breathing technique before a test). Some SEL programs have recommendations for infusion (e.g., *Merrell's Strong Kids* and *Social Decision Making/Social Problems Solving* program). Coordinating SEL content between general and special education settings is recommended (Wiley & Siperstein, 2015).

Effective Instructional Strategies

The most effective SEL instruction follows the acronym SAFE: is *Sequenced* and well-coordinated, uses *Active* learning strategies, is *Focused* on skills, and applies *Explicit* teaching methodology (Durlak et al., 2011). Similar and additional strategies may be particularly relevant for students with LD in academic instruction and can be applied to SEL, such as modeling, using examples to illustrate concepts and skills, cueing, prompting, practice, and feedback (Elias, 2004; Gueldner et al., 2020).

Classroom Organization

Classrooms can be organized to promote an inclusive, positive, and effective learning environment (Thapa et al., 2013) and may include reserving space for SEL activities, decreasing distractions, and providing accommodations for students' unique physical needs (Gueldner et al., 2020). Across tiers, positive behavior supports can be used in tandem with SEL to support classroom climate and students' behavior (Bear et al., 2015) and tailored to SEL instructional periods (e.g., Carrizales-Engelmann et al., 2016). For example, teachers and students can collaboratively agree upon and teach expectations or community agreements such as "listen quietly while another student is sharing" and "avoid giving unsolicited advice."

Adaptations

Adaptations are expected with SEL implementation and can lead to improved outcomes for students (Durlak & DuPre, 2008). Alterations may be made to materials in response to contextual, cultural, and developmental needs. Common adaptations may include shortening or lengthening instruction and discussion, chunking lesson content, substituting examples, and responding to students' and communities' cultural norms and practices (Castro-Olivo & Merrell, 2012; Durlak, 2015). Program instructions may provide guidance regarding ways to adapt materials while maintaining the integrity of the program content and apply implementation procedures that can lead to effective outcomes.

Culturally Responsive Practices

Culturally responsive practices (CRP) have been highly recommended for use with students with LD during customary academic teaching in the classroom (Utley et al., 2011) as well as when implementing SEL (e.g., Castro-Olivo & Merrell, 2012). There is considerable overlap between the research and practices pertaining to CRP with LD and CRP with SEL. Thus, readers are encouraged to review the references and resources provided in this section for further study. In brief, we find the recommendations made for CRP for students with LD regarding general teaching practices (Utley et al., 2011) to be highly applicable to SEL implementation.

Utley et al. (2011) stressed educator behaviors such as understanding how cultural context and experiences inform students' needs, preferences, and behaviors; increasing educators' awareness of personal and systemic biases toward students and community groups that are stereotypic, negative, and discriminatory; actively integrating students' voices and experiences into learning activities to support students' cultural identities; building healthy relationships and partnerships; and adapting instructional materials and interventions to improve goodness-of-fit. Bernal et al. (1995) Ecological Validity Framework includes similar areas of focus and may also support educators at the intersection of SEL, LD, and CRP (see Castro-Olivo & Merrell, 2012, for an example).

SEL Assessment

Despite extensive evidence of the risk of SEL-related challenges for students with LD, largely, the emphasis in school settings has been on the identification and remediation of the academic impacts of LD. The federal definition of LD does not require the assessment of SEL skills, and this may account for why the SEL needs of students with LD are often neither identified nor addressed in schools (Cavioni et al., 2017; Feuerborn & Tyre, 2009).

As it is often said, what we assess we address. The very act of measuring something legitimizes it and communicates it to be a priority, and as a result, we are more likely to take action—be it through systemic planning, professional development, instruction, intervention, and/or more assessment. Ultimately, this punctuates the importance of selecting and using assessment tools responsibly. Currently, there is insufficient coordination between SEL standards and competencies, SEL programming and strategies, and SEL assessment (McKown, 2019). As a result, the onus is on educators—often without sufficient training in this area—to create linkages between the specific skills needed, the appropriate strategies and programming to apply, the constructs and skills to measure, and the appropriate methods and tools to use. This process can be complex, confusing, and problematic. Indeed, in the survey of principals mentioned earlier in this chapter, only a small portion of them reported that SEL was being assessed in their buildings in a coherent, effective manner (DePaoli et al., 2017). In this section, we offer considerations for SEL assessment, including the selection of constructs/skills and tools, along with considerations for culturally and developmentally appropriate assessment, student and family involvement, psychometric merit, and application in MTSS.

Constructs and Competencies

Assessment is influenced by the fact that students with LD are not a homogenous group, and at the same time, understanding group trends can help guide planning and supports. Students with LD can present with diverse exceptionalities, including gifted or "twice exceptional," nonverbal learning disabilities, dyslexia, dyscalculia, and/or dysgraphia. Students with diverse learning attributes bring strengths and assets, such as creativity and innovative problem solving, into the learning environment. They can also bring feelings of shame, hopelessness, anxiety, unrealistic self-expectations, withdrawal, loneliness, and peer rejection (Lackaye et al., 2006; Lambie & Milsom, 2010; Nelson & Harwood, 2011). Carefully selecting tools and methods will allow for valid measurement of constructs and skills mentioned here and in previous sections, including student strengths, needs, and values.

It is important to consider students' developmental trajectories when determining what SEL competency or skill to measure and how to measure it (Denham, 2015). Research reviewing commonly used school-based SEL programs found them to be lacking in developmental sensitivity and differentiation (Malti et al., 2016), so it would behoove those implementing and evaluating SEL to have an understanding of human development and how exceptionalities such as LDs might affect SEL learning trajectories. For instance, typically, SEL in early childhood focuses on self-management, basic self-awareness, and initiating relationship skills, but as children enter elementary school, there is an increased focus on relationship skills as applied in social and academic settings. In middle grades, SEL incorporates more identity development, emotional situations, and social problem solving. In high school, there is increased emphasis on more sophisticated relationships, independence, perspective taking, and the development of values and ethics to guide responsible decision making (Denham, 2018). Some SEL skills are more appropriately measured with older students or students with cognitive complexity (e.g., sophisticated executive functioning skills and responsible decision-making skills). For instance, we would not expect very young children and students without a basic understanding of others to demonstrate an ability to take diverse perspectives and express empathy (McKown, 2019). For readers needing more specific information on SEL development, Denham and colleagues (Denham et al., 2009) have provided a comprehensive outline of developmental social–emotional milestones. Also, state SEL benchmarks and indicators can offer helpful SEL guideposts for SEL assessment. For more information about SEL benchmarks and indicators, see Dusenbury et al. (2015).

Implementation

Assessing implementation is as important as assessing student skills and competencies. If a SEL program is not implemented with fidelity, and only the student response or learning is assessed, we may make erroneous conclusions about the program's effectiveness. Implementation is multifaceted and includes factors such as quality, fidelity, dose, adherence, and student engagement. Current research shows us that some factors are strongly associated with student outcomes, such as implementation quality and student engagement (Humphrey et al., 2018; Vroom et al., 2020). Researchers recommend monitoring these factors via direct methods such as observations whenever feasible because they introduce less error and bias as compared to other methods such as post-implementation self-reports (Domitrovich et al., 2019). Frameworks such as the Quality Implementation Framework

(QIF) (Meyers et al., 2012) and Sanetti and Collier-Meek (2019) offer more in-depth guidance on the topic of implementation.

Student and Family Involvement

Factors related to student involvement, such as receptiveness and engagement, have been found to be associated with improved student outcomes—in some cases, even more than implementation fidelity (e.g., Rojas-Andrade & Bahamondes, 2019). Involving students and families in the development of assessments, analysis of data, and goal development (e.g., IEP goals related to SEL) can increase relevance and help students understand their strengths, set their own goals, and develop self-awareness and self-advocacy—the very skills students with LD often need (Sanderson & Goldman, 2020).

Cultural and Contextual Fit

Best practices point to the importance of collecting and interpreting data with care and consideration of ecological, cultural, and developmental factors and partnering with others in the development, selection, and administration of SEL assessments. Sometimes, the most rigorously developed tools can measure skills that are irrelevant to our communities, and at other times, they can omit skills that are highly valued, thereby failing to accurately depict the strengths of many students (McKown, 2019). Until more culturally responsive SEL tools become available, we can use existing measures and adapt them. However, it is important that we adapt measures in a way that the theoretical underpinnings and original intent are maintained or preserved. The process of making adaptations may include gathering feedback from stakeholders about developmental norms, values, expectations, and priorities; pilot testing; and documenting changes.

SEL Assessment within an MTSS Framework

An MTSS framework supports SEL assessment and data-informed decisions at the student, educator, classroom, and school level. This section overviews assessment methods and resources. Readers interested in a comprehensive list of available tools are encouraged to visit guides such as CASEL's assessment guide (*https://measuringsel.casel.org/access-assessment-guide*).

Tier 1

Assessment practices at the universal level focus on climate (school and classroom), screening to identify students who need additional support, and the effectiveness of Tier 1 practices. Disaggregating Tier 1 data by racial/ethnic, disability, and gender identities can offer opportunities for teams to identify inequities and correct or interrupt the policies, practices, and/or systems causing them. An additional emerging practice in elementary school settings includes the assessment of SEL competencies via software-based technology. As examples, SELweb (McKown et al., 2021) and ZooU (DeRosier & Thomas, 2018) use stories and games to assess self-awareness, self-management (inhibitory control), and social awareness (perspective taking and emotion recognition of others' facial expressions).

Tiers 2 and 3

SEL assessment at the secondary and tertiary levels of prevention includes collecting additional information to examine data gathered at Tier 1, assessing the extent to which students are responding to intervention supports, and collecting data to guide intervention or setting modifications. Advanced tier assessments can be used to connect function or causal explanations to SEL-related challenges and investigate issues related to skills acquisition, performance, and/or fluency. Further, generalization of skills in the intended settings is a hallmark challenge in the field of SEL and for students with LD, so generalization is an important consideration for planning and measurement alike (Walker & Barry, 2018).

Guidelines for assessing growth in competencies or skills include frequent monitoring, adequate skill sampling in a natural context, and direct assessment (Gueldner et al., 2020; Hosp et al., 2016). In many cases, students with LD may already be receiving special education services along with more in-depth assessments that require weekly or daily progress monitoring with instruments sensitive to change. Some researchers assert that this method of gathering and using individual data may be the most accurate and helpful method of data analysis for diverse groups (e.g., Bornstein, 2017), particularly as compared to other commonly used measures of analysis such as normative comparisons (see Riley-Tilman et al., 2020). Direct behavior ratings are validated methods of measuring and monitoring observable SEL competencies and have been developed and tested using SEL-related indicators, such as academic engagement, disruptive behavior, social competence, and anxiety-related behaviors (e.g., von der Embse et al., 2015). Standardized, direct performance assessments can reduce biases often found in other indirect methods such as rating scales (Daneri et al., 2018), and they are being used to assess competencies and skills such as self-management (e.g., persistence, impulse control, and sustained attention via the NEPSY-II [Korkman et al., 2007]; Preschool Self-Regulation Assessment [Smith-Donald et al., 2007]). Direct observations can complement other forms of data and typically occur in the natural context of a school environment, so they offer corresponding information about student SEL, school ecology, classroom context, and adult practices.

Rating Scales

SEL-focused rating scales are widely used to inform comprehensive evaluations, the impact of services and programs, and placement decisions for special programs. Caregivers, teachers, and students all offer unique perspectives and insights into social, emotional, and behavioral development via rating scales, and each has their benefits and limitations. Caregivers can provide a particularly useful perspective as they tend to be more intimately knowledgeable of their child or adolescent's SEL in the home and community environments, and teacher rating scales can offer a valuable perspective as educators can have a broader basis for comparison and interact with students in the instructional environment. However, educators can introduce biases and can rate SEL skills among student identity groups differently, even when direct observations do not reveal these differences (Garcia et al., 2019). Student self-reports can be valuable opportunities to engage student voice and obtain their perspectives on their own SEL strengths, needs, attitudes, and beliefs (e.g., self-esteem), although they can be susceptible to error and bias, too. Although self-reports can be helpful for the assessment of intrapersonal skills and symptomology (self-awareness, social awareness, anxiety, and depression), the information gathered may be limited to the student's awareness of their inner landscape and the ways in which they interact in the world—vulnerabilities particularly pertinent to many students with LD.

Future Directions and Conclusion

Research in SEL has demonstrated the long-standing benefits of SEL programs and strategies (e.g., Taylor et al., 2017). Universal instruction of SEL can be beneficial for students with LD (Cavioni et al., 2017), and integrating such practices with Tier 2 or Tier 3 interventions is believed to be essential (Buckley & Madhavi, 2018; Wiley & Siperstein, 2015). Although the field of SEL has made great strides in recent years, numerous opportunities for growth and unresolved questions remain—especially as we refine SEL practices for students with LD. Although evidence repeatedly demonstrates a need for SEL among many students with LD, research continues to offer discourse centered predominantly on academic deficits. In both research and practice, academic deficits are focal topics for assessment and intervention for students with LD. We advocate for a more inclusive and expanded focus on social and emotional assessment and intervention from a multi-tiered approach. As compared to other student populations, SEL research and practice have overlooked students with LD, giving rise to multiple areas that need further attention, such as isolating and examining responses to universal interventions, creating and evaluating effective programming and methods for adaptation, and developing and examining SEL assessments that are culturally and developmentally appropriate and sensitive to change. Currently, educators are without evidence-based practices for selecting, differentiating, implementing, coordinating, and assessing SEL for diverse students with LD (Daley & McCarthy, 2020; Wiley & Siperstein, 2015).

A more nuanced understanding is vital to address the indicated layers of SEL-related needs, attributes, and strengths for students with LD; yet, as we have discussed in this chapter, there are helpful guidelines and strategies we can apply now. We must use diligence and intentional planning to stay attuned to the needs and values of students and caregivers and consider sociocultural and contextual factors within the school and community—and adapt our practices accordingly. We must work to implement an SEL framework that is coordinated across tiers and service providers and uses data to promote continued improvement. We must also cultivate safe and inclusive educational environments and culturally responsive relationships and partnerships. The need for effective, equity-centered SEL for students with LD is salient and urgent. Students with LD deserve equitable, inclusive, and effective learning environments, and this requires an enhanced presence of this topic in educator preparation programs, quality professional development and supports for educators, and committed attention and advocacy from educators, researchers, and legislators—especially in these challenging and changing times.

REFERENCES

Albright, M. I., & Weissberg, R. P. (2010). School-family partnerships to promote social and emotional learning. In S. L. Christenson & A. L. Reschly (Eds.), *Handbook of school-family partnerships* (pp. 246–265). Routledge.

Alqarni, T. M., & Hammad, M. A. (2021). Effects of mindfulness training program on the impulsivity among students with learning disabilities. *Journal of Educational and Social Research, 11*(4), 190–190.

Al-Yagon, M. (2016). Perceived close relationships with parents, teachers, and peers: Predictors of social, emotional, and behavioral features in adolescents with LD or comorbid LD and ADHD. *Journal of Learning Disabilities, 49*(6), 597–615.

Al-Yagon, M., & Mikulincer, M. (2004). Socioemotional and academic adjustment among children with learning disorders: The mediational role of attachment-based factors. *The Journal of Special Education, 38*(2), 111–123.

American Academy of Pediatrics. (2021). *AAP, AACAP, CHA declaration of a national emergency in children's mental health. www.aappublications.org/news/2021/10/19/children-mental-health-national-emergency-101921*

American Psychiatric Association. (2013). *Diagnostic and statistical manual of mental disorders* (5th ed.). Author.

Atwell, M. N., & Bridgeland, J. M. (2019). *Ready to lead: A 2019 update of principals' perspectives on how social and emotional learning can prepare children and transform schools. A report for CASEL. https://files.eric.ed.gov/fulltext/ED602977.pdf*

Battistich, V. A. (2008). The child development project: Creating caring school communities. In L. P. Nucci & D. Narvaez (Eds.), *Handbook of moral and character education* (pp. 328–351). Routledge.

Baum, D. D., Duffelmeyer, F., & Geelan, M. (1988). Resource teacher perceptions of the prevalence of social dysfunction among students with LD. *Journal of Learning Disabilities, 21*, 380–381.

Bauminger, N., Edelsztein, H. S., & Morash, J. (2005). Social information processing and emotional understanding in children with LD. *Journal of Learning Disabilities, 38*(1), 45–61.

Bear, G. G., & Minke, K. M. (1996). Positive bias in maintenance of self-worth among children with LD. *Learning Disability Quarterly, 19*(1), 23–32.

Bear, G. G., Whitcomb, S., Elias, M., & Blank, J. (2015). SEL and schoolwide positive behavioral interventions and supports. In C. E. Domitrovich, R. P. Weissberg, & T. P. Gullotta (Eds.), *Handbook of social and emotional learning: Research and practice* (pp. 453–467). Guilford Press.

Beauchemin, J., Hutchins, T. L., & Patterson, F. (2008). Mindfulness meditation may lessen anxiety, promote social skills, and improve academic performance among adolescents with learning disabilities. *Complementary Health Practice Review, 13*(1), 34–45.

Beckmann, E., & Minnaert, A. (2018). Non-cognitive characteristics of gifted students with learning disabilities: An in-depth systematic review. *Frontiers in Psychology, 9*, 504.

Bergin, C., & Bergin, D. (2009). Attachment in the classroom. *Educational Psychology Review, 21*(2), 141–170.

Bernal, G., Bonilla, J., & Bellido, C. (1995). Ecological validity and cultural sensitivity for outcome research: Issues for the cultural adaptation and development of psychosocial treatments with Latinos. *Journal of Abnormal Child Psychology, 23*(1), 67–82.

Beyer, L. N. (2017). *Social and emotional learning and traditionally underserved populations. Policy brief.* American Youth Policy Forum. *www.aypf.org/wp-content/uploads/2017/10/SEL-Special-Populations_Final*

Bornstein, M. H. (2017). The specificity principle in acculturation science. *Perspectives on Psychological Science, 12*(1), 3–45.

Bryan, T., Burstein, K., & Ergul, C. (2004). The social–emotional side of learning disabilities: A science-based presentation of the state of the art. *Learning Disability Quarterly, 27*(1), 45–51.

Buckley, M., & Mahdavi, J. N. (2018). Bringing children from the margins to the page: School counselors supporting students with learning disabilities. *Journal of School Counseling 16*(23), 1–40. *https://files.eric.ed.gov/fulltext/EJ1194637.pdf*

Carnazzo, K., Dowdy, E., Furlong, M. J., & Quirk, M. P. (2019). An evaluation of the Social Emotional Health Survey—Secondary for use with students with learning disabilities. *Psychology in the Schools, 56*, 433–446.

Carrizales-Engelmann, D., Feuerborn, L., Gueldner, B. A., & Tran, O. (2016). *Merrell's strong kids: Grades 3–5: A social and emotional learning curriculum* (2nd ed.). Paul H. Brookes Publishing.

Castro-Olivo, S. M., & Merrell, K. W. (2012). Validating cultural adaptations of a school-based social–emotional learning programme for use with Latino immigrant adolescents. *Advances in School Mental Health Promotion, 5*(2), 78–92.

Cavendish, W., & Connor, D. J. (2018). Introduction to special series: Parent voice in educational decision making for students with learning disabilities. *Learning Disability Quarterly, 41*(1), 4–6.

Cavioni, V., Grazzani, I., & Ornaghi, V. (2017). Social and emotional learning for children with learning disability: Implications for inclusion. *International Journal of Emotional Education, 9*(2), 100–109.

Cederlof, M., Maughan, B., Larsson, H., D'Onofrio, B. M., & Plomin, R. (2017). Reading problems and major mental disorders—Co-occurrences and familial overlaps in a Swedish nationwide cohort. *Journal of Psychiatric Research, 91*, 124–129.

Chadi, N., Ryan, N. C., & Georffroy, M. C. (2022). COVID-19 and the impacts on youth mental health: emerging evidence from longitudinal studies. *Canadian Journal of Public Health, 113*, 44–52.

Clarke, A. M., Morreale, S., Field, C. A., Hussein, Y., & Barry, M. M. (2015). *What works in enhancing social and emotional skills development during childhood and adolescence. A review of the evidence on the effectiveness of school-based and out-of-school programmes in the UK.* World Health Organization Collaborating Centre for Health Promotion Research, National University of Ireland, Galway.

Collaborative for Academic, Social, and Emotional Learning. (2020). *What is the CASEL Framework? https://casel.org/fundamentals-of-sel/what-is-the-casel-framework*

Committee for Children. (2008). *Second step: Student success through prevention program.*

Cook, C. R., Gresham, F. M., Kern, L., Barreras, R. B., Thornton, S., & Crews, S. D. (2008). Social skills training for secondary students with emotional and/or behavioral disorders: A review and analysis of the meta-analytic literature. *Journal of Emotional and Behavioral Disorders, 16*(3), 131–144.

Corcoran, R. P., Cheung, A. C., Kim, E., & Xie, C. (2018). Effective universal school-based social and emotional learning programs for improving academic achievement: A systematic review and meta-analysis of 50 years of research. *Educational Research Review, 25*, 56–72.

Curtin, S. C., & Heron, M. P. (2019). Death rates due to suicide and homicide among persons aged 10–24: United States, 2000–2017. *NCHS Data Brief, 352*, 1–8.

Daley, S. G., & McCarthy, M. F. (2020). Students with disabilities in social and emotional learning interventions: A systematic review. *Remedial and Special Education, 42*(6), 384–397.

Daneri, M. P., Sulik, M. J., Raver, C. C., & Morris, P. A. (2018). Observers' reports of self-regulation: Measurement invariance across sex, low-income status, and race/ethnicity. *Journal of Applied Developmental Psychology, 55*, 14–23.

Darrow, A. A. (2014). Promoting social and emotional growth of students with disabilities. *General Music Today, 28*(1), 29–32.

Denham, S. A. (2015). Assessment of social–emotional learning in educational contexts. In J. Durlak, C. E. Domitrovich, R. W. Weissberg, & T. P. Gullotta (Eds.), *The handbook of social and emotional learning* (pp. 285–300). Guilford Press.

Denham, S. A. (2018). *Keeping SEL developmental: The importance of a developmental lens for fostering and assessing SEL competencies.* Measuring SEL: Using Data to Inspire Practice. *https://measuringsel.casel.org/wp-content/uploads/2018/11/Frameworks-DevSEL.pdf*

Denham, S. A., Wyatt, T. M., Bassett, H. H., Echeverria, D., & Knox, S. S. (2009). Assessing social–emotional development in children from a longitudinal perspective. *Journal of Epidemiology & Community Health, 63*(Suppl. 1), i37–i52.

DePaoli, J. L., Atwell, M. N., & Bridgeland, J. (2017). *Ready to lead: A national principal survey on how social and emotional learning can prepare children and transform schools. A report for CASEL. https://files.eric.ed.gov/fulltext/ED579088.pdf*

DeRosier, M. E., & Thomas, J. M. (2018). Establishing the criterion validity of Zoo U's game-based social emotional skills assessment for school-based outcomes. *Journal of Applied Developmental Psychology, 55*, 52–61.

Doll, B., Brehm, K., & Zucker, S. (2014). *Resilient classrooms: Creating healthy environments for learning* (2nd ed.). Guilford Press.

Domitrovich, C. E., Li, Y., Mathis, E. T., & Greenberg, M. T. (2019). Individual and organizational factors associated with teacher self-reported implementation of the PATHS curriculum. *Journal of School Psychology, 76*, 168–185.

Durlak, J. A. (2015). What everyone should know about implementation. In C. E. Domitrovich, R. P. Weissberg, & T. P. Gullotta (Eds.), *Handbook of social and emotional learning: Research and practice* (pp. 395–405). Guilford Press.

Durlak, J. A., & DuPre, E. P. (2008). Implementation matters: A review of research on program outcomes and the factors affecting implementation. *American Journal of Community Psychology, 41*, 327–350.

Durlak, J. A., Weissberg, R. P., Dymnicki, A. B., Taylor, R. D., & Schellinger, K. B. (2011). The impact of enhancing students' social and emotional learning: A meta-analysis of school-based universal interventions. *Child Development, 82*(1), 405–432.

Dusenbury, L., Newman, J. Z., Weissberg, R. P., Goren, P., Domitrovich, C. E., & Mart, A. K. (2015). Developing a blueprint for preschool to high school education in social and emotional learning: The case for state learning standards. In J. A. Durlak, C. E. Domitrovich, R. P. Weissberg, & T. P. Gullotta (Eds.), *Handbook of social and emotional learning: Research and practice* (pp. 532–548). Guilford Press.

Elias, M. J. (2004). The connection between social–emotional learning and learning disabilities: Implications for intervention. *Learning Disability Quarterly, 27*(1), 53–63.

Espelage, D. L., Rose, C. A., & Polanin, J. R. (2015). Social–emotional learning program to reduce bullying, fighting, and victimization among middle school students with disabilities. *Remedial and Special Education, 36*(5), 299–311.

Espelage, D. L., Rose, C. A., & Polanin, J. R. (2016). Social–emotional learning program to promote prosocial and academic skills among middle school students with disabilities. *Remedial and Special Education, 37*(6), 323–332.

Feuerborn, L., & Tyre, A. (2009). Practical social–emotional learning tools for students with specific learning disabilities in the United States of America. *Journal of the International Association of Special Education, 10*(1), 21–25.

Fisher, P. W., Reyes-Portillo, J. A., Riddle, M. A. & Litwin, H. D. (2022). Systemic review: Nonverbal learning disability. *Journal of the American Academy of Child and Adolescent Psychiatry, 61*(2), 159–186.

Fletcher, J. M., Lyon, G. R., Fuchs, L. S., & Barnes, M. A. (2019). *Learning disabilities: From identification to intervention* (2nd ed.). Guilford Press.

Forness, S. R., & Kavale, K. A. (1996). Treating social skill deficits in children with learning disabilities: A meta-analysis of the research. *Learning Disability Quarterly, 19*(1), 2–13.

Garcia, E. B., Sulik, M. J., & Obradović, J. (2019). Teachers' perceptions of students' executive functions: Disparities by gender, ethnicity, and ELL status. *Journal of Educational Psychology, 111*(5), 918.

Garwood, J. D., & Ampuja, A. A. (2019). Inclusion of students with learning, emotional, and behavioral disabilities through strength-based approaches. *Intervention in School and Clinic, 55*(1), 46–51.

Gresham, F. M. (2010). Evidence-based social skills interventions: Empirical foundations for instructional approaches. In M. Shinn & H. M. Walker (Eds.). *Interventions for achievement and behavior problems in a three-tier model including RTI* (pp. 337–362). National Association of School Psychologists.

Gresham, F. M., Van, M. B., & Cook, C. R. (2006). Social skills training for teaching replacement behaviors: Remediating acquisition deficits in at-risk students. *Behavioral Disorders, 31*(4), 363–377.

Grigorenko, E. L., Fuchs, L. S., Willcutt, E. G., Compton, D. L., Wagner, R. K., & Fletcher, J. M. (2019). Understanding, educating, and supporting children with specific learning disabilities: 50 years of science and practice. *American Psychologist, 75*(1), 37–51.

Gueldner, B. A., Feuerborn, L. L., & Merrell, K. W. (2020). *Social and emotional learning in the classroom: Promoting mental health and academic success* (2nd ed.). Guilford Press.

Gus, L., Rose, J., & Gilbert, L. (2015). Emotion coaching: A universal strategy for supporting and promoting sustainable emotional and behavioural well-being. *Educational and Child Psychology, 32*(10), 31–41.

Hatch, T., Shelton, T., & Monk, G. (2009). Making the invisible visible: School counselors empowering students with disabilities through self-advocacy training. *Journal of School Counseling, 7*(14), 14.

Henry, F. M., & Reed, V. A. (1995). Adolescent's perceptions of the relative importance of communication skills. *Language, Speech, & Hearing Services in Schools, 26*, 263–273.

Hosp, M. K., Hosp, J. L., & Howell, K. W. (2016). *The ABCs of CBM: A practical guide to curriculum-based measurement.* Guilford Press.

Humphrey, N., Barlow, A., & Lendrum, A. (2018). Quality matters: Implementation moderates student outcomes in the PATHS curriculum. *Prevention Science, 19*(2), 197–208.

Jagers, R. J., Rivas-Drake, D., & Williams, B. (2018). Transformative social and emotional learning (SEL): Toward SEL in service of educational equity and excellence. *Educational Psychologist, 54*(3), 162–184.

Jennings, P. A. (2018). *The trauma-sensitive classroom: Building resilience with compassionate teaching.* W. W. Norton & Company.

Jones, S. M., Bouffard, S. M., & Weissbourd, R. (2013). Educators' social and emotional skills vital to learning. *Phi Delta Kappan, 94*(8), 62–65.

Jones, S. M., & Doolittle, E. J. (2017). Social and emotional learning: Introducing the issue. *The Future of Children, 27*(1), 3–11.

Kam, C. M., Greenberg, M. T., & Kusché, C. A. (2004). Sustained effects of the PATHS curriculum on the social and psychological adjustment of children in special education. *Journal of Emotional and Behavioral Disorders, 12*(2), 66–78.

Kavale, K. A., & Forness, S. R. (1996). Social skill deficits and learning disabilities: A meta-analysis. *Journal of Learning Disabilities, 29*(3), 226–237.

Kazdin, A. E. (2008). *Parent management training: Treatment for oppositional, aggressive, and antisocial behavior in children and adolescents.* Oxford University Press.

Korkman, M., Kirk, U., & Kemp, S. (2007). *NEPSY—Second Edition (NEPSY-II)* [Database record]. APA PsycTests.

Kusché, C. A., & Greenberg, M. T. (1994). *The PATHS (Promoting Alternative Thinking Strategies) curriculum.* Channing Bete.

Lackaye, T., Margalit, M., Ziv, O., & Ziman, T. (2006). Comparisons of self-efficacy, mood, effort, and hope between students with learning disabilities and their non-LD-matched peers. *Learning Disabilities Research & Practice, 21*(2), 111–121.

Lambie, G. W., & Milsom, A. (2010). A narrative approach to supporting students diagnosed with learning disabilities. *Journal of Counseling & Development, 88*(2), 196–203.

Maag, J. W. (2005). Social skills training for youth with emotional and behavioral disorders and learning disabilities: Problems, conclusions, and suggestions. *Exceptionality, 13*(3), 155–172.

Mahoney, J. L., Durlak, J. A., & Weissberg, R. P. (2019). An update on social and emotional learning outcome research, *Phi Delta Kappan, 100*(4), 18–23.

Malti, T., Chaparro, M. P., Zuffianò, A., & Colasante, T. (2016). School-based interventions to promote empathy-related responding in children and adolescents: A developmental analysis. *Journal of Clinical Child & Adolescent Psychology, 45*(6), 718–731.

McKown, C. (2019). Challenges and opportunities in the applied assessment of student social and emotional learning. *Educational Psychologist, 54*(3), 205–221.

McKown, C., Kharitonova, M., Russo-Ponsaran, N. M., & Aksu-Dunya, B. (2021). Development and validation of a shortened form of SELweb EE, a web-based assessment of children's social and emotional competence. *Assessment*, 10731911211046044.

Meyers, D. C., Durlak, J. A., & Wandersman, A. (2012). The quality implementation framework: A synthesis of critical steps in the implementation process. *American Journal of Community Psychology, 50*(3–4), 462–480.

Moore, B., Smith, C., Boardman, A., & Ferrell, A. (2020). Using video self-reflection to support collaborative learning for students with learning disabilities. *Teaching Exceptional Children, 53*(1), 52–59.

Morgan, P. L., Farkas, G., Cook, M., Strassfeld, N. M., Hillemeier, M. M., Pun, W. H., & Schussler, D., L. (2016). Are black children disproportionately overrepresented in special education? A best-evidence synthesis. *Exceptional Children, 83*(2), 181–192.

Murray, C., & Greenberg, M. T. (2001). Relationships with teachers and bonds with school: Social emotional adjustment correlates for children with and without disabilities. *Psychology in the Schools, 38*(1), 25–41.

Murray, C., & Pianta, R. C. (2007). The importance of teacher–student relationships for adolescents with high incidence disabilities. *Theory into Practice, 46*(2), 105–112.

National Center for Educational Statistics. (2021, May). *Students with disabilities. https://nces.ed.gov/programs/coe/indicator/cgg*

National School Climate Council. (2007). *The School Climate Challenge: Narrowing the gap between school climate research and school climate policy, practice guidelines and teacher education policy. www.schoolclimate.org/climate/advocacy.php*

Nelson, J. M., & Harwood, H. (2011). Learning disabilities and anxiety: A meta-analysis. *Journal of Learning Disabilities, 44*(1), 3–17.

Pennington, B. F. (2009). *Diagnosing learning disorders: A neurological framework* (2nd ed.). Guilford Press.

Peterson, I. T., Bates, J. E., D'Onofrio, B. M., Coyne, C. A., Lansford, J. E., Dodge, K. A., et al. (2013). Language ability predicts the development of behavior problems in children. *Journal of Abnormal Psychology, 122*(2), 542.

Pianta, R. C., & Hamre, B. (2001). *Students, teachers, and relationship support (STARS).* Psychological Assessment Resources.

Radhakrishnan, L., Carey, K., Hartnett, K. P., Kit-Powell, A., Zwald, M., Anderson, K. N., et al. (2022). Pediatric emergency department visits behavior and during the COVID-19 Pandemic—United States, January 2019–January 2022. *Morbidity and Mortality Weekly Report, 71*(8), 313–318. *www.cdc.gov/mmwr/volumes/71/wr/mm7108e1.htm?s*

Riley-Tillman, T. C., Burns, M. K., & Kilgus, S. P. (2020). *Evaluating educational interventions: Single-case design for measuring response to intervention.* Guilford Press.

Rojas-Andrade, R., & Bahamondes, L. L. (2019). Is implementation fidelity important? A systematic review on school-based mental health programs. *Contemporary School Psychology, 23*(4), 339–350.

Sanders, S. M., Durbin, J. M., Anderson, B. G., Fogarty, L. M., Giraldo-Garcia, R. J., & Voight, A. (2018). Does a rising school climate lift all boats? Differential associations of perceived climate and achievement for students with disabilities and limited English proficiency. *School Psychology International, 39*(6), 646–662.

Sanderson, K. A., & Goldman, S. E. (2020). A systematic review and meta-analysis of interventions used to increase adolescent IEP meeting participation. *Career Development and Transition for Exceptional Individuals, 43*(3), 157–168.

Sanetti, L. M. H., & Collier-Meek, M. A. (2019). *Supporting successful interventions in schools: Tools to plan, evaluate, and sustain effective implementation.* Guilford Press.

Shifrer, D., Muller, C., & Callahan, R. (2011). Disproportionality and learning disabilities: Parsing apart race, socioeconomic status, and language. *Journal of Learning Disabilities, 44*(3), 246–257.

Smith, T. E., Sheridan, S. M., Kim, E. M., Park, S., & Beretvas, S. N. (2020). The effects of family–school partnership interventions on academic and social–emotional functioning: A meta-analysis exploring what works for whom. *Educational Psychology Review, 32*(2), 511–544.

Smith-Donald, R., Raver, C. C., Hayes, T., & Richardson, B. (2007). Preschool self-regulation assessment. *Early Childhood Research Quarterly, 22*(2), 173–187.

Taylor, R. D., Oberle, E., Durlak, J. A., & Weissberg, R. P. (2017). Promoting positive youth development through school-based social and emotional learning interventions: A meta-analysis of follow-up effects. *Child Development, 88*(4), 1156–1171.

Thapa, A., Cohen, J., Guffey, S., & Higgins-D'Alessandro, A. (2013). A review of school climate research. *Review of Educational Research, 83*(3), 357–385.

Utley, C. A., Obiakor, F. E., & Bakken, J. P. (2011). Culturally responsive practices for culturally and linguistically diverse students with learning disabilities. *Learning Disabilities: A Contemporary Journal, 9*(1), 5–18.

von der Embse, N. P., Scott, E. C., & Kilgus, S. P. (2015). Sensitivity to change and concurrent validity of direct behavior ratings for academic anxiety. *School Psychology Quarterly, 30*(2), 244.

Vroom, E. B., Massey, O. T., Yampolskaya, S., & Levin, B. L. (2020). The impact of implementation fidelity on student outcomes in the Life Skills Training program. *School Mental Health, 12*(1), 113–123.

Walker, J. D., & Barry, C. (2018). Assessing and supporting social-skill needs for students with high-incidence disabilities. *TEACHING Exceptional Children, 51*(1), 18–30.

Weare, K., & Nind, M. (2011). Mental health promotion and problem prevention in schools: What does the evidence say? *Health Promotion International, 26*(suppl_1), i29–i69.

Weist, M. D., Mellin, E. A., Chambers, K. L., Lever, N. A., Haber, D., & Blaber, C. (2012). Challenges to collaboration in school mental health and strategies for overcoming them. *Journal of School Health, 82*(2), 97–105.

Whitcomb, S., & Feuerborn, L. (2020). Theories of social, emotional, and behavioral development. In *Theories of school psychology* (pp. 96–123). Routledge.

Whitney, D. G., & Peterson, M. D. (2019). US national and state-level prevalence of mental health disorders and disparities of mental health care use in children. *JAMA Pediatrics, 173*(4), 389–391.

Wiley, A. L., & Siperstein, G. N. (2015). SEL for students with high-incidence disabilities. In J. A. Durlak, C. E. Domitrovich, R. P. Weissberg, & T. P. Gullota (Eds.), *Handbook of social and emotional learning: Research and practice* (pp. 213–228). Guilford Press.

Willcutt, E. G., Betjemann, R. S., Pennington, B. F., Olson, R. K., Defries, J. C., & Wadsworth, S. J. (2007). Longitudinal study of reading disability and attention deficit hyperactivity disorder: Implications for education. *Mind, Brain, and Education, 1*(4), 181–192.

Willcutt, E. G., Petrill, S. A., Wu, S., Boada, R., Defries, J. C., Olson, R. K., & Pennington, B. F. (2013). Comorbidity between reading disability and math disability: Concurrent psychopathology, functional impairment, and neuropsychological functioning. *Journal of Learning Disabilities, 46*(6), 500–516.

Woods, L. L., Martin, J. E., & Humphrey, M. J. (2013). The difference a year makes: An exploratory self-directed IEP case study. *Exceptionality, 21*(3), 176–189.

Yard, E., Radhakrishnan, L., Ballesteros, M. F., Sheppard, M. S., Gates, A., Stein, Z., et al. (2021). Emergency department visits for suspected suicide attempts among persons aged 12–25 years before and during the COVID-19 pandemic—United States. *Morbidity and Mortality Weekly Report, 70*, 888–894.

Yoder, N., Dusenbury, L., Martinez-Black, T., & Weissberg, R. P. (2020, March). *Emerging insights: From insights to action redefining state efforts to support social and emotional learning. https://casel.s3.us-east-2.amazonaws.com/CASEL-PR-Insights-to-Action-State-Efforts.pdf*

Zins, J. E. (Ed.). (2004). *Building academic success on social and emotional learning: What does the research say?* Teachers College Press.

CHAPTER 5

Cognitive Processes, Neuroscience, and Learning Disabilities

Emily M. Harriott and Laurie E. Cutting

The National Center for Learning Disabilities (NCLD) estimates that approximately 20% of children in the United States have learning and attention difficulties that could be classified as learning disabilities (Horowitz et al., 2017). Put another way, according to the Learning Disabilities Association of America and the National Center for Education Statistics, approximately 2.3 million students have learning disabilities and receive services in school (Learning Disabilities Association of America, n.d.-a). While these numbers may seem high at first glance, they are actually more likely to be underestimates rather than overestimates; children of racial or ethnic minorities are consistently less likely than White children to be identified as having learning disabilities (Morgan et al., 2015). The Individuals with Disabilities Education Act (IDEA) defines a learning disability as "a disorder in one or more of the basic psychological processes involved in understanding or in using language, spoken or written, which disorder may manifest itself in the imperfect ability to listen, think, speak, read, write, spell, or do mathematical calculations" (IDEA, 2004). These disorders are typically caused by genetic and/or neurobiological factors that alter brain function (Learning Disabilities Association of America, n.d.-b). Included in IDEA's definition of learning disabilities are conditions such as brain injury and dyslexia; excluded from this definition are conditions such as intellectual disabilities or mental health conditions (IDEA, 2004). To be classified as having a learning disability, students must have at least average intelligence (Learning Disabilities Association of America, n.d.-b).

Reading

The most common learning disability is a reading disability; approximately 80% of children who have at least one learning disability also exhibit difficulties with reading (Shaywitz, 2003). Put another way, while they may not all receive a diagnosis, it has been estimated that approximately 16% of students struggle to at least learn to read (Shaywitz et al., 1992). "Reading disability" is synonymous with other similar terms such as "reading difficulty," "reading impairment," and "reading disorder." "Reading disability" is also an umbrella term that encompasses several different types of reading difficulties, including difficulties with sounding out and recognizing words and difficulties with reading comprehension (McArthur & Castles, 2017).

The effects of reading disabilities on personal and public health make the importance of the study of typical and impaired reading development strikingly apparent. Students who struggle to learn to read, failing to achieve their first major milestone in school, are at risk for severe long-term consequences, including school dropout (Daniel et al., 2006), attempted suicide (Daniel et al., 2006), incarceration (Christle & Yell, 2008), anxiety and depression (Carroll et al., 2005), and/or low self-concept (McArthur et al., 2016) compared to their peers reading at grade level (McArthur & Castles, 2017). On a larger scale, these adverse outcomes cost society money; in our present society, special education, public healthcare, incarceration, and underemployment necessitate the use of resources such as extra special education teachers and equipment and systems such as the Supplemental Nutrition Assistance Program and Medicaid, both of which use taxpayer dollars (Center on Budget and Priority Policies, 2022).

Earlier identification of students with reading disabilities and earlier remediation of such disabilities would help lessen the need for these resources and, therefore, lower their costs. Indeed, it is important to study reading and, moreover, reading disabilities in hopes of eventually remediating these disabilities, ultimately alleviating these adverse consequences.

Reading Cognition

After decades of research, reading and reading disabilities are relatively well understood (Fletcher et al., 2007). A framework through which reading is commonly studied and explained (Duke & Cartwright, 2021) is the Simple View of Reading (SVR; Gough & Tunmer, 1986; Hoover & Gough, 1990). The original version of SVR posits that Reading (R), or the comprehension of written text, is the product of two independent, sequential processes: Decoding (D) and Listening Comprehension (LC) (Gough & Tunmer, 1986; Hoover & Gough, 1990). Decoding (D) is defined as the ability to "read isolated words quickly, accurately, and silently" using "letter-sound correspondence rules" (Gough & Tunmer, 1986). Listening comprehension (LC) is the ability to understand the meanings of words (Gough & Tunmer, 1986; Hoover & Gough, 1990). The original version of the SVR can be simplified and reduced to one small but extremely meaningful equation: $D \times LC = R$ (Decoding × Listening Comprehension = Reading). As the product of anything times zero equals zero, this equation involving a product implies that if a student does not have Decoding and/or Listening Comprehension, making at least one of those processes 0, that student is unable to Read.

The original version of the SVR (Gough & Tunmer, 1986) has undergone several revisions and updates in the decades since it was first published. The most recently updated version of the SVR, published in 2020, retains the basic equation but renames the two processes to more appropriately represent their functions (Hoover & Tunmer, 2020). This new version of the SVR broadens "decoding" to "word recognition" and "listening comprehension" to "language comprehension" (Hoover & Tunmer, 2020).

Extensive cognitive research of reading supports and validates the SVR (e.g., Aaron et al., 2008; Carver, 1997, 2003; Catts et al., 2006; Curtis, 1980; Cutting & Scarborough, 2006; Francis et al., 2005; Goff et al., 2005; Joshi et al., 1998; Lervåg et al., 2018; Protopapas et al., 2012; Sabatini et al., 2010; Shankweiler et al., 1999; Vellutino et al., 2007).[1] Neurobiological research also supports the SVR (e.g., Cutting et al., 2013; Hudson et al., 2016; Landi et al., 2013). In the next few sections, we briefly review literature on the cognition and neurobiological correlates of word recognition and reading comprehension and these processes' associated deficits.

Word Recognition Deficits (Dyslexia)

Impairments in word-level processes, such as word recognition and decoding, comprise a common subtype of reading disability: dyslexia. According to Lyon, Shaywitz, Shaywitz, and other members of the International Dyslexia Association, "dyslexia is a specific learning disability that is neurobiological in origin. It is characterized by difficulties with accurate and/or fluent word recognition and by poor spelling and decoding abilities" (Lyon et al., 2003, p. 2), despite at least average intelligence and at least adequate reading instruction (Norton et al., 2015). The fifth edition of the *Diagnostic and Statistical Manual of Mental Disorders* (DSM-5) defines dyslexia as a "specific learning disorder" "with impairment in reading," specifically impairments in word reading accuracy, reading rate, and/or reading fluency (American Psychiatric Association, 2013). It has been estimated that approximately 5–17% of all children and adults in the United States fit these diagnostic criteria (Shaywitz, 2003). Individuals who struggle with word-level processing/dyslexia tend to struggle with those words because they actually have underlying impairments in phonological awareness, or "the conscious ability to detect and manipulate sounds of language" (Marinac, 2008, p. 8; Liberman & Shankweiler, 1985; Wagner & Torgesen, 1987). Phonological deficits contribute to word-level struggles (Snowling & Melby-Lervåg, 2016) because if individuals struggle to segment phonemes in a word, they will also experience difficulty mapping these phonemes onto letters/letter combinations. Then, if individuals struggle

---

[1]Of note, there are many other reading frameworks and theoretical models of discourse processing that are richly developed in the cognitive literature (e.g., Cromley & Azevedo, 2007; Gernsbacher & Faust, 1991; Kintsch, 1988; McKenna & Stahl, 2015; Perfetti, 1999; van den Broek et al., 1999). However, given these other models' relatively limited translation to the neurobiological literature to date, in this chapter, we confine our discussion of reading to the SVR.

to sound out words, they will struggle to read words and eventually commit them to memory as sight words (Harrison & Stewart, 2019).

Word-level impairments can understandably significantly prohibit children's reading development, therefore causing these children to fall behind their peers in terms of their reading abilities. Then, by virtue of being unable to read at grade level, these children also fall behind their peers in terms of their academic content knowledge. Fortunately, there are evidence-based interventions targeting word-level impairments that are beneficial for most children who have dyslexia (see the U.S. Institute of Education Sciences' What Works Clearinghouse for evaluation of evidence-based programs).

Comprehension Deficits (Specific Reading Comprehension Disorder)

Some individuals struggle to understand the meaning of texts they have read, including making inferences and creating mental models of text. This lack of understanding can be independent of or in addition to lower word-level deficits. Individuals who possess at least average word-level skills and at least average intelligence and have been provided with at least adequate reading instruction, but still struggle to comprehend the texts they read, are likely to fit the diagnostic criteria for Specific Reading Comprehension Disorder, or S-RCD (Nation & Snowling, 1997, 1998; Oakhill et al., 1986; Spencer et al., 2014; Stothard & Hulme, 1995; Yuill & Oakhill, 1991).

The DSM-5 defines S-RCD as a "specific learning disorder" "with impairment in reading," specifically in reading comprehension (without word reading accuracy noted as impaired) (American Psychiatric Association, 2013). It has been estimated that up to 10% of children and adults have S-RCD (Catts et al., 2003; Landi, 2010; Nation & Snowling, 1998; Stothard & Hulme, 1995; Yuill & Oakhill, 1991). While S-RCD is relatively prominent in the population, it is relatively understudied, especially when compared to word-level deficits.

However, behavioral studies have revealed that individuals with S-RCD exhibit deficits in oral and written language comprehension, which contribute to their deficits in reading comprehension (Catts et al., 2006; Hulme & Snowling, 2011). More specifically, individuals with S-RCD tend to exhibit deficits in vocabulary (Cain & Oakhill, 2006; Henderson et al., 2013), semantic processing but not phonological processing (Nation et al., 2001), grammar (Goff et al., 2005; Tong et al., 2014), and higher-level language skills such as knowledge of text structure (Cain et al., 2004), inference making (Cain & Oakhill, 1999; Oakhill & Cain, 2000, 2012), and comprehension monitoring (Ehrlich et al., 1999; Oakhill et al., 2005).

That being said, the level of reading comprehension that individuals with S-RCD exhibit is lower than the level of reading comprehension they should be at, as predicted by their oral language skills. This discrepancy in reading comprehension abilities suggests that S-RCD is linked to weaknesses in other areas beyond oral language (Spencer & Wagner, 2018). Additional deficits beyond oral language have been identified in individuals with S-RCD. For example, children with S-RCD tend to also exhibit deficits in executive function (Locascio et al., 2010), suggesting that S-RCD may result from a combination of deficits in both oral language and executive function processes (and possibly other processes, too).

Discourse-level impairments can understandably significantly prohibit children's reading development, therefore causing these children to fall behind their peers in terms of their reading abilities. Then, by virtue of being unable to read and understand at grade level, these children also fall behind their peers in terms of their academic content knowledge. Fortunately, there are evidence-based interventions targeting comprehension impairments that benefit children with S-RCD (Clarke et al., 2010; Hulme & Snowling, 2011).

Regardless of their specific diagnosis, any student with a reading disability requires a timely and appropriate intervention. The longer students with reading disabilities struggle without diagnosis and intervention, the more they fall behind their peers, and the more they must learn and master in order to catch up to grade-level reading ability and grade-level academic content knowledge (Foorman et al., 1997; Fuchs et al., 2014).

Neurobiological Correlates of Reading and Reading Disabilities

Word Recognition

Complementing the large body of research on the cognition of reading, much work has been done to try to understand the neurobiological correlates of reading. The basic neurobiological model of skilled reading proposes the involvement of three major brain areas: (1) the left ventral occipito–temporal region, (2) the left dorsal temporo–parietal region, and (3) the left inferior frontal region (Black et al., 2017; Dehaene et al., 2010; Pugh et al., 2001; Richlan, 2012). The left ventral occipito–temporal region contains the putative "visual word form area" (VWFA). This region is involved in the automatic visual processing of words (McCandliss et al., 2003) and displays a striking preference for processing words and legal pseudowords as compared to illegal pseudowords or other stimuli (Ben-Shachar et al., 2007; Cohen et al., 2002; Cutting et al., 2013; Pammer et al., 2004; Price et al., 1996; Vinckier et al., 2007). The left temporo–parietal region is thought to be involved in the integration of written words and auditory speech sounds (Gabrieli, 2009). The left inferior frontal region has been linked to many aspects of reading, including verbal working memory, phonological and semantic processing, silent reading, and speech planning (Fiez & Petersen, 1998; Poldrack et al., 1999; Price, 2012). While this broad tripartite model has some utility, reading is a complex process that requires the recruitment and coordination of more than just these three broad regions. Using neuroimaging techniques, especially functional MRI, researchers have investigated specific functions of subregions within these three broad regions, resulting in more refined models of word reading (see Kearns et al., 2019). For example, Kearns and colleagues propose that within the left temporo–parietal region, the supramarginal gyrus (SMG) is involved in the translation of decoded written words to auditory speech sounds, or phonemes, while the angular gyrus (AG) is involved in semantic processing, or processing meaning of single words (Kearns et al., 2019).

Word Recognition Deficits (Dyslexia)

With some exceptions, individuals with word recognition deficits generally exhibit reduced functional activation in many regions within the reading network (D'Mello & Gabrieli, 2018). Evidence also suggests that individuals with dyslexia demonstrate greater functional activation in right hemisphere brain regions, possibly indicating use of compensatory strategies for reading (e.g., Grigorenko, 2001; Joseph et al., 2001; Pugh et al., 2008; Waldie, 2002; Waldie et al., 2013). Individuals with dyslexia also tend to exhibit structural brain differences, but those differences will not be discussed in this chapter.

More specifically, compared to that of typical readers, the left occipito–temporal region is underactivated in individuals with dyslexia when processing words (Pugh et al., 2001; Richlan et al., 2009) and other nonreading stimuli such as strings of letters, digits, pseudoletters, or symbols (Lobier & Valdois, 2015). Similarly, individuals with dyslexia tend to show underactivation in the left temporo–parietal cortex during tasks involving phonological processing (Temple et al., 2001), thus supporting the supposition that the temporo–parietal cortex is important for multimodal grapheme–phoneme integration. Compared to the robust findings in the left occipito–temporal cortex and the left temporo–parietal cortex, findings in the left inferior frontal region are rather mixed. As expected, some studies have found decreased activation in the left inferior frontal region in individuals with dyslexia (Landi, 2010; Wimmer et al., 2010). However, other studies have unexpectedly found increased activation in the left inferior frontal region (Hoeft et al., 2007; Shaywitz et al., 1998). This increased activation is hypothesized to reflect the use of compensatory mechanisms and/or an overall increased effort exerted while reading or engaging in reading-related tasks (Hoeft et al., 2007; Price, 2012).

Comprehension

Fewer studies have been conducted beyond word-level reading in developing and/or impaired readers. However, the relatively comprehensive adult literature (e.g., Horowitz-Kraus et al., 2014; Johns et al., 2008; Robertson et al., 2000; Ryherd et al., 2018; Schmithorst et al., 2006; Walenski et al., 2019), along with some studies in developing and/or impaired readers (e.g., Aboud et al., 2016, 2019; Rimrodt et al., 2010; Wang et al., 2020), reveals that comprehension of more complex written material, such as sentences and passages, involves the recruitment and coordination of more widespread and bilateral brain regions. These regions include bilateral superior temporal gyrus (STG), bilateral middle temporal gyrus (MTG), bilateral anterior temporal pole, left AG, and medial structures, such as the ventral medial prefrontal cortex (Horowitz-Kraus et al., 2014; Johns et al., 2008; Robertson et al., 2000; Ryherd et al., 2018; Schmithorst et al., 2006; Wang et al., 2020; Yang et al., 2019). While a comprehensive overview of all the processes involved in comprehension is too complex for the current chapter, understanding neurobiological processes associated with S-RCD sheds light on the neurobiological processes involved in comprehension.

Comprehension Deficits (Specific Reading Comprehension Disorder)

Studies investigating the neurobiological processes associated with reading comprehension in children are relatively sparse. Contributing to this paucity is the use of single-word tasks, instead of sentences or lengthier passages, in most neuroimaging studies investigating reading comprehension (Roe et al., 2018). Furthermore, neuroimaging studies that specifically focus on the S-RCD diagnosis are even fewer (Landi & Ryherd, 2017). However, the studies that do exist support the hypothesis that S-RCD involves intact decoding but weaknesses in comprehension (Cutting et al., 2013; Landi & Perfetti, 2007; Landi & Ryherd, 2017). Here, we elaborate on functional neuroimaging findings linked to S-RCD.

Findings from a functional neuroimaging study conducted by Cutting and colleagues (2013) demonstrate that when reading single words, adolescents with S-RCD exhibit similar patterns of activation to typically reading peers, distinct from peers with dyslexia, in occipital–temporal regions (Cutting et al., 2013). The similarities and differences in activation patterns observed support the behavioral observations that individuals with S-RCD have intact decoding and grapheme–phoneme integration abilities. Additionally, in this study, the presence of S-RCD was linked to context-dependent functional coupling-by-reading group interaction anomaly in the left inferior frontal gyrus. In other words, activity in the left inferior frontal gyrus covaried to a greater extent with activity in the hippocampal, parahippocampal, and prefrontal areas in adolescents with S-RCD than typical readers when reading low-frequency words. This pattern suggests that individuals with S-RCD may have anomalies in systems supporting language and memory processes. Those anomalies may, in turn, contribute to weaknesses in semantic memory and, consequently, reading comprehension.

Ryherd and colleagues (2018) took a different approach to a similar concept, using functional neuroimaging to investigate the functional neural activation to spoken and printed single words and passages in adolescents with a range of reading comprehension abilities. They found that adolescents' reading comprehension abilities were negatively related to functional neural activation in regions associated with executive function and memory, such as the anterior cingulate cortex, insula, and hippocampus. This finding, which supports the finding of Cutting and colleagues (2013), implies that retrieval and, thus, comprehension are more effortful for poor comprehenders, such as those with S-RCD, than good comprehenders. The consistency of these results across spoken and written word modalities supports the idea that S-RCD involves, in part, a language comprehension deficit that also manifests in difficulty with comprehending written text (Ryherd et al., 2018). More research, especially using stimuli that involve lengthier passages, is needed to fully understand the origins of distinct brain patterns observed in individuals with S-RCD.

Neurobiology of Reading: Current and Future Directions

The aforementioned findings briefly reviewed in this chapter offer a window into word recognition and reading comprehension processes in terms of understanding the neurobiological correlates of learning disorders in these areas. Nonetheless, it is notable that most neurobiological models relevant to reading development and disorders have not broken down brain regions linked to word-, sentence-, and discourse-level processes. Admittedly, this is a highly complex task, made even more complex when trying to apply any summarized literature to understanding learning disorders because there are far more studies of word-level versus comprehension-level processes in developing readers/reading impairment. However, it is of value to consider a model that does include word-, sentence-, and comprehension-level processes, especially including more recent studies, which have sought to examine how executive brain regions are involved in the reading process in developing readers. To that end, here in Figure 5.1 (pp. 110–111), we include a model of reading (left hemisphere only) that attempts to incorporate not only those areas commonly noted in word recognition models (e.g., Kearns et al., 2019), but also extends to incorporate comprehension-level processes, as well as begin to think about how executive function regions may be involved in reading. Of note, this model should be viewed as *exploratory* and *underdeveloped*, as it is based largely on meta-analyses with adults along with some specific studies in adolescents; nonetheless, it provides a beginning point for thinking about reading processes that span from word to comprehension-levels and, thus, in turn, begins to set the stage for a reference point for considering neurobiological processes involved with reading development and reading difficulties that include not only word-level but also comprehension-level processes. A fully developed model will need to consider what cognitive processes each core region is engaging in (e.g., lexical processing, phonological processing, semantic integration, etc.) and which regions are anomalous in poor readers, as well as consider how these key regions map onto known brain networks (e.g., fronto–parietal network, default mode network, etc.) (cf., Bailey et al., 2018).

Math

It has been estimated that between 5% and 8% of all students have a math disability (Badian & Ghublikian, 1983; Gross-Tsur et al., 1996; Ostad, 1997; Shalev et al., 2000), with 2.5 million students receiving special education services in United States public schools for math disabilities (Cortiella & Horowitz, 2014). These figures make math disabilities the second-most common learning disability after reading disabilities. However, the literature investigating math disabilities is not nearly as expansive nor as robust in comparison to the literature investigating reading disabilities (Mazzocco, 2005). Math cognition and math disabilities are currently very understudied.

Similar to reading and reading disabilities, the effects of poor math skills on personal and public health make the importance of understanding math development and math disabilities strikingly apparent. Poor math skills have been associated with academic underachievement (Duncan et al., 2007), school dropout (Bynner & Parsons, 1997, 2000), underemployment (Bynner & Parsons, 1997, 2000; Ritchie & Bates, 2013), mental and/or physical illness (Parsons & Bynner, 2005), and/or incarceration (Parsons & Bynner, 2005). Math skills are especially important now more than ever because knowledge of numbers is increasingly required in our increasingly technological, "data-drenched" society (MacKinnon McQuarrie et al., 2014; Steen, 1999). Similar to reading disabilities, all of these aforementioned adverse outcomes cost taxpayer dollars, thus making math disabilities a public health concern; it has even been estimated that math disabilities cost society more money than reading disabilities (Gross et al., 2009; Sheuermann & Pedró, 2010).

Earlier identification of students with math disabilities and earlier intervention for such disabilities would help lessen the need for these resources and therefore lower their costs. Indeed, it is important to study math and, moreover, math disabilities in hopes of eventually remediating these disabilities, ultimately alleviating these adverse consequences. In the following section, we briefly review literature on the cognition and neurobiological correlates of math and math disabilities.

Math Cognition

Math is conceptualized as a domain-specific area of knowledge with distinct cortical correlates (Amalric & Dehaene, 2019). Studies conducted with typically developing/developed populations have established that math relies on both domain-general skills, including spatial skills, visuospatial working memory, and cognitive control, in addition to domain-specific skills, including number sense, quantity manipulation, arithmetic fact retrieval, and problem solving (Menon & Chang, 2021; Soares et al., 2018; Tam et al., 2019). Math can be studied using symbolic stimuli (Arabic numbers), nonsymbolic stimuli (dots), and auditory and visual number words. It is thought that the cognitive mechanisms underlying math, which are both domain-general and domain-specific (to math), account for the link between the processing of nonsymbolic and symbolic magnitudes and their relations to math (Price & Wilkey, 2017).

A foundational concept underlying math is numeracy, or "the universal ability to represent and manipulate numerical magnitudes nonverbally on a spatially oriented mental number line" (von Aster & Shalev, 2007). Put simply, numeracy is one's familiarity and comfort with quantities and numbers. Numeracy extends beyond basic arithmetic, involving the application of math beyond the classroom and in the real world. Somewhat encompassed in numeracy but somewhat unique, two other foundational concepts of math are ordinality and cardinality. Ordinality refers to the ability to place numbers in a sequence (Lyons et al., 2016). Cardinality is the quantity represented by the number symbol (Geary et al., 2018).

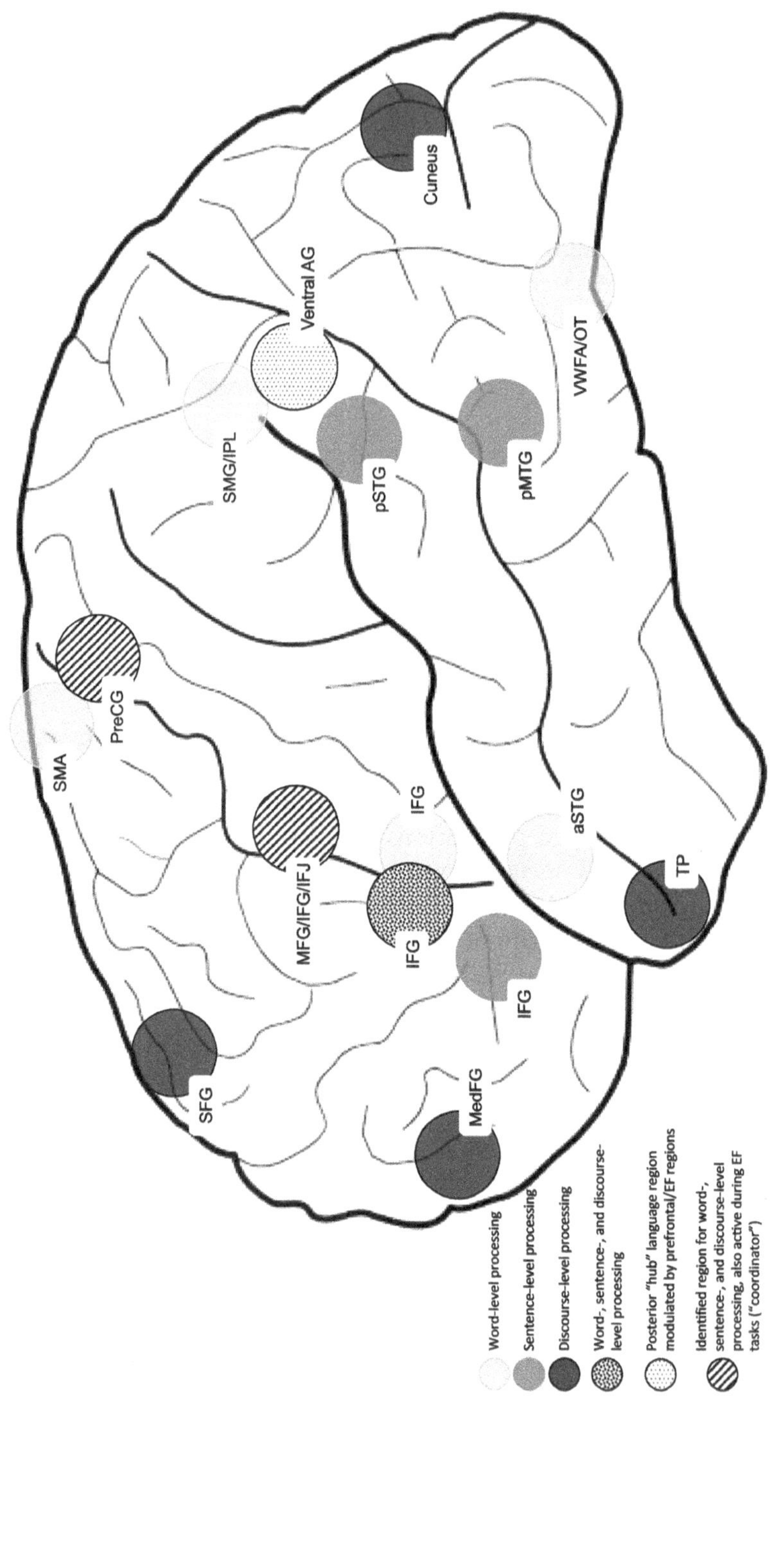
Cuneus
Ventral AG
VWFA/OT
SMG/IPL
pSTG
pMTG
PreCG
SMA
IFG
aSTG
MFG/IFG/IFJ
IFG
TP
IFG
SFG
MedFG
Word-level processing
Sentence-level processing
Discourse-level processing
Word-, sentence-, and discourse-level processing
Posterior "hub" language region modulated by prefrontal/EF regions
Identified region for word-, sentence-, and discourse-level processing, also active during EF tasks ("coordinator")

FIGURE 5.1. Visual depiction of the proposed neurobiological model of reading and executive function. SFG = superior frontal gyrus; MedFG = medial frontal gyrus; MFG = middle frontal gyrus; IFG = inferior frontal gyrus; IFJ = inferior frontal junction; SMA = supplementary motor area; PreCG = precentral gyrus; SMG/IPL = supramarginal gyrus/inferior parietal lobule; AG = angular gyrus; pSTG = posterior superior temporal gyrus; pMTG = posterior middle temporal gyrus; VWFA/OT = visual word form area/occipital-temporal region; aSTG = anterior superior temporal gyrus; TP = temporal pole. Note that the cuneus and MedFG are medial, but for visualization purposes have been placed in more lateral positions.

Note. The proposed neurobiological model of reading and executive function is a synthesis of an activation map derived from Neurosynth (Yarkoni, Poldrack, Nichols, Van Essen, & Wager, 2011), meta-analyses (Martin, Schurz, Kronbichler, & Richlan, 2015; Walenski, Europa, Caplan, & Thompson, 2019; Yang et al., 2019), individual fMRI studies that have tried to understand how executive function may be related to reading processes (Aboud, Bailey, Petrill, & Cutting, 2016; Kim et al., 2022; Wang et al., 2020) and review papers (Banich et al., 2023; Church, Cirino, Miciak, Juranek, Vaughn, & Fletcher, 2019; Kearns, Hancock, Hoeft, Pugh, & Frost, 2019). Using Neurosynth (neurosynth.org), which is a database of fMRI studies across broad topic areas, we searched "reading" using the "term search" function to obtain a synthesized brain activation map from 521 studies of reading and the brain to broadly capture the brain regions proposed to be involved in reading. While this activation map provided a starting point, the 521 studies that comprise it were too diverse (different ages, diagnoses, different levels of reading, etc.) resulting in many brain regions. To narrow down the brain regions involved in word-, sentence- and comprehension-level processes, we used existing meta-analyses for word- (Martin et al., 2015), sentence- (Walenski et al., 2019) and discourse-level processing (Yang et al., 2019). Finally, we identified executive brain regions involved in reading using individual fMRI studies (Aboud et al., 2016; Wang et al., 2020; Kim et al., 2022). For each left lateralized peak coordinate identified in each of the aforementioned meta-analyses and individual studies, we created a region of interest (5mm or 10mm spheres). We then analyzed the overlaps of neurosynth and the masks from each paper for each brain region. From these overlaps, we propose the process(es) that each brain region supports during reading tasks. The proposed ventral AG posterior "hub" language region modulated by prefrontal/EF is largely derived from the results of Kim et al. (2022).

People are thought to mentally represent numbers along a horizontal, imaginary number line, situated from left to right (Galton, 1880). Called the "mental number line representation," this concept is supported by a diverse group of studies, including those of clinical populations with spatial neglect (Vuilleumier et al., 2004), those involving response time (Dehaene et al., 1993), and those involving number comparisons (Moyer & Landauer, 1967). Given the spatial characteristics and setup of the mental number line representation, the mental number line supports the theory that spatial skills underlie math skills (Tam et al., 2019).

Math Disabilities

Math disability is a specific learning disability characterized by difficulties in processing numerical and mathematical information despite at least average intelligence and at least adequate math instruction (Berch & Mazzocco, 2007; Butterworth et al., 2011; Kaufmann et al., 2013; Price & Ansari, 2013). The DSM-5 defines math disability as a "specific learning disorder" "with impairment in mathematics," with noted impairment(s) in number sense, memorization of arithmetic facts, accurate and/or fluent calculation, and/or accurate math reasoning (American Psychiatric Association, 2013). Math disabilities are sometimes referred to as "developmental dyscalculia" (Price & Ansari, 2013).

Researchers have proposed several different models of typical and atypical math learning in attempts to explain the cognitive components of math and math disabilities. These models have not been published long enough for the field to fully test and empirically conclude which singular model or combination of models is likely the most accurate. That being said, the arguably most influential model is currently the triple code model (Skagenholt et al., 2018). The triple code model posits that there are three independent domains of math: (1) numerical quantity representation, (2) visuospatial numerical representation, and (3) auditory verbal representation (Dehaene & Cohen, 1995; Wilson & Dehaene, 2007). This model was based on findings from samples of educated adults, so it has yet to be studied through a developmental or disordered perspective; for this reason and other reasons, further model testing is necessary (Siemann & Petermann, 2018). However, early neuroimaging evidence linking these three domains to three distinct brain regions (intraparietal sulcus, posterior superior parietal lobule, and angular gyrus) provides support for this model (Soares et al., 2018).

While the triple code model is currently arguably the most influential model of math cognition (Skagenholt et al., 2018), there are several other models of typical and atypical math cognition. The "core deficit hypothesis," which can broadly be applied to several disorders, including math disabilities, posits that math disabilities stem from one foundational deficit (Astle & Fletcher-Watson, 2020; Soares et al., 2018). That foundational deficit could be perception and processing of number magnitude (Landerl et al., 2004), general numeracy (Robinson et al., 2002), or something else, but ultimately, it is one foundational deficit that causes all other mathematical difficulties. Another model suggests that math disabilities derive from deficits in domain-general skills that underlie the impaired math skills. In this model, deficits in basic skills, such as verbal working memory, long-term memory, and visuospatial processing, are thought to cause math disabilities (Geary, 2004). Working memory, in particular, plays an integral role in mathematical learning; visuospatial working memory deficits also contribute to dyscalculia (Menon, 2016). Another model, the "procedural deficit hypothesis" of math disability, suggests that abnormalities of brain structures underlying the procedural memory system can lead to difficulties with math skills and other functions associated with these structures (Ullman, 2004). Clinicians have also posited their own models. One of the main clinical models decomposes math disabilities into four main skills/deficits: core number skills, memory, reasoning, and visuospatial skills (Karagiannakis et al., 2014).

Again, all of these models must be viewed with caution as they do not yet have substantial empirical support. For example, emerging evidence indicates that the deficits in numerical magnitude processing and perception previously posited to cause math disabilities may actually be more reflective of deficits in executive function, specifically inhibitory control demands from incongruent visual cues in a nonsymbolic number comparison task (Wilkey et al., 2020). Additionally, a significant portion of math disabilities cannot be explained by the procedural deficit model (Soares et al., 2018). More research into typical and atypical math learning, to ultimately achieve consensus on a theoretical model of math cognition (like the SVR in reading), is needed.

Neurobiological Correlates of Math and Math Disabilities

Canonical research investigating the neurobiological correlates of math indicates that both hemispheres of the brain are involved. However, emerging evidence suggests that during math cognition, the right hemisphere might be more involved than the left (Ashkenazi et al., 2013). Three key brain regions involved in math cognition include: (1) the bilateral intraparietal cortices, (2) the bilateral prefrontal cortices (Dastjerdi et al., 2013; Eger, 2016), and (3) the bilateral inferior temporal cortices (Daitch et al., 2016; Park et al., 2014; Shum et al., 2013). The bilateral intraparietal cortex is involved in the processing of symbolic numerical information and visuospatial working memory (Matejko & Ansari, 2017). The bilateral prefrontal cortex has been linked to cognitive control, attention, inhibition, prospective memory, and cognitive flexibility (Armbruster et al., 2012). The inferior temporal cortex is associated with visual processing and object recognition (Bar et al., 2001; Miyashita, 1993). Recent research suggests that similar to the robust VWFA seen in tasks related to language and reading, math might have its own devoted region. Termed the "number form area" (NFA), this region is located in the right posterior inferior temporal gyrus of the inferior temporal cortex (Abboud et al., 2015; Daitch et al., 2016; Yeo et al., 2017).

The bilateral intraparietal sulci (IPS), located in the bilateral intraparietal cortices, in particular, appear to be the most important brain regions involved in math cognition (Amalric & Dehaene, 2019; Cohen Kadosh et al., 2008; Dehaene et al., 2003; Monti et al., 2012; Pinel et al., 2001; Price et al., 2007). The IPS is thought to support the processing of numerical magnitude (Ansari & Dhital, 2006; Cantlon & Brannon, 2006; Cantlon et al., 2006). However, other brain regions beyond the IPS are also involved in math cognition. There is increasing support for the involvement of the left angular gyrus in math tasks, particularly those involving the processing of numerical symbols (Price & Ansari, 2011) and arithmetic facts (Butterworth et al., 2011; Delazer et al., 2005). The right inferior frontal gyrus is broadly associated with numeracy and, more specifically, with attention to numbers, rendering it important for math cognition (Wilkey & Price, 2019). Other brain regions involved in math-related tasks include (but are not limited to) the bilateral hippocampus, parahippocampal gyrus, perisylvian areas, and fusiform gyrus (Butterworth et al., 2011; Cho et al., 2012; Menon & Chang, 2021; Soares et al., 2018; Wilkey et al., 2017).

The lack of consensus surrounding the brain regions involved in math cognition seems to result from several factors. One such factor is the overall paucity of math studies that use neuroimaging. Another factor is the diversity in the functional neuroimaging tasks used to study brain activation during math-related tasks (examples of tasks include symbolic vs. nonsymbolic tasks, tasks involving magnitude comparisons, tasks involving arithmetic, tasks involving more or less language/reading, etc.) hindering consensus. An additional factor is the widespread use of region-of-interest (ROI) analyses, which involve a priori selection of one specific brain region for intense study. The bilateral intraparietal sulci are understandably commonly used as ROIs in math studies. However, whole-brain analyses that could potentially identify more brain regions involved in math are consequently lacking. More and perhaps more cooperative studies need to be conducted to reach consensus surrounding the brain regions involved in math cognition.

Math Disabilities

The few math-related neuroimaging studies that have been published have generally concluded that individuals with math disabilities exhibit functional differences in both brain hemispheres (Soares et al., 2018), especially the right hemisphere (Ashkenazi et al., 2013), as compared to individuals without math disabilities. These functional differences generally include both underactivation and overactivation in various brain regions (Ashkenazi et al., 2013; Soares et al., 2018). Individuals with math disabilities also tend to exhibit structural brain differences, but those differences will not be discussed in this chapter.

Studies have shown that children with math disabilities have anomalous activation patterns in the bilateral intraparietal sulci compared to their typically developing peers (Mussolin et al., 2010; Price et al., 2007). Some studies demonstrate that children with math disabilities exhibit overactivation of the intraparietal sulci (Kaufmann et al., 2009). Kaufmann and colleagues suggest that overactivation of the intraparietal sulci somehow compensates for the deficits in math subskills (Kaufmann et al., 2009). However, other studies demonstrate that children with math disabilities actually show underactivation in the intraparietal sulci as compared to typically developing children in numeric magnitude differentiation tasks (Mussolin et al., 2010) and performing arithmetic (Kucian et al., 2006). While

Mussolin and colleagues (2010) had initially predicted overactivation in the intraparietal sulci, due to the extra effort exerted by children with math disabilities while completing math tasks as compared to typically developing peers, they actually observed decreased activation in those regions (Mussolin et al., 2010). Mussolin and colleagues therefore broadly conclude that the "lack of IPS sensitivity" in children with math disabilities as compared to typically developing children "concerns domain-specific and domain-general magnitudes" (Mussolin et al., 2010). Similarly, Kucian and colleagues conclude that the weaker activation they observed in the intraparietal sulci in children with math disabilities as compared to typically developing peers was due to a broad lack of recruitment across relevant brain regions (Kucian et al., 2006).

While the findings regarding intraparietal sulci activation are the most commonly reported in those with math disabilities, other brain regions have also been reported to show anomalous activation in children with math disabilities as compared to those without. While findings are relatively inconsistent, children with math disabilities typically exhibit decreased activation in several regions outside the math network (the math network being the intraparietal sulci, angular gyrus, and posterior superior parietal lobule), such as the right middle frontal gyrus and premotor cortex within the prefrontal cortex, the right insula, the right parahippocampal gyrus, and the left cingulate gyrus (Ashkenazi et al., 2012; Kucian et al., 2006; Mussolin et al., 2010) as compared to typically developing peers. Additionally, children with math disabilities exhibit overactivations in the right postcentral gyrus and the right supramarginal gyrus as compared to typically developing peers. Overactivation of the right postcentral gyrus is thought to relate to the increased sensorimotor demands on children with math disabilities when doing math (Mussolin et al., 2010; Pinel et al., 1999). While there are several potential explanations, overactivation of the right supramarginal gyrus is thought to relate to the increased visuospatial working memory required for children with math disabilities to do math (Mussolin et al., 2010). More research is needed to fully understand the origins of distinct brain patterns observed in individuals with math disabilities.

Comorbidity of Reading and Math

Reading and math disabilities are typically studied separately, but they are highly comorbid. A "comorbidity" occurs when another condition or conditions accompanies the primary condition of study (Feinstein, 1970). Reading and math disabilities commonly co-occur and are actually more likely to co-occur than present in isolation (Joyner & Wagner, 2020). Estimates vary based on diagnostic criteria, but approximately 56% of students with reading disabilities also have math disabilities, and approximately 70% of students with math disabilities also have reading disabilities (Barbaresi et al., 2005; Dirks et al., 2008). Indeed, a meta-analysis by Joyner and Wagner (2020) found that there are varying degrees of comorbidity between reading and math disabilities (e.g., Badian, 1999; Barbaresi et al., 2005; Branum-Martin et al., 2013; Dirks et al., 2008; Lewis et al., 1994; Light & DeFries, 1995).

The underlying cognitive skills required for reading and math may provide insight into this comorbidity. Both reading and math are linked to phonological processing (De Smedt & Boets, 2010; Hecht et al., 2001), memory (Hecht et al., 2001; Swanson & Jerman, 2006; Swanson et al., 2009), and executive function (Yeniad et al., 2013). Additionally, there are similarities between letters in alphabetic writing and digits in math (Joyner & Wagner, 2020). Finally, especially as one first learns math through stories and word problems, much of the instruction and computation of math requires language and reading (Joyner & Wagner, 2020). It has actually been suggested that reading disability be included as a diagnostic criterion of math disability (Joyner & Wagner, 2020). Unsurprisingly, comorbidities across both reading and math disabilities include deficits in executive function (Lonergan et al., 2019; Morgan et al., 2017; Yeniad et al., 2013), ADHD (Mayes & Calhoun, 2006; Willcutt & Pennington, 2000), and mental health conditions including anxiety and/or depression (Krinzinger et al., 2009; Mammarella et al., 2016). Discussion of comorbidity is beyond the scope of this chapter (see Willcutt, this volume, for an in-depth review of comorbidity across learning disabilities and psychiatric disorders). However, many of the cognitive studies and most of the neurobiological studies, to date, have not considered the effects of comorbidities. This raises an important caveat of the majority of the neurobiological findings to date; whether the neuroimaging findings reviewed in this chapter vary based on comorbidity status is currently an unanswered question.

Conclusions

Reading and math disabilities are thought to be the most common learning disabilities. Reading has been studied rather extensively, but research in math disabilities lags in comparison. More basic and translational research must be done to understand the core deficits of these types of disabilities, and especially whether comorbid reading and math disabilities have different developmental sequalae and neurobiological origins. Indeed, a better understanding of these disabilities is essential for the improvement of diagnostic criteria and interventions. If individuals with these disabilities can be diagnosed earlier, tailored interventions can be implemented earlier and thus result in better outcomes. Greater specificity and clarity can also refine the nebulous systems of names and diagnostic criteria that muddy the research and clinical practice of these disabilities, which will ultimately help researchers, practitioners, educators, parents, and individuals with the disabilities themselves.

AUTHORS' NOTE

The studies cited throughout this book chapter are quite heterogeneous in their samples, diagnostic criteria, and neuroimaging equipment used (if applicable). Samples of participants include wide age ranges, different age ranges, various comorbidities, and different

English language capabilities. Diagnostic criteria vary widely in percentile (5th to 35th percentile), in criteria (one-third assessments below a certain percentile, all of the assessments below a certain percentile), and in assessment (Woodcock–Johnson, CTOPP, etc.). Neuroimaging studies use different types of equipment and techniques (EEG, structural and functional MRI, PET, etc.); scanners can be a confound when comparing studies. It is therefore of the utmost importance to synthesize information and generalize findings across studies with caution.

REFERENCES

Aaron, P. G., Joshi, R. M., Boulware-Gooden, R., & Bentum, K. (2008). Diagnosis and treatment of reading disabilities based on the component model of reading: An alternative to the discrepancy model of learning disabilities. *Journal of Learning Disabilities, 4*(1), 67–84.

Aboud, K. S., Bailey, S. K., Del Tufo, S. N., Barquero, L. A., & Cutting, L. E. (2019). Fairy tales versus facts: Genre matters to the developing brain. *Cerebral Cortex, 29*(11), 4877–4888.

Aboud, K. S., Bailey, S. K., Petrill, S. A., & Cutting, L. E. (2016). Comprehending text versus reading words in young readers with varying reading ability: Distinct patterns of functional connectivity from common processing hubs. *Developmental Science, 19*(4), 632–656.

Abboud, S., Maidenbaum, S., Dehaene, S., & Amedi, A. (2015). A number-form area in the blind. *Nature Communications, 6*, 6026.

Amalric, M., & Dehaene, S. (2019). A distinct cortical network for mathematical knowledge in the human brain. *NeuroImage, 189*, 19–31.

American Psychiatric Association. (2013). *Diagnostic and statistical manual of mental disorders* (5th ed.). Author.

Ansari, D., & Dhital, B. (2006). Age-related changes in the activation of the intraparietal sulcus during nonsymbolic magnitude processing: An event-related functional magnetic resonance imaging study. *Journal of Cognitive Neuroscience, 18*(11), 1820–1828.

Armbruster, D. J., Ueltzhöffer, K., Basten, U., & Fiebach, C. J. (2012). Prefrontal cortical mechanisms underlying individual differences in cognitive flexibility and stability. *Journal of Cognitive Neuroscience, 24*(12), 2385–2399.

Ashkenazi, S., Black, J. M., Abrams, D. A., Hoeft, F., & Menon, V. (2013). Neurobiological underpinnings of math and reading learning disabilities. *Journal of Learning Disabilities, 46*(6), 549–569.

Ashkenazi, S., Rosenberg-Lee, M., Tenison, C., & Menon, V. (2012). Weak task-related modulation and stimulus representations during arithmetic problem solving in children with developmental dyscalculia. *Developmental Cognitive Neuroscience, 2*(Suppl. 1), S152–S166.

Astle, D. E., & Fletcher-Watson, S. (2020). Beyond the core-deficit hypothesis in developmental disorders. *Current Directions in Psychological Science, 29*(5), 431–437.

Badian, N. A. (1999). Persistent arithmetic, reading, or arithmetic and reading disability. *Annals of Dyslexia, 49*, 45–70.

Badian, N. A., & Ghublikian, M. (1983). The personal-social characteristics of children with poor mathematical computation skills. *Journal of Learning Disabilities, 16*(3), 154–157.

Bailey, S. K., Aboud, K. S., Nguyen, T. Q., & Cutting, L. E. (2018). Applying a network framework to the neurobiology of reading and dyslexia. *Journal of Neurodevelopmental Disorders, 10*, 37.

Banich, M. T., Wang, K., Kim, H., Leopold, D. R., Reineberg, A. E., Thompson, L. A., et al. (2023). The influence of executive processing on reading comprehension during adolescence. *Mind, Brain, and Education, 17*(4), 279–288.

Bar, M., Tootell, R. B., Schacter, D. L., Greve, D. N., Fischl, B., Mendola, J. D., et al. (2001). Cortical mechanisms specific to explicit visual object recognition. *Neuron, 29*(2), 529–535.

Barbaresi, W. J., Katusic, S. K., Colligan, R. C., Weaver, A. L., & Jacobsen, S. J. (2005). Math learning disorder: Incidence in a population-based birth cohort, 1976–82, *Ambulatory Pediatrics: The Official Journal of the Ambulatory Pediatric Association, 5*(5), 281–289.

Ben-Shachar, M., Dougherty, R. F., Deutsch, G. K., & Wandell, B. A. (2011). The development of cortical sensitivity to visual word forms. *Journal of Cognitive Neuroscience, 23*(9), 2387–2399.

Berch, D. B., & Mazzocco, M. M. M. (Eds.). (2007). *Why is math so hard for some children? The nature and origins of mathematical learning difficulties and disabilities.* Brookes.

Black, J. M., Xia, Z., & Hoeft, F. (2017). Neurobiological bases of reading disorder part II: The importance of developmental considerations in typical and atypical reading. *Language and Linguistics Compass, 11*(10), e12252.

Branum-Martin, L., Fletcher, J. M., & Stuebing, K. K. (2013). Classification and identification of reading and math disabilities: The special case of comorbidity. *Journal of Learning Disabilities, 46*(6), 490–499.

Butterworth, B., Varma, S., & Laurillard, D. (2011). Dyscalculia: From brain to education. *Science, 332*(6033), 1049–1053.

Bynner, J., & Parsons, S. (1997). *Does numeracy matter? Evidence from the National Child Development Study on the impact of poor numeracy on adult life.* Basic Skills Agency.

Bynner, J., & Parsons, S. (2000). Impact of poor numeracy on employment and career progression. In C. Tikly & A. Wolf (Eds.), *The maths we need now: Demands, deficits and remedies.* (pp. 26–51). Bedford Way Papers.

Cain, K., & Oakhill, J. V. (1999). Inference making ability and its relation to comprehension failure in young children. *Reading and Writing, 11*, 489–503.

Cain, K., & Oakhill, J. V. (2006). Profiles of children with specific reading comprehension difficulties. *British Journal of Educational Psychology, 76*(4), 683–696.

Cain, K., Oakhill, J. V., & Bryant, P. (2004). Children's reading comprehension ability: Concurrent prediction by working memory, verbal ability, and component skills. *Journal of Educational Psychology, 96*(1), 31–42.

Cantlon, J. F., & Brannon, E. M. (2006). Shared system for ordering small and large numbers in monkeys and humans. *Psychological Science, 17*(5), 401–406.

Cantlon, J. F., Brannon, E. M., Carter, E. J., & Pelphrey, K. A. (2006). Functional imaging of numerical processing in adults and 4-y-old children. *PLOS Biology, 4*(5), e125.

Carroll, J. M., Maughan, B., Goodman, R., & Meltzer, H. (2005). Literacy difficulties and psychiatric disorders: Evidence for comorbidity. *Journal of Child Psychology and Psychiatry, and Allied Disciplines, 46*(5), 524–532.

Carver, R. P. (1997). Reading for one second, one minute, or one year from the perspective of Rauding theory. *Scientific Studies of Reading, 1*(1), 3–43.

Carver, R. P. (2003). The highly lawful relationships among pseudoword decoding, word identification, spelling, listening, and reading. *Scientific Studies of Reading, 7*(2), 127–154.

Catts, H. W., Adlof, S. M., & Ellis Weismer, S. (2006). Language deficits in poor comprehenders: A case for the simple view of reading. *Journal of Speech, Language, and Hearing Research: JSLHR, 49*(2), 278–293.

Catts, H. W., Hogan, T. P., & Fey, M. E. (2003). Subgrouping poor readers on the basis of individual differences in reading-related abilities. *Journal of Learning Disabilities, 36*(2), 151–164.

Center on Budget and Policy Priorities. (2022). *Where do our federal tax dollars go? www.cbpp.org/research/federal-budget/where-do-our-federal-tax-dollars-go.*

Cho, S., Metcalfe, A. W., Young, C. B., Ryali, S., Geary, D. C., & Menon, V. (2012). Hippocampal–prefrontal engagement and dynamic causal interactions in the maturation of children's fact retrieval. *Journal of Cognitive Neuroscience, 24*(9), 1849–1866.

Christle, C. A., & Yell, M. L. (2008). Preventing youth incarceration through reading remediation: Issues and solutions. *Reading & Writing Quarterly, 24*(2), 148–176.

Church, J. A., Cirino, P. T., Miciak, J., Juranek, J., Vaughn, S., & Fletcher, J. M. (2019). Cognitive, intervention, and neuroimaging perspectives on executive function in children with reading disabilities. *New Directions for Child and Adolescent Development, 2019*(165), 25–54.

Clarke, P. J., Snowling, M. J., Truelove, E., & Hulme, C. (2010). Ameliorating children's reading-comprehension difficulties: A randomized controlled trial. *Psychological Science, 21*(8), 1106–1116.

Cohen, L., Lehéricy, S., Chochon, F., Lemer, C., Rivaud, S., & Dehaene, S. (2002). Language-specific tuning of visual cortex? Functional properties of the visual word form area. *Brain: A Journal of Neurology, 125*(Pt. 5), 1054–1069.

Cohen Kadosh, R., Lammertyn, J., & Izard, V. (2008). Are numbers special? An overview of chronometric, neuroimaging, developmental and comparative studies of magnitude representation. *Progress in Neurobiology, 84*(2), 132–147.

Cortiella, C., & Horowitz, S. H. (2014). *The state of learning disabilities: Facts, trends and emerging issues* (3rd ed.). National Center for Learning Disabilities.

Cromley, J. G., & Azevedo, R. (2007). Testing and refining the direct and inferential mediation model of reading comprehension. *Journal of Educational Psychology, 99*(2), 311–325.

Curtis, M. E. (1980). Development of components of reading skill. *Journal of Educational Psychology, 72*(5), 656–669.

Cutting, L. E., Clements-Stephens, A., Pugh, K. R., Burns, S., Cao, A., Pekar, J. J., et al. (2013). Not all reading disabilities are dyslexia: Distinct neurobiology of specific comprehension deficits. *Brain Connectivity, 3*(2), 199–211.

Cutting, L. E., & Scarborough, H. S. (2006). Prediction of reading comprehension: Relative contributions of word recognition, language proficiency, and other cognitive skills can depend on how comprehension is measured. *Scientific Studies of Reading, 10*(3), 277–299.

D'Mello, A. M., & Gabrieli, J. D. E. (2018). Cognitive neuroscience of dyslexia. *Language, Speech, and Hearing Services in Schools, 49*(4), 798–809.

Daitch, A. L., Foster, B. L., Schrouff, J., Rangarajan, V., Kaşikçi, I., Gattas, S., et al. (2016). Mapping human temporal and parietal neuronal population activity and functional coupling during mathematical cognition. *Proceedings of the National Academy of Sciences of the United States of America, 113*(46), E7277–E7286.

Daniel, S. S., Walsh, A. K., Goldston, D. B., Arnold, E. M., Reboussin, B. A., & Wood, F. B. (2006). Suicidality, school dropout, and reading problems among adolescents. *Journal of Learning Disabilities, 39*(6), 507–514.

Dastjerdi, M., Ozker, M., Foster, B., Rangarajan, V., & Parvizi, J. (2013). Numerical processing in the human parietal cortex during experimental and natural conditions. *Nature Communications, 4*, 25–28.

De Smedt, B., & Boets, B. (2010). Phonological processing and arithmetic fact retrieval: Evidence from developmental dyslexia. *Neuropsychologia, 48*(14), 3973–3981.

Dehaene, S., Bossini, S., & Giraux, P. (1993). The mental representation of parity and number magnitude. *Journal of Experimental Psychology: General, 122*(3), 371–396.

Dehaene, S., & Cohen, L. (1995). Towards an anatomical and functional model of number processing. *Mathematical Cognition, 1*(1), 83–120.

Dehaene, S., Pegado, F., Braga, L. W., Ventura, P., Nunes Filho, G., Jobert, A., et al. (2010). How learning to read changes the cortical networks for vision and language. *Science, 330*(6009), 1359–1364.

Dehaene, S., Piazza, M., Pinel, P., & Cohen, L. (2003). Three parietal circuits for number processing. *Cognitive Neuropsychology, 20*(3–6), 487–506.

Delazer, M., Ischebeck, A., Domahs, F., Zamarian, L., Koppelstaetter, F., Siedentopf, C. M., et al. (2005). Learning by strategies and learning by drill—evidence from an fMRI study. *NeuroImage, 25*(3), 838–849.

Dirks, E., Spyer, G., Van Lieshout, E. C. D. M., & De Sonneville, L. (2008). Prevalence of combined reading and arithmetic disabilities. *Journal of Learning Disabilities, 41*(5), 460–473.

Duke, N. K., & Cartwright, K. B. (2021). The science of reading progresses: Communicating advances beyond the Simple View of Reading. *Reading Research Quarterly, 56*(51), S25–S44.

Duncan, G. J., Dowsett, C. J., Claessens, A., Magnuson, K., Huston, A. C., Klebanov, P., et al. (2007). School readiness and later achievement. *Developmental Psychology, 43*(6), 1428–1446.

Eger, E. (2016). Neuronal foundations of human numerical representations. *Progress in Brain Research, 227*, 1–27.

Ehrlich, M. F., Remond, M., & Tardieu, H. (1999). Processing of anaphoric devices in young skilled and less skilled comprehenders: Differences in metacognitive monitoring. *Reading and Writing, 11*, 29–63.

Feinstein, A. R. (1970). The pre-therapeutic classification of co-morbidity in chronic disease. *Journal of Chronic Diseases, 23*(7), 455–468.

Fiez, J. A., & Petersen, S. E. (1998). Neuroimaging studies of word reading. *Proceedings of the National Academy of Sciences of the United States of America, 95*(3), 914–921.

Fletcher, J. M., Lyon, G. R., Fuchs, L. S., & Barnes, M. A. (2007). *Learning disabilities: From identification to intervention.* Guilford Press.

Foorman, B. R., Francis, D. J., Shaywitz, S. E., Shaywitz, B. A., & Fletcher, J. M. (1997). The case for early reading intervention. In B. A. Blachman (Ed.), *Foundations of reading acquisition and dyslexia: Implications for early intervention* (pp. 243–264). Erlbaum.

Francis, D. J., Fletcher, J. M., Catts, H. W., & Tomblin, J. B. (2005). Dimensions affecting the assessment of reading comprehension. In S. G. Paris & S. A. Stahl (Eds.), *Children's reading comprehension and assessment* (pp. 369–394). Erlbaum.

Fuchs, D., Fuchs, L. S., & Vaughn, S. (2014). What is intensive instruction and why is it important? *Teaching Exceptional Children, 46*(4), 13–18.

Gabrieli, J. D. (2009). Dyslexia: A new synergy between education and cognitive neuroscience. *Science, 325*(5938), 280–283.

Galton, F. (1880). Visualised numerals. *Nature, 21*, 252–256.

Geary, D. C. (2004). Mathematics and learning disabilities. *Journal of Learning Disabilities, 37*(1), 4–15.

Geary, D. C., VanMarle, K., Chu, F. W., Rouder, J., Hoard, M. K., & Nugent, L. (2018). Early conceptual understanding of cardinality predicts superior school-entry number-system knowledge. *Psychological Science, 29*(2), 191–205.

Gernsbacher, M. A., & Faust, M. E. (1991). The mechanism of suppression: A component of general comprehension skill. *Journal of Experimental Psychology: Learning, Memory, and Cognition, 17*(2), 245–262.

Goff, D. A., Pratt, C., & Ong, B. (2005). The relations between children's reading comprehension, working memory, language skills and components of reading decoding in a normal sample. *Reading and Writing: An Interdisciplinary Journal, 18*(7–9), 583–616.

Gough, P. B., & Tunmer, W. E. (1986). Decoding, reading, and reading disability. *Remedial and Special Education, 7*(1), 6–10.

Grigorenko, E. L. (2001). Developmental dyslexia: An update on genes, brains, and environments. *Journal of Child Psychology and Psychiatry, 42*(1), 91–125.

Gross, J., Hudson, C., & Price, D. (2009). *The long term costs of numeracy difficulties.* National Numeracy. *www.nationalnumeracy.org.uk/research-and-resources/long-term-costs-numeracy-difficulties-2008*

Gross-Tsur, V., Manor, O., & Shalev, R. S. (1996). Developmental dyscalculia: Prevalence and demographic features. *Developmental Medicine and Child Neurology, 38*(1), 25–33.

Harrison, A. G., & Stewart, M. (2019). Diagnostic implications of the double deficit model for young adolescents with dyslexia. *Dyslexia, 25*(4), 345–359.

Hecht, S. A., Torgesen, J. K., Wagner, R. K., & Rashotte, C. A. (2001). The relations between phonological processing abilities and emerging individual differences in mathematical computation skills: A longitudinal study from second to fifth grades. *Journal of Experimental Child Psychology, 79*(2), 192–227.

Henderson, L., Snowling, M., & Clarke, P. (2013). Accessing, integrating, and inhibiting word meaning in poor comprehenders. *Scientific Studies of Reading, 17*(3), 177–198.

Hoeft, F., Ueno, T., Reiss, A. L., Meyler, A., Whitfield-Gabrieli, S., Glover, G. H., et al. (2007). Prediction of children's reading skills using behavioral, functional, and structural neuroimaging measures. *Behavioral Neuroscience, 121*(3), 602–613.

Hoover, W. A., & Gough, P. B. (1990). The Simple View of Reading. *Reading and Writing, 2*(2), 127–160.

Hoover, W. A., & Tunmer, W. E. (2020). *The cognitive foundations of reading and its acquisition.* Springer.

Horowitz, S. H., Rawe, J., & Whittaker, M. C. (2017). *The state of learning disabilities: Understanding the 1 in 5.* National Center for Learning Disabilities.

Horowitz-Kraus, T., Wang, Y., Plante, E., & Holland, S. K. (2014). Involvement of the right hemisphere in reading comprehension: A DTI study. *Brain Research, 1582*, 34–44.

Hudson, N., Scheff, J., Tarsha, M., & Cutting, L. E. (2016). Reading comprehension and executive function neurobiological findings. *Perspectives on Language and Literacy, 42*(2), 23–29.

Hulme, C., & Snowling, M. (2011). Children's reading comprehension difficulties: Nature, causes, and treatments. *Current Directions in Psychological Science, 20*(3), 139–142.

Individuals with Disabilities Education Act, 20 U.S.C. § 1400 (2004).

Johns, C. L., Tooley, K. M., & Traxler, M. J. (2008). Discourse impairments following right hemisphere brain damage: A critical review. *Language and Linguistics Compass, 2*(6), 1038–1062.

Joseph, J., Noble, K., & Eden, G. (2001). The neurobiological basis of reading. *Journal of Learning Disabilities, 34*(6), 566–579.

Joshi, R. M., Williams, K., & Wood, J. (1998). Predicting reading comprehension from listening comprehension: Is this the answer to the IQ debate? In C. Hulme & R. M. Joshi (Eds.), *Reading and spelling: Development and disorders* (pp. 319–327). Lawrence Erlbaum Associates.

Joyner, R. E., & Wagner, R. K. (2020). Co-occurrence of reading disabilities and math disabilities: A meta-analysis. *Scientific Studies of Reading: The Official Journal of the Society for the Scientific Study of Reading, 24*(1), 14–22.

Karagiannakis, G., Baccaglini-Frank, A., & Papadatos, Y. (2014). Mathematical learning difficulties subtypes classification. *Frontiers in Human Neuroscience, 8*(7), 1–5.

Kaufmann, L., Mazzocco, M. M., Dowker, A., von Aster, M., Göbel, S. M., Grabner, R. H., et al. (2013). Dyscalculia from a developmental and differential perspective. *Frontiers in Psychology, 4*, 516.

Kaufmann, L., Vogel, S. E., Starke, M., Kremser, C., Schocke, M., & Wood, G. (2009). Developmental dyscalculia: Compensatory mechanisms in left intraparietal regions in response to nonsymbolic magnitudes. *Behavioral and Brain Functions, 5*, 35.

Kearns, D. M., Hancock, R., Hoeft, F., Pugh, K. R., & Frost, S. J. (2019). The neurobiology of dyslexia. *Teaching Exceptional Children, 51*(3), 175–188.

Kim, H., Wang, K., Cutting, L. E., Willcutt, E. G., Petrill, S. A., Leopold, D. R., et al. (2022). The angular gyrus as a hub for modulation of language-related cortex by distinct prefrontal executive control regions. *Journal of Cognitive Neuroscience, 34*(12), 2275–2296.

Kintsch, W. (1988). The role of knowledge in discourse comprehension: A construction-integration model. *Psychological Review, 95*(2), 163–182.

Krinzinger, H., Kaufmann, L., & Willmes, K. (2009). Math anxiety and math ability in early primary school years. *Journal of Psychoeducational Assessment, 27*(3), 206–225.

Kucian, K., Loenneker, T., Dietrich, T., Dosch, M., Martin, E., & von Aster, M. (2006).

Impaired neural networks for approximate calculation in dyscalculic children: A functional MRI study. *Behavioral and Brain Functions, 2*, Article 31.

Landerl, K., Bevan, A., & Butterworth, B. (2004). Developmental dyscalculia and basic numerical capacities: A study of 8–9-year-old students. *Cognition, 93*(2), 99–125.

Landi, N. (2010). An examination of the relationship between reading comprehension, higher-level and lower-level reading sub-skills in adults. *Reading and Writing: An Interdisciplinary Journal, 23*(6), 701–717.

Landi, N., Frost, S. J., Menc, W. E., Sandak, R., & Pugh, K. R. (2013). Neurobiological bases of reading comprehension: Insights from neuroimaging studies of word level and text level processing in skilled and impaired readers. *Reading & Writing Quarterly: Overcoming Learning Difficulties, 29*(2), 145–167.

Landi, N., & Perfetti, C. A. (2007). An electrophysiological investigation of semantic and phonological processing in skilled and less-skilled comprehenders. *Brain and Language, 102*(1), 30–45.

Landi, N., & Ryherd, K. (2017). Understanding specific reading comprehension deficit: A review. *Language and Linguistics Compass, 11*(2), 1–24.

Learning Disabilities Association of America. (n.d.-a). *New to LD. https://ldaamerica.org/support/new-to-ld*

Learning Disabilities Association of America. (n.d.-b). *Types of learning disabilities. https://ldaamerica.org/types-of-learning-disabilities*

Lervåg, A., Hulme, C., & Melby-Lervåg, M. (2018). Unpicking the developmental relationship between oral language skills and reading comprehension: It's simple, but complex. *Child Development, 89*(5), 1821–1838.

Lewis, C., Hitch, G. J., & Walker, P. (1994). The prevalence of specific arithmetic difficulties and specific reading difficulties in 9- to 10-year-old boys and girls. *Journal of Child Psychology and Psychiatry, and Allied Disciplines, 35*(2), 283–292.

Liberman, I. Y., & Shankweiler, D. (1985). Phonology and the problems of learning to read and write. *Remedial and Special Education, 6*(6), 8–17.

Light, J. G., & DeFries, J. C. (1995). Comorbidity of reading and mathematics disabilities: Genetic and environmental etiologies. *Journal of Learning Disabilities, 28*(2), 96–106.

Lobier, M., & Valdois, S. (2015). Visual attention deficits in developmental dyslexia cannot be ascribed solely to poor reading experience. *Nature Reviews Neuroscience, 16*, 225.

Locascio, G., Mahone, E. M., Eason, S. H., & Cutting, L. E. (2010). Executive dysfunction among children with reading comprehension deficits. *Journal of Learning Disabilities, 43*(5), 441–454.

Lonergan, A., Doyle, C., Cassidy, C., MacSweeney Mahon, S., Roche, R. A. P., Boran, L., et al. (2019). A meta-analysis of executive functioning in dyslexia with consideration of the impact of comorbid ADHD. *Journal of Cognitive Psychology, 31*(7), 725–749.

Lyon, G. R., Shaywitz, S. E., & Shaywitz, B. A. (2003). A definition of dyslexia. *Annals of Dyslexia, 53*(1), 1–14.

Lyons, I. M., Vogel, S. E., & Ansari, D. (2016). On the ordinality of numbers: A review of neural and behavioral studies. *Progress in Brain Research, 227*, 187–221.

MacKinnon McQuarrie, M. A., Siegel, L. S., Perry, N. E., & Weinberg, J. (2014). Reactivity to stress and the cognitive components of math disability in grade 1 children. *Journal of Learning Disabilities, 47*(4), 349–365.

Mammarella, I. C., Ghisi, M., Bomba, M., Bottesi, G., Caviola, S., Broggi, F., et al. (2016). Anxiety and depression in children with nonverbal learning disabilities, reading disabilities, or typical development. *Journal of Learning Disabilities, 49*(2), 130–139.

Marinac, J. V. (2008). *Phonological core dyslexia in secondary school students: Identification and intervention*. Plural Publishing, Inc.

Martin, A., Schurz, M., Kronbichler, M., & Richlan, F. (2015). Reading in the brain of children and adults: A meta-analysis of 40 functional magnetic resonance imaging studies. *Human Brain Mapping, 36*(5), 1963–1981.

Matejko, A. A., & Ansari, D. (2017). How do individual differences in children's domain specific and domain general abilities relate to brain activity within the intraparietal sulcus during arithmetic? An fMRI study. *Human Brain Mapping, 38*(8), 3941–3956.

Mayes, S. D., & Calhoun, S. L. (2006). Frequency of reading, math, and writing disabilities in children with clinical disorders. *Learning and Individual Differences, 16*(2), 145–157.

Mazzocco, M. M. M. (2005). Challenges in identifying target skills for math disability screening and intervention. *Journal of Learning Disabilities, 38*(4), 318–323.

McArthur, G., & Castles, A. (2017). Helping children with reading difficulties: Some things we have learned so far. *Nature Partner Journals: Science of Learning, 2*, 7.

McArthur, G., Castles, A., Kohnen, S., & Banales, E. (2016). Low self-concept in poor readers: Prevalence, heterogeneity, and risk. *PeerJ, 4*, e2669.

McCandliss, B. D., Cohen, L., & Dehaene, S. (2003). The visual word form area: Expertise for reading in the fusiform gyrus. *Trends in Cognitive Sciences, 7*(7), 293–299.

McKenna, M. C., & Stahl, K. A. D. (2015). *Assessment for reading instruction* (3rd ed.). Guilford Press.

Menon, V. (2016). Working memory in children's math learning and its disruption in dyscalculia. *Current Opinion in Behavioral Sciences, 10*, 125–132.

Menon, V., & Chang, H. (2021). Emerging neurodevelopmental perspectives on mathematical learning. *Developmental Review, 60*, 100964.

Miyashita, Y. (1993). Inferior temporal cortex: Where visual perception meets memory. *Annual Review of Neuroscience, 16*, 245–263.

Monti, M. M., Parsons, L. M., & Osherson, D. N. (2012). Thought beyond language: Neural dissociation of algebra and natural language. *Psychological Science, 23*(8), 914–922.

Morgan, P. L., Farkas, G., Hillemeier, M. M., Mattison, R., Maczuga, S., Li, H., et al. (2015). Minorities are disproportionately underrepresented in special education: Longitudinal evidence across five disability conditions. *Educational Researcher, 44*(5), 278–292.

Morgan, P. L., Li, H., Farkas, G., Cook, M., Pun, W. H., & Hillemeier, M. M. (2017). Executive functioning deficits increase kindergarten children's risk for reading and mathematics difficulties in first grade. *Contemporary Educational Psychology, 50*, 23–32.

Moyer, R. S., & Landauer, T. K. (1967). Time required for judgements of numerical inequality. *Nature, 215*(5109), 1519–1520.

Mussolin, C., De Volder, A., Grandin, C., Schlögel, X., Nassogne, M. C., & Noël, M. P. (2010). Neural correlates of symbolic number comparison in developmental dyscalculia. *Journal of Cognitive Neuroscience, 22*(5), 860–874.

Nation, K., Marshall, C. M., & Snowling, M. J. (2001). Phonological and semantic contributions to children's picture naming skill: Evidence from children with developmental reading disorders. *Language and Cognitive Processes, 16*(2–3), 241–259.

Nation, K., & Snowling, M. J. (1997). Assessing reading difficulties: The validity and utility of current measures of reading skill. *British Journal of Educational Psychology, 67*(3), 359–370.

Nation, K., & Snowling, M. J. (1998). Semantic processing and the development of word-recognition skills: Evidence from children with reading comprehension difficulties. *Journal of Memory and Language, 39*(1), 85–101.

Norton, E. S., Beach, S. D., & Gabrieli, J. D. (2015). Neurobiology of dyslexia. *Current Opinion in Neurobiology, 30*, 73–78.

Oakhill, J. V., & Cain, K. (2000). Children's difficulties in text comprehension: Assessing causal issues. *Journal of Deaf Studies and Deaf Education, 5*(1), 51–59.

Oakhill, J. V., & Cain, K. (2012). The precursors of reading ability in young readers: Evidence from a four-year longitudinal study. *Scientific Studies of Reading, 16*(2), 91–121.

Oakhill, J. V., Hartt, J., & Samols, D. (2005). Levels of comprehension monitoring and working memory in good and poor comprehenders. *Reading and Writing, 18*, 657–686.

Oakhill, J. V., Yuill, N., & Parkin, A. (1986). On the nature of the difference between skilled and less-skilled comprehenders. *Journal of Research in Reading, 9*(2), 80–91.

Ostad, S. A. (1997). Developmental differences in addition strategies: A comparison of mathematically disabled and mathematically normal children. *The British Journal of Educational Psychology, 67(Pt. 3)*, 345–357.

Pammer, K., Hansen, P. C., Kringelbach, M. L., Holliday, I., Barnes, G., Hillebrand, A., et al. (2004). Visual word recognition: The first half second. *NeuroImage, 22*(4), 1819–1825.

Park, J., Li, R., & Brannon, E. M. (2014). Neural connectivity patterns underlying symbolic number processing indicate mathematical achievement in children. *Developmental Science, 17*(2), 187–202.

Parsons, S., & Bynner, J. (2005). *Does numeracy matter more?* National Research and Development Centre for Adult Literacy and Numeracy.

Perfetti, C. A. (1999). Comprehending written language: A blueprint of the reader. In C. Brown & P. Hagoort (Eds.), *The neurocognition of language* (pp. 167–208). Oxford University Press.

Pinel, P., Dehaene, S., Rivière, D., & LeBihan, D. (2001). Modulation of parietal activation by semantic distance in a number comparison task. *NeuroImage, 14*(5), 1013–1026.

Pinel, P., Le Clec, H. G., Van De Moortele, P. F., Naccache, L., Le Bihan, D., & Dehaene, S. (1999). Event-related fMRI analysis of the cerebral circuit for number comparison. *NeuroReport, 10*(7), 1473–1479.

Poldrack, R. A., Wagner, A. D., Prull, M. W., Desmond, J. E., Glover, G. H., & Gabrieli, J. D. (1999). Functional specialization for semantic and phonological processing in the left inferior prefrontal cortex. *NeuroImage, 10*(1), 15–35.

Price, C. J. (2012). A review and synthesis of the first 20 years of PET and fMRI studies of heard speech, spoken language and reading. *NeuroImage, 62*(2), 816–847.

Price, C. J., Moore, C. J., Humphreys, G. W., Frackowiak, R. S. J., & Friston, K. J. (1996). The neural regions sustaining object recognition and naming. *Proceedings of the Royal Society of London. Series B: Biological Sciences, 263*(1376), 1501–1507.

Price, G. R., & Ansari, D. (2011). Symbol processing in the left angular gyrus: Evidence from passive perception of digits. *NeuroImage, 57*(3), 1205–1211.

Price, G. R., & Ansari, D. (2013). Developmental dyscalculia. *Handbook of Clinical Neurology, 111*, 241–244.

Price, G. R., Holloway, I., Räsänen, P., Vesterinen, M., & Ansari, D. (2007). Impaired parietal magnitude processing in developmental dyscalculia. *Current Biology, 17*(24), R1042–R1043.

Price, G. R., & Wilkey, E. D. (2017). Cognitive mechanisms underlying the relation between nonsymbolic and symbolic magnitude processing and their relation to math. *Cognitive Development, 44*, 139–149.

Protopapas, A., Simos, P. G., Sideridis, G. D., & Mouzaki, A. (2012). The components of the simple view of reading: A confirmatory factor analysis. *Reading Psychology, 33*(3), 217–240.

Pugh, K. R., Frost, S. J., Sandak, R., Landi, N., Rueckl, J. G., Constable, R. T., et al. (2008). Effects of stimulus difficulty and repetition on printed word identification: An fMRI comparison of nonimpaired and reading-disabled adolescent cohorts. *Journal of Cognitive Neuroscience, 20*(7), 1146–1160.

Pugh, K. R., Mencl, W. E., Jenner, A. R., Katz, L., Frost, S. J., Lee, J. R., et al. (2001). Neurobiological studies of reading and reading disability. *Journal of Communication Disorders, 34*(6), 479–492.

Richlan, F. (2012). Developmental dyslexia: Dysfunction of a left hemisphere reading network. *Frontiers in Human Neuroscience, 6*, 120.

Richlan, F., Kronbichler, M., & Wimmer, H. (2009). Functional abnormalities in the dyslexic brain: A quantitative meta-analysis of neuroimaging studies. *Human Brain Mapping, 30*(10), 3299–3308.

Rimrodt, S. L., Peterson, D. J., Denckla, M. B., Kaufmann, W. E., & Cutting, L. E. (2010).

White matter microstructural differences linked to left perisylvian language network in children with dyslexia. *Cortex, 46*(6), 739–749.

Ritchie, S. J., & Bates, T. C. (2013). Enduring links from childhood mathematics and reading achievement to adult socioeconomic status. *Psychological Science, 24*(7), 1301–1308.

Robertson, D. A., Gernsbacher, M. A., Guidotti, S. J., Robertson, R. R., Irwin, W., Mock, B. J., et al. (2000). Functional neuroanatomy of the cognitive process of mapping during discourse comprehension. *Psychological Science, 11*(3), 255–260.

Robinson, C. S., Menchetti, B. M., & Torgesen, J. K. (2002). Toward a two-factor theory of one type of mathematics disabilities. *Learning Disabilities Research & Practice, 17*(2), 81–89.

Roe, M. A., Martinez, J. E., Mumford, J. A., Taylor, W. P., Cirino, P. T., Fletcher, J. M., et al. (2018). Control engagement during sentence and inhibition fMRI tasks in children with reading difficulties. *Cerebral Cortex, 28*(10), 3697–3710.

Ryherd, K., Jasinska, K., Van Dyke, J. A., Hung, Y. H., Baron, E., Mencl, W. E., et al. (2018). Cortical regions supporting reading comprehension skill for single words and discourse. *Brain and Language, 186*, 32–43.

Sabatini, J. P., Sawaki, Y., Shore, J. R., & Scarborough, H. S. (2010). Relationships among reading skills of adults with low literacy. *Journal of Learning Disabilities, 43*(2), 122–138.

Schmithorst, V. J., Holland, S. K., & Plante, E. (2006). Cognitive modules utilized for narrative comprehension in children: A functional magnetic resonance imaging study. *NeuroImage, 29*(1), 254–266.

Shalev, R. S., Auerbach, J., Manor, O., & Gross-Tsur, V. (2000). Developmental dyscalculia: Prevalence and prognosis. *European Child & Adolescent Psychiatry, 9*(Suppl. 2), II58–II64.

Shankweiler, D., Lundquist, E., Katz, L., Stuebing, K. K., Fletcher, J. M., Brady, S., et al. (1999). Comprehension and decoding: Patterns of association in children with r7eading difficulties. *Scientific Studies of Reading, 3*(1), 69–94.

Shaywitz, S. E. (2003). *Overcoming dyslexia: A new and complete science-based program of reading problems at any level.* Knopf.

Shaywitz, S. E., Escobar, M. D., Shaywitz, B. A., Fletcher, J. M., & Makuch, R. (1992). Evidence that dyslexia may represent the lower tail of a normal distribution of reading ability. *The New England Journal of Medicine, 326*(3), 145–150.

Shaywitz, S. E., Shaywitz, B. A., Pugh, K. R., Fulbright, R. K., Constable, R. T., Mencl, W. E., et al. (1998). Functional disruption in the organization of the brain for reading in dyslexia. *Proceedings of the National Academy of Sciences of the United States of America, 95*(5), 2636–2641.

Sheuermann, F., & Pedró, F. (Eds.). (2010). Assessing the effects of ICT in education indicators, criteria and benchmarks for international comparisons: Indicators, criteria and benchmarks for international comparisons. *Centre for Educational Research and Innovation* (pp. 21–38). OECD Publishing.

Shum, J., Hermes, D., Foster, B. L., Dastjerdi, M., Rangarajan, V., Winawer, J., et al. (2013). A brain area for visual numerals. *Journal of Neuroscience: The Official Journal of the Society for Neuroscience, 33*(16), 6709–6715.

Siemann, J., & Petermann, F. (2018). Innate or acquired? Disentangling number sense and early number competencies. *Frontiers in Psychology, 9*, 571.

Skagenholt, M., Träff, U., Västfjäll, D., & Skagerlund, K. (2018). Examining the triple code model in numerical cognition: An fMRI study. *PLOS ONE, 13*(6), e0199247.

Snowling, M. J., & Melby-Lervåg, M. (2016). Oral language deficits in familial dyslexia: A meta-analysis and review. *Psychological Bulletin, 142*(5), 498–545.

Soares, N., Evans, T., & Patel, D. R. (2018). Specific learning disability in mathematics: A comprehensive review. *Translational Pediatrics, 7*(1), 48–62.

Spencer, M., Quinn, J. M., & Wagner, R. K. (2014). Specific Reading Comprehension Disability:

Major problem, myth, or misnomer? *Learning Disabilities Research & Practice: A Publication of the Division for Learning Disabilities, Council for Exceptional Children, 29*(1), 3–9.

Spencer, M., & Wagner, R. K. (2018). The comprehension problems of children with poor reading comprehension despite adequate decoding: A meta-analysis. *Review of Educational Research, 88*(3), 366–400.

Steen, L. (1999). Numeracy: The new literacy for a data-drenched society. *Educational Leadership, 57*, 8–13.

Stothard, S. E., & Hulme, C. (1995). A comparison of phonological skills in children with reading comprehension difficulties and children with decoding difficulties. *Child Psychology & Psychiatry & Allied Disciplines, 36*(3), 399–408.

Swanson, H. L., & Jerman, O. (2006). Math disabilities: A selective meta-analysis of the literature. *Review of Educational Research, 76*(2), 249–274.

Swanson, H. L., Zheng, X., & Jerman, O. (2009). Working memory, short-term memory, and reading disabilities: A selective meta-analysis of the literature. *Journal of Learning Disabilities, 42*(3), 260–287.

Tam, Y. P., Wong, T. T., & Chan, W. W. L. (2019). The relation between spatial skills and mathematical abilities: The mediating role of mental number line representation. *Contemporary Educational Psychology, 56*, 14–24.

Temple, E., Poldrack, R. A., Salidis, J., Deutsch, G. K., Tallal, P., Merzenich, M. M., et al. (2001). Disrupted neural responses to phonological and orthographic processing in dyslexic children: An fMRI study. *NeuroReport, 12*(2), 299–307.

Tong, X., Deacon, S. H., & Cain, K. (2014). Morphological and syntactic awareness in poor comprehenders another piece of the puzzle. *Journal of Learning Disabilities, 47*, 22–33.

Ullman, M. T. (2004). Contributions of memory circuits to language: The declarative/procedural model. *Cognition, 92*, 231–270.

Van den Broek, P., Young, M., Tzeng, Y., & Linderholm, T. (1999). The Landscape model of reading: Inferences and the online construction of memory representation. In H. Van Oostendorp & S. R. Goldman (Eds.), *The construction of mental representations during reading* (pp. 71–98). Lawrence Erlbaum Associates.

Vellutino, F. R., Tunmer, W. E., Jaccard, J. J., & Chen, R. (2007). Components of reading ability: Multivariate evidence for a convergent skills model of reading development. *Scientific Studies of Reading, 11*(1), 3–32.

Vinckier, F., Dehaene, S., Jobert, A., Dubus, J. P., Sigman, M., & Cohen, L. (2007). Hierarchical coding of letter strings in the ventral stream: Dissecting the inner organization of the visual word-form system. *Neuron, 55*(1), 143–156.

von Aster, M. G., & Shalev, R. S. (2007). Number development and developmental dyscalculia. *Developmental Medicine and Child Neurology, 49*(11), 868–873.

Vuilleumier, P., Ortigue, S., & Brugger, P. (2004). The number space and neglect. *Cortex: A Journal Devoted to the Study of the Nervous System and Behavior, 40*(2), 399–410.

Wagner, R. K., & Torgesen, J. K. (1987). The nature of phonological processing and its causal role in the acquisition of reading skills. *Psychological Bulletin, 101*(2), 192–212.

Waldie, K. E. (2002). Reading with the right hemisphere: From normal development to dysphonetic dyslexia. In S. P. Shohov (Ed.), *Advances in psychology research* (pp. 157–183). Nova Science.

Waldie, K. E., Haigh, C., Badzakova-Trajkov, G., Buckley, J., & Kirk, I. (2013). Reading the wrong way with the right hemisphere. *Brain Sciences, 3*(4), 1060–1075.

Walenski, M., Europa, E., Caplan, D., & Thompson, C. K. (2019). Neural networks for sentence comprehension and production: An ALE-based meta-analysis of neuroimaging studies. *Human Brain Mapping, 40*(8), 2275–2304.

Wang, K., Banich, M. T., Reineberg, A. E., Leopold, D. R., Willcutt, E. G., Cutting, L. E., et al. (2020). Left posterior prefrontal regions support domain-general executive processes needed for both reading and math. *Journal of Neuropsychology, 14*(3), 467–495.

What Works Clearinghouse. Institute of Education Sciences. *https://ies.ed.gov/ncee/wwc.*

Wilkey, E. D., Barone, J. C., Mazzocco, M. M. M., Vogel, S. E., & Price, G. R. (2017). The effect of visual parameters on neural activation during nonsymbolic number comparison and its relation to math competency. *NeuroImage, 159*, 430–442.

Wilkey, E. D., Pollack, C., & Price, G. R. (2020). Dyscalculia and typical math achievement are associated with individual differences in number-specific executive function. *Child Development, 91*(2), 596–619.

Wilkey, E. D., & Price, G. R. (2019). Attention to number: The convergence of numerical magnitude processing, attention, and mathematics in the inferior frontal gyrus. *Human Brain Mapping, 40*(3), 928–943.

Willcutt, E. G., & Pennington, B. F. (2000). Psychiatric comorbidity in children and adolescents with reading disability. *Journal of Child Psychology and Psychiatry, 41*(8), 1039–1048.

Wilson, A. J., & Dehaene, S. (2007). Number sense and developmental dyscalculia. In D. Coch, G. Dawson, & K. W. Fischer (Eds.), *Human behavior, learning, and the developing brain: Atypical development* (pp. 212–238). Guilford Press.

Wimmer, H., Schurz, M., Sturm, D., Richlan, F., Klackl, J., Kronbichler, M., et al. (2010). A dual-route perspective on poor reading in a regular orthography: An fMRI study. *Cortex, 46*(10), 1284–1298.

Yang, X., Li, H., Lin, N., Zhang, X., Wang, Y., Zhang, Y., et al. (2019). Uncovering cortical activations of discourse comprehension and their overlaps with common large-scale neural networks. *NeuroImage, 203*, 116200.

Yarkoni, T., Poldrack, R. A., Nichols, T. E., Van Essen, D. C., & Wager, T. D. (2011). Large-scale automated synthesis of human functional neuroimaging data. *Nature Methods, 8*(8), 665–670.

Yeniad, N., Malda, M., Mesman, J., Van IJzendoorn, M. H., & Pieper, S. (2013). Shifting ability predicts math and reading performance in children: A meta-analytical study. *Learning and Individual Differences, 23*, 1–9.

Yeo, D. J., Wilkey, E. D., & Price, G. R. (2017). The search for the number form area: A functional neuroimaging meta-analysis. *Neuroscience and Biobehavioral Reviews, 78*, 145–160.

Yuill, N., & Oakhill, J. V. (1991). *Children's problems in text comprehension: An experimental investigation.* Cambridge University.

CHAPTER 6

Genetics, Learning Abilities, and Disabilities

Stephen A. Petrill and Alexa Levison

Decades of quantitative genetic research using twin and adoption designs have convincingly shown that learning disabilities, such as reading disability, math disability, and language impairment, demonstrate significant heritability, substantial genetic stability across time, and significant genetic overlap across traits (e.g., Daucourt et al., 2020; Plomin et al., 2016). For the past 20 years, molecular genetic research has developed increasingly replicable DNA-based models of learning disabilities (e.g., Doust et al., 2021; Gialluisi et al., 2021; Andres et al., 2020). These efforts have more recently been integrated with plausible models linking genes, brain, and behavior (e.g., Centanni, 2020; Thomas et al., 2021). Alongside these findings, a robust discussion has emerged concerning the present utility of genetically sensitive studies in the identification, prevention, and treatment of learning disabilities in education. Some have begun to examine the utility and dangers of using genetic information as part of educational practice (e.g., Asbury & Plomin, 2013; Shero et al., 2021; Harden, 2021; Martschenko et al., 2019; Martschenko & Smith, 2021).

This chapter discusses the genetics of learning disabilities in the following ways. First, the chapter summarizes and integrates quantitative and molecular genetic studies of learning disabilities. Second, the chapter presents the methods employed in these approaches, analyzing their strengths and weaknesses. Third, the issue of using genetics in educational decision making is discussed. Finally, possible pathways for advancing basic and applied genetic studies on learning disabilities are proposed. Throughout, the chapter focuses primarily on reading ability and disability, drawing additional examples from mathematics, attention-deficit/hyperactivity disorder (ADHD), and language disability.

Overview of Genetic Models

Genes are stretches of DNA located throughout the genome. Some genes code for protein products that constitute or impact cellular functions, whereas other genes moderate the function or production of proteins. Genes can have different forms or variants (each called an allele) at particular places (loci) on the genome. Some of these alleles impact individual differences in learning disability, along with environmental variation (see Knopik et al., 2017). Others impact multiple traits of interest (pleiotropy), while most genetic variants have no known function and may have no consequences. Genes are dynamically expressed and turn on and turn off as a function of development, the regulation of biological function, and the response to the environment (collectively called *gene expression*). Table 6.1 presents a glossary of definitions and terms that will be used throughout the chapter.

Genetic variation is distributed across two dimensions: (1) *effect size*—how much variance a given allele from a particular gene accounts for in a measured trait and (2) *frequency*—how often a given allele from that gene is found in a population (see Figure 6.1). At one end of the continuum, the one gene–one disorder (OGOD) model explains situations where alleles at a gene or small set of genes are large in effect size but rare. The genes responsible for conditions that fall into the OGOD model are both necessary and sufficient for diagnosis. Down syndrome, also called trisomy 21 (three copies of chromosome 21), Prader–Willi syndrome (deletion of genes on chromosome 15), and Williams syndrome (deletion of genes on chromosome 7) are all examples associated with the OGOD model that impact intellectual disability and, hence, downstream to learning disabilities (see Knopik et al., 2017). At the other end of the continuum, the common disease–common variant (CDCV) model suggests that diseases and disorders are not etiologically distinct from the rest of the population. Instead, conditions such as learning disabilities constitute the lower tail of the overall distribution of learning skills, or a threshold of negatively modulating variants was reached in order to present with clinical symptoms. In this situation, a large set of genes is necessarily operative, with alleles within those genes individually contributing very small amounts of variance (see Manolio et al., 2009). These genetic risk and protective factors act together, along with the environment, across the distribution. For traits such as learning disabilities, the assumption has been that most genetic variance in the population arises from the CDCV model, with some rare/severe cases emanating from the OGOD model. That said, as indicated by the oval in Figure 6.1 (p. 132), there may also be genes of lower frequency and moderate effect size that are operative.

Quantitative Genetic Studies of Learning Disabilities

Figure 6.2 (p. 133) presents the relations among the varying genetically sensitive designs that have been employed in the field of learning disabilities. Figure 6.2 also

TABLE 6.1. Terms and Definitions

Term	Definition
Alleles	Different variations of a gene that can be measured at a given place on the genome.
Association study	Examines whether DNA markers correlate with the differences between groups selected for absence of presence of a trait and/or individual differences in a trait. Employs unrelated individuals. Best suited for the CDCV model.
Candidate gene	A gene hypothesized as influencing a particular trait based on its function or position in the genome.
Common disease common variant model	Also called the *quantitative trait locus hypothesis.* Holds when genetic effects are small in effect size and are noncausal. Genetic factors operate as probabilistically as risk/protective factors.
Dizyogotic twin	Fraternal twins. Share 50% of genes inherited from parents (on average). Full siblings from a genetic perspective.
DNA marker	A stretch of DNA at a particular location that varies between persons. DNA markers can be within a candidate gene or may be a stretch of DNA that is close to/co-inherited with a candidate gene.
G × E Interaction	Gene × environment interaction. Heritability on a trait or set of traits is moderated by a measure of the environment. This will be reflected by higher/lower levels of heritability depending on level of the environment.
Gene–environment correlation	Genetic factors increase or decrease the probability of exposure to an environment. There are three types of G–E correlation: active = genetic factors on a trait are associated with the seeking out of environments; reactive = genetic factors on a trait are associated with others providing environments; passive = genetic factors contribute to the correlation between a trait and an environment as a "third variable."
Gene expression	The extent to which a gene is "on," that is, production of RNA being made that can influence other genes or be used in the production of proteins.
GCTA	Genomewide complex trait analysis. Unlike twin and adoption designs that infer genetic resemblance from familial relationships alone, GCTA uses measured genetic resemblance between unrelated individuals to estimate heritability.
GWAS	Genomewide association study. An association study performed systematically across the entire genome.
Heritability (h^2)	Ref. The proportion of variance in a trait that is due to genetic differences.

(continued)

TABLE 6.1. *(continued)*

Term	Definition
Linkage design	Examines the co-inheritance of DNA markers and measured traits within a pedigree of genetically related family members. Best suited for the OGOD model.
Locus	Particular location on the genome.
Monozygotic twin	Identical twins, who share 100% of the genes inherited from parents.
Multivariate quantitative genetics	Examines the genetic and environmental contribution to the covariance among a set of measures. This approach can address a broad range of questions, such as the relationship between variables at a given time point, as well as longitudinally across time points.
Nonshared environment (e^2)	Environments that make family members different from one another.
OGOD model	Also called the *one gene–one disorder hypothesis*. Genes are causal but are also rare.
Phenotype	Observed trait. Can be behavioral, neurobiological, metabolic, or any other outcome that can be measured.
Polygenetic risk score	Using genomewide SNP data or whole genome sequencing, identified genomic differences across multiple genes are combined to yield an overall measure of risk.
Polymorphism	Differences in DNA between persons at a particular location in the genome that may affect differences in outcomes.
Shared environment (c^2)	Also called *common environment*. Any experience that makes family members similar (same prenatal environment, same school, same parents, etc.).
SNP-based heritability	The proportion of variance in a trait that is explained by measured genetic differences using (common) SNP variants.
Quantile regression	One of a set of approaches used to examine whether genetic, shared environmental, and nonshared environmental factors are higher or lower depending on level of ability/skill/performance. DeFries–Fulker and liability threshold approaches have also been employed to address this general question.
Univariate quantitative genetics	Examines the genetic, shared environmental, and nonshared environmental contribution to variance on a single variable.

forms the framework of the discussion of genetics, genetically sensitive designs, and learning disabilities going forward. The largest triangle in Figure 6.2 refers to the total variance in the population. Inside that triangle, twin designs, adoption designs, and other quantitative genetic methods leverage the differences in genetic relatedness among family members. Identical (MZ) twins, for example, share 100% of the same genes inherited by their parents, whereas fraternal (DZ) twins share 50% of the same genes, on average. In a twin study, heritability (h^2, or the proportion of variance due to genetics) is inferred if identical twins are more similar in a trait than fraternal twins. In an adoption study, heritability is inferred if biological siblings are more similar than adoptive siblings or biological parent–child relationships are more similar than adoptive parent–child relationships. Quantitative genetic methods can also estimate shared environment (c^2) when family members experiencing the same environment are similar, irrespective of their genetic relationships. Finally, nonshared environment (e^2), which includes measurement error, is inferred when identical twins are different from one another.

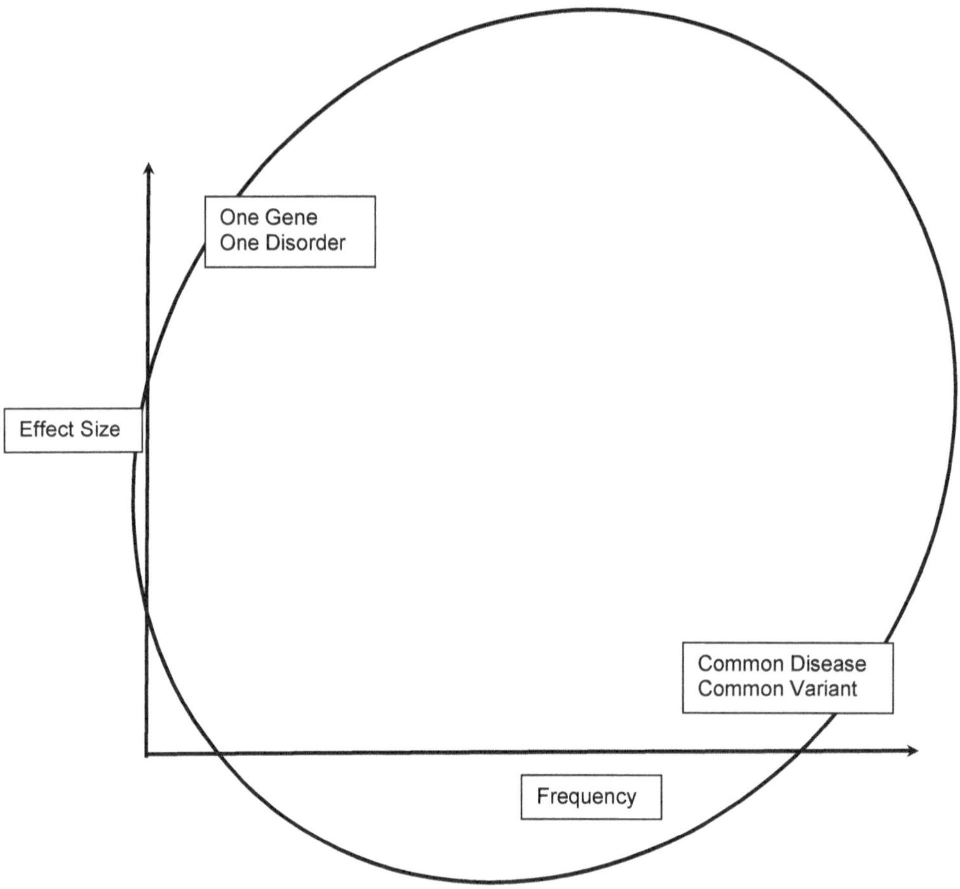

FIGURE 6.1. Genetic influences on behavior vary by frequency and effect size.

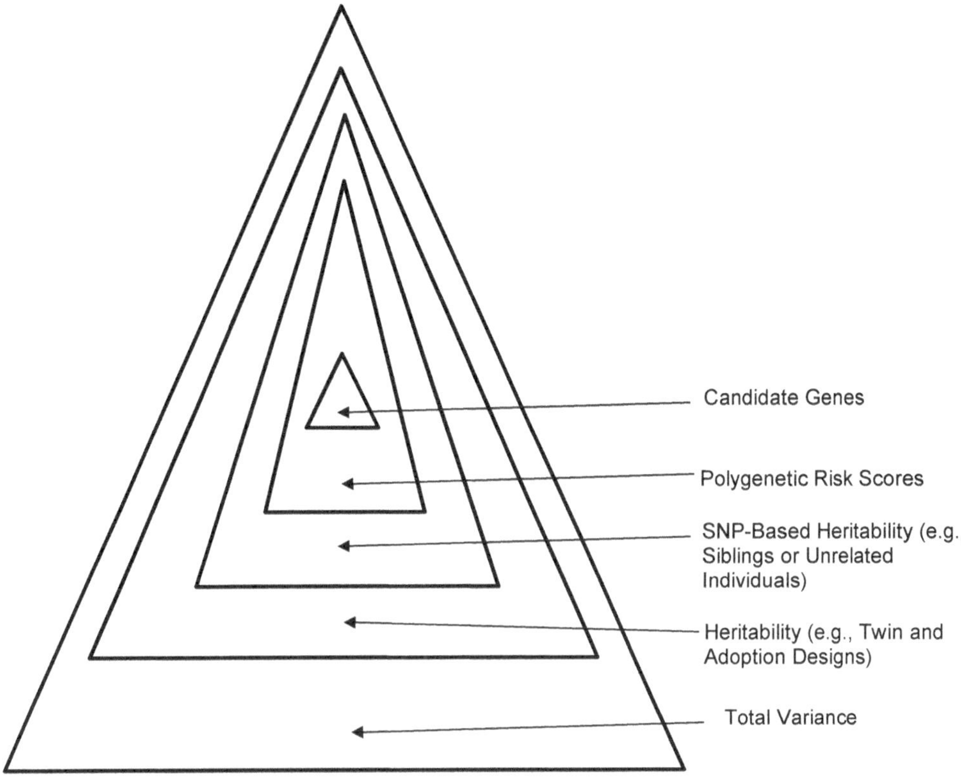

FIGURE 6.2. Variance accounted for by various genetic designs employed to examine learning disabilities.

Univariate Quantitative Genetic Studies

The most basic question addressed by quantitative genetics is the extent to which genetic, shared environmental, and nonshared environmental factors impact outcomes associated with learning disability. For example, Adrcola ct al. (2021) presented a meta-analysis of 49 twin studies, representing 38,000 individuals ranging in age from 4 to 18 years of age. Their results suggested that the overall heritability of general reading was h^2 = .66, with c^2 = .13 and e^2 = .21. In other words, two-thirds of the variance in general reading can be accounted for by genetic differences. Nonshared environment accounted for 13% of the variance. Finally, 21% of the variance was due to nonshared environment + error, with evidence for increasing heritability at higher ages. Significant heritability was also found for components of reading, such as letter word knowledge, phonological decoding, phonological awareness, spelling, rapid automatized naming, and language. Significant shared environmental effects were found for all components except for spelling. Nonshared environment was significant in all variables. These findings are consistent with decades of quantitative genetic studies of reading and related cognition, such as language and mathematics (see de Zeeuw et al., 2015; Rice et al., 2020; Little et al., 2017). The reading findings are therefore unsurprising given the overall significance of genetic factors generally across a wide range of complex human traits (see Harden 2021).

Multivariate Genetic Studies

This univariate approach has been extended using structural equation modeling to examine multivariate sets of outcomes within twin and adoption designs (beginning with Martin & Eaves, 1977). Using this general approach, it becomes possible to examine the extent to which genetic and environmental factors contribute to the covariance among a set of variables. For example, if the covariance between early language in twin 1 and later reading in twin 2 is higher in identical versus fraternal twins, then genetic factors are significant. Conversely, if the covariance between early language in twin 1 and reading in twin 2 is significant but similar in identical and fraternal twins, then shared environmental influences are inferred. If the covariance between twin 1 early language and twin 1 reading is significant but there is no significant covariance with twin 2, then nonshared environmental factors are inferred.

Daucourt et al. (2020) examined 38 multivariate twin studies of reading, mathematics, and ADHD, finding that domain-general genetic factors support the covariance between reading and mathematics, but not necessarily the covariance between reading and ADHD. This work builds on a long-standing literature suggesting that genetic effects, particularly for reading, math, and language, tend to be generalist (Plomin & Kovas, 2005; Hart et al., 2009; see Grigorenko et al., 2020, for a more recent discussion). Similar results have been obtained with respect to longitudinal quantitative genetic studies. For example, in our own work (Soden et al., 2015), we examined the longitudinal stability of reading comprehension in two twin studies: our own Western Reserve Reading and Math Project (WRRMP) and the U.S. sample of the Colorado International Twin Study (ILTS). Reading comprehension was assessed in grades 1–6 in WWRMP and grades 1, 2, and 4 in ILTS. Results suggested that the longitudinal stability of reading comprehension was completely accounted for by shared genetic factors. These findings are consistent with other studies (e.g., Harlaar et al., 2007; Oliver et al., 2007; Greven et al., 2012; Christopher et al., 2015).

Thus, alongside the substantial average growth in reading skills due to formal and non-formal instruction, there are wide individual differences at any given time point in the development of learning skills. These individual differences are correlated with one another across longitudinal time points. The correlation is influenced largely by genetics, suggesting a core of genetically influenced individual differences that span the wide longitudinal period of reading growth. On the other hand, children move up or down on the distribution of learning skills relative to their peers over time, and this instability appears to be largely due to the environment.

Quantitative Genetic Studies of Low versus Typically Developing Ability

The studies described earlier examine the genetic and environmental contributions to learning skills across the entire range of ability. However, genetic and/or environmental influences may be higher or lower at the extremes of ability. Additional genes may be operative at the extremes, increasing heritability. Conversely, extreme environments may overshadow genetic differences, increasing shared or nonshared environments. As discussed more fully in Logan et al. (2012), several statistical approaches have been employed, including liability threshold models (Gottesman & Shields, 1979), DeFries–Fulker analysis (DeFries & Fulker, 1985, 1988; LaBuda et al., 1990; Cherny et al., 1992), and quantile regression (Logan et al., 2012). For example, Plomin and Kovas (2005) examine the etiology of low language, reading, and mathematics performance as compared to the unselected range of ability. In all three traits, the heritability at the end was not only significant but similar in magnitude to the heritability across the entire range of ability.

In our own work (Logan et al., 2012), we developed an application of quantile regression to address the question of which simultaneously estimates effects at separate points across the distribution. This method offers not only more precise statistical estimates than subgroup analyses since it estimates all parameters using all the data, while subgroups are always less than the total dataset. This method has been employed not only in quantitative genetic studies but also in learning disabilities research more broadly (see Petscher & Logan, 2014).

Using this approach, we examined whether multivariate genetic and environmental relations vary as a function of performance level. In particular, Shero et al. (2021) built on Daucourt's (2020) meta-analysis described earlier. Multivariate quantile regression was employed to examine the genetic and environmental contributions to the correlation between ADHD and reading comprehension. At issue was whether the relative importance of genetics and environment varied depending on whether ADHD and/or reading comprehension was low or high. Using data from the Florida Twin Project, the Colorado International Longitudinal Twin Study, and the Western Reserve Reading and Math Projects, Shero et al. (2021) found that shared environment effects were more important in explaining the correlation between ADHD and reading comprehension at lower quantiles. This suggests that either genetic effects are suppressed or that additional shared environmental influences emerge at the lower end of performance.

Quantitative Genetics and Measured Environments

The approaches described earlier estimate shared and nonshared environments at a statistical factorial level. Another set of approaches has examined measures of the environment directly. For example, van Bergen et al. (2018) examined the etiology of the relationship between print exposure and reading in a sample of n = 11,559 twins aged 7.5, drawn from the Netherlands Twin Register. They found reading ability led to higher levels of print exposure. Moreover, identical twins were more similar than fraternal twins with respect to the correlation between reading and print exposure, suggesting genetic influences related to reading are largely responsible for the correlation between reading and print exposure. These findings suggest that gene–environment correlation was operative: (1) identical twins may have more similarly sought out higher levels of print exposure (active gene–environment correlation), (2) others in the environment (parents/teachers) may have reacted to the identical twins' genetically driven similarity in reading with more similar print exposure (evocative gene–environment correlation), and/or (3) genes may generally increase or lower the level of both reading and print exposure (passive gene–environment correlation).

An important take-home message of this work is that the high heritability for reading and other learning-related outcomes likely involves both direct effects (e.g., genetic factors directly impacting individual differences in brain development) and indirect effects (e.g., genetic factors that increase or decrease the probability of coming into contact with environments that affect reading). Most twin and adoption studies are based on sibling correlations that cannot parse out direct and indirect effects due to gene–environment correlation (see Pittner et al., 2019, from the parenting literature, which uses designs that can). Significant and high heritability and significant genetic stability are not determinative or immutable. Instead, they contain environmental factors that may be yoked to genetic variance, but those tendencies to experience certain environments can be disrupted, enhanced, or redirected through intervention.

Moreover, as described more fully by Selita and Kovas (2019), gene × environment effects have also been indicated for learning disabilities. In this case, genetic factors may be higher or lower as a function of environmental moderation. In general, heritability is higher for educational outcomes in higher SES versus lower SES groups. This is consistent with the larger cognitive literature (e.g., Giangrande & Turkheimer, 2022; Tucker-Drob & Bates, 2016), suggesting that heritability may be higher at the high end of SES and lower at the lower end of SES. Economic advantage may increase the impact of the evocative and active gene–environment effects described earlier because children from advantaged environments have a higher ceiling in terms of supportive, self-directed, and personalized environments. These personalized and self-directed opportunities can move the higher-performing children to even greater performance but may also more effectively attend to the needs of lower-performing individuals as well. Conversely, these personalized and self-directed environmental factors may be less available to children from lower SES backgrounds, which will reduce the impact of evocative and active gene–environment effects, depressing heritability. These kinds of possibilities are poorly understood and offer important opportunities to understand the contexts in which supportive and unsupportive educational environments may be unequally applied in the context of genetic risk and protective factors for learning disabilities.

In summary, quantitative genetic studies of reading and other learning-related outcomes suggest that genetic effects are significant; they account for the relations among reading, math, language, and, to a lesser extent, ADHD. Moreover, genetic effects are significant longitudinally. Shared environmental effects, although significant, tend to attenuate with development. Genetic effects are also significant in measures of the environment and between measures of the environment and learning outcomes (see Olson et al., 2019, for another recent discussion). That said, there is also evidence to suggest that genetic effects are lower at the lower end of ability (especially for reading and measures of general cognitive ability) and in lower SES. Shared environmental factors seem to be more important early in the development of reading and math, at the lower end of ability, and at the lower end of SES.

Taken together, quantitative genetic studies have done much to demonstrate the importance of genetic influences in learning and learning disabilities. Quantitative genetics has also delineated how genetic and environmental influences impact concurrent and longitudinal models of the constructs important to learning disabilities and their development. Twin and adoption studies have also afforded better models of the environment: those that vary between families (shared environment) and those that vary within families (nonshared environment). Quantitative genetics has also helped illuminate how levels of the environment moderate the importance of genetic influences. Finally, like other literatures, quantitative genetics has begun to make good use of meta-analysis and simultaneous analysis of primary datasets to allow for better-tested and more generalizable findings.

However, there are aspects of quantitative genetic studies that limit their utility in the study of learning disabilities and educational outcomes. First, quantitative genetic studies rely on special populations that incur assumptions such as the equal environments assumption in twins or the unselected placement assumption in adoption studies. More importantly, quantitative genetic studies do not identify the genes that account for the genetic variance being estimated. As a result, quantitative genetic studies do not shed light on the bioinformatics of the genetic influence of (neuro)biological pathways: they cannot directly test genetic models presented in Figure 6.1; nor can they yield genetic markers of risk and resilience that may be usable in the prevention, identification, and treatment of learning disabilities.

Molecular Genetic Studies of Learning Disabilities

Whereas quantitative genetic studies indirectly estimate genetic, shared environmental, and nonshared environmental factors on constructs or sets of constructs, molecular genetic studies directly examine the impact of measured DNA differences, individually or *en masse*, on complex human traits. Molecular genetic efforts have grown up alongside quantitative genetic studies of learning abilities and disabilities described earlier (see Smith et al., 1983; Plomin et al., 1994; Morris et al., 2000; Stromswold, 2001, for examples of earlier studies). Up until the Human Genome Project released the first reference sequence of the human genome in 2003, efforts to examine the impact of differences in DNA polymorphisms on human traits were hampered by several limitations. There were relatively few DNA markers to measure differences in the human genome, the cost to genotype was high, both in terms of money and time, and the statistical tools to analyze the data were less developed by today's standards. Returning to Figure 6.2, molecular genetic research prior to 2003 was focused almost exclusively on finding candidate genes (defined as a gene that varies in the population that was hypothesized to impact differences in measured outcomes). Moreover, at that time, the number of candidate genes and statistical methodologies available restricted the search for genetic markers to the extremes of the OGOD and CDCV models presented in Figure 6.1. In the case of the OGOD model, researchers would employ the linkage design, which involves comparison of genetically related family members in multigenerational pedigrees. Linkage is implied to the extent that the DNA markers (defined as the candidate gene itself of a stretch of DNA close to that gene) were inherited in members of the same family pedigree alongside the inheritance of the trait of study. In the case of the CDCV model, researchers employed the association design, which involved unrelated individuals selected into groups based on the presence or absence of a trait. Association is implied to the extent that DNA markers explained a portion of the difference between the groups. Combining across these approaches, replicated candidate genes for dyslexia were identified on chromosomes 15, 6, and 3, with potential findings at chromosomes 2, 18, 11, 1, and X (see Paracchini et al., 2007; Paracchini et al., 2016). Consistent with the CDCV model, the regions identified at that time individually accounted for a very small proportion of the heritability of dyslexia and an even smaller proportion of the variance in dyslexia overall.

These initial efforts have been transformed by what has been called the "postgenomic era," which was ushered in by the completion of the first reference sequence of the human genome in 2003. Because the human genome has been fully sequenced now in many more individuals from across the globe, it is now possible to identify the regions on the genome that vary and their frequency across the full spectrum of rare and common variants. Moreover, continuing advances in high-throughput genotyping and statistical genetics have made it possible to look systematically for DNA differences across the genome. One approach, called whole genome sequencing, attempts to literally assay every base pair in a person's genome. The cost is around $1000 per person. Genome-wide single-nucleotide polymorphism arrays (sometimes called SNP arrays or SNP chips) have been more widely employed. For around $60 per participant, using SNP arrays, it is now possible to look for several million locations on the genome where genetic differences between people exist. These advances have led to three molecular genetic approaches that are currently being employed in the field of learning disabilities: genome-wide association studies (GWAS), SNP-based heritability, and polygenic risk scores. Each will be discussed in turn.

Genome-wide Association Studies

GWAS emerged directly from the Human Genome Project. Essentially, GWAS looks for places across the entire genome (often using SNP arrays) where significant associations exist between genetic locations of interest and measured outcomes. It was thought that the CDCV model held for most complex human traits. Therefore, the increased capacity to identify differences efficiently and cheaply across the genome was expected to yield an increased number of candidate genes beyond the relatively small numbers that existed prior to 2003. This larger number of identified candidate genes would, in turn, account for more of the heritability and thus lead to clinically meaningful amounts of variance in measured behavior overall.

New scientific instruments lead to new discoveries, and GWAS changed the understanding of genetics in fundamental ways (see Duncan et al., 2019). First, the impact of individual genes appears to be exceedingly small for most polymorphisms and most phenotypes. The number of genes required to account for the heritability and genetic overlap discussed earlier in quantitative genetics is very large, requiring very large samples to interrogate. Second, because GWAS looks systematically across the genome, it is now possible to identify significant genetic effects across multiple gene regions and across multiple gene systems. Other advances in neuroimaging and bioinformatics allow for very sensitive studies examining gene–brain–cognition–behavior. As a result, there has been a general movement away from single-candidate gene studies (Figure 6.1) to systemic analyses of the whole genome through GWAS and other methods (see Buniello, 2019). This is not to say that there are no candidate genes. As described earlier, there are many candidate genes within the OGOD model. However, genetics has moved away from candidate genes as a gene-discovery paradigm and introduced SNP-based heritability and polygenic risk scores to capture genetic variance from the CDCV model.

SNP-Based Heritability

In 2006, Visscher and colleagues developed a methodology to estimate heritability and multivariate genetic parameters without special populations like twins and adoptees. SNP arrays systematically measure genetic differences across the genome, which means they can be used to directly estimate genetic variance in a sample. Visscher's original imputation of the approach involved directly estimating the genetic relationship among siblings (which are 50% genetically related on average, but Visscher was able to estimate the actual amount of resemblance using SNP arrays). Later versions of the approach have examined unrelated individuals (see Yang et al., 2017), who will also naturally vary in their genetic relatedness across the SNP array. This variability in genetic relatedness can then be used to estimate heritability and genetic covariance on and between behavioral outcomes. The proportion of variance in outcomes accounted for by these SNP-based measures of genetic variability is called SNP-based heritability. Note that whole genome sequencing can also be used to directly measure genetic variance (see Yang et al., 2015).

For example, Eising et al. (2022) conducted a GWAS meta-analysis of language skills, reading skills, and neuroimaging measures in samples drawn from the GeneLang consortium (N = 34,000 individuals). Results suggested genome-wide significant association and significant SNP-based heritability. Results also suggested significant SNP heritability-based genetic association with cortical surface area of the banks of the left superior temporal sulcus, a region important for both reading and language.

Interestingly, estimates of heritability using SNP-based approaches tend to be lower than the estimates obtained from twin/adoption-based quantitative genetic designs. This has been called the "missing heritability problem" (Manolio et al., 2009; Young, 2019) and has been a topic of great interest within genetics. Although advances in genetics and statistical genetics have narrowed the gap between SNP- and twin/adoption-based heritability, the issue persists, eliciting questions as to why. One possibility is that, as noted in Figure 6.1, the frequency and effect sizes of genes associated with complex human traits operate across a continuum, between the OGOD and CDCV models. These somewhat rare, mildly deleterious genes are captured by twin/adoption designs (by virtue of familial relationships) more readily than SNP-based heritability studies. This would increase the heritability from twin/adoption studies relative to SNP-based studies. Moreover, returning to the discussion of gene–environment effects, SNP-based heritability studies are less likely to conflate gene–environment effects, which would reduce heritability in SNP-based studies as compared with twin/adoption studies.

Moreover, returning to Figure 6.1, between the few OGOD genes of high effect size and low frequency and the multitude of genes that influence genetic variability along the lines of the CDCV model lie moderately infrequent genes of smaller effect size. These may be clustered in such a way that they operate through identifiable biological mechanisms to raise or lower risk for learning difficulties. Put another way, individuals may demonstrate the same reading score, but there may be many different genetic/biological pathways to that score that are yet to be discovered.

Polygenic Risk Scores

Polygenic risk scores use SNP arrays to identify sets of SNPs across multiple genes (hence polygenic), which, when combined, yield an overall measure of risk for an outcome of interest. This tends to be achieved through a multistep process involving (1) GWAS and identification of loci of interest, (2) SNP-based heritability, and (3) deriving an overall index of genetic risk based on the loci of interest, often across multiple datasets or independent portions of the same dataset.

Since the first published study (Purcell et al., 2009), there has been a proliferation of studies examining polygenic risk scores. For example, Lee et al. (2018) examined educational attainment in a sample of 1.1 million individuals. Using genome-wide SNP data, they were able to estimate a polygenetic risk score that accounted for 7–10% of the variance in cognitive performance and 11–13% of the variance in educational attainment. Polygenic risk scores have also been estimated for learning-related outcomes, such as general cognitive ability (see Plomin & Von Stumm, 2018), ADHD (Ronald et al., 2021), and mathematics (Lee et al., 2018) with effect sizes roughly similar to what has been found in many medical conditions (see Wray et al., 2021).

In another representative study, Gialluisi et al. (2019) combined multiple datasets to examine multiple measures of reading, including rapid automatized naming

(RAN), phonological awareness, spelling, and word reading. Gialluisi et al. found that certain regions within chromosome 18 were particularly important for RAN but that other regions within chromosome 18 contributed to the genetic overlap across all reading tasks. Polygenetic risk score analysis across all SNPs yields a significant association with years of education.

Turning to reading disability, Doust et al. (2021) examined 51,000 adults self-reporting with dyslexia and over 1 million control subjects. Using GWAS, they found 42 independent loci (locations on the genome), 17 in genes that overlapped with educational attainment/cognition, and 25 that were unique to dyslexia. From these general findings, Doust et al. conducted fine-grained mapping to better understand how these loci operate. They estimated SNP-based heritability and, within that context, examined how these loci contributed to the covariance between dyslexia and other traits, including neuroimaging measures. Finally, Doust et al. (2021) estimated a polygenic risk score that accounted for 6% of the variance in dyslexia.

Summary and New Directions

Taken together, human genetics has been moving extremely rapidly over the past 20 years. New technologies and approaches have allowed the field to directly estimate genetic variance, removing the need for twins and adoptees, and have made the classic candidate gene study obsolete (see Duncan et al., 2019). The Human Genome Project has also stimulated advances in bioinformatics, computing, and molecular biology (see Lesk, 2019). What has emerged is not only a deeper ability to investigate the genome and how it functions within biological systems, but also an appreciation for the incredible complexity of genomics, especially when considering the intersection with molecular biology and the environment (see Pan et al., 2021). Quantitative genetics sets the stage, demonstrating that genetics is important to learning disabilities and the relations among learning disabilities, but also shows the importance of the environment. The more conservative estimates from SNP-based heritability studies (because they directly measure genetic variance without the assumptions of twin and adoption studies) further suggest that the heritability of learning-related outcomes is substantial and that the genetic correlation among different learning outcomes is significant. More fine-grained molecular genetic studies attempt to characterize that genetic variance, which opens the possibility to better understand the biological pathways through which genes function, directly, and in the context of the environment.

This increased understanding of etiology and process has led some to advocate using new genetic diagnostic tools to prevent, identify, and remediate learning disabilities (Plomin & Von Stumm, 2018; Erbeli, 2019). On the one hand, there is great positivity in this promise. A heritable trait like reading, for example, that demonstrates significant genetic stability across time and with other learning outcomes is likely to have different biological pathways leading to the same measured reading problems. Using genetically sensitive information could help identify risk pathways sooner, utilize environments that mediate or moderate those risks, and tailor educational practices/interventions to remediate or prevent the onset of biological risk for reading disability. These would be positive developments.

Yet challenges remain. First, the utility of genomics is dependent not only on the quality of the genomics but also on the quality of the phenotypes being measured. Individual gene variants have very small effect sizes, particularly for those falling into the CDCV model. This means that gene-discovery efforts require extremely large samples for purposes of power. Moreover, there has been a general movement toward larger teams of scientists, larger datasets, and systems variables (e.g., "Big Science"), evidenced by the accelerating number of meta-analyses and data consortia that have emerged in the past decade in learning disabilities and in other fields. These are important and necessary advances, but moving to extremely large samples and combining across multiple datasets hinders the ability to conduct deep measurements of behavior/performance. This is the very kind of measurement necessary to understand the components of language, reading, and math; their growth; and how they may vary in persons with difficulties or disabilities. Similarly, the increased reliance on meta-analyses and consortia of primary datasets also requires the harmonization and comparison of sets of studies that employ overlapping but nonidentical constructs or measures of those constructs. New approaches are needed to offset this erosion of the phenotype at the expense of the sample size in genetics. In our own work, we have developed an approach that accomplishes this called ROSETTA (Bartlett et al., 2019). This approach estimates a common set of latent factors across datasets with overlapping constructs but with nonoverlapping measures. This has allowed us to not only utilize the power afforded by increased sample sizes but also conduct deep levels of measurement using primary data.

Other challenges emanate from what will likely be an increased profusion of polygenic risk scores examining an increasing number of educationally relevant phenotypes. Statistically, polygenic risk scores account for similar amounts of variance in complex traits, as do broad social variables like SES. Given low genotypic costs, studies within learning disabilities can cheaply add polygenic risk scores to their research protocols using the results of gene-discovery studies (which require thousands or tens of thousands of participants to develop those propensity scores). This situation is similar to the early 2000s, when researchers began to collect candidate genes as part of psychological or educational studies. As these findings proliferated in the literature, the use of candidate gene outcome or candidate gene × environment interactions in substantive studies became increasingly detached from the field of genetics and molecular biology. The result was many nonreplicated findings (see Duncan et al., 2014), due in part to the emergence of GWAS, but also due to a lack of attention to plausible models for gene systems, gene function, and how environments could plausibly impact gene function.

Polygenic risk scores are developed far more systematically and account for far more variance than candidate genes did. However, without careful attention to ongoing molecular genetic gene-discovery and gene-function research on learning disability, efforts by nongenetic studies using polygenic risk scores could publish studies that are statistically significant but are not biologically plausible. If this happens, studies using polygenic risk scores will fall into the same non-replication trap, as did candidate gene studies.

At the same time, mainstream psychological, neuroscience, and educational research on learning disabilities examines the kinds of deep phenotypes genetic studies need. Therefore, genetic studies would be well served to pay close attention to mainstream studies that offer theoretically, clinically, and educationally meaningful phenotypes. In this way, gene-discovery and gene-function research will reflect the best phenotypes and will generate better polygenic risk scores.

As noted by Harden (2021) and Martschenko (2021), another obstacle is that, with some exceptions (e.g., Rabinowitz et al., 2019), most genetic research has been nonrepresentative, based almost exclusively on populations of European ancestry (see Martin et al., 2019). There are subtle genetic differences between populations of different ancestries that are independent from traits being studied. These differences can confound genetic studies and make the results of genetic studies, including polygenic risk scores, less predictive in ancestries that were not part of the original analysis (see Duncan et al., 2019; Martin et al., 2019; Wojcik et al., 2019). This means that polygenic risk scores could be incorrectly generalized to segments of the population at risk for learning disabilities for the purpose of making educational/treatment decisions.

There are also phenotypic considerations; for example, the impact of dialect or English language learner status on achievement measures, as well as the language of instruction (e.g., Washington et al., 2018; Francis et al., 2019), which may also impact the relations among polygenic risk scores and outcomes. Underperforming polygenic risk scores due to original study underrepresentation in genetics and phenotype is a major concern empirically but is also a social issue due to potential health disparities and a general unfairness of the situation. Finally, as noted by Shero et al. (2021), the practical utility of polygenic risk scores is limited in isolation but may be useful in concert with other screening tools reflecting the environment and child skills and learning. Given a lack of representation within the community of researchers conducting genetic research and the historical mistrust of genetic approaches, a great deal of caution and dialogue is warranted before using polygenic risk scores in a diagnostic manner.

Conclusions

In summary, the study of genetics continues to grow alongside the field of learning disabilities and offers the potential to more fully elucidate how learning disabilities arise and develop. Recent advances in genetics offer a great deal of promise for basic research. The tools for translating this work into practice are beginning to emerge, which will be aided by better sampling, phenotyping, as well as the careful weighing of the pros and cons of making educational and clinical decisions based on genetic information.

REFERENCES

Andreola, C., Mascheretti, S., Belotti, R., Ogliari, A., Marino, C., Battaglia, M., & Scaini, S. (2021). The heritability of reading and reading-related neurocognitive components: A multi-level meta-analysis. *Neuroscience & Biobehavioral Reviews, 121*, 175–200.

Andres, E. M., Earnest, K. K., Smith, S. D., Rice, M. L., & Raza, M. H. (2020). Pedigree-based gene mapping supports previous loci and reveals novel suggestive loci in specific language impairment. *Journal of Speech, Language, and Hearing Research, 63*(12), 4046–4061.

Asbury, K., & Plomin, R. (2013). *G is for genes: The impact of genetics on education and achievement* (Vol. 24). John Wiley & Sons.

Bartlett, C. W., Klamer, B. G., Buyske, S., Petrill, S. A., & Ray, W. C. (2019). Forming big datasets through latent class concatenation of imperfectly matched database features. *Genes, 10*(9), 727.

Buniello, A., MacArthur, J. A. L., Cerezo, M., Harris, L. W., Hayhurst, J., Malangone, C., & Parkinson, H. (2019). The NHGRI-EBI GWAS Catalog of published genome-wide association studies, targeted arrays and summary statistics 2019. *Nucleic Acids Research, 47*(D1), D1005–D1012.

Centanni, T. M. (2020). Neural and genetic mechanisms of dyslexia. In G. P. D. Argyropoulos (Ed.), *Translational neuroscience of speech and language disorders* (pp. 47–68). Springer Nature Switzerland AG.

Cherny, S. S., Cardon, L. R., Fulker, D. W., & DeFries, J. C. (1992). Differential heritability across levels of cognitive ability. *Behavior Genetics, 22*(2), 153–162.

Christopher, M. E., Hulslander, J., Byrne, B., Samuelsson, S., Keenan, J. M., Pennington, B., et al. (2015). Genetic and environmental etiologies of the longitudinal relations between prereading skills and reading. *Child Development, 86*(2), 342–361.

Daucourt, M. C., Erbeli, F., Little, C. W., Haughbrook, R., & Hart, S. A. (2020). A meta-analytical review of the genetic and environmental correlations between reading and attention-deficit/hyperactivity disorder symptoms and reading and math. *Scientific Studies of Reading, 24*(1), 23–56.

Daucourt, M. C., Haughbrook, R., Van Bergen, E., & Hart, S. A. (2020). The association of parent-reported executive functioning, reading, and math is explained by nature, not nurture. *Developmental Psychology, 56*(12), 2246.

de Zeeuw, E. L., de Geus, E. J., & Boomsma, D. I. (2015). Meta-analysis of twin studies highlights the importance of genetic variation in primary school educational achievement. *Trends in Neuroscience and Education, 4*(3), 69–76.

DeFries, J. C., & Fulker, D. W. (1985). Multiple regression analysis of twin data. *Behavior Genetics, 15*(5), 467–473.

DeFries, J. C., & Fulker, D. W. (1988). Multiple regression analysis of twin data: Etiology of deviant scores versus individual differences. *Acta Geneticae Medicae et Gemellologiae: Twin Research, 37*(3–4), 205–216.

Doust, C., Fontanillas, P., Eising, E., Gordon, S. D., Wang, Z., Alagöz, G., et al. (2021). Discovery of 42 genome-wide significant loci associated with dyslexia. *Nature Genetics, 54*(11), 1621–1629.

Duncan, L. E., Ostacher, M., & Ballon, J. (2019). How genome-wide association studies (GWAS) made traditional candidate gene studies obsolete. *Neuropsychopharmacology, 44*(9), 1518–1523.

Duncan, L. E., Pollastri, A. R., & Smoller, J. W. (2014). Mind the gap: Why many geneticists and psychological scientists have discrepant views about gene–environment interaction (G × E) research. *American Psychologist, 69*(3), 249.

Duncan, L., Shen, H., Gelaye, B., Meijsen, J., Ressler, K., Feldman, M., et al. (2019). Analysis of polygenic risk score usage and performance in diverse human populations. *Nature Communications, 10*(1), 1–9.

Eising, E., Mirza-Schreiber, N., De Zeeuw, E. L., Wang, C. A., Truong, D. T., Allegrini, A. G., et al. (2022). Genome-wide analyses of individual differences in quantitatively assessed reading- and language-related skills in up to 34,000 people. *Proceedings of the National Academy of Sciences, 119*(35), e2202764119.

Erbeli, F. (2019). Translating research findings in genetics of learning disabilities to special education instruction. *Mind, Brain, and Education, 13*(2), 74–79.

Francis, D. J., Rojas, R., Gusewski, S., Santi, K. L., Khalaf, S., Hiebert, L., & Bunta, F. (2019). Speaking and reading in two languages: On the identification of reading and language disabilities in Spanish-speaking English learners. *New Directions for Child and Adolescent Development, 2019*(166), 15–41.

Gialluisi, A., Andlauer, T. F., Mirza-Schreiber, N., Moll, K., Becker, J., Hoffmann, P., et al. (2019). Genome-wide association scan identifies new variants associated with a cognitive predictor of dyslexia. *Translational Psychiatry, 9*(1), 1–15.

Gialluisi, A., Andlauer, T. F., Mirza-Schreiber, N., Moll, K., Becker, J., Hoffmann, P., et al. (2021). Genome-wide association study reveals new insights into the heritability and genetic correlates of developmental dyslexia. *Molecular psychiatry, 26*(7), 3004–3017.

Giangrande, E., & Turkheimer, E. (2022). Race, ethnicity, and the Scarr–Rowe hypothesis: A cautionary example of fringe science entering the mainstream. *Perspectives on Psychological Science, 17*(3), 696–710.

Gottesman, I. I., & Shields, J. (1973). Genetic theorizing and schizophrenia. *British Journal of Psychiatry, 122*(566), 15–30.

Greven, C. U., Rijsdijk, F. V., Asherson, P., & Plomin, R. (2012). A longitudinal twin study on the association between ADHD symptoms and reading. *Journal of Child Psychology and Psychiatry, 53*(3), 234–242.

Grigorenko, E. L., Compton, D. L., Fuchs, L. S., Wagner, R. K., Willcutt, E. G., & Fletcher, J. M. (2020). Understanding, educating, and supporting children with specific learning disabilities: 50 years of science and practice. *American Psychologist, 75*(1), 37.

Harden, K. P. (2021). "Reports of my death were greatly exaggerated": Behavior genetics in the postgenomic era. *Annual Review of Psychology, 72*, 37–60.

Harlaar, N., Dale, P. S., & Plomin, R. (2007). From learning to read to reading to learn: Substantial and stable genetic influence. *Child Development, 78*(1), 116–131.

Hart, S. A., Petrill, S. A., Thompson, L. A., & Plomin, R. (2009). The ABCs of math: A genetic analysis of mathematics and its links with reading ability and general cognitive ability. *Journal of Educational Psychology, 101*(2), 388.

Knopik, V. S., Neiderhiser, J. M., DeFries, J. C., & Plomin, R. (2017). *Behavioral genetics*. Worth Publishers, Macmillan Learning.

LaBuda, M. C., DeFries, J. C., & Pennington, B. F. (1990). Reading disability: A model for the genetic analysis of complex behavioral disorders. *Journal of Counseling & Development, 68*(6), 645–651.

Lee, J. J., Wedow, R., Okbay, A., Kong, E., Maghzian, O., Zacher, M., et al. (2018). Gene discovery and polygenic prediction from a genome-wide association study of educational attainment in 1.1 million individuals. *Nature Genetics, 50*(8), 1112–1121.

Lesk, A. (2019). *Introduction to bioinformatics*. Oxford University Press.

Little, C. W., Haughbrook, R., & Hart, S. A. (2017). Cross-study differences in the etiology of reading comprehension: A meta-analytical review of twin studies. *Behavior Genetics, 47*(1), 52.

Logan, J. A., Petrill, S. A., Hart, S. A., Schatschneider, C., Thompson, L. A., Deater-Deckard, K., et al. (2012). Heritability across the distribution: An application of quantile regression. *Behavior Genetics, 42*(2), 256–267, 76.

Manolio, T. A., Collins, F. S., Cox, N. J., Goldstein, D. B., Hindorff, L. A., Hunter, D. J., et al. (2009). Finding the missing heritability of complex diseases. *Nature, 461*(7265), 747–753.

Martin, A. R., Kanai, M., Kamatani, Y., Okada, Y., Neale, B. M., & Daly, M. J. (2019). Clinical use of current polygenic risk scores may exacerbate health disparities. *Nature Genetics, 51*(4), 584–591.

Martin, N. G., & Eaves, L. J. (1977). The genetical analysis of covariance structure. *Heredity, 38*(1), 79–95.

Martschenko, D. O., & Smith, M. (2021). Genes do not operate in a vacuum, and neither should our research. *Nature Genetics, 53*(3), 255–256.

Martschenko, D., Trejo, S., & Domingue, B. W. (2019). Genetics and education: recent developments in the context of an ugly history and an uncertain future. *AERA Open, 5*(1), 2332858418810516.

Morris, D. W., Robinson, L., Turic, D., Duke, M., Webb, V., Milham, C., et al. (2000). Family-based association mapping provides evidence for a gene for reading disability on chromosome 15q. *Human Molecular Genetics, 9*(5), 843–848.

Oliver, B. R., & Plomin, R. (2007). Twins' Early Development Study (TEDS): A multivariate, longitudinal genetic investigation of language, cognition and behavior problems from childhood through adolescence. *Twin Research and Human Genetics, 10*(1), 96–105.

Olson, R. K., Keenan, J. M., Byrne, B., & Samuelsson, S. (2019). Etiology of developmental dyslexia. In L. Verhoeven, C. Perfetti, & K. Pugh (Eds.), *Developmental dyslexia across languages and writing systems* (pp. 391–412). Cambridge University Press.

Pan, Y., Lei, X., & Zhang, Y. (2021). Association predictions of genomics, proteinomics, transcriptomics, microbiome, metabolomics, pathomics, radiomics, drug, symptoms, environment factor, and disease networks: A comprehensive approach. *Medicinal Research Reviews, 42*(1), 441–461.

Paracchini, S., Diaz, R., & Stein, J. (2016). Advances in dyslexia genetics—New insights into the role of brain asymmetries. *Advances in Genetics, 96*, 53–97.

Paracchini, S., Scerri, T., & Monaco, A. P. (2007). The genetic lexicon of dyslexia. *Annual Review of Genomics and Human Genetics, 8*, 57–79.

Petscher, Y., & Logan, J. A. (2014). Quantile regression in the study of developmental sciences. *Child Development, 85*(3), 861–881.

Pittner, K., Van Ijzendoorn, M. H., Alink, L. R., Buisman, R. S., Compier-de Block, L. H., Van Den Berg, L. J., et al. (2019). The genetic and environmental etiology of child maltreatment in a parent-based extended family design. *Development and Psychopathology, 31*(1), 157–172.

Plomin, R., DeFries, J. C., Knopik, V. S., & Neiderhiser, J. M. (2016). Top 10 replicated findings from behavioral genetics. *Perspectives on Psychological Science, 11*(1), 3–23.

Plomin, R., & Kovas, Y. (2005). Generalist genes and learning disabilities. *Psychological Bulletin, 131*(4), 592.

Plomin, R., Owen, M. J., & McGuffin, P. (1994). The genetic basis of complex human behaviors. *Science, 264*(5166), 1733–1739.

Plomin, R., & Von Stumm, S. (2018). The new genetics of intelligence. *Nature Reviews Genetics, 19*(3), 148–159.

Purcell, S. M., Wray, N. R., Stone, J. L., Visscher, P. M., O'Donovan, M. C., & Sullivan, P. F. (2009). Common polygenic variation contributes to risk of schizophrenia and bipolar disorder. *Nature, 460*, 748–752.

Rabinowitz, J. A., Kuo, S. I. C., Felder, W., Musci, R. J., Bettencourt, A., Benke, K., et al. (2019). Associations between an educational attainment polygenic score with educational attainment in an African American sample. *Genes, Brain and Behavior, 18*(5), e12558.

Rice, M. L., Taylor, C. L., Zubrick, S. R., Hoffman, L., & Earnest, K. K. (2020). Heritability of specific language impairment and nonspecific language impairment at ages 4 and 6 years across phenotypes of speech, language, and nonverbal cognition. *Journal of Speech, Language, and Hearing Research, 63*(3), 793–813.

Ronald, A., de Bode, N., & Polderman, T. J. (2021). Systematic review: How the attention-deficit/

hyperactivity disorder polygenic risk score adds to our understanding of ADHD and associated traits. *Journal of the American Academy of Child & Adolescent Psychiatry, 60*(10), 1234–1277.

Selita, F., & Kovas, Y. (2019). Genes and Gini: What inequality means for heritability. *Journal of Biosocial Science, 51*(1), 18–47.

Shero, J., van Dijk, W., Edwards, A., Schatschneider, C., Solari, E. J., & Hart, S. A. (2021). The practical utility of genetic screening in school settings. *NPJ Science of Learning, 6*(1), 1–10.

Smith, S. D., Kimberling, W. J., Pennington, B. F., & Lubs, H. A. (1983). Specific reading disability: Identification of an inherited form through linkage analysis. *Science, 219*(4590), 1345–1347.

Soden, B., Christopher, M. E., Hulslander, J., Olson, R. K., Cutting, L., Keenan, J. M., et al. (2015). Longitudinal stability in reading comprehension is largely heritable from grades 1 to 6. *PLOS One, 10*(1), e0113807.

Stromswold, K. (2001). The heritability of language: A review and meta-analysis of twin, adoption, and linkage studies. *Language, 77*(4), 647–723.

Thomas, T., Khalaf, S., & Grigorenko, E. L. (2021). A systematic review and meta-analysis of imaging genetics studies of specific reading disorder. *Cognitive Neuropsychology, 38*(3), 179–204.

Tucker-Drob, E. M., & Bates, T. C. (2016). Large cross-national differences in gene × socioeconomic status interaction on intelligence. *Psychological Science, 27*(2), 138–149.

van Bergen, E., Snowling, M. J., de Zeeuw, E. L., van Beijsterveldt, C. E., Dolan, C. V., & Boomsma, D. I. (2018). Why do children read more? The influence of reading ability on voluntary reading practices. *Journal of Child Psychology and Psychiatry, 59*(11), 1205–1214.

Visscher, P. M., Medland, S. E., Ferreira, M. A. R., Morley, K. I., Zhu, G., et al. (2006). Assumption-free estimation of heritability from genome-wide identity-by-descent sharing between full siblings. *PLOS Genetics, 2*(3), e4.

Washington, J. A., Branum-Martin, L., Sun, C., & Lee-James, R. (2018). The impact of dialect density on the growth of language and reading in African American children. *Language, Speech, and Hearing Services in Schools, 49*(2), 232–247.

Wojcik, G. L., Graff, M., Nishimura, K. K., Tao, R., Haessler, J., Gignoux, C. R., et al. (2019). Genetic analyses of diverse populations improves discovery for complex traits. *Nature, 570*(7762), 514–518.

Wray, N. R., Lin, T., Austin, J., McGrath, J. J., Hickie, I. B., Murray, G. K., & Visscher, P. M. (2021). From basic science to clinical application of polygenic risk scores: A primer. *JAMA Psychiatry, 78*(1), 101–109.

Yang, J., Bakshi, A., Zhu, Z., Hemani, G., Vinkhuyzen, A. A., Lee, S. H., et al. (2015). Genetic variance estimation with imputed variants finds negligible missing heritability for human height and body mass index. *Nature Genetics, 47*(10), 1114–1120.

Yang, J., Zeng, J., Goddard, M. E., Wray, N. R., & Visscher, P. M. (2017). Concepts, estimation and interpretation of SNP-based heritability. *Nature Genetics, 49*(9), 1304–1310.

Young, A. I. (2019). Solving the missing heritability problem. *PLOS Genetics, 15*(6), e1008222.

CHAPTER 7

Executive Functions and Learning Disabilities

Marcia A. Barnes and Peng Peng

Studies of executive functions (EFs) are abundant in the literature on the development of academic skills, including in studies of individuals with learning disabilities. In this chapter, we discuss what is meant by EFs and why understanding their relationship to learning disabilities (LDs) is important. The origins of the concept of EFs and theoretical perspectives on EFs are briefly presented, followed by a review of the literature on the relation of EFs to academic performance, relying principally on well-controlled longitudinal studies and systematic reviews. We then focus on what is known about EFs in relation to intervention and response to intervention for individuals with LDs. Throughout, we discuss the types of research involving EFs that might be useful for better understanding, preventing, and treating LDs.

EFs broadly refer to the control of thoughts, actions, and emotions (Miyake & Friedman, 2012). The study of EFs, using the term *EFs*, has a relatively recent history, with relatively few articles published before 1990, followed by striking growth over the next three decades (Müller & Kearns, 2015). Furthermore, this rapid increase in research on EFs has occurred in several disciplines, including cognitive science and neuroscience, developmental science, psychiatry, clinical and health psychology (Müller & Kearns, 2015), and the education sciences, including special education. To give a few examples, of the most cited articles since 2018 in the *Journal of Experimental Child Psychology*, one-third of them included EFs. Of the articles published in the *Journal of Learning Disabilities* between January 2021 and May 2022, 22% measured EFs and related them to reading, spelling, or math.

The ubiquitous nature of EFs across these literatures reflects the fact that EFs vary between individuals, change with development, and are generally lower across a large variety of adult and child clinical, neurological, neurodevelopmental, and learning and behavioral disorders. Because EFs are correlates of many disorders, including LDs, this presents a scientific challenge. On the one hand, it questions the usefulness of the EF construct in the identification of learning disabilities (see Chapter 1 by Miciak and Fletcher, this volume). On the other hand, given that EFs are involved in so many aspects of cognition, their consideration might be important in the design of interventions for children with LDs. This is the focus of the second half of the chapter. First, we present a brief history of EFs, along with conceptual and measurement models of EFs, followed by what is known about the relation of EFs to academic achievement for individuals with LDs.

Early History of Executive Functions

Despite the relatively recent use of the term *EF*, the types of functions captured by this term have their origins in much older literature on changes in behavior as a function of lesions to the frontal lobes. Lesions to the frontal lobes in adults (Stuss & Benson, 1984) were long known to be associated with changes in personality and certain habits of mind (the classic case of Phineas Gage from the mid-1800s is often cited). In their seminal article on the frontal lobes, Stuss and Benson (1984) summarized frontal lobe dysfunctions as involving *separation of action from knowledge, impairment of sequential memory, impairment in the ability to establish or change a set resulting in random or perseverative behaviors, difficulties in maintaining a set in the presence of interference, problems in monitoring personal behavior,* and *attitudes of lack of concern, apathy.* One sees parallels between several, though not all, of these "frontal lobe symptoms" and how we currently think about EFs in children whose difficulties in cognition, learning, and behavior arise through development rather than frank insult to the brain (note: current conceptions of EF and brain involve more than frontal lobes, see Chapter 5 by Harriott and Cutting).

The idea of executive functions (if not the specific term EFs), while often cited as emerging from the adult neuropsychology lesion literature, is also found in memory systems research in cognitive psychology and in research on metacognition in developmental psychology. In cognitive psychology, older sequential information processing models (e.g., Broadbent, 1957) sought to describe the route from sensation and perception to short-term and long-term memory. These *pipeline* models (Cowan, 1988) eventually incorporated working memory as an expansion of the short-term memory component of the memory system. The Baddeley and Hitch (1974) model hypothesized a *central executive*, or CE, that gates and coordinates encoding of verbal and visual–spatial information and retrieval from long-term memory in the service of current information processing (see Parkin, 1998, for a critique of the notion of the CE).

In developmental psychology, Flavell's (1970) and Ann Brown's (1975) work described the increasing ability with development to understand and reflect on *one's own* and *other's* cognition, called metacognition. Flavell distinguished between metacognitive knowledge and metacognitive behavior, the latter overlapping with current views of EFs, that is, processes and behaviors involving monitoring, planning, self-regulation, and the strategic use of cognitive resources and knowledge.

Metacognitive theory was quickly applied to education and to interventions in reading, writing, and math for children with LDs (see 1992 special issue of the *Journal of Learning Disabilities;* Borkowski, 1992; review in Baker et al., 2020).

Both the developmental and cognitive psychology paradigms included the study of factors that could make the limited capacity human information processing system more or less functional, including one's long-term store of knowledge, which allowed for more "chunking" of information in working memory, and faster processing of visual or verbal materials, "freeing" limited capacity resources to be devoted to mental operations requiring more strategic, effortful thinking and behaviors (reviewed in Torgesen, 1994).

Contemporary Models of Executive Functions

In 1994, Torgesen noted similarities but also significant differences in EF concepts and measurement arising from cognitive psychology, developmental psychology, and neuropsychology (Denckla, 1994). Two decades later, Barkley (2012) noted the lack of agreement about both the definition and measurement of EF; this state of affairs remains to this day. In terms of the *definition* of EFs, consider that similar EF-like constructs may have different names depending on the research tradition. Also consider that what is identified as an EF has considerably expanded over time. For example, one review (Packwood et al., 2011) reported over 60 hypothesized subcomponents of EF. In terms of the *measurement* of EFs, the two main critiques are that EF tasks cluster together less because they have an EF component in common than because they share method variance (Karr et al., 2018) and that EF tasks are multidimensional, requiring many cognitive skills for their performance—the task impurity issue. These issues pose significant challenges for theories and measurement of EFs.

One approach to some of these measurement issues was the confirmatory factor analytic work undertaken by Miyake and colleagues (2000). Their latent structural modeling approach found evidence for three separable but related factors (memory updating or working memory, inhibition, and attention switching) with a common underlying factor (see Miyake & Freidman, 2012, for a more recent treatment). Given this is a predominant model in studies relating EFs and academic achievement (Butterfuss & Kenedeou, 2020), what is the evidence for this structural or component skills account of EFs?

A systematic review (Karr et al., 2018) investigated different types of factor structures for EF models. No one model provided a consistent fit to the data. Karr and colleagues suggested that low rates of model acceptance and selection might have resulted from the publication of well-fitting models whose findings are not replicable (i.e., publication bias). Consistent with theories that EFs develop out of more basic cognitive functions such as attention and differentiate with increasing age (e.g., Posner & Rothbart, 2007; Garon et al., 2008), they found that model solutions showed somewhat greater unidimensionality of EFs in children; however, these effects were not as strong as expected based on developmental theory, possibly due to limited construct-specific variance in the models as a function of lack of valid and reliable EF measures in younger children and time constraints on testing children compared to adults.

Other models that have been used to guide theoretical framing and measurement in studies of EFs in children with LDs include the working memory/attention control framework provided by Engle (e.g., 2018) and Sweller's (2010) cognitive load theory. Both deal with the role that individual differences in EFs play in performance, including academics. We describe Sweller's theory in more detail because it was explicitly designed for instructional purposes. According to this theory, most learning involves complex processing of several interactive elements; learners have limited capacity to accomplish this complex processing; instruction should be designed to take the learner's working memory limitations into account, reducing extraneous load (i.e., that which does not contribute to learning) while also optimizing germane load, which is the type of load that promotes learning (Sweller, 2010). In this theory, domain knowledge (e.g., from fluency in word recognition to one's store of world knowledge) acts as a "load reducer." In cognitive load theory, there is a focus on working memory as a characteristic of persons, cognitive load as a characteristic of learning tasks, and their interaction.

One additional recent theoretical account of EF deserves mention, given our focus in the latter part of this chapter on EFs in the context of interventions for students with LDs. This is the bidirectional hypothesis outlined by Peng and Kievit (2020), in which it is proposed that not only are EFs important for academic skills development, but also that learning and practicing academic skills influence the development of EFs. This approach contrasts with more typical unidirectional hypotheses, also called *milk-and-jug* type of thinking (Share et al., 1989), in which EF capacity determines or places limitations on academic skill learning.

Despite some of their differences, most models of EF, whether deriving from the neuropsychological or cognitive tradition and whether structural or more process-based in nature, rely on the basic assumption that some aspects of human information processing in some situations are limited in capacity; it is under such conditions that the temporary storage of information and the ability to control potentially interfering information in order to accomplish task goals comes into play. In the remainder of this chapter, we take a fairly agnostic approach to what EF is and is not, relying on this broad conceptualization. To read more comprehensively, Müller and Kerns (2015) provide a treatment of the coherence and validity of the construct of EFs specific to development, Doebel (2020) proposes a knowledge-, belief-, and values-based perspective on the development of EFs, and Evans and Stanovich (2013) have a dual-processing approach that invokes slower working memory-demanding processing when rapid autonomous responding based on prior learning needs to be overridden for higher-order reasoning.

Relations of EFs and Learning Disabilities

As noted, the three-factor model of Miyake et al. (2000) has been the predominant model of EFs used in the developmental and educational literature. The choice of models is important because it determines the constructs and tasks that make their way into empirical studies of the relations of EFs to academic development and disability. In their review of the relations between EFs and academic achievement based on this three-factor model, Jacob and Parkinson (2015) argued that the evidence for causal relations of EF and academic achievement are not "compelling": experimental studies in which EFs are trained had not shown far transfer effects to academic outcomes (also see Melby-Lervåg et al., 2016; Sala & Gobet, 2020; Shipstead et al., 2012). Furthermore, of the over 20 longitudinal studies they reviewed, which might provide evidence of the temporal precedence of EFs' relationships to academic achievement, studies were found wanting in terms of internal validity because they did not control for potentially confounding factors. We took these Jacob and Parkinson (2015) critiques into account to select studies for our review that investigate the relation of EFs to academic outcomes.

Disabilities in Word-Level Reading and Reading Comprehension

Models of word reading and reading comprehension both propose a role for auditory working memory. For word reading acquisition, the assembly of letter-sound correspondences into words is thought to draw on working memory (Perfetti, 1985), although connectionist theories need not invoke working memory in the learning process (Perfetti & Helder, 2022). For reading comprehension, some cognitive models implicitly or explicitly include working memory, inhibition, and switching as mechanisms accounting for the construction and revision of the textbase and situation model and for individual differences in reading comprehension. For a review of these models and connections to EFs, see Butterfuss and Kendeou (2018). Although it is often presumed that working memory is more relevant for reading comprehension, similar-sized relations with working memory have been found for word reading and comprehension (Peng, Barnes, et al., 2018). The following section reviews findings from longitudinal and meta-analytic studies conducted with samples of children with LDs in word reading and reading comprehension.

Morgan and colleagues (2017) used the ECLS-K data and included several control variables in their analyses (e.g., prior academic achievement) to test whether kindergarten working memory and cognitive flexibility/attention switching predict end-of-first-grade word reading outcomes. Using both categorical (i.e., deficit vs. no deficit in EF) and continuous EF predictors, they found that cognitive flexibility and working memory independently predicted risk for poor progress in reading by the end of first grade, with a larger effect of working memory. These findings replicated in third grade (Morgan et al., 2019).

Three meta-analyses provide summaries of findings for the relation of EFs and reading disabilities. Note that there are other meta-analyses (e.g., Peng, Barnes, et al., 2018, for working memory and component skills of reading; Jacob & Parkinson, 2015, for EFs and academic achievement) looking at effect sizes for EFs and academic outcomes, but because they do not focus solely or largely on individuals with reading disabilities, they are not included in this review.

Lonergan et al. (2019) used the three-factor model to look at differences in updating/working memory, inhibition, and attention switching/flexibility in individuals with word-level reading disabilities (WLRD) compared to typically developing (TD) children and children with both WLRD and ADHD. This latter contrast is of interest because it has been proposed that while WLRD is most often associated with deficits in verbal working memory (Willcutt et al., 2001), inhibition is a cognitive marker of ADHD (Schachar et al., 2000), even though it is also associated with deficits in working memory (e.g., Martinussen et al., 2005). Thus, children with WLRD+ADHD might have more widespread deficits in EFs.

Effects of inhibition and attention switching for both WLRD-only and WLRD+ADHD were medium sized compared to TD children and not statistically different from each other. Effects for auditory working memory were large and medium in size for the WLRD and WLRD+ADHD groups, respectively. Because the addition of comorbid ADHD did not change the size of these EF effects, ADHD might not confer additional deficits in EF over and above those associated with WLRD. Findings also further underline the fact that fairly broad EF deficits are linked to several neurodevelopmental conditions (Müller & Kerns, 2015).

Another meta-analysis looked at one EF—working memory—in individuals with specific reading comprehension disabilities without WRLD. Across 18 studies, Carretti et al. (2009) found large effects compared to TD individuals on working memory tasks, particularly those that drew more on central executive aspects of working memory (i.e., versus just memory storage) and for those that were verbal–auditory in nature.

These two meta-analyses provide important information on the relation of EFs to reading in individuals with various types of reading disabilities. However, there are two aspects of the findings that deserve further scrutiny. First, some of the findings may reflect a gradient of severity, such that the more severe the reading disability, the larger the effect sizes are for EF differences between groups with and without WLRD or reading comprehension disabilities. It would be helpful to know whether the type and size of the relations of EF and reading vary across the distribution of reading level. Second, there was a great deal of variability in effect sizes across studies for some EF components in the Lonergan et al. (2019) meta-analysis.

A meta-analysis on effects for EFs and different types of reading outcomes by Peng, Zhang, et al. (2022) explored this variability as well as potential moderating effects of severity of reading difficulties, age, and the verbal/nonverbal nature of the materials used to measure EFs. They found statistically similar mean effect sizes for all of the EFs and EF-related constructs measured (working memory, updating, processing speed, short-term memory, attention, inhibition, switching, and spatial skills). However, working memory and updating were the only EFs that did not show a great degree of individual variation amongst reading disability groups, suggesting that working memory/updating are more central to reading disabilities (RDs) than are other EFs.

A second finding of interest was that the more severe the RD, the larger the effects for some (but not all) EFs. Third, students with RD who were identified on the basis of reading comprehension disabilities *or* on the basis of WLRD were similar in terms of the EFs that distinguished them from TD readers. Fourth, deficits in EFs were larger for older individuals with RD than for younger individuals. Peng, Zhang, et al. (2022) saw this as fitting with the idea that later-identified individuals have had less access to reading intervention (itself a type of cognitive intervention); however, studies with older students contain readers with more persistent, severe reading deficits, which would also be associated with larger effect sizes. These are not necessarily mutually exclusive explanations and require longitudinal studies to disentangle. Finally, they tested whether the relation of EFs to reading comprehension was mediated by components of the Simple View of Reading (Gough & Tunmer, 1986). Word reading and linguistic comprehension largely, but did not completely, mediate the relation of EFs to reading (though they did for working memory; also see Peng, Barnes, et al., 2018). These findings are compatible with the idea of bidirectional effects of EFs on reading and of reading experience on EF development (Peng & Kievit, 2020; Zhang & Peng, 2023b). They are also compatible with structural models of reading comprehension showing that simple view skills—word reading and linguistic comprehension—themselves have EF processing requirements, so EFs may have substantial indirect if not direct effects on reading (Kim, 2020).

Disabilities in Written Expression

Meta-analyses of EFs and writing are not currently available, so the following discussion focuses on theoretical models and individual studies investigating these relationships, some in individuals with writing difficulties and some in samples not selected for LDs. Although writing involves many of the same linguistic, code-based, and cognitive processes involved in reading and reading comprehension, the need to generate text according to an internal mental model is thought to draw heavily on EFs, including higher-level skills such as planning and reviewing processes (e.g., Flower & Hayes, 1981). Planning and reviewing have been proposed to draw on more basic EF skills, such as working memory, attention switching, and inhibition. The expanded Simple View of Writing (e.g., Berninger & Winn, 2006) was the first to explicitly include EFs and working memory as component skills of writing. However, we note that the writing interventions designed by Graham and Harris have long focused on explicitly supporting and remediating difficulties in regulatory skills in beginning and disabled writers (Graham & Harris, Chapter 15, this volume). Outside of the context of this intervention research, contemporary studies have shown that EFs are related to writing, as described in the following discussion.

Similar to the Peng, Zhang, et al. (2022) reading meta-analysis, studies testing a component skills model of writing, the Direct Indirect Effects model of Writing (or DIEW; Kim & Park, 2019), have shown that the effect of EFs (particularly working memory) on writing are entirely statistically mediated (in the elementary grades; reviewed in Kim, 2020) by oral language and transcription skills, which are the component skills in the Simple View of Writing. Even though EFs were not directly related to writing after accounting for higher-order cognitive processes such as inference-making, monitoring, and perspective-taking, the indirect effects of EFs on writing were substantial. However, in a study of third- to fifth-grade English learners receiving English-only instruction, working memory, measured in both English and Spanish, had large effects on writing in English even with English and Spanish phonological and oral language skills in the model (Peng, Orosco, et al., 2022). EFs may be more directly implicated in written expression when more foundational component skills are still developing and lacking in fluency.

Although overlap in reading and writing disabilities is not complete (Willcutt et al., 2019), longitudinal twin studies suggest that disabilities in written expression wholly share variance with other learning disabilities (Peterson et al., 2021). Longitudinal studies (first to fourth grade; Ahmed et al., 2014; and third to sixth grade; Kim et al., 2018) show directionality in development from reading to writing, but not vice versa. Together, these findings suggest that the EFs that have been related to WLRD and reading comprehension disabilities are likely to be similar to those implicated in disabilities in written expression, which is important to know given the much larger number of studies measuring EF constructs in reading compared to writing.

Disabilities in Mathematics

For reading, we discussed EFs in relation to word reading and reading comprehension, all of which one can measure in some form very early in schooling or earlier for developmentally unconstrained knowledge and skills such as language comprehension (Paris, 2005). For mathematics, the situation is rather different. There are different domains within mathematics (whole number concepts/calculation, rational number and fractions concepts/calculations, algebra, geometry, math word problems that can include these previously mentioned aspects of math, and so forth), and although informal knowledge in some of these domains may develop early (Ginsburg et al., 1998), conceptual and procedural knowledge in these domains are strongly linked to school-based formal instruction (Rittle-Johnson et al., 2015). With this in mind, we discuss what is known about the relation of EFs to overall math achievement and also to various domains of mathematics, for children with and without mathematics learning disabilities (MLD).

The longitudinal studies using ECLS-K data, as reported earlier for reading (Morgan et al., 2017, 2019), also found that cognitive flexibility and working memory independently predicted risk for poor progress in mathematics by the end of first and third grades. Similar to reading, the effects of working memory were larger than they were for cognitive flexibility. Interestingly, the size of the effects for both EFs was larger for mathematics versus reading, which is similar to that reported in a meta-analysis comparing effect sizes for EF in reading and math (Cortés Pascual et al., 2019). In a meta-analysis of longitudinal studies that measured predictors of mathematics achievement over time, controlling for prior mathematical performance, Lin and Powell (2021) found that prior mathematical achievement, reading achievement, and working memory were unique predictors of later math achievement, albeit with a smaller effect of working memory.

Meta-analyses find that working memory has moderate-sized relations with several aspects of math, with the largest effect sizes for calculations and math word problem solving (Peng et al., 2016; Spiegel et al., 2021). Spiegel et al. (2021) also looked at inhibitory control and attention switching based on the three-factor model. They found small to moderate effect sizes for inhibitory control that were similar for different domains of math. Attention shifting was more strongly related to calculations and word problem solving than to other aspects of math.

Although most meta-analyses in mathematics contain studies comprised largely of TD individuals, some meta-analyses have either considered MLD as a moderator or have specifically focused on students with MLD. Peng et al. (2016) did not find that MLD moderated effect sizes for the relation of working memory and math achievement, although this relationship was bigger among children with MLD comorbid with other neurodevelopmental disabilities. The Friso-Van den Bos et al. (2013) meta-analysis found that math achievement showed the strongest relation with working memory compared to inhibition and switching. Children with MLD, psychological disorders, or physical disabilities all showed higher associations between math achievement and working memory functioning than TD children. In another meta-analysis, Peng, Wang, et al. (2018) found significant effects for a large number of variables, including EFs, when comparing individuals with MLD to TD peers. For EFs, working memory, attention, and other EFs were all significant, though some had larger effect sizes than others. One hypothesis for these larger effect sizes for children with MLD is that these children rely more heavily on EF to help perform mathematics to compensate for their relatively poorer math problem-solving strategies and weaker retrieval of math knowledge from long-term memory (Peng et al., 2016; Friso-Van den Bos et al., 2013).

Summary and Future Research Directions

The review of EFs and their relation to LDs reveals two general findings. First, there is more information available for the relation of RDs and EFs than for other types of learning disabilities; this larger evidence base for RDs is, of course, not unique to EFs. Second, regardless of academic domain, there are more studies of working memory versus other types of EFs in relation to LDs; however, when these other EFs are measured, inhibitory control and attention switching are related to LDs across academic domains and to particular skills within domains. The robust findings for working memory may partly be a function of its having been most frequently measured, using common tasks with strong psychometric properties. Findings for inhibition and attention switching are more variable across studies, which may be related to less use of common measures and use of measures less reliable than those assessing working memory (see Lee & Lee, 2019, for a discussion of inhibition).

One EF construct we think deserves additional research in relation to LDs is inhibition. Inhibition plays a central role in theories of general cognitive development (Cragg, 2016; Posner & Rothbart, 2007), is considered to be foundational for the development of more complex EFs (Garon et al., 2008), and is a central mechanism and source of individual differences in some cognitive models of reading comprehension (Gernsbacher, 1997). However, empirical evidence is mixed on the role of inhibition in academic skills. For example, within the domain of reading, some studies show relations of inhibition to reading comprehension (Mason et al., 2020), others to reading fluency, but not comprehension (Arrington et al., 2014), others show no relation to reading comprehension (Barnes et al., 2016; Christopher et al., 2012), and yet others suggest that the relation of inhibition to reading comprehension is mediated by mind wandering, a difficulty with the internal control of attention (Kane & McVay, 2012).

We suggest that this mixed picture may be related to a lack of theory-driven hypotheses connecting inhibition to specific academic skills as well as a lack of precision in measuring inhibition. Studies of LDs that measure inhibitory control often fail to distinguish between types of inhibition. Inhibitory control is not a unitary construct (Cragg, 2016); it encompasses both behavioral control as well as interference control, which is an internal form of attentional control applied to minimize cognitive interference from distracting information in stimuli and tasks. Take the Lonergan et al. (2019) meta-analysis as an example—the studies that measured inhibition almost exclusively measured behavioral control, likely because the Stop Signal Response Time task is the predominant measure of inhibition in ADHD studies. We also do not know much about whether different types of inhibition are related to different types of academic learning and performance within an academic domain. Consider, for example, hypothetical needs for interference control for specific academic skills: when space and quantity are in conflict; when math word problems contain irrelevant information (see Ng et al., 2017, for a monitoring vs. inhibitory account of this issue); in beginning reading where frequent pronunciations may interfere with low-frequency exceptional pronunciations; in reading comprehension when the situation model requires revision (Gernsbacher & Faust, 1991); or when what is read conflicts with one's prior knowledge or beliefs (e.g., Mason et al., 2020). The most comprehensive treatment to date of these issues can be found in Table 2 of Spiegel et al. (2021). In contrast to reading, Wilkey and colleagues have developed a theoretical account for the putative relationship of both general inhibition and domain-specific (i.e., quantity-specific) inhibition to mathematical cognition (Wilkey et al., 2020). Whether and how domain-general and domain-specific inhibition are related to difficulties in various aspects of mathematics remains to be studied.

In sum, we extend the Lee and Lee (2019) proposal to rethink studies of the relation of inhibition and mathematics to include studies of the relation of inhibition to reading and writing, in which attention is paid to both the types of inhibition as well as the types of academic subskills that are being assessed. Given that different types of attention switching may also exist and be differentially related to different aspects of cognition (von Bastian & Druey, 2017), these suggestions for inhibition could be equally applied to switching.

Another topic for additional research has to do with testing whether EFs have direct or indirect (i.e., mediated) effects on math performance. These types of analyses are rare in mathematics (but see Cirino et al., 2022) in comparison to those in reading and writing that were discussed earlier. Whether EFs mediate the relations of more foundational or component skills of math to higher-level math skills or vice versa has not been well-studied and has prompted a call for more such longitudinal studies and meta-analytic path models (De Smedt, 2022).

EFs in the Context of Interventions

Moderation Effects: The Interaction of Child and Intervention Characteristics

Cronbach (1957) argued that psychology would advance by combining experimental and correlational traditions to study the interactions of person and treatment variables. These interactions, moderation effects, are thought to be important for understanding for whom a treatment works best. Thus, one potential contribution of EFs to understanding intervention effects for individuals with LDs has to do with whether or not EFs, which might be thought of as supporting many different types of learning, might be important *moderators* of intervention effects. In other words, might one's level of EFs at the start of an intervention have predictive value for whether that individual will respond in more or less positive ways to that intervention?

We use the lens of cognitive load theory to argue that moderation effects force one to scrutinize not only the EF characteristics of the child, but also the EF requirements of the intervention. We include studies of individuals with LDs that tested EFs as moderators of intervention effects. We adopt the view of Stuebing et al. (2015) that conditional models (i.e., controlling for initial status on academic outcomes) are most pertinent to education because they ask whether there are child characteristics (EF) that predict response to intervention amongst children performing at the same initial level on the academic skill targeted by the intervention.

Reading

Within the domain of reading, there is not much evidence for EFs as moderators of treatment effects for school-age children. In one meta-analysis of struggling readers in third grade and below, Stuebing et al. (2015) looked at several non-EF cognitive predictors, as well as working memory. Most of the studies focused on word reading instruction. In conditional models, reading-related cognitive variables, such as phonological awareness and RAN, showed small effects in predicting response, while working memory did not show effects. In a study of older readers with reading comprehension disabilities receiving a multicomponent reading intervention, Miciak and colleagues (2019) used a latent EF factor to predict responders and non-responders and did not find moderation effects for latent EF;

however, Miciak et al. (2019) categorized responders and non-responders based on standardized reading scores at post-intervention, making it difficult to compare these findings to studies that test moderation effects across the distribution of outcomes conditionalizing on pretest.

In a literacy intervention for at-risk preschoolers, Goodrich et al. (2023) found that EF (latent factor) significantly moderated intervention effects such that children with relatively lower EF at pretest benefited more from the literacy intervention compared to those with average or high pretest EF. Conversely, in an intervention designed to improve young children's behavioral and emotional control (PATHS), Bierman and colleagues (2008) found that PreK children in PATHS who started lower in EFs showed larger effects on print knowledge compared to similar children in control classrooms at the end of the PreK year. Findings from these two studies are consistent with models of developmental mutualism, that is, bidirectional effects of EFs and reading for children early in the development of literacy and EF.

Stuebing et al. (2015) point out that many baseline measures of abilities used to assess moderation effects are intercorrelated. For example, phonological awareness tasks include a working memory component. The Peng, Zhang, et al. (2022) meta-analysis showed that simple view components largely accounted for the relations of EFs to reading comprehension. Halverson and colleagues (2021) found that inference-making, which is the strongest direct predictor of reading comprehension in adolescents (Ahmed et al., 2016), completely mediated the relation of working memory to reading comprehension. Perhaps it is not surprising, then, that EFs have not been found to predict response to reading interventions in conditional models in which baseline levels of word reading and/or reading comprehension are included.

Although there are few studies testing moderating effects of EFs on outcomes of reading interventions, the implication of moderation findings (or lack thereof) thus far for assessment, at least for school-age children, is clear. EF measures are unlikely to add value to the prediction of response to intervention over and above initial reading status. However, this is not the same as asking whether it is valuable to attend to the cognitive or EF load of interventions or to try and use reading interventions to also promote growth in EFs. These are issues that we come back to when discussing studies on these two approaches to intervention design.

Mathematics

To our knowledge, there is no published meta-analysis of moderation effects in mathematics intervention research; however, we report on a systematic review in progress that included only studies of children with math learning disabilities, which is summarized in Barnes et al. (2023). Based on a systematic search of peer-reviewed publications up to the end of 2021, we found 13 studies that measured one or more EFs, most published in the last decade. Types of interventions varied with math word problem solving and fractions interventions accounting for close to 70% of the interventions, and with 12 of the 13 studies measuring working memory, 4 assessed attention using a behavioral checklist, and only 1 assessed inhibitory control. Most studies used single indicators of EF variables in their analyses. General findings were that (1) of the 12 studies that measured working memory, 10 found moderating effects; (2) more complex working memory measures were associated with moderated treatment effects regardless of modality (i.e., verbal vs. visual–spatial); (3) the most consistent pattern was that children with relatively higher working memory at baseline gained more from the intervention; and (4) studies that tested more than one form of a math intervention produced more nuanced findings. For example, one study showed that conceptually based practice embedded in a fractions intervention was more beneficial for children with MLD with relatively lower working memory at baseline, while fluency-based practice embedded in the same fractions intervention was more beneficial for children with MLD and relatively higher working memory (Fuchs et al., 2013). In another example, Swanson (2016) investigated the effects of systematically increasing working memory load (by increasing interfering information) in word-problem-solving instruction for third graders with MLD. This was a multi-arm experiment in which different instructional conditions also either required the use of verbal and/or visual (diagramming) strategies or no strategies. Compared to the control group, children with relatively higher working memory benefited in word problem and calculation outcomes if they practiced problems that gradually increased in their working memory load but did not require them to also use verbal or visual strategies. Children with lower WM capacity performed better in the control group, suggesting that none of the experimental conditions were a good fit for them, even though these conditions used word-problem-solving strategies common to many interventions for MLD. In other words, all of the conditions in this study overtaxed the cognitive capacity of students with MLD and low working memory.

Implications for Future Research

Based on the findings from studies employing moderator analyses of EFs in both reading and mathematics and the gaps in this research, recommendations for additional research are straightforward. They include: (1) the expansion beyond working memory of the EFs that are tested for moderation; (2) the use of latent EF measures in samples of sufficient size to test moderation hypotheses; and (3) a theory-driven approach to posing moderator hypotheses within each academic domain. For example, in mathematics, are there some types of skill learning that particularly require inhibitory control, and do some intervention materials and procedures draw heavily on inhibition?

Explanations of moderation effects have tended to focus more on child-level characteristics as the important ingredient in the aptitude by treatment interaction and less on understanding that interventions also have characteristics that can increase cognitive load in both detrimental (extraneous-load) and positive (germane-load) ways. Furthermore, what is extraneous or germane load might also depend on what the child with LD brings to the learning context, including their level of EF skills as well as their domain knowledge. A good illustration of this is the study by Fuchs et al. (2013) in which different types of practice differentially advantaged children with higher versus lower working memory and vice versa. Thus, in interpreting EF moderator effects, it is important to think more carefully about the *fit* between the child's EF and the intervention's EF requirements than about the EF status of the child alone.

Interventions for children with LDs often try to minimize what are considered to be aspects of instruction that are taxing on EFs. For example, the use of direct, simple, and precise language in mathematical interventions is prescribed to lessen the burden on both WM and language comprehension. The CRA (concrete–representational–abstract) sequence is similarly thought to reduce capacity limitations by sequencing instruction from more concrete representations to more abstract symbolic representations. The use of manipulatives is presumed to help with working memory offloading. However, our assumptions about what reduces or increases cognitive load for children with LDs may require more systematic study. For example, manipulatives are not always load-reducing (Petersen & McNeil, 2013), and rich perceptual detail in illustrations that accompany academic concepts may be helpful for some children but interfere with processing for others (Menendez et al., 2022). Similarly, instructional principles presumed to be universally helpful for learning (e.g., the use of examples and non-examples in vocabulary learning to produce contextual interference; Barnes et al., 2021) may pose too great a load on EF for some learners, particularly when domain knowledge is low (Barnes et al., 2022). Moderation effects, such as those we discussed, may prompt experimental studies that manipulate design features of our interventions in a theoretically motivated manner to determine which features or components of our interventions best fit the needs of children with LDs.

Causal Evidence for the Relation of EFs and Academic Skill Learning

In this section, we ask whether: (1) training EFs in concert with academic interventions improves academic skills; (2) whether academic interventions improve EFs; and (3) if the answer is "yes" to either of these questions, what the mechanism(s) are that account for these effects. Although there are a number of studies that have trained EFs and looked for far transfer to academic outcomes, particularly in children without LDs, we do not review these studies, as there is ample evidence for the lack of such far transfer effects (Melby-Lervåg et al., 2016; Sala & Gobet, 2020; Shipstead et al., 2012). We confine our review to studies in which EF and academic interventions are combined and where the populations of interest are children with LDs.

Reading

A few studies have integrated EFs within content-based reading instruction for children with or at risk for RDs (Fuchs et al., 2018; Goodrich et al., 2023). Fuchs et al. (2018) tested working memory–reading training with a three-group design among at-risk readers: a reading instruction-only group, a working memory–reading group that received the same reading intervention with an additional working memory practice component, and a business-as-usual control group. In addition to reading instruction, the working memory–reading group received about 5 to 10 minutes of working memory–reading task training in each session. For example, in a cloze span task, students completed the cloze task and then recalled, in order, words they had selected to fill in the blanks in the cloze task. In a working memory–main idea task, students recalled, in order, main ideas from previous paragraphs together with the one that they had just created. For third graders, both treatment groups significantly outperformed controls on researcher-developed vocabulary and reading comprehension measures (Hedges' g = 0.31–1.46), but differences between treatment groups were not significant.

Goodrich et al. (2023) conducted a randomized controlled trial with preschool English learners at risk for language and reading difficulties with three conditions: EF–reading training, reading instruction-only, and business-as-usual control. EF–reading tasks tapped working memory, inhibition, and switching. For example, in one working memory–reading task, students identified the initial sound/letter of words and recalled the relevant sounds/letters in order. In an inhibition–reading task, students performed a task that conflicted with what the word rhymed with; if they heard the word *hose*, they touched their ear, and if they heard the word *gear*, they were required to touch their nose. Goodrich et al. (2023) found that the EF–reading training group significantly outperformed controls on standardized vocabulary and syntax measures (Hedges' g = 0.67 ~ 1.30) and also showed higher performance on syntax than the reading instruction-only group (Hedges' g = 0.78), although this effect was not significant.

Mathematics

There are also a few mathematics intervention studies that have embedded EFs. Kroesbergen et al. (2014) randomly assigned 51 5-year-old children with below-average mathematics skills to three study groups: domain-general working memory training, domain-specific working memory training, and a business-as-usual control. The difference between domain-general working memory training and domain-specific working memory training is that the latter used numerical materials. For example, in a "Counting Recall" activity, children saw a set of triangles and circles on a screen, counted the circles, remembered the count for each set, and recalled the (count) number from each set in order. In a "linear board game," children took turns to throw a die with the numbers one, two, and three and remembered the number they threw. When all the children had thrown the die, they recalled the number they threw and attempted to take the right number of steps on the board. Results showed that the domain-specific WM group significantly outperformed the control group on numeracy (Hedges' g = .93) and outperformed the domain-general working memory group on both researcher-developed and standardized numeracy measures, Hedges' g = .49 ~.53, although none of these comparisons between active treatment groups were statistically significant.

In the Swanson (2016) study discussed earlier with respect to moderator effects for working memory, EF was embedded in the word-problem-solving intervention by slowly increasing working memory load with the incremental presentation of irrelevant propositions. Recall that practice with problem solving that increased load without introducing additional verbal or visual strategies was beneficial, but only for children with relatively higher working memory (for word problem performance, Hedges' $g = .47$, $p < .05$, and for calculations, Hedges' $g = .80$, $p < .05$), Findings from this study suggest that systematically increasing working memory load within an intervention is helpful to some children with MLD, but not others.

In Muñez et al. (2022), children at risk of MLD were assigned to one of four different treatment groups: working memory training, working memory plus numeracy training, numeracy training, and active control (same activities as in working memory training, but without the recall component). In the working memory plus numeracy training, children were tasked with working memory activities such as updating, n-back, and complex span tasks with numerical stimuli. Compared to the working memory training and the active control groups, the numeracy training and working memory plus numeracy training groups showed improvements in various early numeracy skills as well as math achievement. In comparison to the active control group, both numeracy and working memory plus numeracy training groups showed improvements in various early numeracy skills as well as math achievement after accounting for training exposure. However, because none of the treatment groups improved on working memory, the effects on math for both groups are likely specific to numeracy training rather than working memory.

Barnes et al. (2016) randomized 518 children in prekindergarten with very low math knowledge to one of three groups: a business-as-usual control, an intensive math intervention, and the same intensive math intervention with a brief (8-minute) weekly attention training session (training focused attention, inhibition, and task switching). There were positive effects compared to controls on early mathematics skills for the two math intervention groups, but no additional benefit of attention training on mathematics. There were small, significant effects of attention training on attention, but no effects of math intervention alone on attention. The low dosage of the attention intervention may have precluded synergistic effects of attention training on math.

Finally, Fuchs et al. (2022) compared various conditions with and without working memory training in an intensive math word-problem-solving intervention study for second graders with MLD. Children ($N = 240$) were randomized to one of four conditions: general working memory training (CogMed); word-problem-solving intervention; word-problem-solving intervention with an embedded working memory training component; and a business-as-usual control. Children in all active treatment conditions had 30-minute sessions, with the last 5 minutes of each session devoted to calculation and math word problem practice. What distinguished the math word problems instruction from the math word problems instruction with working memory training was a 6-minute session in which the former group played arithmetic and word-problem-solving games and the latter group played math games with an added working memory (i.e., serial order recall) requirement. Compared to the controls, the group that received general working memory training with short, contiguous math practice showed a small, significant effect on math word problems (Cohen's d = .23) and a large effect on latent working memory (Cohen's d = 1.22). The two groups receiving the math word problems intervention showed large effects on math word problems (Cohen's d = 1.36 and 1.51) as well as a moderate and significant effect on latent working memory (Cohen's d = .30 and .62). The two math intervention groups did not differ in the size of their effects on either math or working memory.

The mechanism for these findings was tested using longitudinal mediation analyses. The effects on word problem solving were mediated in every case by improvements in working memory; in contrast, the positive effects on calculation did not show mediation by working memory. These findings are consistent with bidirectional models of EF and academic skills development (Peng & Kievit, 2020; Zhang & Peng, 2023a, 2023b) and with knowledge-based developmental models (Doebel, 2020); however, there was also specificity in that the largest effects for both math and working memory were associated with more intensive interventions in math and working memory, respectively, suggesting domain-specific interventions are necessary for children with MLD.

Summary and Future Research

If we had written this chapter for the previous edition of the *Handbook*, we would have concluded that there was no evidence that causally links EFs to academic skills development in individuals with LDs. Times have changed; however, for several of the studies we reviewed, there were often no significant differences in academic outcomes when comparing academic skills intervention versus academic skills intervention with an EF component, even though effect sizes sometimes favored the combined academic and EF interventions. Thus, it is the academic skills intervention in the various conditions across several of these studies that can be credited with positive effects on academic outcomes. Keeping this caveat in mind, we present some takeaways as well as suggestions for future work in this area.

First, it is clearly possible to embed components into academic instruction that require the learner to draw on EFs, and there is some evidence that such manipulations are associated with positive effects on learning and performance in both reading and math; however, the research base is thin, it is not clear whether embedding EFs into academic skills interventions provides added value over and above traditional academic interventions when instructional time is held constant, and it is not clear for whom and when in learning such EF intervention components might be most beneficial. Second, the findings from some of these experimental studies provide causal evidence for the hypothesis that there is mutualism in the development of academic and EF skills, and they are inconsistent with jug-and-milk-type thinking that one's EF capacity is the limiting factor in academic learning. Third, the testing of mediation hypotheses (in Fuchs et al., 2022) strengthens the degree to which we can infer that the relationship between one EF (working memory) and one type of mathematics (word problem solving) is a causal one.

Our suggestions for future research follow from these general takeaways. They are to (1) encourage additional experimental studies in which EFs are explicitly embedded in academic skills interventions or are trained contiguous with academic skills; (2) test whether incoming level of EF moderates the effects of interventions in which EFs are either trained or embedded in academic interventions; (3) design studies in such a way that mechanisms of hypothesized effects can be empirically tested (i.e., using longitudinal mediation models); and (4) determine whether academic interventions with EF components mitigate common limitations associated with traditional interventions, that is, whether they do anything to promote transfer of learning across time, materials, and tasks. In relation to this latter point, Peng and Swanson (2022) proposed a domain-specific approach to WM training in which they suggested that training tasks should closely link the central executive (attentional control) with the use of long-term memory through retrieval practice in a specific academic domain and that training tasks should promote strategy use that can be effectively applied (i.e., transferred) to different academic tasks.

Concluding Comments

Continued uncertainty regarding the definition and measurement of EFs, and the fact that deficits in EFs are not specific to LDs, makes us question the usefulness of EFs for assessment and identification purposes. We think that the utility of EFs in the field of learning disabilities lies in considering their potential importance for interventions. In particular, we proposed that when EFs moderate intervention effects, it helps us to understand not only for whom certain interventions may be most effective, but also whether there are unintended EF requirements in interventions that provide less than optimal *fit* for children with LDs. We suggested that an emerging body of experimental work that embeds EFs in or combines EFs with academic skills interventions has implications for theory and practice. Implications for theory are that experimental methods may elucidate the nature and direction of relationships between EFs and academic skills development. Implications for practice are that these embedded and combined interventions provide a novel approach to intensifying academic interventions (Fuchs & Fuchs, 2014); however, whether this approach has promise requires considerably more investigation.

ACKNOWLEDGMENTS

The writing of this chapter was supported by Grants R324A200101 to Vanderbilt University and R324A220268 to the University of Texas at Austin, from the National Center for Special Education Research (NCSER), Institute of Education Sciences, U.S. Department of Education, and by Grants 2100328 to Vanderbilt University and 2405797 to the University of Texas at Austin from the National Sciences Foundation. The contents of this chapter are solely the responsibility of the authors and do not necessarily reflect the official views of the Department of Education or the National Sciences Foundation.

REFERENCES

Ahmed, Y., Francis, D. J., York, M., Fletcher, J. M., Barnes, M. A., & Kulesz, P. (2016). Validation of the direct and inferential mediation (DIME) model of reading comprehension in grades 7 through 12. *Contemporary Educational Psychology, 44–45*, 68–82.

Ahmed, Y., Wagner, R. K., & Lopez, D. (2014). Developmental relations between reading and writing at the word, sentence, and text levels: A latent change score analysis. *Journal of Educational Psychology, 106*(2), 419–434.

Arrington, C. N., Kulesz, P. A., Francis, D. J., Fletcher, J. M., & Barnes, M. A. (2014). The contribution of attentional control and working memory to reading comprehension and decoding. *Scientific Studies of Reading, 18*(5), 325–346.

Baddeley, A. D., & Hitch, G. J. (1974). Working memory. In G. H. Bower (Ed.), *Psychology of learning and motivation* (pp. 47–89). Academic Press.

Baker, L., Millman, Z. B., & Singer Trakhman, L. M. (2020). How the construct of metacognition has contributed to translational research in education, mental health, and beyond. *Translational Issues in Psychological Science, 6*(1), 1–7.

Barkley, R. A. (2012). *Executive functions: What they are, how they work, and why they evolved.* Guilford Press.

Barnes, M. A. (2023). Executive functions: What are they good for? A perspective from intervention research. *Mind, Brain, and Education, 17*(4), 238–245.

Barnes, M. A., Clemens, N. H., & Miller, A. H. (2022). Historical context, current influences, and future directions. In T. W. Farmer, E. Talbott, K. McMaster, D. Lee, & T. C. Aceves (Eds.), *Handbook of special education research, Vol. I: Theory, methods, and developmental processes* (pp. 24–39). Routledge.

Barnes, M. A., Davis, C., Kulesz, P., & Francis, D. (2021). Effects of semantic reinforcement, semantic discrimination, and affix frequency on new word learning in skilled and less skilled readers in grades 6 to 12. *Journal of Experimental Child Psychology, 205*, 105083.

Barnes, M. A., Klein, A., Swank, P., Starkey, P., McCandliss, B., Flynn, K., et al. (2016). Effects of tutorial interventions in mathematics and attention for low-performing preschool children. *Journal of Research on Educational Effectiveness, 9*(4), 577–606.

Barnes, M. A., Stuebing, K., Fletcher, J. M., Barth, A., & Francis, D. (2016). Investigating cognitive difficulties in struggling comprehenders: A comparison of group selection and regression-based models. *Journal of Research on Educational Effectiveness, 9*(2), 153–172.

Berninger, V. W., & Winn, W. (2006). Implications of advancements in brain research and technology for writing development, writing instruction, and educational evolution. In C. A. MacArthur, S. Graham, & J. Fitzgerald (Eds.), *Handbook of writing research* (pp. 96–114). Guilford Press.

Bierman, K. L., Nix, R. L., Greenberg, M. T., Blair, C., & Domitrovich, C. E. (2008). Executive functions and school readiness intervention: Impact, moderation, and mediation in the Head Start REDI program. *Development and Psychopathology, 20*(3), 821–843.

Borkowski, J. G. (1992). Metacognitive theory: A framework for teaching literacy, writing, and math skills. *Journal of Learning Disabilities, 25*(4), 253–257.

Broadbent, D. E. (1957). A mechanical model for human attention and immediate memory. *Psychological Review, 64*(3), 205–215.

Brown, A. L. (1975). The development of memory: Knowing, knowing about knowing, and knowing how to know. *Advances in Child Development and Behavior, 10*, 103–152.

Butterfuss, R., & Kendeou, P. (2018). The role of executive functions in reading comprehension. *Educational Psychology Review, 30*(3), 801–826.

Butterfuss, R., & Kendeou, P. (2020). Reducing interference from misconceptions: The role of inhibition in knowledge revision. *Journal of Educational Psychology, 112*(4), 782–794.

Carretti, B., Borella, E., Cornoldi, C., & De Beni, R. (2009). Role of working memory in explaining the performance of individuals with specific reading comprehension difficulties: A meta-analysis. *Learning and Individual Differences, 19*(2), 246–251.

Christopher, M. E., Miyake, A., Keenan, J. M., Pennington, B., DeFries, J. C., Wadsworth, S. J., et al. (2012). Predicting word reading and comprehension with executive function and speed measures across development: A latent variable analysis. *Journal of Experimental Psychology: General, 141*(3), 470–488.

Cirino, P. T., Tolar, T. D., & Fuchs, L. S. (2022). Domain general and specific contributions to algebra: A sequenced longitudinal path model. *Contemporary Educational Psychology, 68*, 102026.

Cortés Pascual, A., Moyano Muñoz, N., & Quilez Robres, A. (2019). The relationship between executive functions and academic performance in primary education: Review and meta-analysis. *Frontiers in Psychology, 10*, 1582.

Cowan, N. (1988). Evolving conceptions of memory storage, selective attention, and their mutual constraints within the human information-processing system. *Psychological Bulletin, 104*(2), 163–191.

Cragg, L. (2016). The development of stimulus and response interference control in midchildhood. *Developmental Psychology, 52*(2), 242–252.

Cronbach, L. J. (1957). The two disciplines of scientific psychology. *American Psychologist, 12*(11), 671–684.

De Smedt, B. (2022). Individual differences in mathematical cognition: A Bert's eye view. *Current Opinion in Behavioral Sciences, 46*, 101175.

Denckla, M. B. (1994). Measurement of executive function. In G. R. Lyon (Ed.), *Frames of reference for the assessment of learning disabilities: New views on measurement issues* (pp. 117–142). Paul H. Brookes.

Doebel, S. (2020). Rethinking executive function and its development. *Perspectives on Psychological Science, 15*(4), 942–956.

Engle, R. W. (2018). Working memory and executive attention: A revisit. *Perspectives on Psychological Science, 13*(2), 190–193.

Evans, J. S. B., & Stanovich, K. E. (2013). Dual-process theories of higher cognition: Advancing the debate. *Perspectives on Psychological Science, 8*(3), 223–241.

Flavell, J. H. (1970). Cognitive changes in adulthood. In L. R. Goulet & P. B. Baltes (Eds.), *Life-span developmental psychology* (pp. 247–253). Academic Press.

Flower, L., & Hayes, J. R. (1981). A cognitive process theory of writing. *College Composition and Communication, 32*(4), 365–387.

Friso-Van den Bos, I., Van der Ven, S. H. G., Kroesbergen, E. H., & van Luit, J. E. H. (2013). Working memory and mathematics in primary school children: A meta-analysis. *Educational Research Review, 10*, 29–44.

Fuchs, D., & Fuchs, L. S. (2014). Rethinking service delivery for students with significant learning problems: Developing and implementing intensive instruction. *Remedial and Special Education, 36*(2), 105–111.

Fuchs, D., Patton, S., Fuchs, L. S., Gilbert, J., Walsh, M., Lute, N., et al. (2018). Combining reading comprehension instruction with cognitive training to provide intensive intervention to at-risk students. In P. C. Pullen & M. J. Kennedy (Eds.), *Handbook of response to intervention and multi-tiered systems of support* (pp. 198–217). Routledge.

Fuchs, L. S., Fuchs, D., Sterba, S. K., Barnes, M. A., Seethaler, P. M., & Changas, P. (2022). Building word-problem solving and working memory capacity: A randomized controlled trial comparing three intervention approaches. *Journal of Educational Psychology.* Advance online publication.

Fuchs, L. S., Schumacher, R. F., Long, J., Namkung, J., Hamlett, C. L., Cirino, P. T., et al. (2013). Improving at-risk learners' understanding of fractions. *Journal of Educational Psychology, 105*(3), 683–700.

Garon, N., Bryson, S. E., & Smith, I. M. (2008). Executive function in preschoolers: A review using an integrative framework. *Psychological Bulletin, 134*(1), 31–60.

Gernsbacher, M. A. (1997). Two decades of structure building. *Discourse Processes, 23*(3), 265–304.

Gernsbacher, M. A., & Faust, M. E. (1991). The mechanism of suppression: A component of general comprehension skill. *Journal of Experimental Psychology: Learning, Memory, and Cognition, 17*(2), 245–262.

Ginsburg, H. P., Klein, A., & Starkey, P. (1998). The development of children's mathematical thinking: Connecting research with practice. In W. Damon, I. E. Sigel, & K. A. Renninger (Eds.), *Handbook of child psychology: Child psychology in practice* (pp. 401–476). John Wiley & Sons, Inc.

Goodrich, J. M., Peng, P., Bohaty, J., Leiva, S., & Thayer, L. (2023). Embedding executive function training into early literacy instruction for dual language learners: A pilot study. *Journal of Speech, Language, and Hearing Research, 66*(2), 573–588.

Gough, P. B., & Tunmer, W. E. (1986). Decoding, reading, and reading disability. *Remedial and Special Education, 7*(1), 6–10.

Halverson, K. K., Derrick, J. L., Medina, L. D., & Cirino, P. T. (2021). Executive functioning with the NIH EXAMINER and inference making in struggling readers. *Developmental Neuropsychology, 46*(3), 213–231.

Jacob, R., & Parkinson, J. (2015). The potential for school-based interventions that target executive function to improve academic achievement: A review. *Review of Educational Research, 85*(4), 512–552.

Kane, M. J., & McVay, J. C. (2012). What mind wandering reveals about executive-control abilities and failures. *Current Directions in Psychological Science: A Journal of the American Psychological Society, 21*(5), 348–354.

Karr, J. E., Areshenkoff, C. N., Rast, P., Hofer, S. M., Iverson, G. L., & Garcia-Barrera, M. A. (2018). The unity and diversity of executive functions: A systematic review and re-analysis of latent variable studies. *Psychological Bulletin, 144*(11), 1147–1185.

Kim, Y. S. G. (2020). Interactive dynamic literacy model: An integrative theoretical framework for reading-writing relations. In R. A. Alves, T. Limpo, & R. M. Joshi (Eds.), *Reading-writing connections: Towards integrative literacy science* (pp. 11–34). Springer.

Kim, Y. S. G., & Park, S. H. (2019). Unpacking pathways using the direct and indirect effects model of writing (DIEW) and the contributions of higher order cognitive skills to writing. *Reading and Writing, 32*(5), 1319–1343.

Kim, Y. S. G., Petscher, Y., Wanzek, J., & Al Otaiba, S. (2018). Relations between reading and writing: A longitudinal examination from grades 3 to 6. *Reading and Writing, 31*(7), 1591–1618.

Kroesbergen, E. H., van't Noordende, J. E., & Kolkman, M. E. (2014). Training working memory in kindergarten children: Effects on working memory and early numeracy. *Child Neuropsychology, 20*(1), 23–37.

Lee, K., & Lee, H. W. (2019). Inhibition and mathematical performance: Poorly correlated, poorly measured, or poorly matched? *Child Development Perspectives, 13*(1), 28–33.

Lin, X., & Powell, S. R. (2021). Examining the relation between whole numbers and fractions: A meta-analytic structural equation modeling approach. *Contemporary Educational Psychology, 67*, 102017.

Lonergan, A., Doyle, C., Cassidy, C., Mahon, S. M., Roche, R. A. P., Boran, L., & Bramham, J. (2019). A meta-analysis of executive functioning in dyslexia with consideration of the impact of comorbid ADHD. *Journal of Cognitive Psychology, 31*(7), 725–749.

Martinussen, R., Hayden, J., Hogg-Johnson, S., & Tannock, R. (2005). A meta-analysis of working memory impairments in children with attention-deficit/hyperactivity disorder. *Journal of the American Academy of Child & Adolescent Psychiatry, 44*(4), 377–384.

Mason, L., Borella, E., Diakidoy, I. N., Butterfuss, R., Kendeou, P., & Carretti, B. (2020). Learning from refutation and standard expository science texts: The contribution of inhibitory functions in relation to text type. *Discourse Processes, 57*(10), 921–939.

Melby-Lervåg, M., Redick, T. S., & Hulme, C. (2016). Working memory training does not improve performance on measures of intelligence or other measures of "far transfer": Evidence from a meta-analytic review. *Perspectives on Psychological Science, 11*(4), 512–534.

Menendez, D., Rosengren, K. S., & Alibali, M. W. (2022). Detailed bugs or bugging details? The influence of perceptual richness across elementary school years. *Journal of Experimental Child Psychology, 213*, 105269.

Miciak, J., Cirino, P. T., Ahmed, Y., Reid, E., & Vaughn, S. (2019). Executive functions and response to intervention: Identification of students struggling with reading comprehension. *Learning Disability Quarterly, 42*(1), 17–31.

Miyake, A., & Friedman, N. P. (2012). The nature and organization of individual differences in executive functions: Four general conclusions. *Current Directions in Psychological Science, 21*(1), 8–14.

Miyake, A., Friedman, N. P., Emerson, M. J., Witzki, A. H., Howerter, A., & Wager, T. D. (2000). The unity and diversity of executive functions and their contributions to complex "frontal lobe" tasks: A latent variable analysis. *Cognitive Psychology, 41*(1), 49–100.

Morgan, P. L., Farkas, G., Wang, Y., Hillemeier, M. M., Oh, Y., & Maczuga, S. (2019). Executive function deficits in kindergarten predict repeated academic difficulties across elementary school. *Early Childhood Research Quarterly, 46*, 20–32.

Morgan, P. L., Li, H., Farkas, G., Cook, M., Pun, W. H., & Hillemeier, M. M. (2017). Executive functioning deficits increase kindergarten children's risk for reading and mathematics difficulties in first grade. *Contemporary Educational Psychology, 50*, 23–32.

Müller, U., & Kerns, K. (2015). The development of executive function. In L. S. Liben, U. Müller, & R. M. Lerner (Eds.), *Handbook of child psychology and developmental science: Cognitive processes* (pp. 571–623). John Wiley & Sons.

Muñez, D., Lee, K., Bull, R., Khng, K. H., Cheam, F., & Rahim, R. A. (2022). Working memory and numeracy training for children with math learning difficulties: Evidence from a large-scale implementation in the classroom. *Journal of Educational Psychology, 114*(8) 1866–1880.

Ng, J., Lee, K., & Khng, K. H. (2017). Irrelevant information in math problems need not be inhibited: Students might just need to spot them. *Learning and Individual Differences, 60*, 46–55.

Packwood, S., Hodgetts, H. M., & Tremblay, S. (2011). A multiperspective approach to the conceptualization of executive functions. *Journal of Clinical and Experimental Neuropsychology, 33*(4), 456–470.

Paris, S. G. (2005). Reinterpreting the development of reading skills. *Reading Research Quarterly, 40*(2), 184–202.

Parkin, A. J. (1998). The central executive does not exist. *Journal of the International Neuropsychological Society, 4*(5), 518–522.

Peng, A., Orosco, M. J., Wang, H., Swanson, H. L., & Reed, D. K. (2022). Cognition and writing development in early adolescent English learners. *Journal of Educational Psychology, 114*(5), 1136–1155.

Peng, P., Barnes, M. A., Wang, C., Wang, W., Li, S., Swanson, H. L., et al. (2018). A meta-analysis on the relation between reading and working memory. *Psychological Bulletin, 144*(1), 48–76.

Peng, P., & Kievit, R. A. (2020). The development of academic achievement and cognitive abilities: A bidirectional perspective. *Child Development Perspectives, 14*(1), 15–20.

Peng, P., Namkung, J., Barnes, M. A., & Sun, C. (2016). A meta-analysis of mathematics and working memory: Moderating effects of working memory domain, type of mathematics skill, and sample characteristics. *Journal of Educational Psychology, 108*(4), 455–473.

Peng, P., & Swanson, L. (2022). The domain-specific approach of working memory training. *Developmental Review.* [Epub ahead of print]

Peng, P., Wang, C., & Namkung, J. (2018). Understanding the cognition related to mathematics difficulties: A meta-analysis on the cognitive deficit profiles and the bottleneck theory. *Review of Educational Research, 88*(3), 434–476.

Peng, P., Zhang, Z., Wang, W., Lee, K., Wang, T., Wang, C., et al. (2022). A meta-analytic review of cognition and reading difficulties: Individual differences, moderation, and language mediation mechanisms. *Psychological Bulletin, 148*(3–4), 227–272.

Perfetti, C. A. (1985). *Reading ability.* Oxford University Press.

Perfetti, C., & Helder, A. (2022). Progress in reading science: Word identification, comprehension, and universal perspectives. In M. J. Snowling, C. Hulme, & K. Nation (Eds.), *The science of reading: A handbook* (2nd ed., pp. 5–35). Wiley-Blackwell.

Petersen, L. A., & McNeil, N. M. (2013). Effects of perceptually rich manipulatives on preschoolers' counting performance: Established knowledge counts. *Child Development, 84*(3), 1020–1033.

Peterson, R. L., McGrath, L. M., Willcutt, E. G., Keenan, J. M., Olson, R. K., & Pennington, B. F. (2021). How specific are learning disabilities? *Journal of Learning Disabilities, 54*(6), 466–483.

Posner, M. I., & Rothbart, M. K. (2007). Research on attention networks as a model for the integration of psychological science. *Annual Review of Psychology, 58*(1), 1–23.

Rittle-Johnson, B., Schneider, M., & Star, J. R. (2015). Not a one-way street: Bidirectional relations between procedural and conceptual knowledge of mathematics. *Educational Psychology Review, 27*(4), 587–597.

Sala, G., & Gobet, F. (2020). Working memory training in typically developing children: A multilevel meta-analysis. *Psychonomic Bulletin & Review, 27*(3), 423–424.

Schachar, R., Mota, V. L., Logan, G. D., Tannock, R., & Klim, P. (2000). Confirmation of an inhibitory control deficit in attention-deficit/hyperactivity disorder. *Journal of Abnormal Child Psychology, 28*(3), 227–235.

Share, D. L., McGee, R., & Silva, P. A. (1989). IQ and reading progress: A test of the capacity notion of IQ. *Journal of the American Academy of Child and Adolescent Psychiatry, 28*(1), 97–100.

Shipstead, Z., Redick, T. S., & Engle, R. W. (2012). Is working memory training effective? *Psychological Bulletin, 138*(4), 628–654.

Spiegel, J. A., Goodrich, J. M., Morris, B. M., Osborne, C. M., & Lonigan, C. J. (2021). Relations between executive functions and academic outcomes in elementary school children: A meta-analysis. *Psychological Bulletin, 147*(4), 329–351.

Stuebing, K. K., Barth, A. E., Trahan, L. H., Reddy, R. R., Miciak, J., & Fletcher, J. M. (2015). Are child cognitive characteristics strong predictors of responses to intervention? A meta-analysis. *Review of Educational Research, 85*(3), 395–429.

Stuss, D. T., & Benson, D. F. (1984). Neuropsychological studies of the frontal lobes. *Psychological Bulletin, 95*(1), 3–28.

Swanson, H. L. (2016). Word problem solving, working memory and serious math difficulties: Do cognitive strategies really make a difference? *Journal of Applied Research in Memory and Cognition, 5*(4), 368–383.

Sweller, J. (2010). Element interactivity and intrinsic, extraneous, and germane cognitive load. *Educational Psychology Review, 22*(2), 123–138.

Torgesen, J. K. (1994). Issues in the assessment of executive function: An information-processing perspective. In G. R. Lyon (Ed.), *Frames of reference for the assessment of learning disabilities: New views on measurement issues* (pp. 143–162). Paul H. Brookes Publishing Co.

von Bastian, C. C., & Druey, M. D. (2017). Shifting between mental sets: An individual differences approach to commonalities and differences of task switching components. *Journal of Experimental Psychology: General, 146*(9), 1266–1285.

Wilkey, E. D., Pollack, C., & Price, G. R. (2020). Dyscalculia and typical math achievement are associated with individual differences in number-specific executive function. *Child Development, 91*(2), 596–619.

Willcutt, E. G., McGrath, L. M., Pennington, B. F., Keenan, J. M., DeFries, J. C., Olson, R. K., & Wadsworth, S. J. (2019). Understanding comorbidity between specific learning disabilities. *New Directions for Child and Adolescent Development, 2019*(165), 91–109.

Willcutt, E. G., Pennington, B. F., Boada, R., Ogline, J. S., Tunick, R. A., Chhabildas, N. A., & Olson, R. K. (2001). A comparison of the cognitive deficits in reading disability and attention-deficit/hyperactivity disorder. *Journal of Abnormal Psychology, 110*(1), 157–172.

Zhang, Z., & Peng, P. (2023a). Co-development among reading, math, science, and verbal working memory in the elementary stage. *Child Development, 94*(6), e328–e343.

Zhang, Z., & Peng, P. (2023b). Longitudinal reciprocal relations among reading, executive function, and social-emotional skills: Maybe not for all. *Journal of Educational Psychology, 115*(3), 475–501.

CHAPTER 8

Memory Difficulties in Children with Specific Learning Disabilities

H. Lee Swanson and Jennifer E. Kong

Memory reflects the ability to encode, process, and retrieve information that one has been exposed to. As a skill, it is inseparable from intellectual functioning and learning. Individuals deficient in memory skills, such as children with learning disabilities (LD), would be expected to have difficulty with several academic and cognitive tasks. Although memory is linked to performance in several academic (e.g., reading) and cognitive areas (e.g., inhibition), it is a critical area of focus in the field of LD for three reasons. First, it reflects applied cognition; that is, memory functioning affects all aspects of learning. Second, several studies suggest that the memory skills used by students with LD do not appear to exhaust, or even to tap, their ability; therefore, we need to discover instructional procedures that capitalize on their potential. Finally, several cognitive intervention programs that attempt to enhance the overall cognition of persons with LD rely on principles derived from memory research (see Swanson et al., 2004, for a review). In this chapter, we highlight foundational and current studies, as well as selectively review our recent research on working memory (WM). The reader is referred to earlier reviews that provide a historical context of memory research as applied to LD (e.g., Cooney & Swanson, 1987; Swanson et al., 2004) and emerging models linking WM to LD (Swanson & Siegel, 2001a, 2001b). Our previous chapters in the earlier editions of the *Handbook on Learning Disabilities* focused on applications of WM performance to academic domains, longitudinal outcomes, guidelines for strategy instruction (e.g., reading comprehension) (Swanson & Sáez, 2004; Swanson & Zheng, 2013), and, more recently, a theoretical view of WM and LD, competing models, and competing interpretations of a WM deficit (Swanson, 2020).

This chapter provides an update on a model that suggests that specific processes related to the phonological and executive system of WM underlie specific LD in reading (RD) and/or math (MD). Before discussing the research linking learning disabilities in reading and/or math to WM, we review our operational definition of specific LD and WM. We next review syntheses of the literature linking WM to RD and/or MD and then review work from our lab, linking specific LD in reading and/or math to specific components of WM. Finally, we review some of our recent work that briefly covers two areas: identifying LD among English language learners (ELLs) and intervention work focused on WM and math.

Definition of Terms

Specific Learning Disabilities

In general, the concept of specific LD rests on two assumptions: (1) academic difficulties are not due to inadequate opportunity to learn, general intelligence, or physical or emotional disabilities, but to basic disabilities in specific psychological processes; and (2) these specific processing deficits are a reflection of neurological, constitutional, and/or biological factors. Thus, to assess specific LD at the cognitive level, systematic efforts are made to detect (1) normal psychometric intelligence, (2) consistently below normal achievement in a specific academic skill across grade levels, (3) below normal performance in specific cognitive processes (i.e., phonological awareness, WM), (4) systematic opportunity to learn (documentation that optimal instruction has been presented but deficits in isolated processes remain) has occurred; and (5) processing deficits are not directly caused by environmental factors (e.g., poor instruction) or contingencies (e.g., SES, lack of English proficiency, and child-rearing).

We operationally defined specific LD as those children and adults who have general intelligence scores on standardized tests above 85 and who have reading scores and/or math scores below the 25th percentile (90 standard score) on a standardized norm-referenced reading/and or mathematics achievement measure. This operational definition is not unique to our work but is captured in a plethora of studies (e.g., Cirino et al., 2015; Martin et al., 2013; Passolunghi & Siegel, 2004; Siegel & Ryan, 1989). While variability exists within the field in how students are identified with LD in previous research and practice, the growing consensus among researchers has indicated that a cutoff score on achievement is appropriate to determine LD (e.g., Swanson et al., 2014, 2018). For example, our recent classification studies that utilize latent class and latent transition analysis suggest that a discrete class of children with RD and MD emerges that is consistent with our cutoff points (e.g., Swanson et al., 2016; Swanson et al., 2018).

We have also identified children with specific LD in reading and math who are ELLs with Spanish as a first language (Swanson et al., 2016, 2019a, 2019b, 2020). Children with specific LD exhibit low reading and/or math achievement on normative tests in each language system (in our case, normative tests in both English and Spanish). The conundrum, of course, in our studies is that children yielded clear variations in English and Spanish language proficiency. The literature varies in methodology for operationalizing variations in bilingualism (e.g., Peña et al., 2016; Rosselli et al., 2016), with some studies suggesting a focus on proficiency within each language system that, in turn, yields a total score and/or focus on conceptual proficiency (tests that allow for responses in either language that yields the highest score in the preferred language, see Peña et al., 2016; for a comprehensive review). At present, conceptual scoring has been used in our studies because it combines children's vocabulary knowledge across languages (Swanson et al., 2019a, 2019b, 2020)

Working Memory

Working memory consists of a limited capacity system of temporary stores and functions related to the preservation of information while simultaneously processing other information, as well as maintaining attention control related to these functions (e.g., Baddeley, 2012; Cowan, 2014; Unsworth & Engle, 2007; see Swanson, 1999, 2017, for review). Cowan (2014) defines WM "as the small amount of information that can be held in the mind and used in the execution of cognitive tasks, in contrast with long-term memory, which is the vast amount of information saved in one's life" (p. 197). Working memory or complex span tasks share the same processes (e.g., rehearsal, updating, and controlled search) as short-term memory (STM) or simple span tasks. However, simple tasks (e.g., recalling words or digits in the order of presentation) have a greater reliance on phonological processes than WM or complex span tasks (e.g., recalling words or digits in the context of interference/distraction) (see Unsworth & Engle, 2007, pp. 1045–1046, for a review). WM tasks, on the other hand, assess an individual's ability to maintain task-relevant information in an active state and regulate controlled processing. Individuals performing WM tasks must remember some task elements and ignore, or inhibit, other elements as they complete task-relevant operations (e.g., Miyake et al., 2000). In contrast, STM tasks typically involve situations that do not vary from initial encoding (e.g., Unsworth & Engle, 2007). In elaborating on the distinction between STM and WM, Cowan (1997) emphasized the role of attentional processes. WM is depicted as a subset of items of information stored in STM that are, in turn, submitted to limited attentional control processing (see also Engle et al., 1999). This assumes that when the contents of STM are separated from WM, what is left of WM is some form of controlled attention or processing related to the central executive system (also referred to as the central executive component of WM). As will be reviewed, several of our studies find that children with RD and/or MD suffer difficulties with both types of tasks across various age ranges (e.g., Swanson & Ashbaker, 2000; Swanson & Fung, 2016; Swanson & Jerman, 2006; Swanson et al., 2008; Swanson, Kudo, et al., 2019). No doubt, the distinction between STM and WM is less clear in younger children (e.g., Hutton & Towse, 2001) but becomes more distinct as children approach the upper middle grades (Gathercole et al., 2004). Our regression modeling finds that both types of tasks (STM and WM) uniquely contribute to reading and math performance among children at risk for RD and/or MD (Swanson et al., 2008; Swanson & Fung, 2016). The independent contribution of these two memory systems (STM and WM) to reading and math will be further detailed later in the chapter.

Theoretical Foundation

By far, the most utilized framework for understanding the role of WM as it applies to specific LD is Baddeley's multiple-components model (Baddeley, 2012; Baddeley & Logie, 1999). In this model, WM consists of three components: visual–spatial sketchpad, phonological loop, and central executive. The visual–spatial sketchpad is for the temporary storage of visual and spatial information, which is important for the manipulation of mental images, such as symbols and shapes. The phonological loop is for the temporary storage of verbal information, and it is important for the temporary storage of text and verbal information, such as the story within a text reading. The central executive coordinates activities between the two subsystems (i.e., visual–spatial sketchpad and phonological loop) and increases the amount of information that can be stored in the two subsystems.

In general, we find (e.g., Swanson, 1992, 1993c; Swanson & Jerman, 2007; Swanson & Fung, 2016; Swanson et al., 2020), as do others, that children with average intelligence but have specific LD in reading (RD) and/or math (MD) experience considerable difficulties on WM tasks (e.g., Attout & Majerus, 2015; Brandenburg et al., 2015; De Weerdt et al., 2013; Passolunghi & Siegel, 2004; Peng et al., 2012; Wang & Gathercole, 2013). An explanation for these findings (Swanson, 2020) is embedded within Baddeley's (2012) multicomponent model.

Research on Working Memory

Synthesis of Literature

Before selectively reviewing some of our work, a quantitative overview of the literature on WM is necessary to provide a context for our findings. We briefly summarize our quantitative syntheses of the published literature on LD as it applies to reading (RD), math (MD), and memory (e.g., Kudo et al., 2015; Johnson et al., 2010; Peng et al., 2017; Swanson & Jerman, 2006). A common metric utilized in these meta-analyses is referred to as effect size (ES) and reported as a d-index. To make ds more interpretable, statisticians have adopted Cohen's (1988) system for classifying *d*s in terms of their size (i.e., .00–.19 is described as trivial; .20–.49, small; .50–.79, moderate; .80 or higher, large).

Reading Disabilities

Our recent synthesis has found a strong relationship between WM and reading in average achievers (Peng et al., 2017). This meta-analysis investigated the relationship between reading and WM among average readers. Overall, the relation between reading and WM was moderate (r = .29) and was significantly influenced by grade level. The importance of this finding was that WM made unique contributions to reading performance even when decoding and vocabulary were controlled for in the analysis. Further meta-analyses by Peng and his colleagues have synthesized research on WM among children with RD, children with MD, and children with reading and mathematics difficulties (RD/MD). As expected, typically developing children outperformed all learning difficulty groups on WM tasks. Children with MD and children with RD showed comparable verbal WM deficits, whereas children with combined RD/MD showed the most severe WM deficits. Although there was no clear demarcation between STM and WM tasks, the results are consistent with an earlier analysis (Swanson et al., 2009) that found difficulties in both STM and WM tasks for children with RD. This earlier meta-analysis provided a more differentiated analysis of performance on STM (simple span tasks) and WM (complex span) tasks and found that children with RD vary from their average reading counterparts on STM and WM tasks. ESs across a broad age, reading, and IQ range yielded a mean ES (children with RD vs. average readers) across memory studies of –.89 (SD = 1.03) in favor of their chronologically matched average reading counterparts. The moderate range for STM measures consisted of 255 ESs (M = –.61, 95% confidence range of –.65 to –.58), and 320 ESs were in the moderate range for WM measures (M = –.67, 95% confidence range of –.68 to –.64). The synthesis indicated that children with RD were distinctively disadvantaged compared to average readers on (1) STM measures requiring the recall of phonemes and digit sequences and (2) WM measures requiring the simultaneous processing and storage of digits and words within sentence sequences and final words from unrelated sentences. The results of this synthesis also indicated, via a meta-regression analysis, no significant moderating effects related to age, IQ, or reading level emerged when predicting memory ESs. In general, the findings indicated STM and WM differences between ability groups persisted across age, suggesting that both phonological (STM) and components of the executive system (WM) underlie RD.

Math Disabilities

Of interest is whether MD and RD share the same and/or different WM problems. Peng and Fuchs (2016) meta-analysis indicated that both groups suffer WM difficulties compared to average achievers, but the RD group tends to have deficits primarily on verbal WM tasks, whereas the MD group experiences deficits on verbal and numerical WM tasks. To address this question directly as it applies to STM and WM tasks, Swanson and Jerman (2006) performed an earlier quantitative synthesis of the literature comparing the cognitive functioning of children with MD with (1) average-achieving children, (2) children with RD, and (3) children with comorbid disabilities (RD + MD) on this issue. When focusing on children with MD, approximately 194 effect sizes compared children with MD with average achievers (M ES = –.52, SE = .01), 58 effect sizes compared MD and children with RD (M = –.10, SE = .03), and 102 effect sizes compared children with MD to children with MD/RD (*M* = .26, *SE* = .02) on various cognitive measures. Overall, average achievers outperformed children with MD on measures of verbal problem solving (*M* = –.58), naming speed (*M* = –.70), STM (*M* = –.71), verbal WM (*M* = –.70), visual–spatial WM (*M* = –.63), and long-term memory (LTM, *M* = –.72). These moderate to high ESs were consistent across age and severity of MD. The results indicated that children with MD could only be differentiated on measures of naming speed (*M* = –.23) and visual WM (*M* = –.30). More importantly, both children with MD and RD share similar difficulties on measures of STM (*M* = .16) and WM (*M* = .07) tasks. The results further indicated that children with MD outperformed children with comorbid disabilities (MD/RD) on measures of literacy (*M* = .75), visual–spatial problem solving (*M* = .51), LTM (*M* = .44), STM for words (*M* = .71), and verbal WM (*M* = .30). Interestingly, as also found by Peng and Fuchs (2016), children with MD could only be differentiated (although weakly) from children with RD on measures of naming speed and visual–spatial WM. Both children with RD or MD outperformed the comorbid group on STM and WM measures. More importantly, hierarchical linear modeling of the data showed that the magnitude of ESs in overall cognitive functioning (criterion measure) between MD and average achievers was primarily related to WM deficits when the effects of all other variables (e.g., age, IQ, reading level, and other domain categories) were partialed out in the analysis.

Shared Memory Difficulties?

The takeaway message from the previously described syntheses of the literature is that children with RD and/or MD share common WM and STM problems. Thus, the question emerges: "How is it that both groups can share STM and WM deficits but manifest themselves as reading or math deficits?" Recall that a neurological inefficiency is assumed to underlie RD and MD in the fifth edition of the *Diagnostic and Statistical Manual of Mental Disorders* (DSM-5; American Psychiatric Association, 2013); however, finding the commonality is still under investigation. Because RD and/or MD are assumed to have a neurological basis in learning problems (DSM-5), it is important to note there are correlates in the neuropsychological literature that complement the tripartite WM structure of Baddeley and Logie's (1999) model, suggesting that some functional independence exists among the systems (e.g., Acheson et al., 2011; Bledowski et al., 2010; Chein & Fiez, 2010; Nee et al., 2013; Smith & Jonides, 1997, 1999). Neuropsychological evidence suggests that children with RD and/or MD experience difficulties related to these structures (e.g., Beneventi et al., 2009; Beneventi et al., 2010; Rosenberg-Lee et al., 2009). Further, recent meta-analyses of functional magnetic resonance imaging (fMRI) studies of children with RD and/or MD may provide some light on this issue. Neuroimaging studies have indicated that math and reading processes tap several common areas of the brain (e.g., Evans et al., 2016) and that manifestations of these deficits reflect *hypoactivation* (underactivation) of these common areas of the brain. For example, Kaufmann et al. (2011) meta-analysis of fMRI studies focusing on children with MD (dyscalculia) showed observable *hypoactivation* in number processing in the prefrontal and occipital cortex when compared to children without MD. Likewise, Richlan et al. (2011) meta-analysis of fMRI studies that included children with dyslexia (RD) also found a *hypoactivation* in the anterior portion of the left occipito–temporal cortex for dyslexic children. Richlan's (2012) reanalysis of the data also found little support for the assumption that standard neural anatomical models of developmental dyslexia are localized to problems primarily related to phonological decoding deficits in the left temporo–parietal regions. Rather, Richlan found evidence that points to dysfunction in dyslexics in the left hemisphere, reflecting a larger reading network that included the "hypoactivation" of the occipital–temporal, inferior frontal, and inferior parietal regions. In general, the sharing of common problems in STM and WM suggests that "hypoactivation" (underactivation) may occur in common areas of the brain for children with RD and/or MD.

Some recent work supports this assumption. An fMRI study (Wang et al., 2020) found that both math and reading, as well as WM, overlap in brain regions. The fMRI study of 231 adolescents with LD found activation of reading (sentence-level reading comprehension), math (line estimation), and executive processing (WM was measured as an N-back task) on the left ventrolateral prefrontal cortex, left inferior frontal junction, and left precentral gyrus. This neuroimaging study was followed up with a meta-analytic database (referred to as Neurosynth, a brain-mapping procedure) that deduced from hundreds of fMRI studies aspects of mathematical processing, reading, and WM, respectively. Common brain activation areas across reading, math, and WM performance were the left prefrontal regions (inferior frontal junction, premotor regions, and ventral lateral prefrontal cortex), thus identifying regions that play an overlapping role in reading and math performance. Taken together, there is evidence that reading and math are supported by the same brain regions as WM (executive processing), suggesting children with RD and/or MD have a shared domain-general WM component that underlies their LD.

Given this overview of a multicomponent view of WM, we will now briefly review some of our findings linking RD and/or MD to specific components of WM. The links between the components of WM to various achievement measures have been reviewed previously (e.g., Swanson, 2020; Swanson & Alloway, 2012; Swanson & Kong, 2018; Swanson & Zheng, 2013) and, because of space limitations, are not reviewed here. Instead, some selective studies are reviewed that have included children with specific LD in reading and/or math under each WM component.

Executive Component of WM

A crucial activity of the central executive of WM as it applies to children with RD and/or MD is controlled attention. The involvement of controlled attention in children with RD and/or MD is inferred from three outcomes: (1) depressed performance across both verbal and visual–spatial tasks that require concurrent storage and processing, (2) poor performance on complex divided attention tasks (attention to relevant and irrelevant information), and (3) poor concurrent monitoring of attention on high-demand tasks.

Combined Processing and Storage Demands

The majority of our recent studies (Swanson, 2012, 2017; Swanson & Jerman, 2007; Swanson et al., 2008) on executive processing have included tasks that follow the format of Daneman and Carpenter's (1980) Sentence Span measure, a task strongly related to achievement measures (see Swanson & Alloway, 2012, for a review). For example, three unrelated sentences are presented, and the child is asked to recall the last word of each sentence. Before the recall of last words, however, the child is asked a process question. Our WM studies typically engage participants in at least two activities after initial encoding: (1) a response to questions about the material or retrieval of related material and (2) a response to recall item information that increases in set size.

These laboratory tasks have an analog to everyday learning (Uppal & Swanson, 2016). Some everyday examples include holding a person's address in mind while listening to instructions about how to get there, listening to a sequence of events in a story while trying to understand what the story means, locating a sequence of landmarks on a map while determining the correct route, and listening to specific word features among several in one ear and suppressing the same features in the other ear. All of these tasks have some aspects of interference (a competing memory trace that draws away from the targeted memory trace) and monitoring (decisions related to the allocation of attention to the stimulus that is under consideration simultaneously with the active consideration of several other stimuli whose current status is essential for completing the task).

An example of the difficulties experienced by children and adults with RD on these complex span tasks can be found in an earlier cross-sectional study (Swanson, 2003). The study compared four age groups (7, 10, 13, and 20) on phonological, semantic, and visual–spatial WM measures administered under a variety of conditions (also see Swanson, 1992, 1996): initial (no probes or cues), gain (cues that bring performance to an asymptotic level), and maintenance conditions (asymptotic conditions without cues). The general findings of the Swanson (2003) study were that both participants with and without RD showed continuous growth in verbal and visual–spatial WM. The results suggested that initial constraints in WM can be modified under gain conditions. However, the study provided little evidence that participants with RD catch up in WM skills with average readers as they age, suggesting that a deficit model rather than a developmental lag model best captured such readers' age-related performance.

In terms of MD, a longitudinal study (Swanson et al., 2008) examined the influence of growth in WM on growth in mathematical problem solution accuracy in elementary school children with and without MD across 3 years. Their results showed that children identified with MD in wave 1 showed less growth and lower levels of performance on WM measures than children not at risk at wave 3 (3 years later). More importantly, the results indicated that WM contributed unique variance to problem solving beyond what phonological processes (e.g., phonological knowledge), fluid intelligence, reading skill, inhibition, and processing speed contributed. Thus, there was clear evidence that WM contributed important variance to math performance 3 years later beyond processes related to speed, phonological knowledge, fluid intelligence, and reading skills.

COMPLEX DIVIDED ATTENTION TASKS

Our earlier research showed that children with RD can be distinguished from average achievers in how they handled attentional demands (Swanson, 1989). For example, Swanson (1989) compared central and incidental recall on WM tasks between children with RD, children with low verbal IQ, average achievers, and intellectually gifted children. In general, the results suggested that children with low verbal IQ and children with RD recalled less information as a function of encoding conditions than higher-ability groups on both central and incidental memory tasks. However, the results also indicated that lower-ability groups differed from higher-ability groups in executive processing (how they shared, discriminated, and selectively allocated resources between the central and secondary recall tasks). Children with low verbal IQ compensated for their executive processing deficiencies by maintaining a constant resource supply (recall was comparable between central and secondary tasks), whereas children with RD failed to effectively prioritize items (recall fluctuated between central and secondary tasks) despite having a higher verbal IQ.

General Monitoring Difficulties

In another one of our earlier experiments (Swanson, 1993b, Exp. 1), a concurrent memory task adapted from Baddeley (Baddeley et al., 1984) was administered to children with RD and average readers. The task required subjects to remember digit strings (e.g., 9, 4, 1, 7, 5, and 2) while they concurrently sorted blank cards, cards with pictures of nonverbal shapes, or cards with pictures of items that fit into semantic categories (e.g., vehicles—car, bus, truck; clothing—dress, socks, belt). Demands on the central executive capacity system were manipulated through the level of difficulty (three- vs. six-digit strings) and type of sorting required (e.g., nonverbal shapes, semantic categories, and blank cards). Sorting activities that placed demands on the verbal storage (phonological system) included the categorization of pictures into semantic categories, whereas sorting activities that made demands on the visual store (i.e., visual–spatial sketchpad) included discrimination among complex nonverbal shapes. Baddeley et al. (1984) found that in such activities, the main task difficulty (sorting) interacted with concurrent memory load, but only with a memory load of six digits. Performance for the six-digit memory load condition placed processing demands on the central executive, thereby interfering with the main task. Swanson's (1993b) results indicated a clear effect on memory load. The results showed that children with RD can perform comparably to their chronological age (CA)-matched counterparts on verbal and visual–spatial sorting conditions that included three-digit strings (low demands) and that only when the coordination of tasks becomes more difficult (six-digit strings) do ability group differences emerge. More importantly, the results for the high memory load condition (six-digit strings) showed that children with RD were inferior to the CA-matched readers (and reading-matched controls for ordered recall) in their ability to recall digits during both verbal and nonverbal sorting. Because recall performance for children with RD was not restricted to a particular storage system (i.e., verbal storage), compared with the performance of CA-matched average readers, one can infer that processes other than a language-specific system accounted for the results.

Summary

We have selectively reviewed some of our research findings that show that children with RD and/or MD manifest WM deficits that, depending on the task and information processing demand, reflect problems related to an executive processing system. Although our research suggests that difficulties related to the executive component of WM underlie RD and/or MD, we also want to emphasize that several activities that involve executive processing are very much intact for children with RD/MD. Depending on the task, of course, some of these intact executive processes relate to planning (Swanson, 1993a). For example, although planning (such as mapping out a sequence of moves to solve a problem) is considered a component of the executive system (e.g., see Miyake et al., 2000, p. 91), we have not found overall solution differences between children with RD (and/or MD) and average-achieving students on problem-solving tasks (see Swanson, 1988, 1993a). Thus, only a few activities related to executive processing underlie RD and/or MD.

Phonological Loop

The previous section highlighted the role of the executive system of WM in the academic performance of children with RD and/or MD. However, previous regression analyses have found that both STM and WM also contribute unique variance to academic performance in children with RD and/or MD (e.g., Swanson & Ashbaker, 2000; Swanson et al., 2008). Thus, the role of STM, referred to as the phonological loop, is reviewed. The phonological loop is specialized for the retention of verbal information over short periods of time. A cognitive process consistently implicated in RD is phonological awareness (e.g., Melby-Lervåg et al., 2012). Phonological awareness is "the ability to attend explicitly to the phonological structure of spoken words" (Scarborough, 1998, p. 95). This difficulty in forming and accessing phonological representations impairs the ability to retrieve verbal information from STM. A substantial number of studies support the notion that children with RD experience deficits in phonological processing (e.g., see the synthesis of Kudo et al., 2015), such as forming or accessing phonological representations of information. These findings build on research that has shown that the manifestations of this phonological deficit are poor word recognition, poor performance on phonological awareness tasks, computation, slow naming speed, and impaired verbal STM.

Several studies have attributed arithmetic skills to the phonological loop (e.g., Logie et al., 1994) or to a combination of both the phonological and executive systems (e.g., Fürst & Hitch, 2000). The research to date indicates that some children who are less proficient in math appear to rehearse less and perform more poorly on tasks requiring short-term retention of order information than children proficient in math, especially on measures of digits (Geary, 2011, 2013; Geary et al., 2012; McLean & Hitch, 1999), suggesting inefficient utilization of the phonological rehearsal process. Swanson and Kim (2007) found that both STM and WM tasks each uniquely predicted individual differences in mathematical performance. WM was independent of the contribution of STM and naming speed in predicting children's mathematical performance. The results were interpreted as support for the notion that both the central executive system (controlled attention) and storage system of WM (i.e., phonological loop) predict children's math performance.

A key finding in several of our studies is that the contribution of STM (phonological loop) and WM (storage + controlled attention) can contribute unique variance to achievement measures and, therefore, can operate independently of one another. Swanson and Ashbaker (2000) directly tested whether the operations related to STM and WM operated independently of one another. In this study, they compared children with and without RD and younger reading level-matched children on a battery of WM and STM tests to assess executive and phonological processing, respectively. The study found that reading group differences were pervasive across verbal and visual–spatial WM tasks, even when the influence of verbal STM was statistically removed, suggesting that reading group differences are domain-general. These results suggested that the executive component of WM predicted reading problems independent of specific problems related to the phonological component of WM.

Visual–Spatial Sketchpad

The visual–spatial sketchpad is specialized for the processing and storage of visual material, spatial material, or both and for linguistic information that can be recoded into imaginable forms (see Baddeley, 2012, for a review). Our work linking RD to visual–spatial memory deficits is mixed. For example, when visual–spatial WM (combined storage and processing demands) performance is considered, some studies find that visual–spatial WM in students with RD is intact when compared with their same-age counterparts (e.g., Swanson et al., 1996, Exp. 1), whereas others suggest problems in various visual–spatial tasks (e.g., Mammarella et al., 2018; Swanson et al., 1996, Exp. 2). Most studies suggest, however, that depending on the type of academic disability, greater problems in performance are more likely to occur on verbal than visual–spatial WM tasks for children with RD and/or MD (Peng et al., 2017; Swanson & Jerman, 2007). Likewise, our meta-analysis synthesizing research on the cognitive studies of MD (Kudo et al., 2015; Swanson & Jerman, 2006) suggests that memory deficits are more apparent in the verbal than visual–spatial domain. In general, our studies suggest that the visual–spatial system of children with RD is generally intact, but when excessive demands are placed on the executive system, their visual–spatial performance is depressed compared with chronological age-matched average achievers (Swanson, 2000).

Summary

When performance demands on various tasks directly tax the WM capacity of individuals with RD and/or MD, deficiencies related to the accessing of speech-based information and/or the monitoring of attentional processes emerge. Thus, these two areas of deficiency are related to components of WM referred to in Baddeley's model (Baddeley & Logie, 1999) as the phonological loop and the executive system. Individuals with RD and/or MD do not exhibit deficits in all aspects of the phonological loop (e.g., they have relatively normal abilities in producing spontaneous speech and have few difficulties in oral language comprehension) or the executive system (e.g., they have relatively normal abilities in planning). Those aspects of the phonological system that appear particularly problematic for individuals with RD and/or MD relate to the accurate and speedy access of speech codes in STM, whereas those aspects of the executive system that appear faulty are related to the concurrent monitoring of processing and storage demands in addition to the suppression of conflicting (e.g., irrelevant) information.

Taken together, we place our findings within a multicomponent model of WM. Two components are viewed as critical. The model views children with RD and/or MD as manifesting deficits related to the phonological loop, a component of WM that specializes in the retention of speech-based information. However, in situations that place high demands on processing, individuals with RD and/or MD have deficits related to the executive component of WM, primarily related to controlled attentional processes (e.g., updating and/or maintaining task-relevant information in the face of distraction or interference) that can operate independently of their problems in the phonological system.

Future Directions

We have two directions in our current research. One focuses on the need to separate fundamental deficits in WM from fundamental deficits related to language acquisition. Our current research focuses on ELLs with RD and MD whose first language is Spanish. We feel this line of work is important because ELL children with Spanish as a first language in the United States have been found to yield low reading and mathematics scores when compared to other ELL groups on national assessments across several years (e.g., National Assessment of Education Progress, 2017, 2020). Our recent studies have focused on the role of WM in predicting children at risk for RD (e.g., Swanson et al., 2016; Swanson et al., 2015) and MD

(Swanson et al., 2019a, 2019b) within ELL samples. Past and more recent studies (Lanfranchi & Swanson, 2005; Swanson et al., 2004; Swanson et al., 2011) have attempted to determine (1) whether the memory processes implicated in reading and second language acquisition extend beyond the phonological domain and (2) whether the cognitive processes that underlie difficulties in second language acquisition are the same as those that underlie difficulties in reading and/or math for monolingual students.

In one of our earlier studies of reading (Swanson et al., 2004), bilingual and nonbilingual elementary school children were administered a battery of cognitive measures [STM, WM, rapid naming, random letter and number generation, vocabulary, and reading (real word and pseudoword reading)] in both Spanish and English. The results showed that English word identification performance was best predicted by a general verbal WM latent factor (a factor that reflected loading from both English and Spanish WM measures) and a Spanish STM factor, whereas English pseudoword reading performance was best predicted by Spanish pseudoword reading and a WM factor. The results also showed that WM and STM performance differed among ELL children with and without RD (Swanson et al., 2004).

In terms of math, our recent study (Swanson et al., 2019a, 2019b) determined those components of WM that played a significant role in predicting math growth in children who are ELLs with MD. A battery of tests was administered in English and Spanish that assessed computation, reading, vocabulary, inhibition, and components of WM in grade 1 children, with follow-up testing in grades 2 and 3. The results indicated that growth in the executive component of WM was significantly related to growth in math performance even when covariates (STM, vocabulary, reading, and fluid intelligence) were entered into the latent growth models.

In our attempts to isolate fundamental processing difficulties in reading and math, the question emerges, however, as to whether the tripartite structure of WM fits with ELLs. Swanson, Kudo, et al. (2019) tested the tripartite structure (e.g., executive, phonological, and visual–spatial) on five age groups (6-, 7-, 8-, 9-, and 10-year-olds) of ELLs. The tasks were administered in Spanish and English on separate occasions. Confirmatory factor analysis showed that a three-factor structure of WM emerged in both L1 and L2 administrations for each age group. Thus, there are three important implications for our work with ELL children: (1) the theoretical framework for WM fits the data in both English and Spanish for children who are ELLs, (2) the distinction between the phonological loop and executive system in young children becomes stronger with increases in age, and (3) the cross-language structure of measures is stronger for the executive component of WM than for the phonological loop. Taken together, this cross-sectional study found that Baddeley's tripartite model of WM is an adequate conceptualization for ELLs and that the construct of WM can be measured within both English and Spanish language systems.

The second area of research focuses on identification of children with WM difficulties and providing appropriate interventions. Previous research has indicated that teachers' ratings of WM accurately predicted student performance on latent measures of Spanish STM and the executive component of WM (Uppal & Swanson, 2016). As teachers are one of the primary sources for screening for children with learning and memory problems, accurately identifying these constructs in the classroom would be an early first step in identification and prompt intervention to address WM challenges in young children who are ELLs. Although our previous work found that WM can be modified via dynamic testing conditions (Swanson, 1992, 2003, 2011; Swanson et al., 1996), whether such modifications improve academic performance is unclear. That is, WM training studies as a means to improve academic performance have yielded mixed results (e.g., Melby-Lervåg & Hulme, 2013; Schwaighofer et al., 2015), and few studies have shown any direct influence of WM training on academic performance (e.g., see Melby-Lervåg & Hulme, 2013; Shipstead et al., 2010, for a review of this literature). Instead of trying to modify WM directly, we are taking a different approach in our studies by embedding WM demands within classroom curriculum materials. Our more recent intervention studies have been directed toward focusing on math word problem-solving strategies and including WM demands within these lesson plans (e.g., Swanson, 2014, 2016; Swanson et al., 2015; Swanson et al., 2013; Swanson et al., 2014). That is, we have been focusing on how strategies can enhance math problem solving as a function of variations of both the WM demands within the curriculum and the WM capacity of the individual child.

For example, a study (see Swanson, 2016), which replicated an earlier study (Swanson et al., 2013), included randomized control/experimental conditions, which investigated the role of cognitive strategy instruction on problem-solving solution accuracy in elementary school children (grade 3) with MD ($N = 162$). Comparisons were made on three popular cognitive strategy conditions. These included verbal and/or visual–spatial schema activities + controlled attention training and a controlled attention training condition (referred to as MOC, materials-only condition in the article). The MOC conditions included the same materials, practice, small group setting, and teacher feedback as the other conditions. The materials included practice with solving word problems that systematically increased into a five-sentence "load" condition. For example, Load 1 included seven lessons of four sentences and one irrelevant sentence. In contrast, Load 5 (lessons 18 through 20) required solving problems of eight sentences that included five irrelevant sentences. We found all intervention conditions were effective relative to the control condition (e.g., Swanson et al., 2013). However, we also found that the controlled attention condition (MOC) yielded higher ESs relative to the other strategy conditions at posttest on measures of problem solving and WM. Our rationale for the controlled attention condition (referred to in the article as MOC) was that some of our pilot work found that various activities (e.g., underlining keywords, circling the question, placing numbers in the diagram, etc.) placed unnecessary cognitive demands on the processing of materials for children with MD. The challenge, of course, is developing intervention materials that can be used in L1, L2, or dual-language settings.

Summary

Our preliminary work with ELL children at risk for LD has suggested that growth in reading and math is directly tied to the development of the executive WM system. We would not argue at this point that this system acts independently of cross-language skills across grades. Likewise, although our preliminary intervention work that has embedded WM training within the curriculum materials has yielded some positive outcomes, its application has been applied only to English monolingual children. Thus, additional research is necessary before substantive conclusions can be drawn in terms of its application to ELL children at risk for RD and/or MD.

Conclusion

We conclude that WM deficits are fundamental problems of children with a specific LD in reading and/or math (i.e., RD and/or MD). Students with RD and/or MD exhibit STM deficits related to the phonological loop, a component of WM that specializes in the retention of speech-based information. However, this subsystem is not the only aspect of WM that underlies RD and/or MD. We find that in situations that place high demands on processing, which in turn place demands on controlled attentional processing (e.g., monitoring limited resources, suppressing conflicting information, and updating information), children with RD and/or MD are at a clear disadvantage when compared with their chronological aged counterparts. Further, these deficits are sustained when articulation speed, phonological processing, fluid intelligence, and verbal STM are partialed from the analysis.

No doubt, a limitation of our work is that only two components (executive and phonological loop) of the tripartite model (Baddeley & Logie, 1999) have been thoroughly explored as playing a fundamental role in specific LD in reading and/or math. We find weak support that the visual–spatial sketchpad plays a primary role in specific LD, but this is in conflict with other researchers (e.g., Mammarella et al., 2018). These differences in findings may be related to the limitations of our visual–spatial WM tasks. Recently, the tripartite model has been revised to include an episodic buffer (Baddeley, 2012), which captures the binding of visual and verbal information. However, its application to specific LD has yielded mixed results as an area of focus, as some see the episodic buffer as a strength (Dawes et al., 2015), while others view it as a weakness (Masoura et al., 2021) in children with reading problems. No studies we are aware of have compared children with MD on tasks assumed to capture the episodic buffer. More important, consistent support for the tripartite model has been found across various age groups of children (e.g., Alloway et al., 2004; Gathercole et al., 2004; Gray et al., 2017). The tripartite model has also been supported in studies that include samples of children with RD and/or MD (e.g., Swanson, 2008; Swanson & Jerman, 2007; Swanson, Kudo, et al., 2019; Swanson & Fung, 2016).

Although couching our findings within a tripartite model unifies the results of several of our studies at present, we recognize there are gaping holes in our knowledge about how WM and learning problems are related to specific LD. For example, our classroom research has not identified all factors of WM amenable to particular manipulations, such as extended practice, specific instructions, and strategy use. Additional research needs to be directed toward explaining why WM tasks are good predictors of academic performance. Although, for example, it makes sense that controlled attention ability (e.g., the ability to switch attention between processing and storage requirements) may be particularly good for reading comprehension but not necessarily for simple sight word recognition, this has not been tested experimentally. No doubt, the complexity of the task determines whether general or domain-specific factors come into play.

ACKNOWLEDGMENTS

This chapter draws liberally from previous discussions in the final report to U.S. Department of Education, Institute of Education Sciences (R305H020055; R324A09002), Swanson (2011, 2017, 2020), Swanson and Zheng (2013), and Swanson and Siegel (2001a, 2001b), and the reader is referred to those sources for additional information.

REFERENCES

Acheson, D. J., Hamidi, M., Binder, J. R., & Postle, B. R. (2011). A common neural substrate for language production and verbal working memory. *Journal of Cognitive Neuroscience, 23*(6), 1358–1367.

Alloway, T. P., Gathercole, S. E., Willis, C., & Adams, A. (2004). A structural analysis of working memory and related cognitive skills in young children. *Journal of Experimental Child Psychology, 87,* 85–106.

American Psychiatric Association (2013). *Diagnostic and statistical manual of mental disorders* (5th ed.). Author.

Attout, L., & Majerus, S. (2015). Working memory deficits in developmental dyscalculia: The importance of serial order. *Child Neuropsychology, 21*(4), 432–450.

Baddeley, A. D. (2012). Working memory: Theories, models, and controversies. *Annual Review of Psychology, 63,* 1–29.

Baddeley, A. D., Eldridge, M., Lewis, V., & Thomson, N. (1984). Attention and retrieval from long-term memory. *Journal of Experimental Psychology: General, 113,* 518–540.

Baddeley, A. D., & Logie, R. H. (1999). The multiple-component model. In A. Miyake & P. Shah (Eds.), *Models of working memory: Mechanisms of active maintenance and executive control* (pp. 28–61). Cambridge University Press.

Beneventi, H., Tønnessen, F. E., & Ersland, L. (2009). Dyslexic children show short-term memory deficits in phonological storage and serial rehearsal: An fMRI study. *International Journal of Neuroscience, 119*(11), 2017–2043.

Beneventi, H., Tønnessen, F. E., Ersland, L., & Hugdahl, K. (2010). Executive working memory processes in dyslexia: Behavioral and fMRI evidence. *Scandinavian Journal of Psychology, 51*(3), 192–202.

Bledowski, C., Kaiser, J., & Rahm, B. (2010). Basic operations in working memory: Contributions from functional imaging studies. *Behavioural Brain Research, 214*(2), 172–179.

Brandenburg, J., Klesczewski, J., Fischbach, A., Schuchardt, K., Büttner, G., & Hasselhorn, M. (2015). Working memory in children with learning disabilities in reading versus spelling: Searching for overlapping and specific cognitive factors. *Journal of Learning Disabilities, 48*(6), 622–634.

Chein, J. M., & Fiez, J. A. (2010). Evaluating models of working memory through the effects of concurrent irrelevant information. *Journal of Experimental Psychology: General, 139*(1), 117–137.

Cirino, P. T., Fuchs, L. S., Elias, J. T., Powell, S. R., & Schumacher, R. F. (2015). Cognitive and mathematical profiles for different forms of learning difficulties. *Journal of Learning Disabilities, 48*(2), 156–175.

Cohen, J. (1988). *Statistical power analysis for the behavioral sciences* (2nd ed.). L. Erlbaum Associates.

Cooney, J. B., & Swanson, H. L. (1987). Memory and learning disabilities: An overview. In H. L. Swanson (Ed.), *Advances in learning and behavioral disabilities: Memory and learning disabilities* (Suppl. 2, pp. 1–40). JAI Press.

Cowan, N. (1997). *The development of working memory.* In N. Cowan (Ed.), *The development of working memory in childhood* (pp. 163–199). Psychology Press/Erlbaum.

Cowan, N. (2014). Working memory underpins cognitive development, learning, and education. *Educational Psychology Review, 26*(2), 197–223.

Daneman, M., & Carpenter, P. A. (1980). Individual differences in working memory and reading. *Journal of Verbal Learning and Verbal Behavior, 19*(4), 450–466.

Dawes, E., Leitão, S., Claessen, M., & Nayton, M. (2015). A profile of working memory ability in poor readers. *Australian Psychologist, 50*(5), 362–371.

De Weerdt, F., Desoete, A., & Roeyers, H. (2013). Working memory in children with reading disabilities and/or mathematical disabilities. *Journal of Learning Disabilities, 46*(5), 461–472.

Engle, R. W., Tuholski, S. W., Laughlin, J. E., & Conway, A. R. (1999). Working memory, short-term memory, and general fluid intelligence: A latent variable approach. *Journal of Experimental Psychology: General, 128,* 309–331.

Evans, T. M., Flowers, D. L., Luetje, M. M., Napoliello, E., & Eden, G. F. (2016). Functional neuroanatomy of arithmetic and word reading and its relationship to age. *NeuroImage, 143,* 304–315.

Fürst, A. J., & Hitch, G. J. (2000). Separate roles for executive and phonological components of working memory in mental arithmetic. *Memory & Cognition, 28*(5), 774–782.

Gathercole, S. E., Pickering, S. J., Ambridge, B., & Wearing, H. (2004). The structure of working memory from 4 to 15 years of age. *Developmental Psychology, 40,* 177–190.

Geary, D. C. (2011). Cognitive predictors of achievement growth in mathematics: A 5-year longitudinal study. *Developmental Psychology, 47*(6), 1539–1552.

Geary, D. C. (2013). Learning disabilities in mathematics: Recent advances. In H. L. Swanson, K. Harris, & S. Graham (Eds.). *Handbook of learning disabilities* (pp. 239–256). Guilford Press.

Geary, D. C., Hoard, M. K., Nugent, L., & Bailey, D. H. (2012). Mathematical cognition deficits in children with learning disabilities and persistent low achievement: A five-year prospective study. *Journal of Educational Psychology, 104*(1), 206–223.

Gray, S., Green, S., Alt, M., Hogan, T., Kuo, T., Brinkley, S., & Cowan, N. (2017). The structure of working memory in young children and its relation to intelligence. *Journal of Memory and Language, 92,* 183–201.

Hutton, U. M. Z., & Towse, J. N. (2001). Short-term memory and working memory as indices of children's cognitive skills. *Memory, 9*(4–6), 383–394.

Kaufmann, L., Wood, G., Rubinsten, O., & Henik, A. (2011). Meta-analyses of developmental fMRI studies investigating typical and atypical trajectories of number processing and calculation. *Developmental Neuropsychology, 36*(6), 763–787.

Kudo, M. F., Lussier, C. M., & Swanson, H. L. (2015). Reading disabilities in children: A selective meta-analysis of the cognitive literature. *Research in Developmental Disabilities, 40,* 51–62.

Johnson, E. S., Humphrey, M., Mellard, D. F., Woods, K., & Swanson, H. L. (2010). Cognitive processing deficits and students with specific learning disabilities: A selective meta-analysis of the literature. *Learning Disability Quarterly, 33*(1), 3–18.

Lanfranchi, S., & Swanson, H. L. (2005). Short-term memory and working memory in children as a function of language-specific knowledge in English and Spanish. *Learning and Individual Differences, 15*(4), 299–319.

Logie, R. H., Gilhooly, K. J., & Wynn, V. (1994). Counting on working memory in arithmetic problem solving. *Memory & Cognition, 22*(4), 395–410.

Mammarella, I. C., Caviola, S., Giofrè, D., & Szűcs, D. (2018). The underlying structure of visuospatial working memory in children with mathematical learning disability. *British Journal of Developmental Psychology, 36,* 220–235.

Martin, R. B., Cirino, P. T., Barnes, M. A., Ewing-Cobbs, L., Fuchs, L. S., Stuebing, K. K., & Fletcher, J. M. (2013). Prediction and stability of mathematics skill and difficulty. *Journal of Learning Disabilities, 46*(5), 428–443.

Masoura, E., Gogou, A., & Gathercole, S. E. (2021). Working memory profiles of children with reading difficulties who are learning to read in greek. *Dyslexia: An International Journal of Research and Practice, 27*(3), 312–324.

McLean, J. F., & Hitch, G. J. (1999). Working memory impairments in children with specific arithmetic learning difficulties. *Journal of Experimental Child Psychology, 74*(3), 240–260.

Melby-Lervåg, M., & Hulme, C. (2013). Is working memory training effective? A meta-analytic review. *Developmental Psychology, 49*(2), 270–291.

Melby-Lervåg, M., Lyster, S. H., & Hulme, C. (2012). Phonological skills and their role in learning to read: A meta-analytic review. *Psychological Bulletin, 138*(2), 322–352.

Miyake, A., Friedman, N. P., Emerson, M. J., Witzki, A. H., & Howerter, A. (2000). The unity and diversity of executive functions and their contributions to complex "frontal lobe" tasks: A latent variable analysis. *Cognitive Psychology, 41,* 49–100.

National Assessment of Educational Progress. (2017). *The condition of education (update 2017).* U.S. Department of Education.

Nee, D. E., Brown, J. W., Askren, M. K., Berman, M. G., Demiralp, E., Krawitz, A., & Jonides, J. (2013). A meta-analysis of executive components of working memory. *Cerebral Cortex, 23*(2), 264–282.

Passolunghi, M. C., & Siegel, L. S. (2004). Working memory and access to numerical information in children with disability in mathematics. *Journal of Experimental Child Psychology, 88*(4), 348–367.

Peña, E. D., Bedore, L. M., & Kester, E. S. (2016). Assessment of language impairment in bilingual children using semantic tasks: Two languages classify better than one. *International Journal of Language & Communication Disorders, 51*(2), 192–202.

Peng, P., Barnes, M., Wang, C., Wang, W., Li, S., Swanson, H. L., & Tao, S. (2017). A meta-analysis on the relation between reading and working memory. *Psychological Bulletin, 144*(1), 48–76.

Peng, P., Congying, S., Beilei, L., & Sha, T. (2012). Phonological storage and executive function deficits in children with mathematics difficulties. *Journal of Experimental Child Psychology, 112*(4), 452–466.

Peng, P., & Fuchs, D. (2016). A meta-analysis of working memory deficits in children with learning difficulties: Is there a difference between verbal domain and numerical domain? *Journal of Learning Disabilities, 49*(1), 3–20.

Richlan, F. (2012). Developmental dyslexia: Dysfunction of a left hemisphere reading network. *Frontiers in Human Neuroscience, 6,* 120.

Richlan, F., Kronbichler, M., & Wimmer, H. (2011). Meta-analyzing brain dysfunctions in dyslexic children and adults. *NeuroImage, 56*(3), 1735–1742.

Rosenberg-Lee, M., Lovett, M. C., & Anderson, J. R. (2009). Neural correlates of arithmetic calculation strategies. *Cognitive, Affective & Behavioral Neuroscience, 9(3),* 270–285.

Rosselli, M., Ardila, A., Lalwani, L. N., & Vélez-Uribe, I. (2016). The effect of language proficiency on executive functions in balanced and unbalanced Spanish–English bilinguals. *Bilingualism: Language and Cognition, 19*(3), 489–503.

Scarborough, H. S. (1998). Early identification of children at risk for reading disabilities: Phonological awareness and some other promising predictors. In B. Shapiro, P. Accardo, & A. Capute (Eds.), *Specific reading disability: A view of the spectrum* (pp. 75–119). York Press.

Schwaighofer, M., Fischer, F., & Bühner, M. (2015). Does working memory training transfer? A meta-analysis including training conditions as moderators. *Educational Psychologist, 50*(2), 138–166.

Shipstead, Z., Redick, T. S., & Engle, R. W. (2010). Does working memory training generalize? *Psychologica Belgica, 50*(3&4), 245–276.

Siegel, L. S., & Ryan, E. B. (1989). The development of working memory in normally achieving and subtypes of learning disabled children. *Child Development, 60*(4), 973–980.

Smith, E. E., & Jonides, J. (1997). Working memory: A view from neuroimaging. *Cognitive Psychology, 33*(1), 5–42.

Smith, E. E., & Jonides, J. (1999). Storage and executive processes in the frontal lobes. *Science, 283*(5408), 1657–1661.

Swanson, H. L. (1988). Learning disabled children's problem solving: Identifying mental processes underlying intelligent performance. *Intelligence, 12*(3), 261–278.

Swanson, H. L. (1989). The effects of central processing strategies on learning disabled, mildly retarded, average, and gifted children's elaborative encoding abilities. *Journal of Experimental Child Psychology, 47*(3), 370–397.

Swanson, H. L. (1992). Generality and modifiability of working memory among skilled and less skilled readers. *Journal of Educational Psychology, 84*(4), 473–488.

Swanson, H. L. (1993a). An information processing analysis of learning disabled children's problem solving. *American Educational Research Journal, 30*(4), 861–893.

Swanson, H. L. (1993b). Executive processing in learning-disabled readers. *Intelligence, 17*(2), 117–149.

Swanson, H. L. (1993c). Working memory in learning disability subgroups. *Journal of Experimental Child Psychology, 56*(1), 87–114.

Swanson, H. L. (1996). Individual and age-related differences in children's working memory. *Memory & Cognition, 24,* 70–82.

Swanson, H. L. (1999). What develops in working memory? A life span perspective. *Developmental Psychology, 35*(4), 986–1000.

Swanson, H. L. (2000). Are working memory deficits in readers with learning disabilities hard to change? *Journal of Learning Disabilities, 33*(6), 551–566.

Swanson, H. L. (2003). Age-related differences in learning disabled and skilled readers' working memory. *Journal of Experimental Child Psychology, 85*(1), 1–31.

Swanson, H. L. (2008). Working memory and intelligence in children: What develops? *Journal of Educational Psychology, 100*(3), 581–602.

Swanson, H. L. (2011). The influence of working memory growth on reading and math performance in children with math and/or reading disabilities. In P. Barrouillet & V. Gaillard (Eds.), *Cognitive development and working memory: A dialogue between neo-Piagetian theories and cognitive approaches* (pp. 203–231). Psychology Press.

Swanson, H. L. (2012). Intellectual growth in children as a function of domain specific and domain general working memory subgroups. *Intelligence, 39,* 481–492.

Swanson, H. L. (2014). Does cognitive strategy training on word problems compensate for working memory capacity in children with math difficulties? *Journal of Educational Psychology, 106*(3), 831–848.

Swanson, H. L. (2016). Word problem solving, working memory and serious math difficulties: Do cognitive strategies really make a difference? *Journal of Applied Research in Memory and Cognition, 5*(4), 368–383.

Swanson, H. L. (2017). Verbal and visual-spatial working memory: What develops over a life span? *Developmental Psychology, 53*(5), 971–995.

Swanson, H. L. (2020). Learning disabilities as a working memory deficit: A revised model. In R. Sperling, A. Martin, & K. Newton (Eds.), *Handbook of educational psychology & students with special needs* (pp. 19–51). Routledge.

Swanson, H. L., & Alloway, T. P. (2012). Working memory, learning, and academic achievement. In K. Harris, T. Urban, & S. Grahm (Eds.), *APA educational psychology handbook, vol 1: Theories, constructs, and critical issues* (pp. 327–366). American Psychological Association.

Swanson, H. L., & Ashbaker, M. H. (2000). Working memory, short-term memory, speech rate, word recognition and reading comprehension in learning disabled readers: Does the executive system have a role? *Intelligence, 28*(1), 1–30.

Swanson, H. L., Ashbaker, M. H., & Lee, C. (1996). Learning-disabled readers' working memory as a function of processing demands. *Journal of Experimental Child Psychology, 61*(3), 242–275.

Swanson, H. L., Cooney, J. B., & McNamara, J. K. (2004). Learning disabilities and memory. In B. Y. L. Wong (Ed.), *Learning about learning disabilities* (pp. 41–92). Elsevier Academic Press.

Swanson, H. L., & Fung, W. (2016). Working memory components and problem-solving accuracy: Are there multiple pathways? *Journal of Educational Psychology, 108*(8), 1153–1177.

Swanson, H. L., & Jerman, O. (2006). Math disabilities: A selective meta-analysis of the literature. *Review of Educational Research, 76*(2), 249–274.

Swanson, H. L., & Jerman, O. (2007). The influence of working memory on reading growth in subgroups of children with reading disabilities. *Journal of Experimental Child Psychology, 96*(4), 249–283.

Swanson, H. L., Jerman, O., & Zheng, X. (2008). Growth in working memory and mathematical problem solving in children at risk and not at risk for serious math difficulties. *Journal of Educational Psychology, 100*(2), 343–379.

Swanson, H. L., Jerman, O., & Zheng, X. (2009). Math disabilities and reading disabilities: Can they be separated? *Journal of Psychoeducational Assessment, 27*(3), 175–196.

Swanson, H. L., & Kim, K. (2007). Working memory, short-term memory, and naming speed as predictors of children's mathematical performance. *Intelligence, 35*(2), 151–168.

Swanson, H. L., & Kong, J. E. (2018). Working memory and reading: Is there evidence for an executive processing deficit. In I. L. Meltzer (Ed.), *Executive function in education* (pp. 218–239). Guilford Press.

Swanson, H. L., Kong, J. E., & Petcu, S. (2018). Math difficulties and working memory growth in English language learner children: Does bilingual proficiency play a significant role? *Language, Speech, and Hearing Services in Schools, 49*(3), 379–394.

Swanson, H. L., Kong, J. E., & Petcu, S. D. (2019a). Growth in math computation among monolingual and English language learners: Does the executive system have a role? *Developmental Neuropsychology, 44*(8), 566–593.

Swanson, H. L., Kong, J. E., & Petcu, S. D. (2019b). Individual differences in math problem solving and executive processing among emerging bilingual children. *Journal of Experimental Child Psychology, 187*, 25.

Swanson, H. L., Kong, J. E., & Petcu, S. (2020). Emerging bilingual children at risk and not at risk for math difficulties. *Child Neuropsychology, 26*(4), 489–517.

Swanson, H. L., Kudo, M., & Guzman-Orth, D. (2016). Cognition and literacy in English language learners at risk for reading disabilities: A latent transition analysis. *Journal of Educational Psychology, 108*(6), 830–856.

Swanson, H. L., Kudo, M. F., & Van Horn, M. L. (2019). Does the structure of working memory in EL children vary across age and two language systems? *Memory, 27*(2), 174–191.

Swanson, H. L., Lussier, C. M., & Orosco, M. J. (2015). Cognitive strategies, working memory, and growth in word problem solving in children with math difficulties. *Journal of Learning Disabilities, 48*(4), 339–358.

Swanson, H. L., Moran, A. S., Bocian, K., Lussier, C., & Zheng, X. (2013). Generative strategies, working memory, and word problem solving accuracy in children at risk for math disabilities. *Learning Disability Quarterly, 36*(4), 203–214.

Swanson, H. L., Moran, A., Lussier, C., & Fung, W. (2014). The effect of explicit and direct generative strategy training and working memory on word problem-solving accuracy in children at risk for math difficulties. *Learning Disability Quarterly, 37*(2), 111–122.

Swanson, H. L., Olide, A. F., & Kong, J. E. (2018). Latent class analysis of children with math difficulties and/or math learning disabilities: Are there cognitive differences? *Journal of Educational Psychology, 110*(7), 931–951.

Swanson, H. L., Orosco, M. J., & Lussier, C. M. (2015). Growth in literacy, cognition, and working memory in English language learners. *Journal of Experimental Child Psychology, 132,* 155–188.

Swanson, H. L., Orosco, M. J., Lussier, C. M., Gerber, M. M., & Guzman-Orth, D. (2011). The influence of working memory and phonological processing on English language learner children's bilingual reading and language acquisition. *Journal of Educational Psychology, 103*(4), 838–856.

Swanson, H. L., & Sáez, L. (2004). Memory difficulties in children and adults with learning disabilities. In H. L. Swanson, K. Harris, & S. Graham (Eds), *Handbook of learning disabilities* (pp. 182–198). Guilford Press.

Swanson, H. L., Sáez, L., Gerber, M., & Leafstedt, J. (2004). Literacy and cognitive functioning in bilingual and nonbilingual children at or not at risk for reading disabilities. *Journal of Educational Psychology, 96*(1), 3–18.

Swanson, H. L., & Siegel, L. (2001a). Elaborating on working memory and learning disabilities: A reply to commentators. *Issues in Education: Contributions from Educational Psychology, 7,* 107–129.

Swanson, H. L., & Siegel, L. (2001b). Learning disabilities as a working memory deficit. *Issues in Education: Contributions from Educational Psychology, 7,* 1–48.

Swanson, H. L., & Zheng, X. (2013). Memory difficulties in children and adults with learning disabilities. In H. L. Swanson, K. Harris, & S. Graham (Eds), *Handbook of learning disabilities* (2nd ed., pp. 214–238). Guilford Press.

Swanson, H. L., Zheng, X., & Jerman, O. (2009). Working memory, short-term memory, and reading disabilities: A selective meta-analysis of the literature. *Journal of Learning Disabilities, 42*(3), 260–287.

Unsworth, N., & Engle, R. W. (2007). On the division of short-term and working memory: An examination of simple and complex span and their relation to higher order abilities. *Psychological Bulletin, 133*(6), 1038–1066.

Uppal, H. K., & Swanson, H. L. (2016). Teachers' ratings of working memory in English language learners: Do laboratory measures predict classroom analogues? *Applied Cognitive Psychology, 30*(6), 871–884.

Wang, K., Banich, M. T., Reineberg, A. E., Leopold, D. R., Willcutt, E. G., Cutting, L. E., & Petrill, S. A. (2020). Left posterior prefrontal regions support domain-general executive processes needed for both reading and math. *Journal of Neuropsychology, 14*(3), 467–495.

Wang, S., & Gathercole, S. E. (2013). Working memory deficits in children with reading difficulties: Memory span and dual task coordination. *Journal of Experimental Child Psychology, 115*(1), 188–197.

CHAPTER 9

Language Development, Developmental Language Disorder, and Reading Disabilities

Suzanne M. Adlof and Lesly Wade-Woolley

Spoken language development sets the foundation for reading and writing and, by extension, overall academic achievement. However, there is limited public awareness about how different aspects of language ability relate to observations of reading performance at different points in development. We open this chapter with descriptions of three children who experienced significant challenges related to reading and writing in school and for whom testing revealed different profiles of difficulty. We argue that all of them could have been identified earlier as being at risk for reading difficulties and that earlier identification and differentiated instruction could have prevented—or at least mitigated—their academic struggles. To this end, we provide a brief overview of the connections between language and reading development and disorders, contextualized in the Simple View of Reading (Gough & Tunmer, 1986). Next, we compare and contrast commonly used frameworks for identifying children with oral language versus reading disabilities in schools. Finally, we advocate for better integration of identification and intervention frameworks for children with oral language and reading difficulties. We believe that all professionals serving children with language or learning disabilities need to be aware of the importance of oral language to academic achievement and of the high rate of comorbidity between language disorders and learning disabilities.

I. Case Descriptions

Amy, David, and Josh are pseudonyms for children we have encountered in our research. Each child completed a battery of assessments to characterize their strengths and weaknesses related to oral language and reading skills.

I. A. "Amy"

We met Amy in the spring of her second-grade year. Amy's parents reported no prior concerns about her speech, language, or academic performance, but they noticed a significant decline in her scores on the school's most recent standardized tests. Previously, Amy had always scored in the average range, and in the fall of second grade, she scored at the 48th percentile in reading. However, in the spring, the school reported that her overall reading achievement had dropped to the 18th percentile compared to her peers. Our testing revealed that Amy had relatively strong word-reading and decoding abilities (she scored between the 50th and 63rd percentiles relative to age-based norms on measures of word and nonword reading accuracy and fluency) but substantial challenges with reading comprehension (she scored at the 22nd and 23rd percentiles on two different assessments). Further assessment of Amy's oral language abilities indicated significant difficulties with morphology, syntax, and narrative comprehension (5th–9th percentiles) and low-average scores in receptive and expressive vocabulary (27–34th percentiles).

I. B. "David"

We met David when he was 11 years old and in the fifth grade. His mother had concerns about his spelling, his ability to understand what he read, and his ability to remember and follow directions. David had received speech therapy in preschool. In kindergarten, he met his speech goals and was dismissed. She recalled that he enjoyed school in kindergarten and first grade, but as he got older, he began struggling to keep up. When we assessed David, the results indicated significant difficulties with word reading and decoding, scoring at the 1st and 12th percentiles compared to age norms on word and pseudoword reading fluency, respectively. A spelling assessment revealed that David spelled words the way they sounded but with the wrong letter patterns (e.g., "unifie" vs. "unify"), and his spelling score corresponded to the 8th percentile for his age. He also scored at the 12th percentile on a timed measure of reading comprehension. David scored in the low-average range on a phonological awareness assessment (25th percentile), and his overall score on a diagnostic assessment of oral language was at the 9th percentile relative to age norms.

I. C. "Josh"

We met Josh when he was 13 years old and in eighth grade. Josh's mother reported that he had struggled somewhat throughout middle school, and each year was harder than the last. Although he was previously an A and B student, his grades had slipped considerably, and his mother was concerned about his transition to high school. She reported that Josh had received speech therapy from preschool through second grade, but she did not really have concerns about his reading before middle school. However, she thought that he now struggled the most in classes that required a lot of reading. When asked about a family history of reading difficulties, Josh's mother recalled that she completed a brief reading intervention program herself when she was in fourth or fifth grade. She thought it had been helpful because she enjoys reading and does not find reading and writing challenging anymore. Josh disagreed with his mother's concern about his reading skills. He said he could read fine; he just didn't like it. Josh was willing to undergo an evaluation to learn more about his skills, but we also sensed that he didn't want to be viewed differently from other students. Josh showed a scattered pattern of scores on norm-referenced assessments. On measures of untimed single-word and nonword reading accuracy, Josh scored at the 47th percentile. He also scored at the 45th percentile on a measure of text reading fluency. However, on timed measures of single-word and nonword reading fluency, Josh scored at the 10th and 13th percentiles. On an untimed measure of reading comprehension involving no more than three sentences per passage, Josh scored at the 27th percentile. However, on a grade-level, criterion-referenced passage, Josh was not able to answer open-ended comprehension questions. Josh scored at the 25th percentile on a measure of phonological awareness, at the 3rd percentile on a measure of phonological memory, and at the 1st percentile on a measure of rapid automatized naming (RAN). He scored at the 50th percentile on a measure of syntactic knowledge.

II. Connections Between Oral Language and Reading Development and Difficulties

A point of commonality within Amy, David, and Josh's cases is that they all experienced reading comprehension difficulties that impacted their ability to keep up with schoolwork. Additionally, their academic struggles seemed to increase with time. However, our testing revealed different sources of difficulty for each child. To understand these differing sources of concern, we turn to the Simple View of Reading (Gough & Tunmer, 1986) and relations between different learning disorders, including dyslexia and developmental language disorder (DLD).

II.A. Simple View of Reading

The "Simple View" is a simplified model of reading comprehension in which reading comprehension is the product of two general classes of skills. First, "decoding" is the ability to quickly and accurately translate printed strings of letters into spoken words (Gough & Tunmer, 1986; Hoover & Tunmer, 2018). Second, "linguistic comprehension" is the ability to understand the sentences and paragraphs of the text if the spoken words are provided. It is often measured by asking individuals to listen to a text read aloud and answer questions about it, and the terms "listening comprehension" and "linguistic comprehension" are often used interchangeably in studies of the Simple View. Importantly, decoding and listening comprehension are correlated but separate skills. The multiplicative relationship between decoding and listening comprehension with reading comprehension emphasizes that both components are necessary, and neither alone is sufficient, for successful reading comprehension. In the last 40 years, over 100 studies have provided empirical support for the Simple View as an explanatory model of concurrent reading comprehension across ages and levels of proficiency (García & Cain, 2014).

Although it is a simple conceptual model, the skills that comprise the components of the Simple View are quite complex, language-based skills. As shown in Figure 9.1, skilled decoding relies on phonological, orthographic, and morphological knowledge, which are all interrelated with each other, and with broader language skills, including vocabulary. Listening comprehension relies on understanding the vocabulary and sentence structures (i.e., syntax), as well as higher-level language skills (e.g., inferences) and background knowledge about the topic. According to Gough and Tunmer (1986), "The simple view presumes that, once the printed matter is decoded, the reader applies to the text exactly the same mechanisms which he or she would bring to bear on its spoken equivalent" (p. 9). However, it is important to note that written language differs from spoken language in several ways, such that text comprehension requires higher levels of linguistic skills than conversation. For example, spoken language employs syntax and vocabulary that is simpler than that seen in written language (Dawson et al., 2021; Montag, 2019). Spoken utterances are shorter than written sentences, feature more deictic terms (*here/there*; *this/that*) that make reference to the immediate environment or situation, and are bolstered by body language and facial expressions that are not available in print. New or contrastive aspects of the spoken discourse are highlighted by prosodic accenting. Typographical elements, such as bold or italic font, can mimic prosodic emphasis in text, but they are optional and used sparingly in formal written contexts. Speech is produced and processed in the context of "in the moment"

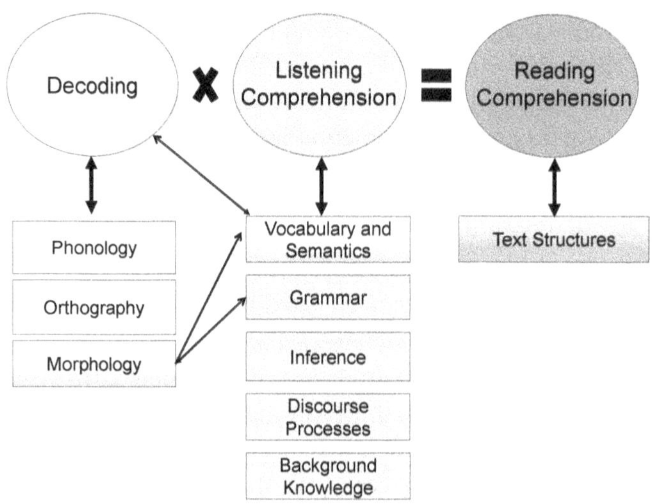

FIGURE 9.1. Language abilities contributing to the components of the Simple View of Reading. Bidirectional arrows signify reciprocal relations between the constructs of the simple view and their component skills. Adapted by permission from Figure 21.1 in Adlof et al. (2022). Copyright © 2022 Wiley.

interpersonal exchanges by interlocutors who often have established relationships (Horowitz & Samuels, 1987). This allows fluid shifts in conversational topics, and any breakdown in the exchange can be rectified immediately by asking for clarification. In the absence of these extralinguistic characteristics of spoken language, authors of printed texts rely on logical and coherent organization of ideas, connecting propositions and paragraphs with abstract cohesive devices rarely found in speech (e.g., *hence* and *therefore*). These features, in addition to the greater lexical diversity in written texts, exert greater cognitive and linguistic demands on readers than spoken language does on listeners. Thus, individuals with language impairments are likely to find written language—particularly the written academic language of textbooks and school material—more challenging than spoken language.

Longitudinal studies have demonstrated that early measures of the foundational language skills that support decoding and listening comprehension predict future reading comprehension skills (Kendeou et al., 2009; Language and Reading Research Consortium & Chiu, 2018) and that the relative contributions of word-reading and listening comprehension skills to reading comprehension shift across the development (Adlof et al., 2006; Foorman et al., 2018). Spoken language abilities develop before children learn to decode. Thus, when children are first learning to read in the primary school grades, individual differences in reading comprehension are largely explained by their decoding skills. Once most children have developed fluent decoding skills, which is around third grade for students in the United States, listening comprehension is the stronger predictor of reading comprehension.

In addition to explaining individual differences in reading comprehension, the Simple View is useful for understanding profiles of struggling readers who need support in different areas to improve their literacy. Under the Simple View, reading comprehension difficulties may be traced back to problems with decoding, listening comprehension, or both. Children with decoding difficulties will need support to develop phonological awareness, orthographic knowledge, and an understanding of how morphology influences spelling patterns. In contrast, children with listening comprehension difficulties will need support to increase their understanding of academic vocabulary, complex syntax, and text structures and the ability to use these skills to increase their general knowledge.

II.B. Dyslexia and DLD

The Simple View is also a useful conceptual framework for understanding relations between severe deficits in reading and oral language, including dyslexia and DLD. Severe difficulties with decoding and spelling are the chief hallmark of dyslexia (Carrol et al., 2025; Lyon et al., 2003; National Institute on Child Health and Human Development [NICHD], 2020), whereas the primary characteristic of DLD is difficulty understanding and producing spoken language. Although dyslexia and DLD are different disorders, there are some similarities in how they are defined. Both disorders are diagnosed by excluding factors that would otherwise explain observed poor performance in reading or oral language. That is, both disorders rule out factors such as hearing or vision impairment, brain injury, intellectual disability, or a lack of stimulation or instruction. Both disorders have a genetic and neurobiological basis (Landi & Perdue, 2019; Nudel et al., 2023). Both disorders may be described as dimensional disorders, reflecting the low end of a range of normally distributed abilities. Thus, prevalence rates for each disorder will depend on the specific cut point that is used for diagnosis (Fletcher, 2009; Norbury et al., 2016). Additionally, the terminology used for each of these disorders has evolved over time. For example, other terms used for children with dyslexia have included *congenital word blindness* and *strephosymbolia* (Henry & Brickley, 1999), and past terms for DLD include *congenital aphasia* and *developmental dysphasia* (Leonard, 2014).

According to contemporary definitions, dyslexia is characterized by significant difficulties with accurate and fluent word reading and spelling abilities caused by core deficits in the phonological component of language (Carroll et al., 2025; NICHD, 2020). Prevalence estimates vary, depending on the specific cut scores used for diagnosis, ranging from 3–20% in past studies (e.g., Rutter et al., 2004; Shaywitz, 1996; Spencer et al., 2014). Weak mental representations of the sounds of oral language inhibit children's ability to flexibly map phonemes to graphemes and decode words (Vellutino et al., 2004). Following the Simple View, a secondary consequence of dyslexia is poor reading comprehension, which, in combination with reduced reading experience, may negatively impact growth in vocabulary and general knowledge.

DLD is a significant and persistent impairment in the ability to understand and produce spoken language that does not have a known biomedical cause (Bishop et al., 2017). Children with DLD usually display weakness across multiple aspects of language, including phonology, morphology, syntax, vocabulary, and discourse. Delays in early language milestones indicate a risk for developing DLD, but many children with early language delays eventually catch up to their peers. Oral language impairments that are identified after 5 years of age—or after children have entered formal schooling—are likely to persist (Rice & Hoffman, 2015; Stothard et al., 1998). Epidemiologic studies in the United States and United Kingdom estimate the prevalence of DLD as 7–9% of 5-year-old children, but most of these children are not identified and do not receive speech–language services (Norbury et al., 2016; Tomblin et al., 1997). Until recently, DLD was most commonly referred to as "specific language impairment" (SLI) (Leonard, 2014). As part of an effort to raise awareness of the disorder, an international consortium selected the label "developmental language disorder" (Bishop et al., 2017), now commonly referred to by the acronym "DLD." Given broad language weaknesses, the Simple View predicts reading comprehension difficulties for children with DLD. Accordingly, DLD is associated with increased risk of reading and academic difficulties (Duff et al., 2023; Snowling et al., 2019; Ziegenfusz et al., 2022) as well as mood disorders and broader psychosocial difficulties (Goh et al., 2021; McGregor, 2020; Snow, 2019; Winstanley et al., 2021).

Just as individual differences in decoding and listening comprehension are moderately correlated, DLD and dyslexia are separate disorders, but they frequently co-occur. Clarity on the nature of the relationship between these disorders has been impeded partly due to the fact that investigations into dyslexia and DLD have been conducted by researchers with different disciplinary orientations. At a practical level, students with these disorders have been served by different professionals. Over time, it was noted that children with DLD in preschool or kindergarten often displayed difficulties learning to read words. Additionally, retrospective longitudinal studies of children with dyslexia found they had slower development of vocabulary and morphosyntax in preschool. Such observations led researchers to question whether the disorders were indeed unique (Bishop & Snowling, 2004; Catts et al., 2005; McArthur et al., 2000). However, evidence from multiple studies has accumulated indicating that DLD and dyslexia are different disorders (Bishop et al., 2009; Catts et al., 2005; Ehrhorn et al., 2021; Snowling et al., 2020). Such studies show that within each disorder, a wide range of abilities in the complementary skills are observed, including average and high ranges. Such a pattern would not be predicted if DLD and dyslexia were the same disorder. Current research now focuses on greater precision in the early discrimination of the two disorders, that is, what cognitive, biological, environmental, or other factors determine whether a child will have DLD but good word reading, dyslexia but good oral language, or both DLD and dyslexia?

II.C. Return to Cases

We return now to the cases of Amy, David, and Josh. All three experienced difficulties with reading comprehension that increased over time. A close inspection of their case histories reveals important differences between the cases, but each of them can be productively interpreted in the context of the Simple View of Reading.

Amy's reading achievement showed a significant decline at the end of second grade, despite scoring well within the average range at previous assessments. Further analysis of her reading revealed relatively strong word-reading and decoding skills. The Simple View of Reading predicts that, in the presence of strong decoding skills, poor reading comprehension is likely to result from poor linguistic comprehension, and this was borne out in Amy's case. Her difficulties were found to lie in the domain of oral language, with significant weakness in morphology, syntax, and narrative comprehension: a profile consistent with DLD. Her grade-level reading performance in earlier grades reflects the fact that reading comprehension in beginning readers is carried by decoding ability, a relative strength for Amy. As her school texts became more challenging, containing more complex language, Amy's performance began to drop relative to same-age peers. Thus, we conclude that Amy needs support in developing academic language skills as well as reading comprehension strategies to support her reading comprehension growth. Ideally, Amy would receive support from a speech–language pathologist who collaborates with her classroom teachers.

Josh's case tells the story of a student, like Amy, whose reading performance decreased over time. Until middle school, Josh had managed the demands of reading. However, at the time of assessment in eighth grade, Josh was experiencing difficulty with reading comprehension and decreased motivation to read. Unlike Amy, Josh's oral language skills were largely intact except for phonological awareness. Further assessment of Josh's reading skills, however, revealed some notable weaknesses in word reading and decoding. When allowed to take his time to read isolated words and nonwords, Josh demonstrated grade-level performance. Likewise, when reading connected text, his fluency was in the low-average range. However, when pressed to read single words and nonwords quickly, Josh scored in the 10th and 13th percentiles. The skills that are known to support word-reading development, namely phonological awareness, phonological memory, and rapid naming, were also significantly below age-expected norms. Consistent with the Simple View of Reading, slow and inaccurate decoding is a proximal cause of reading comprehension difficulties. Josh's profile is consistent with that of a child with dyslexia who has been able to compensate for some reading tasks by memorizing words and relying on strong language skills and background knowledge. Students with poor decoding skills can succeed to a certain degree by memorizing words; this is not, however, an effective long-term strategy. As Josh progressed in school, his academic reading is likely to have contained a greater proportion of unfamiliar words, and his underlying deficits in decoding and working memory combined to impede comprehension. Josh's case was further complicated by socio-emotional factors that are common in adolescent struggling readers, including feelings of anxiety and a need to protect his self-image and avoid feelings of failure (McArthur et al., 2022). Additionally, Josh needed help to make progress within his high school curriculum right away. Thus, for a student like Josh, recommendations include (1) counseling strategies and socio-emotional supports to reinforce his self-concept and build motivation to practice reading; (2) systematic, explicit, and intensive instruction in word-level reading skills to improve decoding and fluency; and (3) accommodations to help him access the curriculum and make progress in his academic courses, including additional time for written tests, outlines for note-taking, recorded lectures, audiobooks, and text-to-speech and speech-to-text software.

Whereas Amy and Josh exemplify the reading comprehension difficulties that result when the linguistic comprehension and decoding components of the Simple View of Reading, respectively, are weak, David shares the weaknesses of both Amy and Josh. Like them, David displayed markedly low reading comprehension, with a score at the 12th percentile. One likely contributing factor to his comprehension was his slow and inaccurate word and nonword reading. His uncertainty around orthographic patterns was also reflected in his very low spelling skills. Both reading and spelling were impacted by his low phonological awareness, assessed at the 25th percentile. These features are consistent with dyslexia. David's comprehension was also affected by his history of speech and language difficulties. David was dismissed from school speech and language services in kindergarten, so we assume he was competent in managing conversational language and social interactions. However, his score at the 9th percentile on a diagnostic assessment of oral language is consistent with a diagnosis of DLD. This would be expected to impact both listening and reading comprehension. Thus, we conclude that David needs support in both components of the Simple View at a high level of intensity in order to make progress. Like Josh and Amy, David may benefit from accommodations to help him access and make progress within the curriculum. Some instructional time may be used to help him learn to access and use compensatory tools and strategies, such as visual supports and graphic organizers, audiobooks and video summaries of course content, text-to-speech and speech-to-text software, and spelling and grammar checking software.

III. Frameworks for Identifying Oral versus Written Language Disorder

Currently, school systems use different frameworks to identify children with spoken language disorders versus reading disorders. In most schools, a formal assessment of oral language skills begins after a parent or teacher raises concerns about a child's speech or language abilities and requests an evaluation from a speech–language pathologist. The evaluation process generally includes informal assessments of the child's functioning in their classroom and at home, as well as formal testing to determine whether the child's comprehension and production of different language units (e.g., phonemes, words, sentences, and discourse) is commensurate with developmental norms. For the most part, the outcome of the evaluation is binary: The child is determined to have a disorder that qualifies them for speech or language services, or it is determined that the child does not have a disorder and does not receive services.

In contrast to current approaches in the identification of language disorders, most school systems in the United States use tiered assessment and intervention frameworks, such as response to intervention (RTI) or multi-tiered systems of support (MTSS), to identify and serve children with reading disabilities in the elementary grades. In tiered frameworks, universal screening of all students is used to identify risk for reading difficulties, and students' progress in meeting reading benchmarks is monitored several times per year. The results of these assessments are used to identify students who may need higher levels of support and more frequent progress monitoring. For example, students placed in Tier 2 of an RTI system for reading may receive additional small-group instruction, and their progress will be monitored more frequently (e.g., weekly or monthly vs. quarterly). Students who demonstrate a need for the highest levels of support (e.g., due to inability to reach progress monitoring goals) may be evaluated for a learning disability and considered for special education services.

The rationale for these tiered systems for reading is that it is difficult to diagnose dyslexia before children have received reading instruction that is sufficient in terms of both amount and quality. Instructional programs vary in their systematicity, explicitness, and evidence of effectiveness. If students have received evidence-based reading instruction from the beginning, their failure to make progress is more likely to be due to a learning disability. Because most children enter school unable to read many words, poor performance on assessments of early word-reading and precursor skills like phonemic awareness is as likely to reflect floor effects in measurement as evidence of disability (Catts et al., 2009). As children progress in school, greater variation in reading performance can be observed among students, allowing for clearer interpretation of poor performance and better identification of children who are struggling. An unfortunate trade-off results in waiting for unequivocal signs of poor performance, as early intervention is reliably more effective at improving reading outcomes (Al Otaiba et al., 2014; Lovett et al., 2017).

High-quality implementation of RTI can reduce the risk that a student will fall through the cracks, a result not uncommonly observed in previous systems, which have been referred to as "wait to fail" models. RTI is a whole-school prevention model designed to serve all students, inclusive of culturally and linguistically diverse students who have been traditionally simultaneously over- and underidentified with diagnostic labels (cf. Marencin et al., 2024; Morgan et al., 2017; Morgan et al., 2016). RTI is relatively agnostic to diagnostic labels; indeed, a child whose reading behavior meets the criteria for dyslexia may not be identified for public school special education services in the United States if they are making appropriate educational progress within their RTI tier. At the same time, RTI should not be used to delay or deny an evaluation for special education eligibility (Musgrove, 2011). A prevention focus means an emphasis on *early* intervention that closes gaps as swiftly as possible. Within RTI, assessment should measure progress related to curricular standards, and assessment tools should be sensitive to both student progress and instructional change. A child's movement in and out of the RTI tiers is determined by their own performance data, and under optimal implementation conditions, this movement is smooth and efficient. There is strong evidence for the use of RTI to improve word-reading skills for struggling and at-risk readers in the primary grades when interventions are implemented consistently and with fidelity (Coyne et al., 2018; Gersten et al., 2017; Wanzek et al., 2016). If Josh and David's schools had used RTI in this way, their word-reading difficulties may have been addressed sooner. Most elementary schools in the United States now use tiered frameworks for reading. However, the quality of core reading instruction, the quality of implementation of RTI, and the outcomes of reading instruction are quite variable across schools (Balu et al., 2015; Fuchs & Fuchs, 2017). A problem at any of these levels can have negative consequences for students like Josh and David. Additionally, most RTI frameworks are not set up to support students like Amy, who develop good word-reading skills but struggle with comprehension related to language difficulties.

IV. Current Challenges for Identifying and Serving Children with DLD

There are several challenges related to current methods of identifying and serving children with DLD. One challenge is underidentification. Epidemiologic studies indicate that as many as two-thirds of kindergarten-aged children with DLD are not identified and are not receiving speech–language intervention services (Norbury et al., 2016; Tomblin et al., 1997). This underidentification may be related to a general lack of awareness of DLD (Bishop, 2010; McGregor, 2020) as well as to difficulties recognizing the signs of delayed language development in children who seem to be developing normally in all other areas. Although most adults can recognize a child who produces speech sounds differently than same-age peers, the signs of language difficulty may be less obvious. Even though children with DLD make more grammatical errors than their peers, most of what they say is grammatically correct (Rice et al., 2004), and parents may pay more attention to the content of the child's message than its grammaticality. There are also many contextual supports in conversational language that support mutual understanding even when utterances contain errors. It is difficult to determine what a child has understood without directly assessing it, and without such assessment, a lack of understanding might be misperceived as shyness, inattention, or forgetfulness. Although parents tailor their communication to their children's level, they may not be aware of what is "typical" for their developmental stage. For example, two recent studies reported very low rates of parent-reported concerns about language development among children meeting research criteria for DLD (Adlof et al., 2017; Hendricks et al., 2019; see also Chan et al., 2022). On the other hand, although teachers may be in a position to compare students to their peers, large class sizes may make it difficult for them to attend to individual students' oral language skills. Recent evidence indicates that classroom teachers also have difficulty discriminating normal from disordered language abilities (Christopulos & Kean, 2020; Jessup et al., 2008; Williams, 2006). Amy's case, in which assessment in a research project showed significant language deficits in the absence of any concerns expressed by school personnel or family members, represents a typical underidentified student.

In addition to general underidentification, a second challenge is disproportionalities in which children are identified and do receive services (see review by McGregor, 2020). Boys are more likely to receive school-based speech and language services than girls, and the difference in service receipt between males and females is greater than the difference in rates of affectedness (Lindsay & Strand, 2016; Morgan et al., 2017; see also Nudel et al., 2023; Peterson & Pennington, 2015). Children from historically minoritized groups, including Black and Hispanic children, have significantly lower odds of receiving services than White, non-Hispanic children (Morgan et al., 2017; Robinson & Norton, 2019; see also Samson & Lesaux, 2009). Children whose mothers have higher education levels are more likely to receive services (Wittke & Spaulding, 2018). Most children with DLD do not have co-occurring conditions, but those with co-occurring conditions, especially those with more overt characteristics, are most likely to receive services. Often, language impairment is uncovered during the assessment for these more noticeable conditions. For example, most children with DLD have normal speech articulation abilities, but those with overt speech difficulties are more likely to receive language services (Zhang & Tomblin, 2000). Likewise, the language deficits of children with DLD and co-occurring executive function deficits (Wittke & Spaulding, 2018) and those with combined DLD and dyslexia (Catts et al., 2005; Duff et al., 2022) are more likely to be served.

A third challenge for the current system is the limited availability of resources for the accurate assessment of language ability in children who speak more than one language or who speak a dialect that differs from general American English

(GAE) (Karem et al., 2019; Muñoz et al., 2014), although some progress has been made for Spanish–English bilingual children (Peña et al., 2018) and those who speak African American English (Seymour et al., 2005). Using assessments normed for children who speak GAE with children with a different linguistic background can increase diagnostic errors, including both over- and underidentification (Peña et al., 2023; Hendricks & Diehm, 2020; Marencin et al., 2024). Both types of errors are problematic.

Fourth, the current binary system is poorly equipped to identify and support children with subclinical *spoken* language difficulties—those who score just above the eligibility criterion for speech–language services—who are likely to have significant difficulties with *written* language, including reading comprehension. This is complicated by the fact that, while language difficulties can be detected before reading instruction begins, the impact of those difficulties might not be apparent until the middle to late elementary grades. For example, several studies have examined the phenomenon of "late-emerging poor readers," that is, children who score within normal limits on reading assessments in the early grades and below normal limits later on (Catts et al., 2012; Leach et al., 2003; Psyridou et al., 2020). Both word-reading and reading comprehension difficulties may be late to emerge, but late-emerging reading comprehension difficulties are much more common (Catts et al., 2012; Psyridou et al., 2020), and both types have been linked to weak—but not necessarily within clinical ranges—oral language skills in earlier grades. For example, a longitudinal study of kindergarten children with DLD found that 70% exhibited significant reading difficulties by tenth grade, but 40% of those emerged in fourth grade or later (Catts et al., 2012; see also Fong & Ho, 2019; Snowling et al., 2020). In a retrospective study of fifth graders with good word reading but poor reading comprehension, Justice, Mashburn, and Petscher (2013) found that these students had significantly poorer oral language skills than their same-age peers at 15 months of age. Furthermore, their oral language skills continued to decline relative to peers between 15 and 54 months. The case of David, whose language skills were not monitored after dismissal from early services, exemplifies problems that arise when the demands of written language in later grades outstrip oral language abilities. These challenges have impacts on students, as can be seen in the three cases we presented earlier. Both David and Amy demonstrated significant oral language difficulties that ultimately impacted reading progress. Amy's language difficulties remained undetected until her reading comprehension difficulties emerged. David's broad language deficits impacted both word reading and reading comprehension. Although David and Josh both had a history of early speech–language services, it appears that their skills were not monitored after dismissal, allowing them both to still "fall through the cracks."

V. Recommendations and Conclusions

Whereas the frameworks used to identify children in need of reading support are intended to be *preventive*, they do not currently include sufficient consideration of language abilities. For example, recommended universal screening measures for reading in the primary grades generally do not include measures of oral language ability beyond phonological awareness and occasionally vocabulary knowledge (Gersten et al., 2008; International Dyslexia Association, 2020). Current frameworks to identify children with language disorders may be described as *reactive* because they rely on someone to notice symptoms before an assessment will be initiated. We argue that integrating identification and service delivery for spoken language within the tiered systems that exist for reading would be advantageous for several reasons.

First, incorporating sensitive measures of broader language abilities, including semantics, syntax, and higher-level language skills, into universal screening and progress monitoring frameworks can help to identify language difficulties before their impact on reading comprehension is realized. This may help to improve the identification of children with DLD as well as those with subclinical oral language difficulties who may need support to achieve adequate comprehension of written language. Under current frameworks, subclinical language difficulties that are present from an early age often manifest as "late-emerging" poor reading comprehension in middle school grades (Catts et al., 2012; Justice et al., 2013). Additionally, a systematic approach to monitoring academic language skills over time can be helpful for differentiating between normal variations in language production related to linguistic and cultural identity and signs of a language disorder that are likely to impact educational progress. Including language measures in universal screening may also help understand some children's slower response to targeted word-reading interventions. Research indicates that children with broad language deficits, including vocabulary and grammar as well as phonological awareness, tend to make less progress in reading than children with deficits only in the phonological domain (Denton et al., 2013; Duff et al., 2008; Vadasy et al., 2008).

As just described, there is much to be gained by monitoring language development over time. We also contend that there can be further benefits with a systematic, explicit approach to language instruction in Tier 1. Many individual states' standards, as well as the Common Core standards, set expectations for what students should know at each grade level. For example, in the Common Core standards, kindergarten students are expected to "use verbs to convey a sense of past, present, and future" (CCSS.ELA-Literacy.L.1.1.e), and second-grade students should be able to "Produce, expand, and rearrange complete simple and compound sentences" (CCSS.ELA-Literacy.L.2.1.f). However, while these examples focus on what children produce, there is room for better integration within the standards for language comprehension and expression. Additionally, in our experience, instruction of these standards does not receive full priority and often varies according to the choice of language arts curriculum and teacher knowledge and preferences. Having an explicit and systematic core language curriculum in place affords the development and implementation of Tier 2 instruction to provide support for children with subclinical language difficulties who are not served in current frameworks and who are likely to experience reading comprehension difficulties in the future. As with tiered frameworks for word reading, the goal is to provide support for language as early as possible, with more flexibility than the current binary system provides. This is an important topic in need of research.

The existing literature base related to the effects of language interventions to support reading comprehension for students in all tiers is promising but limited in the number and scope of studies. The majority of extant intervention studies focus on preschoolers or kindergarten students, and in those studies, students are not usually followed long enough to demonstrate impacts on reading comprehension (Rogde et al., 2019). Additionally, in this literature overall, the range of treatment targets is heavily skewed toward vocabulary and narratives, with less attention to other aspects of language, including syntax. Overall, these studies reveal small, positive effects of language intervention, particularly when the intervention is delivered to small groups (Herrera et al., 2021; Rogde et al., 2019). Two recent studies highlight the promise of systematic, explicit language instruction for students in Tier 1 and Tier 2. In Tier 1, a randomized control trial of the *Let's Know* curriculum in the United States led to significant improvements in first-, second-, and third-grade students' oral language skills. Further analysis revealed significant impacts of instruction on reading comprehension, mediated by vocabulary, in all three grades (Language and Reading Research Consortium et al., 2019). Turning to Tier 2, West et al. (2021) found significant positive effects from a scaled evaluation of the *Nuffield Early Language Intervention*, a 20-week small-group language intervention for students in their reception year (ages 4–5 years) in the United Kingdom. Students were identified for the small-group intervention based on their performance on a universally administered language screen (West et al., 2021). Such results are encouraging and suggest the potential for tiered frameworks to monitor and support language development in school-aged children and, by extension, their reading comprehension and overall academic achievement.

One final observation is that the recommendations we have outlined here require the collaboration of all school personnel to support children with language-based learning disabilities. As we have seen, current service models that assign students with dyslexia to the care of educators and those with DLD to the speech–language pathologist contribute to the fractionalization of special education. We advocate, therefore, for better integration of identification and intervention frameworks for children with oral language and reading difficulties that increases collaboration among professionals and places students' needs at the center.

REFERENCES

Adlof, S. M., Catts, H. W., & Little, T. D. (2006). Should the Simple View of Reading include a fluency component? *Reading and Writing: An Interdisciplinary Journal, 19*, 933–958.

Adlof, S. M., Chan, J., Werfel, K., & Catts, H. W. (2022). Learning to read with a language or hearing impairment. In M. J. Snowling, C. Hulme, & K. Nation (Eds.), *The science of reading* (pp. 460–485). Wiley.

Adlof, S. M., Scoggins, J., Brazendale, A., Babb, S., & Petscher, Y. (2017). Identifying children at risk for language impairment or dyslexia with group-administered measures. *Journal of Speech, Language, and Hearing Research, 60*, 3507–3522.

Al Otaiba, S., Kim, Y. S., Wanzek, J., Petscher, Y., & Wagner, R. K. (2014). Long-term effects of first-grade multitier intervention. *Journal of Research on Educational Effectiveness, 7*(3), 250–267.

Balu, R., Zhu, P., Doolittle, F., Schiller, E., Jenkins, J., & Gersten, R. (2015). *Evaluation of response to intervention practices for elementary school reading.* U.S. Department of Education. *https://files.eric.ed.gov/fulltext/ED560820.pdf*

Bishop, D. V. M. (2010). Which neurodevelopmental disorders get researched and why? *PLOS One, 5*(11), e15112.

Bishop, D. V. M., McDonald, D., Bird, S., & Hayiou-Thomas, M. (2009). Children who read words accurately despite language impairment: Who are they and how do they do it? *Child Development, 80*, 593–605.

Bishop, D. V. M., & Snowling, M. J. (2004). Developmental dyslexia and specific language impairment: Same or different? *Psychological Bulletin, 130*(6), 858–886.

Bishop, D. V., Snowling, M. J., Thompson, P. A., Greenhalgh, T., Consortium, C.-2, Adams, C., & Bellair, J. (2017). Phase 2 of CATALISE: A multinational and multidisciplinary Delphi consensus study of problems with language development: Terminology. *Journal of Child Psychology and Psychiatry, 58*(10), 1068–1080.

Carroll, J. M., Holden, C., Kirby, P., Thompson, P. A., Snowling, M. J., & Dyslexia Delphi Panel. (2025). Toward a consensus on dyslexia: Findings from a Delphi study. *Journal of Child Psychology and Psychiatry, 66*, 1065–1076.

Catts, H. W., Adlof, S. M., Hogan, T. P., & Weismer, S. (2005). Are specific language impairment and dyslexia distinct disorders? *Journal of Speech, Language, and Hearing Research, 48*, 1378–96.

Catts, H. W., Compton, D., Tomblin, J. B., & Bridges, M. S. (2012). Prevalence and nature of late-emerging poor readers. *Journal of Educational Psychology, 104*, 166–181.

Catts, H. W., Petscher, Y., Schatschneider, C., Bridges, M. S., & Mendoza, K. (2009). Floor effects associated with universal screening and their impact on the early identification of reading disabilities. *Journal of Learning Disabilities, 42*(2), 163–176.

Chan, J., Adlof, S. M., Duff, D. M., Mitchell, A., Ragunathan, M., & Ehrhorn, A. (2022). Examining the associations between parent concerns and school-age children's language and reading abilities: A comparison of samples recruited for in-school vs. online participation. *Language Speech and Hearing Services in Schools, 53*(2), 431–444.

Christopulos, T., & Kean, J. (2020). General education teachers' contribution to the identification of children with language disorders. *Perspectives of the ASHA Special Interest Groups, 5*(4), 770–777.

Coyne, M. D., Oldham, A., Dougherty, S. M., Leonard, K., Koriakin, T., Gage, N. A., & Gillis, M. (2018). Evaluating the effects of supplemental reading intervention within an MTSS or RTI reading reform initiative using a regression discontinuity design. *Exceptional Children, 84*(4), 350–367.

Dawson, N., Hsiao, Y., Tan, A. W. M., Banerji, N., & Nation, K. (2021). Features of lexical richness in children's books: Comparisons with child-directed speech. *Language Development Research, 1.*

Denton, C. A., Tolar, T. D., Fletcher, J. M., Barth, A. E., Vaughn, S., & Francis, D. J. (2013). Effects of Tier 3 intervention for students with persistent reading difficulties and characteristics of inadequate responders. *Journal of Educational Psychology, 105*(3), 633–648.

Duff, D., Hendricks, A. E., Fitton, L., & Adlof, S. M. (2022). Reading and math achievement in children with dyslexia, developmental language disorder, or typical development: Achievement gaps persist from second through fourth grades. *Journal of Learning Disabilities, 56*(5), 371–391.

Duff, F. J., Fieldsend, E., Bowyer-Crane, C., Hulme, C., Smith, G., Gibbs, S., & Snowling, M. J. (2008). Reading with vocabulary intervention: Evaluation of an instruction for children with poor response to reading intervention. *Journal of Research in Reading, 31*(3), 319–336.

Ehrhorn, A., Adlof, S. M., Fogerty, D., & Laing, S. (2021). Probing phonological processing differences in nonword repetition for children with separate or co-occurring dyslexia and developmental language disorder. *Scientific Studies of Reading, 25*(6), 486–503.

Fletcher, J. M. (2009). Dyslexia: The evolution of a scientific concept. *Journal of the International Neuropsychological Society, 15*, 501–508.

Fong, C. Y.-C., & Ho, C. S. H. (2019). Poor oral discourse skills are the key cognitive-linguistic weakness of Chinese poor comprehenders: A three-year longitudinal study. *First Language, 39*(3), 281–297.

Foorman, B. R., Petscher, Y., & Herrera, S. (2018). Unique and common effects of decoding and language factors in predicting reading comprehension in grades 1–10. *Learning and Individual Differences, 63*, 12–23.

Fuchs, D., & Fuchs, L. S. (2017). Critique of the national evaluation of response to intervention: A case for simpler frameworks. *Exceptional Children, 83*(3), 255–268.

García, J. R., & Cain, K. (2014). Decoding and reading comprehension: A meta-analysis to identify which reader and assessment characteristics influence the strength of the relationship in English. *Review of Educational Research, 84*(1), 74–111.

Gersten, R., Compton, D., Connor, C. M., Dimino, J., Santoro, L., Linan-Thompson, S., & Tilly, W. D. (2008). *Assisting students struggling with reading: Response to intervention and multi-tier intervention for reading in the primary grades: A practice guide* (NCEE 2009-4045). National Center for Education Evaluation and Regional Assistance, Institute of Education Sciences, U.S. Department of Education. *http://ies.ed.gov/ncee/wwc/publications/practiceguides*

Gersten, R., Jayanthi, M., & Dimino, J. (2017). Too much, too soon? Unanswered questions from national response to intervention evaluation. *Exceptional Children, 83*(3), 244–254.

Goh, S. K. Y., Griffiths, S., Norbury, C. F., & SCALES Team. (2021). Sources of variability in the prospective relation of language to social, emotional, and behavior problem symptoms: Implications for developmental language disorder. *Journal of Abnormal Psychology, 130*(6), 676–689.

Gough, P. B., & Tunmer, W. E. (1986). Decoding, reading, and reading disability. *RASE: Remedial and Special Education, 7*, 6–10.

Hendricks, A. E., Adlof, S. M., Alonzo, C. N., Fox, A. B., & Hogan, T. P. (2019). Identifying children at risk for developmental language disorder using a brief, whole-classroom screen. *Journal of Speech, Language, and Hearing Research, 62*(4), 896–908.

Hendricks, A. E., & Diehm, E. A. (2020). Survey of assessment and intervention practices for students who speak African American English. *Journal of Communication Disorders, 83*, 105967.

Henry, M. K., & Brickley, S. G. (1999). *Dyslexia . . . Samuel T. Orton and his legacy.* International Dyslexia Association.

Herrera, S., Phillips, B. M., Newton, Y., Dombek, J. L., & Hernandez, J. A. (2021). *Effectiveness of early literacy instruction: Summary of 20 years of research* (REL 2021–084). U.S. Department of Education, Institute of Education Sciences, National Center for Education Evaluation and Regional Assistance, Regional Educational Laboratory Southeast. *http://ies.ed.gov/ncee/edlabs*

Hoover, W. A., & Tunmer, W. E. (2018). The Simple View of Reading: Three assessments of its adequacy. *Remedial and Special Education, 39*(5), 304–312.

Horowitz, R., & Samuels, S. (1987). *Comprehending oral and written language.* Emerald Group.

International Dyslexia Association. (2020). *Universal screening: K–2 reading. https://dyslexiaida.org/universal-screening-k-2-reading*

Jessup, B., Ward, E., Cahill, L., & Keating, D. (2008). Teacher identification of speech and language impairment in kindergarten students using the Kindergarten Development Check. *International Journal of Speech-Language Pathology, 10*(6), 449–459.

Justice, L., Mashburn, A., & Petscher, Y. (2013). Very early language skills of fifth-grade poor comprehenders. *Journal of Research in Reading, 36*(2), 172–185.

Karem, R. W., Washington, K. N., Crowe, K., Jenkins, A., Leon, M., Kokotek, L., et al. (2019). Current methods of evaluating the language abilities of multilingual preschoolers:

A scoping review using the International Classification of Functioning, Disability and Health–Children and Youth Version. *Language, Speech, and Hearing Services in Schools, 50*(3), 434–451.

Kendeou, P., van den Broek, P., White, M. J., & Lynch, J. S. (2009). Predicting reading comprehension in early elementary school: The independent contributions of oral language and decoding skills. *Journal of Educational Psychology, 101*(4), 765–778.

Landi, N., & Perdue, M. V. (2019). Neuroimaging genetics studies of specific reading disability and developmental language disorder: A review. *Language and Linguistics Compass, 13*, e12349.

Language and Reading Research Consortium, & Chiu, Y. D. (2018). The Simple View of Reading across development: Prediction of grade 3 reading comprehension from prekindergarten skills. *Remedial and Special Education, 39*(5), 289–303.

Language and Reading Research Consortium, Jiang, H., & Logan, J. (2019). Improving reading comprehension in the primary grades: Mediated effects of a language-focused classroom intervention. *Journal of Speech, Language, and Hearing Research, 62*(8), 2812–2828.

Leach, J. M., Scarborough, H. S., & Rescorla, L. (2003). Late-emerging reading disabilities. *Journal of Educational Psychology, 95*(2), 211–224.

Leonard, L. B. (2014). *Children with specific language impairment* (2nd ed.). MIT Press.

Lindsay, G., & Strand, S. (2016). Children with language impairment: Prevalence, associated difficulties, and ethnic disproportionality in an English population. *Frontiers in Education, 1*(2).

Lovett, M. W., Frijters, J. C., Wolf, M., Steinbach, K. A., Sevcik, R. A., & Morris, R. D. (2017). Early intervention for children at risk for reading disabilities: The impact of grade at intervention and individual differences on intervention outcomes. *Journal of Educational Psychology, 109*(7), 889–914.

Lyon, G. R., Shaywitz, S. E., & Shaywitz, B. A. (2003). A definition of dyslexia. *Annals of dyslexia, 53*(1), 1–14.

Marencin, N. C., Edwards, A. A., & Terry, N. P. (2024). African American preschoolers' performance on norm-referenced language assessments: Examining the effect of dialect density and the use of scoring modifications. *Language, Speech, and Hearing Services in Schools, 55*(3), 918–937.

McArthur, G., Badcock, N., Castles, A., & Robidoux, S. (2022). Tracking the relations between children's reading and emotional health across time: Evidence from four large longitudinal studies. *Reading Research Quarterly, 57*(2), 555–585.

McArthur, G. M., Hogben, J. H., Edwards, V. T., Heath, S. M., & Mengler, E. D. (2000). On the "specifics" of specific reading disability and specific language impairment. *Journal of Child Psychology and Psychiatry, 41*(7), 869–874.

McGregor, K. K. (2020). How we fail children with developmental language disorder. *Language, Speech, and Hearing Services in Schools, 51*(4), 981–992.

Montag, J. L. (2019). Differences in sentence complexity in the text of children's picture books and child-directed speech. *First Language, 39*(5), 527–546.

Morgan, P. L., Farkas, G., Hillemeier, M. M., & Maczuga, S. (2017). Replicated evidence of racial and ethnic disparities in disability identification in U.S. schools. *Educational Researcher, 46*(6), 305–322.

Morgan, P. L., Hammer, C. S., Farkas, G., Hillemeier, M. M., Maczuga, S., Cook, M., & Morano, S. (2016). Who receives speech/language services by 5 years of age in the United States? *American Journal of Speech-Language Pathology, 25*(2), 183–199.

Muñoz, M. L., White, M., & Horton-Ikard, R. (2014). The identification conundrum. *The ASHA Leader, 19*(11), 48–53.

Musgrove, M. (2011). *A response to intervention (RtI) process cannot be used to delay–deny an evaluation for eligibility under the Individuals with Disabilities Education Act (IDEA).* United States Department of Education Office of Special Education and Rehabilitative Services. *www2.ed.gov/policy/speced/guid/idea/memosdcltrs/osep11-07rtimemo.pdf*

National Institute on Child Health and Human Development. (2020). *What are reading disorders? www.nichd.nih.gov/health/topics/reading/conditioninfo/disorders*

Norbury, C. F., Gooch, D., Wray, C., Baird, G., Charman, T., Simonoff, E., et al. (2016). The impact of nonverbal ability on prevalence and clinical presentation of language disorder: Evidence from a population study. *Journal of Child Psychology and Psychiatry, 57*(11), 1247–1257.

Nudel, R., Christensen, R. V., Kalnak, N., Schwinn, M., Banasik, K., Dinh, K. M., et al. (2023). Developmental language disorder—A comprehensive study of more than 46,000 individuals. *Psychiatry Research, 323*, 115171.

Peña, E. D., Bedore, L. M., & Vargas, A. G. (2023). Exploring assumptions of the bilingual delay in children with and without developmental language disorder. *Journal of Speech, Language, and Hearing Research, 66*(12), 4739–4755.

Peña, E. D., Gutiérrez-Clellen, V. F., Iglesias, A., Goldstein, B., & Bedore, L. M. (2018). *Bilingual English–Spanish Assessment (BESA)*. Brookes.

Peterson, R. L., & Pennington, B. F. (2015). Developmental dyslexia. *Annual Review of Clinical Psychology, 11*, 283–307.

Psyridou, M., Tolvanen, A., Lerkkanen, M.-K., Poikkeus, A.-M., & Torppa, M. (2020). Longitudinal stability of reading difficulties: Examining the effects of measurement error, cutoffs, and buffer zones in identification. *Frontiers in Psychology, 10*, 2841.

Rice, M. L., & Hoffman, L. (2015). Predicting vocabulary growth in children with and without specific language impairment: A longitudinal study from 2;6 to 21 years of age. *Journal of Speech, Language, and Hearing Research, 58*, 345–359.

Rice, M. L., Tomblin, J. B., Hoffman, L., Richman, W. A., & Marquis, J. (2004). Grammatical tense deficits in children with SLI and nonspecific language impairment. *Journal of Speech, Language, and Hearing Research, 47*, 816–834.

Robinson, G. C., & Norton, P. C. (2019). A decade of disproportionality: A state-level analysis of African American students enrolled in the primary disability category of speech or language impairment. *Language, Speech, and Hearing Services in Schools, 50*(2), 267–282.

Rogde, K., Hagen, Å. M., Melby-Lervåg, M., & Lervåg, A. (2019). The effect of linguistic comprehension instruction on generalized language and reading comprehension skills: A systematic review. *Campbell Systematic Reviews, 15*, e1059.

Rutter, M., Caspi, A., Fergusson, D., Horwood, L. J., Goodman, R., Maughan, B., et al. (2004). Sex differences in developmental reading disability: New findings from 4 epidemiological studies. *Journal of the American Medical Association, 291*, 2007–2012.

Samson, J. F., & Lesaux, N. K. (2009). Language-minority learners in special education: Rates and predictors of identification for services. *Journal of Learning Disabilities, 42*(2), 148–162.

Seymour, H. N., Roeper, T., de Villiers, J. G., & de Villiers, P. A. (2005). *Diagnostic Evaluation of Language Variation–Norm Referenced* (DELV-NR). Pearson.

Shaywitz, S. E. (1996). Dyslexia. *Scientific American, 275*(5), 98–104.

Snow, P. C. (2019). Speech-language pathology and the youth offender: Epidemiological overview and roadmap for future speech-language pathology research and scope of practice. *Language, Speech, and Hearing Services in Schools, 50*(2), 324–339.

Snowling, M. J., Hayiou-Thomas, M. E., Nash, H. M., & Hulme, C. (2020). Dyslexia and developmental language disorder: Comorbid disorders with distinct effects on reading comprehension. *The Journal of Child Psychology and Psychiatry, 61*, 672–680.

Snowling, M. J., Nash, H., Gooch, D. C., Hayiou-Thomas, M. E., & Hulme, C. (2019). Developmental outcomes for children at high risk of dyslexia and children with developmental language disorder. *Child Development*, e548–e564.

Spencer, M., Wagner, R. K., Schatschneider, C., Quinn, J. M., Lopez, D., & Petscher, Y. (2014). Incorporating RTI in a hybrid model of reading disability. *Learning Disability Quarterly, 37*(3), 161–171.

Stothard, S. E., Snowling, M. J., Bishop, D. V. M., Chipchase, B. B., & Kaplan, C. A. (1998).

Language-impaired preschoolers: A follow-up into adolescence. *Journal of Speech, Language, and Hearing Research, 41*(2), 407–418.

Tomblin, J. B., Records, N. L., Buckwalter, P., Zhang, X., Smith, E., & O'Brien, M. (1997). Prevalence of specific language impairment in kindergarten children. *Journal of Speech, Language, and Hearing Research, 40*(6), 1245–1260.

Vadasy, P. F., Sanders, E. A., & Abbott, R. D. (2008). Effects of supplemental early reading intervention at 2-year follow up: Reading skill growth patterns and predictors. *Scientific Studies of Reading, 12*(1), 51–89.

Vellutino, F. R., Fletcher, J. M., Snowling, M. J., & Scanlon, D. M. (2004). Specific reading disability (dyslexia): What have we learned in the past four decades? *Journal of Child Psychology and Psychiatry, 45*(1), 2–40.

Wanzek, J., Vaughn, S., Scammacca, N., Gatlin, B., Walker, M. A., & Capin, P. (2016). Meta-analyses of the effects of tier 2 type reading interventions in grades K–3. *Educational Psychology Review, 28*(3), 551–576.

West, G., Snowling, M. J., Lervåg, A., Buchanan-Worster, E., Duta, M., Hall, A., et al. (2021). Early language screening and intervention can be delivered successfully at scale: evidence from a cluster randomized controlled trial. *Journal of Child Psychology and Psychiatry, and Allied Disciplines, 62*(12), 1425–1434.

Williams, C. (2006). Teacher judgements of the language skills of children in the early years of schooling. *Child language teaching and therapy, 22*(2), 135–154.

Winstanley, M., Webb, R. T., & Conti-Ramsden, G. (2021). Developmental language disorders and risk of recidivism among young offenders. *Journal of Child Psychology and Psychiatry, 62*(4), 396–403.

Wittke, K., & Spaulding, T. J. (2018). Which preschool children with specific language impairment receive language intervention? *Language, Speech, and Hearing Services in Schools, 49*(1), 59–71.

Zhang, X., & Tomblin, J. B. (2000). The association of intervention receipt with speech-language profiles and social-demographic variables. *American Journal of Speech-Language Pathology, 9*(4), 345–357.

Ziegenfusz, S., Paynter, J., Flückiger, B., & Westerveld, M. F. (2022). A systematic review of the academic achievement of primary and secondary school-aged students with developmental language disorder. *Autism & Developmental Language Impairments, 7*, 23969415221099397.

CHAPTER 10

Learning Disabilities and Comorbidity

Prevalence, Etiology, and Implications

Erik G. Willcutt

Current definitions of specific learning disability (SLD) in the 5th edition of the *Diagnostic and Statistical Manual of Mental Disorders* (DSM-5; American Psychiatric Association, 2013), the 10th edition of the *International Classification of Diseases* (ICD-10; World Health Organization, 1992), and the 2004 Individuals with Disabilities Education Improvement Act (IDEA) identify a heterogeneous population that includes individuals with weaknesses in different aspects of reading, math, or writing (American Psychiatric Association, 2013). While some individuals with SLD exhibit a specific weakness in a single academic domain, SLDs in reading (RD), mathematics (MD), and writing (WD) co-occur more often than expected by chance with one another and with other disorders such as attention-deficit/hyperactivity disorder (ADHD), a phenomenon known as *comorbidity* (e.g., Badian, 1999; Landerl & Moll, 2010; Olson et al., 2013; Willcutt, Betjemann, et al., 2010; Willcutt et al., 2013).

It is important to understand the frequency, implications, and causes of comorbidity for several reasons. The presence of more than one disorder in the same individual makes it difficult to interpret research studies reporting an association between a variable and a specific SLD because it is not clear whether an undetected comorbidity could be contributing to the association. High rates of comorbidity also raise practical questions about whether treatment of one disorder will also improve symptoms of comorbid disorders or whether treatment approaches should be modified to account for comorbidities. Further, individuals with comorbid disorders often differ in important ways from individuals with a disorder in isolation, with the comorbid group frequently experiencing greater symptom severity, more extensive and severe functional impairment, and poorer long-term outcomes (e.g., Waschbusch, 2002; Willcutt, Betjemann, Pennington, et al., 2007; Willcutt,

Pennington, et al., 2010). Finally, the high rates of comorbidity between putatively distinct SLDs directly challenge simple theoretical models of SLDs and the overall concept of *specific* learning disabilities.

The current chapter summarizes the existing literature and new results from two of our ongoing studies to provide an overview of current knowledge regarding the prevalence, causes, and implications of comorbidity between RD, MD, and WD and between these SLDs and ADHD and other internalizing and externalizing psychopathology. After a brief overview of our ongoing studies to set the stage for the new analyses described in this chapter, the first section of the chapter summarizes existing knowledge regarding the frequency of comorbidity between RD, MD, and WD, along with the rates of comorbidity between each of these SLDs and psychological disorders such as ADHD, anxiety and depression, and conduct disorder. The second section then reviews the potential impact of comorbidity on academic functioning and other important developmental outcomes in our studies and the broader literature, including new analyses of the early adult outcomes of individuals who were identified with RD or MD during childhood or adolescence. The third section then briefly reviews studies of the etiology of comorbidity between RD, MD, and ADHD and summarizes studies of the shared neurocognitive weaknesses that may lead to comorbidity. The chapter concludes by providing a number of recommendations to help clinicians address comorbidity most effectively in applied settings and then proposes several key directions for future research.

New Data Analyses for the Current Chapter

In addition to summarizing the existing literature, this chapter includes several new analyses of different aspects of comorbidity in samples drawn from two of our ongoing studies. To set the stage for these analyses, these two samples are described briefly in this section.

Colorado Learning Disabilities Research Center

The Colorado Learning Disabilities Research Center (CLDRC) twin study is an ongoing study of the etiology of learning disorders that has included nearly 6,000 participants since the study was first initiated (e.g., DeFries et al., 1997; McGrath et al., 2011; Olson et al., 2017; Peterson et al., 2017, 2021; Willcutt et al., 2019; Willcutt, Pennington, et al., 2010). In collaboration with administrators in over 20 Colorado school districts, parents of all twin pairs in each district were contacted and invited to complete a screening for learning difficulties (for a full description of recruitment procedures, see Willcutt et al., 2013, 2019). If either member of a twin pair exhibited significant learning difficulties, the pair was then invited to participate in the full study, along with a matched comparison sample of twins without learning or attentional difficulties. All twins then completed an extensive assessment that included a comprehensive battery of standardized measures of academic achievement in reading, math, writing, and spelling, and parents and teachers also completed measures of ADHD and internalizing and externalizing symptoms.

In addition to the primary cross-sectional data collection, a subsample of approximately 1,000 participants from the initial twin study returned for a follow-up assessment that was completed approximately 5 years after their initial participation (e.g., Wadsworth et al., 2007, 2015, 2016; Wakeman et al., 2023; Willcutt, Betjemann, Pennington, et al., 2007). The new analyses conducted for this chapter focus on the subsample of participants who completed the longitudinal follow-up study.

International Longitudinal Twin Study of Early Reading and Attention (ILTSERD)

The ILTSERD is a longitudinal twin study of the development of reading, math, and attention (e.g., Becker et al., 2018; Byrne et al., 2002; Leopold et al., 2016; Willcutt, Betjemann, Wadsworth, et al., 2007). An unselected sample of 928 twins completed measures of reading achievement and ADHD symptoms during the summer prior to the start of kindergarten and then again during the summer after the twins completed kindergarten, first grade, second grade, fourth grade, and ninth grade (measures of mathematics achievement were added as part of the ninth-grade assessment). A subset of the sample ($N = 742$) then recently completed an online survey of outcomes when they were approximately 25 years of age. The current chapter includes new analyses of these measures to begin to assess the impact of comorbidity between RD, MD, and ADHD on important developmental outcomes in emerging adulthood.

Prevalence of Comorbidity between SLD and Other Disorders

Comorbidity between RD, MD, and WD

The majority of studies of comorbidity among SLDs have examined comorbidity between RD and MD, and these studies consistently suggest that RD and MD co-occur in 30–70% of individuals with either disorder (e.g., Badian, 1999; Katusic et al., 2009; Landerl & Moll, 2010; Willcutt et al., 2013; Yoshimasu et al., 2011). While comorbidity between RD and MD is common no matter how each group is defined, recent results from the CLDRC suggest that the relative frequency of comorbidity may vary for different definitions of RD and MD (Willcutt, McGrath, et al., 2019). When RD was defined by a deficit in word reading, nearly half of the probands with RD also met criteria for MD, whether it was defined by a deficit in mathematics calculations (47%), mathematics fluency (50%), or word problems (51%). However, when RD was defined by a deficit in reading fluency, rates of comorbidity were significantly higher when MD was defined by a deficit in mathematics fluency (63%) than by a weakness in mathematics calculations (47%) or word problems (41%). The stronger association between deficits in fluency may potentially reflect the impact of slow processing speed across different aspects of academic fluency. In contrast, individuals with a deficit in reading comprehension were more likely to have a deficit in word problems (69%) versus calculations (49%) or mathematics fluency (38%), reflecting the importance of language comprehension for these academic skills. While these results should be interpreted with caution until they are replicated in an independent sample, these preliminary findings suggest that the frequency and implications of comorbidity between RD and MD may potentially differ as a function of the specific aspects of reading or mathematics difficulties that are used to define each SLD.

Difficulties in writing are also significantly correlated with weaknesses in both reading and mathematics (e.g., Woodcock et al., 2001). In comparison to studies of RD and MD, however, far fewer studies have examined comorbidity between WD and other SLDs, and virtually no studies have examined the overlap between MD and WD or among all three SLDs. To address this gap in the literature, new analyses were completed for this chapter to estimate the rates of comorbidity between RD, MD, and WD in the ongoing CLDRC twin study (Table 10.1).

Groups with RD, MD, and WD were defined by a cutoff score at the 10th percentile of the population on reading, math, and writing composite measures. Rates of comorbidity were significantly higher than expected by chance for RD and MD (44%), RD and WD (50–53%), and WD and MD (42–45%), and approximately 30% of individuals with WD, RD, or MD met criteria for *both* of the other SLDs. In contrast, only a minority of the individuals in each group met criteria for an SLD in that single academic domain alone (34–36% of cases with RD and WD and 42% of cases with MD). Taken together, these results illustrate the frequent comorbidity between RD, MD, and WD and underscore that few individuals meet criteria for a "specific" LD that is truly restricted to a single academic domain. Instead, comorbidity between SLDs appears to be the rule rather than the exception.

TABLE 10.1. Rates of Comorbidity between RD, MD, and WD in the Colorado Learning Disabilities Research Center Twin Study

		Rates of comorbidity with other SLDs				
Selected SLD	Total *N*	LD in selected domain only *N* (%)	Comorbid RD only *N* (%)	Comorbid MD only *N* (%)	Comorbid WD only *N* (%)	Comorbidity with both other SLDs *N* (%)
RD	62	21 (34%)	N/A	8 (13%)	23 (23%)	19 (31%)
MD	62	26 (42%)	8 (13%)	N/A	9 (15%)	19 (31%)
WD	65	23 (36%)	14 (22%)	9 (14%)	N/A	19 (29%)

Note. RD = reading disorder, MD = math disorder, WD = disorder of written expression.

Comorbidity between SLDs and Psychopathology

In addition to comorbidity with other LDs, results from the CLDRC and multiple other studies indicate that many individuals with RD or MD also meet criteria for at least one additional emotional or behavioral disorder (e.g., Badian, 1999; Goldston et al., 2007; Maughan et al., 2003; Sexton et al., 2012; Visser et al., 2020; Wakeman et al., 2023; White et al., 1992; Willcutt & Pennington, 2000b; Willcutt et al., 2013). Figure 10.1 summarizes results of the most recent analyses of the CLDRC twin sample that were completed for the current chapter to estimate rates of comorbidity in groups with RD-only, MD-only, both RD and MD, and neither RD nor MD (the sample with WD was too small to be included in these analyses).

The latest data from both the CLDRC (Figure 10.1) and other community samples indicate that ADHD is the most frequent comorbid psychological disorder in groups with RD or MD (e.g., Sexton et al., 2012; Visser et al., 2020; Willcutt et al., 2012, 2013; Willcut, McGrath, et al., 2019; Willcutt, Pennington, et al., 2010). Further, the results from the CLDRC clearly indicate that the rate of ADHD is significantly higher in the group with both RD and MD than in the group with either RD or MD alone.

The results in Figure 10.1 indicate that individuals with RD and MD are also at higher risk for externalizing disorders such as oppositional defiant disorder (ODD) and conduct disorder (CD). However, results from our group and several others suggest that associations between RD and these aspects of antisocial behavior may largely be restricted to the subset of individuals with comorbid ADHD (e.g., Frick et al., 1991; Maughan et al., 2003; Willcutt, McGrath, et al., 2019; Willcutt & Pennington, 2000b), and our initial results suggest that this pattern is similar for MD (Figure 10.1) (for a more detailed discussion, see Willcutt et al., 2013).

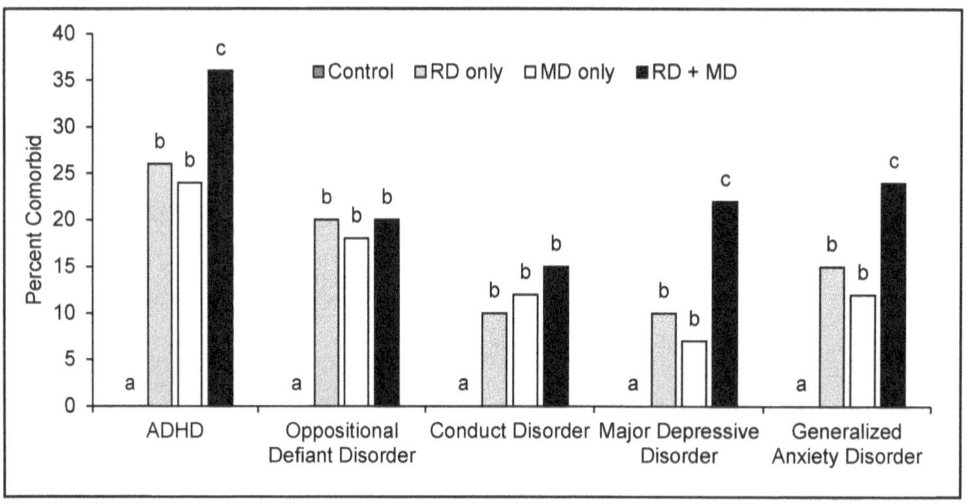

FIGURE 10.1. Rates of comorbid psychopathology in groups with and without RD and MD in the CLDRC twin sample. Bars with different letters indicate a significant difference between groups ($p < .05$).

Finally, RD and MD are each associated with higher rates of anxiety and depression (Daniel et al., 2006; Fortes et al., 2016; Goldston et al., 2007; Maughan et al., 2003; Wakeman et al., 2023; Willcutt & Pennington, 2000b), and rates of these internalizing disorders are highest in the group with both RD and MD (Figure 10.1). In contrast to the results for externalizing disorders, however, our results consistently indicate that both RD and MD are associated with significant elevations of anxiety and depression even after symptoms of ADHD are controlled.

Summary and Conclusions from Studies of the Prevalence of Comorbidity

The results summarized in this section indicate that RD, MD, and WD frequently co-occur with one another and that RD and MD are often comorbid with ADHD and a range of externalizing and internalizing disorders. While additional research is needed to assess rates of comorbidity in groups with WD and to clarify whether results differ in groups with RD or MD that are defined by measures beyond word reading and mathematics calculations, the existing literature clearly indicates that comorbidity is nearly ubiquitous and important to understand. The next section summarizes studies of the functional implications of comorbidity.

Functional Implications of Comorbidity between RD, MD, and ADHD

The studies reviewed in the previous section clearly demonstrate that comorbidity occurs more often than expected by chance between different SLDs and between these SLDs and other developmental psychopathologies. The next critical question is whether this comorbidity matters. We can begin to address this question by examining whether the presence of a comorbid disorder leads to different or greater impairment in functioning in comparison to individuals without the comorbid disorder. This section reviews studies that tested the impact of comorbidity on important aspects of functioning, including both short-term and long-term academic outcomes and a broader range of measures of social, adaptive, and global functioning. Because very few studies have used this approach to examine the impact of comorbidity with WD or internalizing and externalizing disorders, this section focuses on the functional implications of comorbidity between RD, MD, and ADHD.

Impact of Comorbidity on Academic Functioning and Outcomes

Cross-Sectional Analyses

Cross-sectional analyses in our samples and others consistently demonstrate that RD and MD are associated with significant impairment on virtually all measures of "real world" academic functioning, including lower grades, greater difficulty understanding assignments and completing daily academic responsibilities, and significantly higher rates of academic difficulties that were sufficiently severe to

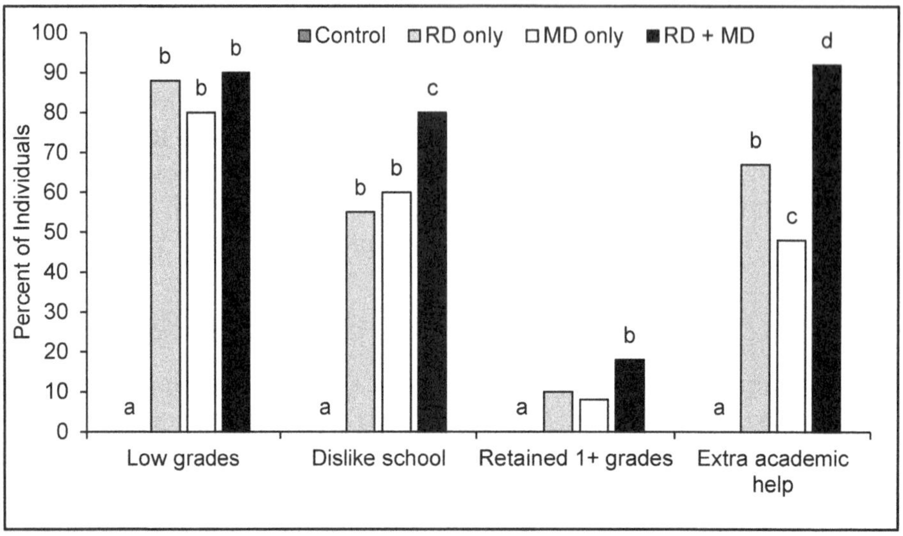

FIGURE 10.2. Academic functioning in groups with and without RD and MD in the CLDRC twin sample. Bars with different letters indicate a significant difference between groups ($p < .05$).

require extra support (Willcutt et al., 2013; Willcutt, McGrath, et al., 2019). Importantly, analyses of the latest data from the CLDRC twin study indicate that many of these academic difficulties are most pronounced in the group with both RD and MD (Figure 10.2). Individuals with RD-only, MD-only, and RD + MD were all very likely to receive low grades, dislike school, and receive extra academic help. However, the comorbid group was significantly more likely to dislike school and receive academic services than the groups with RD or MD alone, and only the group with comorbid RD + MD was more likely than the control group to have been retained at least one grade. Similarly, our earlier analyses indicated that RD or MD groups with comorbid ADHD were more likely than groups with RD or MD alone to exhibit significant academic impairment and be retained in school (Willcutt, McGrath, et al., 2019).

Longitudinal Analyses of Academic Outcomes

Longitudinal analyses of the CLDRC and ILTSERD samples further underscore the impact of comorbidity on more distal academic outcomes later in development. Results of a 5-year follow-up study of the CLDRC sample indicated that 65–70% of all individuals who met criteria for RD in late childhood continued to meet criteria for RD at the follow-up assessment in late adolescence (Willcutt, McGrath, et al., 2019). Importantly, the stability of RD was significantly higher among individuals who also met criteria for MD at the time of the initial assessment (82% continued to meet criteria for RD) than among individuals with RD alone (54% met criteria for RD at the follow-up assessment), and similar results were observed for comorbidity with ADHD (it was not yet possible to test the stability of MD alone because mathematics achievement measures were only recently added to our longitudinal follow-up battery in the CLDRC study). Further, in comparison to the groups with RD or MD alone at initial testing, the group with both RD and MD reported lower grades and greater difficulty keeping up with assignments and were significantly more likely to have received ongoing additional academic support.

The recently completed online follow-up assessment of the ILTSERD sample provides an important opportunity to extend the initial findings in the CLDRC by examining the impact of comorbidity between RD and MD on a broader range of academic outcomes over an even longer period of time. Groups with and without RD and MD were defined based on a score below the 10th percentile of the population on measures of reading and mathematics achievement in ninth grade, and participants then completed the follow-up survey approximately 10 years later when they were in their mid-20s. Initial results for academic outcomes are presented in Figure 10.3. Because the outcome measures are dimensional, the bars in the figure represent the effect size for the comparison between each SLD group and the comparison group without an SLD (Cohen's *d*; Cohen, 1988). An effect size of 1 indicates a difference of one standard deviation between the two groups, and Cohen recommends that effects of 0.3 or less be interpreted as "small" effect sizes, whereas effects between 0.4 and 0.6 are considered medium effect sizes, and effects greater than 0.7 are interpreted as large effects.

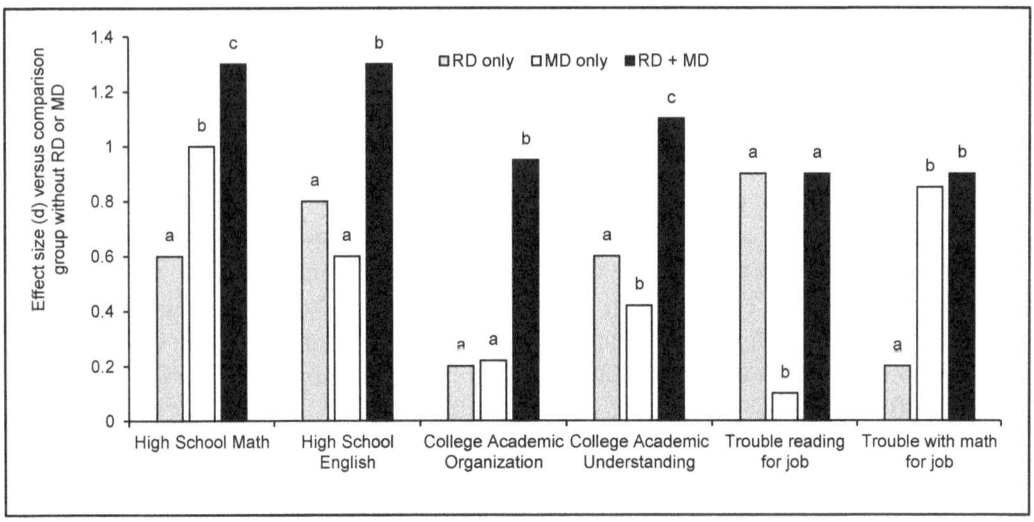

FIGURE 10.3. Academic and educational outcomes in early adulthood for groups that met criteria for RD or MD in ninth grade. Bars indicate the effect size (Cohen's *d*) for a comparison between the group with RD, MD, or RD + MD and a comparison group without RD or MD. Groups with RD, MD, and RD + MD were significantly different from the comparison group without RD or MD on all measures with the exception of "trouble reading for job" in the group with MD-only and "trouble with math for job" in the group with RD-only. Bars with different letters indicate a significant difference between groups with RD, MD, or RD + MD ($p < .05$).

The three groups who met criteria for RD or MD in ninth grade reported significant difficulties on nearly all measures of academic functioning later in development (Figure 10.3). Interestingly, the one exception to this pattern was observed on questions that asked about the specific impact of reading and mathematics demands in the workplace. Specifically, individuals with MD (with or without RD) reported significant difficulties when their job required them to use mathematics as part of their assigned duties, whereas individuals with RD alone did not report any difficulty when required to use mathematics for their job. In contrast, individuals with RD-only and RD + MD reported significant difficulties when duties for their job required them to read.

However, on measures of overall functioning, the group that met criteria for both RD and MD in ninth grade was significantly more impaired than the groups with RD or MD alone on measures of high school grades and college academic performance, with effect sizes that were large in magnitude on all four of these measures. These results add to a growing literature that underscores the impact of comorbidity on the immediate and long-term academic outcomes of individuals with SLDs.

Impact of Comorbidity on Functioning in Nonacademic Domains

Cross-Sectional Studies

While the association with long-term academic outcomes is one of the most critical questions regarding the developmental course of LDs, cross-sectional analyses by our group and others indicate that RD and MD are also associated with a broader range of difficulties that extend beyond academic functioning. For example, individuals with RD and MD experience more frequent peer rejection and social isolation, have greater difficulty completing daily responsibilities, and have lower overall functioning, and our initial results suggest that each of these difficulties is most pronounced in the group with both RD and MD (e.g., Willcutt et al., 2013; Willcutt, McGrath, et al., 2019). A similar pattern of results was observed in our earlier analyses of the impact of comorbid ADHD on the functioning of individuals with RD or MD (e.g., Willcutt, Betjemann, Pennington, et al., 2007; Willcutt et al., 2013).

Longitudinal Outcomes

New analyses were also completed in the ILTSERD sample to examine the association between RD and MD and a broad range of development outcomes in early adulthood (Figure 10.4). In comparison to individuals without RD or MD, individuals who met the criteria for RD or MD in ninth grade reported greater impairment in early adulthood in nearly all domains of functioning. Both RD and MD are associated with lower ratings of life satisfaction and higher levels of stress and anxiety, greater difficulties in social relationships with family and friends, and specific impairment in work performance, driving, and money management. However,

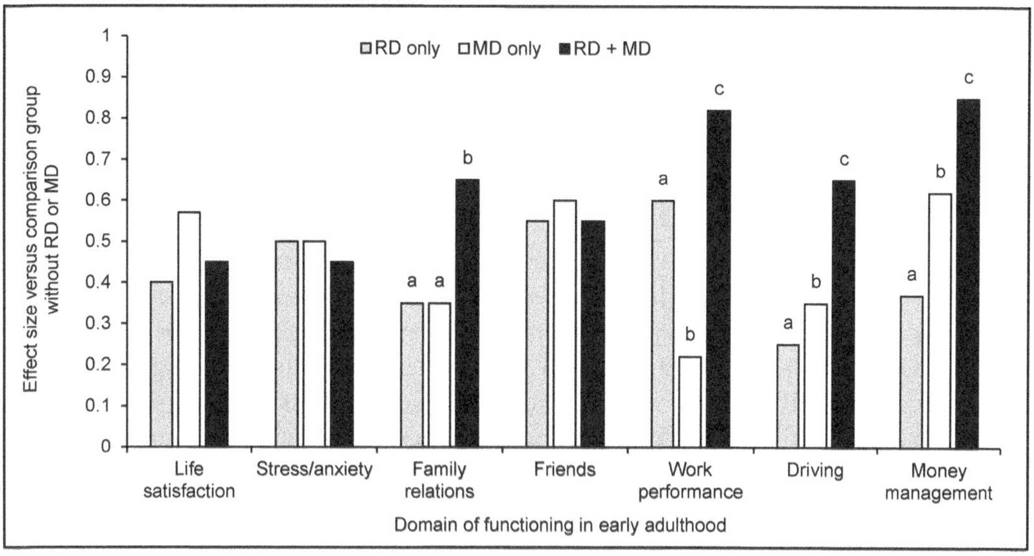

FIGURE 10.4. Functional outcomes in early adulthood for groups that met criteria for RD or MD in ninth grade. Bars indicate the effect size (Cohen's *d*) for a comparison between the group with RD, MD, or RD + MD and a comparison group without RD or MD. Groups with RD, MD, and RD + MD were significantly different from the comparison group without RD or MD on all measures with the exception of work performance in the group with MD only. Bars with different letters indicate a significant difference between groups with RD, MD, or RD + MD ($p < .05$).

it is also important to point out that most of these effects are medium in magnitude, in contrast to the very large effect sizes observed for academic outcomes.

Although both RD and MD were associated with less positive outcomes in most domains, several interesting and potentially important differences emerged in the functional outcomes of the groups. Specifically, individuals with RD in childhood were more likely than those with MD to report difficulties in work performance, whereas MD was more strongly associated with difficulties with driving and money management. Finally, most relevant to the current chapter, the group with comorbid RD + MD exhibited greater impairment than the groups with RD or MD alone on measures of social relationships with family members, work performance, driving, and money management. Individuals with RD + MD were also most likely to be fired from a job or to drop out of college before completing a degree.

Summary and Conclusions from Studies of the Functional Impact of Comorbidity

Both cross-sectional and longitudinal studies clearly underscore the short-term and long-term impact of comorbidity between RD and MD. Similarly, while additional longitudinal research is needed, initial studies suggest that individuals with RD or

MD who also meet criteria for ADHD exhibit greater impairment in a range of important functional domains. The next section summarizes results of studies that have begun to test why these comorbidities may occur.

Etiology of Comorbidity between RD, MD, and ADHD

The results summarized in the previous sections clearly underscore the frequency and importance of comorbidity, but these findings do not explain why comorbidity occurs. Over 20 different hypotheses have been proposed as competing theoretical explanations for the comorbidity between developmental disorders (e.g., Neale & Kendler, 1995; Rhee et al., 2005). Due to space constraints, this chapter focuses on the theoretical models that have received the strongest support from previous studies. As in previous sections, I focus primarily on the etiology of comorbidity between RD and MD but also describe studies that included measures of ADHD or other psychopathologies when these are available.

Artifactual Explanations of Comorbidity

As a first step toward understanding the etiology of comorbidity, it is essential to first test whether comorbidity is observed in all samples or if it may simply be an artifact of a biased sampling procedure or measurement problem. Therefore, the first part of this section summarizes the results of studies that tested and ruled out several different artifactual explanations for comorbidity between RD, MD, and ADHD.

Clinic Sampling Bias

Many influential early studies of comorbidity between RD, MD, and ADHD used samples recruited through LD or ADHD assessment clinics (e.g., Semrud-Clikeman et al., 1992), leaving open the possibility that comorbidity might only be observed in more severely affected samples that are referred for clinical assessment and intervention. However, subsequent analyses by our group and others consistently showed that the rates of comorbidity between RD, MD, and ADHD are similar in community samples and samples recruited through clinics, providing strong evidence that the elevated rates of comorbidity between RD, MD, and ADHD do not simply reflect clinic sampling bias (e.g., Badian, 1999; Bauermeister et al., 2005; Knopik et al., 1997; Kovas et al., 2007; Landerl & Moll, 2010; Sexton et al., 2012; Visser et al., 2020; Willcutt, Betjemann, et al., 2010; Willcutt & Pennington, 2000a).

Shared Method Variance

Another way that artifactual comorbidity could occur is if the same method is used to assess both disorders, and something about that method of assessment impacts a child's performance across domains (Angold et al., 1999). RD and MD could potentially co-occur due to shared method variance because they are often defined by scores on reading and mathematics subtests from the same achievement test battery. However, significant covariance has also been reported between parent and teacher ratings of reading or mathematics difficulties and scores on standardized tests of the other domain (e.g., Kovas et al., 2005; Willcutt et al., 2011), suggesting that the significant association between reading and mathematics difficulties is robust across different methods of assessment and is not simply an artifact of the use of similar academic achievement measures to assess RD and MD. Further, because RD and MD are assessed by psychometric achievement tests, whereas ADHD is assessed by behavioral ratings, comorbidity between SLDs and ADHD cannot be explained by shared method variance.

Common Etiology Models as Explanations for Comorbidity between RD, MD, and ADHD

As noted earlier, at least 20 different theoretical models have been proposed to account for true comorbidity between complex disorders (Angold et al., 1999; Neale & Kendler, 1995; Rhee et al., 2005), and a number of these hypotheses have been tested as explanations for comorbidity of RD, MD, and ADHD. Due to space constraints, this section focuses on the *common etiology model*, the theoretical model that has received the most consistent support in the studies that have been completed to date (for more detailed reviews, see Willcutt, 2014, 2019a). This model suggests that two disorders co-occur more often than expected by chance due to shared genetic or environmental influences that increase risk for both disorders, whereas the disorders are distinguished by other etiological influences that are specific to each disorder.

The optimal methods to test the common etiology model are etiologically informative designs such as twin and molecular genetic studies. Twin studies compare pairs of identical (monozygotic, or MZ) versus fraternal (dizygotic, or DZ) twins to estimate the relative importance of genetic and environmental influences on individual differences or group deficits in a trait. Because MZ twins share all of their genes, whereas DZ twins share half of their segregating genes on average, this comparison is used to estimate the extent to which individual differences or extreme scores are due to genetic or environmental influences (Plomin et al., 2013). *Heritability* is defined as the proportion of the total phenotypic variance in a trait that is attributable to genetic influences. *Shared environmental influences* are environmental factors that increase the similarity of individuals within a family in comparison to unrelated individuals in the population. These effects may potentially include environmental influences within the home or any other shared experiences, such as mutual friends or shared teachers. In contrast, *nonshared environmental influences* specifically affect only one member of a twin pair or affect the two twins differently. Examples of nonshared environmental risk factors could include a head injury or other accident, a traumatic event, or exposure to physical or sexual abuse (if the other twin was not similarly exposed).

Our review of all published twin studies of reading, mathematics, and ADHD indicated that heritability estimates were moderate to high for both individual differences and group deficits on these measures (e.g., Willcutt, 2014; Willcutt, Pennington, et al., 2010). These reviews indicated that approximately 50–70% of the risk for MD, 60–70% of the risk for RD, and 70–75% of the risk for ADHD is explained by genetic influences. Shared environmental influences account for an additional 10–15% of the variance in reading and mathematics but play a minimal role in the etiology of ADHD symptoms. Nonshared environmental influences and measurement errors typically explain 20–25% of the risk for all three disorders.

Our group and others then extended these univariate results to examine the etiology of covariance between ADHD, math, and reading (Ebejer et al., 2010; Greven et al., 2011, 2012; Hart et al., 2010; Paloyelis et al., 2010; Willcutt, 2014, 2019b; Willcutt, Betjemann, et al., 2010; Willcutt, Betjemann, Wadsworth, et al., 2007). These studies indicate that common genetic influences explain the majority of the comorbidity between RD, MD, and ADHD, with the important caveat that few studies have examined measures of reading and mathematics beyond word decoding and mathematics calculations.

Neuropsychological and Neuroimaging Approaches

Until recently, neuropsychological models of RD, MD, ADHD, and other developmental disorders often proposed that a single primary neurocognitive deficit was necessary and sufficient to explain all of the symptoms of the disorder. However, data from our group and a number of other studies have consistently challenged the validity of simple single-deficit models, most importantly by demonstrating that nearly all disorders are associated with multiple neuropsychological weaknesses (see Pennington, 2006, for a comprehensive review and discussion).

These converging results have precipitated a significant reconceptualization of neuropsychological models of SLDs and other developmental disorders. Rather than attempting to identify a single neuropsychological weakness that is a necessary and sufficient cause of each disorder, more recent theoretical models from our group and others have explicitly hypothesized that RD, MD, ADHD, and other developmental disorders arise from the additive and interactive effects of multiple neuropsychological weaknesses (e.g., Geary, 2010; McGrath et al., 2011; Pennington et al., 2012; Peterson et al., 2017; Willcutt, 2015; Willcutt, Betjemann, et al., 2010; Willcutt et al., 2008). For example, while weakness in phonological processing is clearly the strongest neuropsychological correlate of reading difficulties in our sample and the overall literature (e.g., Wagner, 1986; Willcutt et al., 2013), not all children with RD have phonological weaknesses (Pennington et al., 2012), and RD is also independently associated with weaknesses in verbal reasoning, naming speed, and processing speed (e.g., McGrath et al., 2011; Peterson et al., 2017; Willcutt, Betjemann, et al., 2010). Similarly, MD is associated with weaknesses in number sense, phonological processing, executive functions, verbal reasoning, and processing speed in our sample and others, and ADHD is independently associated with weaknesses in processing speed, sustained attention, and aspects of executive functions that include response inhibition and working memory (e.g., McGrath et al., 2011; Peterson et al., 2017; Willcutt, 2015; Willcutt et al., 2005).

In addition to providing a more comprehensive explanation of each individual disorder, these multiple deficit models provide a potentially compelling theoretical framework to understand the neurocognitive mechanisms of the significant comorbidity between RD, MD, and ADHD. Rather than qualitatively distinct neuropsychological weaknesses, SLDs and other related disorders may be distinguished by quantitative differences in the specific profile or severity of neuropsychological weaknesses across multiple domains that are impaired to some extent in most or all disorders. For example, it is possible that shared weaknesses in processing speed or verbal working memory may be domain-general risk factors that increase risk for RD, MD, ADHD, and potentially other disorders, whereas other neurocognitive weaknesses distinguish between the disorders.

Summary and Conclusions from Studies of the Etiology of Comorbidity

Analyses of twins consistently indicate that comorbidity between RD, MD, and ADHD is primarily explained by shared genetic influences, whereas other genetic and environmental influences are uniquely associated with each disorder. Studies that incorporated neuropsychological measures suggest that these shared genetic influences may be associated with weaknesses in cognitive processing speed or executive functions that contribute to comorbidity between these SLDs and ADHD.

Conclusions and Future Directions for Studies of Comorbidity and LDs

Clinical Implications

Diagnostic Formulation

The existing literature strongly supports a model in which RD, MD, and ADHD are distinct disorders that frequently co-occur. Consistent with this overarching framework, each disorder is independently associated with important aspects of functional impairment in a range of domains, and their combined impact often leads to the greatest impairment among individuals with comorbidity. Therefore, rather than attempting to determine which disorder is "primary" when RD, MD, or ADHD co-occur in the same individual, clinicians should conceptualize both conditions as primary disorders that may each benefit from targeted intervention.

Clinical Assessment Procedures

The high prevalence of comorbidity described in this chapter suggests that comprehensive assessments of SLDs should always assess all domains of academic functioning, along with symptoms of ADHD and other psychopathology. Similarly, assessments of ADHD should at least screen for difficulties in reading, math, and writing. Any comorbidities that are observed should then be considered carefully when developing recommendations for interventions or accommodations.

Having said that, it is also important to recognize that a key barrier to this recommendation is the time required to complete a full battery of individually administered measures of academic achievement or to complete interviews or obtain comprehensive ratings of symptoms of ADHD and other psychopathology from parents and teachers. Therefore, while these comprehensive assessment approaches provide the most valid assessment of SLDs, ADHD, and related socioemotional and behavioral difficulties, these may not be feasible in some research or clinical settings, and more streamlined procedures may be needed.

If time constraints do not allow a clinician to complete a full diagnostic interview with parents and teachers, a number of more abbreviated instruments can be used to at least identify individuals who may need a referral for a more comprehensive psychological evaluation. Similarly, if it is not feasible to administer a full academic achievement battery in an assessment of ADHD, it may be possible to at least include a brief screening measure to identify individuals who may need a referral for a more comprehensive evaluation of academic functioning. Nearly all standardized achievement tests include a very brief (3–5 minutes) measure of single-word reading or mathematics calculations (and often writing and spelling) that can be used effectively to screen for significant learning difficulties. Alternatively, we have developed and validated the freely available Colorado Learning Difficulties Questionnaire, a 20-item parent-report rating scale that was specifically designed as a screening measure to identify individuals who may require additional academic assessment (Willcutt et al., 2011).

Intervention

Despite the voluminous literature describing treatment of RD, MD, and ADHD in isolation, surprisingly few intervention studies of either disorder have examined the impact of comorbidity. A study of comorbidity between RD and MD suggested that students with RD respond similarly to reading interventions whether or not they also meet criteria for MD (Fuchs et al., 2013), whereas the group with RD + MD responded differently than the group with MD alone (Fuchs et al., 2013). Similarly, an initial study of RD and ADHD suggested that treatment of reading difficulties may not be as effective for children with concurrent attentional difficulties (Rabiner & Malone, 2004), but a second demonstrated that children with both RD and ADHD benefited from treatments that specifically targeted both reading and ADHD (Denton et al., 2020). Overall, much more work is needed to fill the important gap in the literature on the potential impact of comorbidity on intervention outcomes.

Implications of Comorbidity for the Developmental Stability and Outcomes of SLDs

Consistent with the procedures used in most previous studies, RD and MD were defined in our studies by deficits in measures of word reading and mathematics calculations. Existing data indicate that deficits in these domains and in symptoms of ADHD are stable over time and associated with a range of negative outcomes, with the worst outcomes often occurring for individuals with more than one of these disorders. In contrast, little is known about the stability of deficits in more complex aspects of reading or mathematics, such as reading comprehension or word problems, nor the relation between these deficits and difficulties with writing or symptoms of ADHD. Incorporation of these measures in future studies will provide important new information about the developmental course and prognosis of SLDs, including aspects of impairment due to difficulties in higher-order academic skills that may only become apparent later in development. For example, difficulties in writing or reading comprehension may predict greater academic impairment later in development due to the increased demands that students encounter in high school and postsecondary education.

Future Directions for Studies of Comorbidity between SLDs and ADHD

Early Shared Risk Factors

Longitudinal twin studies of preschool samples provide important verification that early reading weaknesses and inattention symptoms are significantly correlated prior to the beginning of formal reading instruction (Willcutt, Betjemann, Wadsworth, et al., 2007). Similarly, while early skills related to mathematics and reading are correlated from an early age (e.g., Purpura et al., 2011), few longitudinal studies to date have prospectively examined early risk factors prior to the beginning of school that may play a role in the development of comorbidity between RD, MD, and ADHD.

Understanding Shared Cognitive Weaknesses in RD, MD, and ADHD

The neuropsychological studies discussed in this chapter clearly suggest that RD, MD, and ADHD are associated with slow processing speed on standard psychometric measures. However, interpretation of these results is not always straightforward, as slow processing speed could potentially be associated with RD, MD, and ADHD for different reasons. For example, this pattern could reflect general slow processing across all trials in groups with RD, MD, or other learning disabilities but intermittent lapses in attention on a subset of trials in groups with ADHD. Because the coarse measures of processing speed used in previous studies are not sensitive to these different possibilities, future research is needed using more sensitive measures of trial-level processing efficiency or alternative methodologies such as event-related potentials or functional neuroimaging.

Neuroimaging

Finally, we recently completed a structural and functional neuroimaging study of a subsample of CLDRC participants with RD-only, MD-only, both RD and MD, and neither disorder, providing the largest sample to date for a neuroimaging study of RD and MD. This study will allow us to test for the first time which neural markers are uniquely associated with reading and math and which neural correlates may help to explain the shared variance that underlies comorbidity between RD and MD.

Conclusions

This chapter provided an overview of current knowledge regarding the frequency, implications, and etiology of comorbidity between RD, MD, ADHD, and other developmental disorders. In comparison to individuals with each disorder alone, individuals with more than one of these disorders exhibit increased functional impairment and have less positive developmental outcomes. Etiologically informative analyses indicate that nearly all of the phenotypic covariance between RD, MD, and ADHD is due to shared genetic influences that may be associated with slower and more variable cognitive processing speed and weaknesses in some aspects of executive functions. Future research is needed to continue to examine the potential implications of comorbidity for interventions for SLDs, ADHD, and other related disorders.

ACKNOWLEDGMENTS

Primary funding for the Colorado Learning Disabilities Research Center was provided by grant P50 HD27802 from the *Eunice Kennedy Shriver* National Institute of Child Health and Human Development. The content is solely the responsibility of the authors and does not necessarily reflect the official views of the *Eunice Kennedy Shriver* National Institute of Child Health and Human Development or the National Institutes of Health.

REFERENCES

American Psychiatric Association. (2013). *Diagnostic and statistical manual of mental disorders* (5th ed.). Author.

Angold, A., Costello, E. J., & Erkanli, A. (1999). Comorbidity. *Journal of Child Psychology and Psychiatry and Allied Disciplines, 40*, 57–87.

Badian, N. A. (1999). Persistent arithmetic, reading, or arithmetic and reading disability. *Annals of Dyslexia, 49*, 45–70.

Bauermeister, J. J., Matos, M., Reina, G., Salas, C. C., Martinez, J. V., Cumba, E., & Barkley, R. A. (2005). Comparison of the DSM-IV combined and inattentive types of ADHD in a school-based sample of Latino/Hispanic children. *Journal of Child Psychology and Psychiatry, 46*, 166–179.

Becker, S. P., Burns, G. L., Leopold, D. R., Olson, R. K., & Willcutt, E. G. (2018). Differential impact of trait sluggish cognitive tempo and ADHD inattention in early childhood on adolescent functioning. *Journal of Child Psychology and Psychiatry, 59*, 1094–1104.

Byrne, B., Delaland, C., Fielding-Barnsley, R., Quain, P., Samuelsson, S., Hoien, T., et al. (2002). Longitudinal twin study of early reading development in three countries: Preliminary results. *Annals of Dyslexia, 52*, 49–73.

Cohen, J. (1988). *Statistical power analyses for the behavioral sciences.* Erlbaum.

Daniel, S. S., Walsh, A. K., Goldston, D. B., Arnold, E. M., Reboussin, B. A., & Wood, F. B. (2006). Suicidality, school dropout, and reading problems among adolescents. *Journal of Learning Disabilities, 39*, 507–514.

DeFries, J. C., Filipek, P. A., Fulker, D. W., Olson, R. K., Pennington, B. F., Smith, S. D., & Wise, B. W. (1997). Colorado Learning Disabilities Research Center. *Learning Disabilities: A Multidisciplinary Journal, 8*, 7–19.

Denton, C. A., Tamm, L., Schatschneider, C., & Epstein, J. N. (2020). The effects of ADHD treatment and reading intervention on the fluency and comprehension of children with ADHD and word reading difficulties: A randomized clinical trial. *Scientific Studies of Reading, 24*, 72–89.

Ebejer, J. L., Coventry, W. L., Byrne, B., Willcutt, E. G., Olson, R. K., Corley, R., & Samuelsson, S. (2010). Genetic and environmental influences on inattention, hyperactivity-impulsivity, and reading: Kindergarten to grade 2. *Scientific Studies of Reading, 14*, 293–316.

Fortes, I. S., Paula, C. S., Oliveira, M. C., Bordin, I. A., de Jesus Mari, J., & Rohde, L. A. (2016). A cross-sectional study to assess the prevalence of DSM-5 specific learning disorders in representative school samples from the second to sixth grade in Brazil. *European Child and Adolescent Psychiatry, 25*, 195–207.

Frick, P. J., Kamphaus, R. W., Lahey, B. B., Loeber, R., Christ, M. A., Hart, E. L., & Tannenbaum, L. E. (1991). Academic underachievement and the disruptive behavior disorders. *Journal of Consulting and Clinical Psychology, 59*, 289–294.

Fuchs, L. S., Fuchs, D., & Compton, D. L. (2013). Intervention effects for students with comorbid forms of learning disability: Understanding the needs of nonresponders. *Journal of Learning Disabilities, 46*, 534–548.

Geary, D. C. (2010). Mathematical disabilities: Reflections on cognitive, neuropsychological, and genetic components. *Learning and Individual Differences, 20*, 130–133.

Goldston, D. B., Walsh, A., Mayfield, A. E., Reboussin, B., Sergent, D. S., Erkanli, A., et al. (2007). Reading problems, psychiatric disorders, and functional impairment from mid- to late adolescence. *Journal of the American Academy of Child and Adolescent Psychiatry, 46*, 25–32.

Greven, C. U., Harlaar, N., Dale, P., & Plomin, R. (2011). Genetic overlap between attention-deficit hyperactivity disorder and reading is largely driven by inattentiveness rather than by hyperactivity-impulsivity. *Journal of the Canadian Academy of Child and Adolescent Psychiatry, 20*, 6–14.

Greven, C. U., Rijsdisjk, F. V., Asherson, P., & Plomin, R. (2012). A longitudinal twin study of associations between ADHD symptoms and reading. *Journal of Child Psychology and Psychiatry, 53*, 234–242.

Hart, S. A., Petrill, S. A., Willcutt, E. G., Thompson, L. A., Schatschneider, C., Deater-Deckard, K., & Cutting, L. E. (2010). Exploring how ADHD symptoms are related to reading and mathematics performance: General genes, general environments. *Psychological Science, 21*, 1708–1715.

Katusic, S. K., Colligan, R. C., Weaver, A. L., & Barbaresi, W. J. (2009). The forgotten learning disability: Epidemiology of written-language disorder in a population-based birth cohort (1976–1982), Rochester, Minnesota. *Pediatrics, 125*, 1306–1313.

Knopik, V. S., Alarcon, M., & DeFries, J. C. (1997). Comorbidity of mathematics and reading deficits: evidence for a genetic etiology. *Behavior Genetics, 27*, 447–453.

Kovas, Y., Harlaar, N., Petrill, S. A., & Plomin, R. (2005). "Generalist genes" and mathematics in 7-year-old twins. *Intelligence, 33*, 473–489.

Kovas, Y., Haworth, C. M., Harlaar, N., Petrill, S. A., Dale, P. S., & Plomin, R. (2007). Overlap and specificity of genetic and environmental influences on mathematics and reading disability in 10-year-old twins. *Journal of Child Psychology and Psychiatry, 48*, 914–922.

Landerl, K., & Moll, K. (2010). Comorbidity of learning disorders: prevalence and familial transmission. *Journal of Child Psychology and Psychiatry, 51*, 287–294.

Leopold, D. R., Christopher, M. E., Burns, G. L., Becker, S. P., Olson, R. K., & Willcutt, E. G.

(2016). Attention-deficit/hyperactivity disorder and sluggish cognitive tempo throughout childhood: temporal invariance and stability from preschool through ninth grade. *Journal of Child Psychology and Psychiatry, 57*, 1066–1074.

Maughan, B., Rowe, R., Loeber, R., & Stouthamer-Loeber, M. (2003). Reading problems and depressed mood. *Journal of Abnormal Child Psychology, 31*, 219–229.

McGrath, L. M., Pennington, B. F., Shanahan, M. A., Santerre-Lemmon, L. E., Barnard, H. D., Willcutt, E. G., et al. (2011). A multiple deficit model of reading disability and attention-deficit/hyperactivity disorder: Searching for shared cognitive deficits. *Journal of Child Psychology and Psychiatry, 52*, 547–557.

Neale, M. C., & Kendler, K. S. (1995). Models of comorbidity for multifactorial disorders. *American Journal of Human Genetics, 57*, 935–953.

Olson, R. K., Hulslander, J., Christopher, M., Keenan, J. M., Wadsworth, S. J., Willcutt, E. G., et al. (2013). Genetic and environmental influences on writing and their relations to language and reading. *Annals of Dyslexia, 63*(1), 25–43.

Olson, R. K., Keenan, J. M., Byrne, B., & Samuelsson, S. (2017). Genetic and environmental influences on the development of reading and related skills. In K. Cain, D. Compton, & R. Parilla (Eds.), *Theories of reading development* (pp. 33–53): John Benjamins Publishing Co.

Paloyelis, Y., Rijsdijk, F., Wood, A. C., Asherson, P., & Kuntsi, J. (2010). The genetic association between ADHD symptoms and reading difficulties: The role of inattentiveness and IQ. *Journal of Abnormal Child Psychology, 38*, 1083–1095.

Pennington, B. F. (2006). From single to multiple deficit models of developmental disorders. *Cognition, 101*, 385–413.

Pennington, B. F., Santerre-Lemmon, L., Rosenberg, J., MacDonald, B., Boada, R., Friend, A., et al. (2012). Individual prediction of dyslexia by single versus multiple deficit models. *Journal of Abnormal Psychology, 121*, 212–224.

Peterson, R. L., Boada, R., McGrath, L., Willcutt, E. G., Olson, R. K., & Pennington, B. F. (2017). Cognitive prediction of reading, math, and attention: Shared and unique influences. *Journal of Learning Disabilities, 50*, 408–421.

Peterson, R. L., McGrath, L. M., Willcutt, E. G., Keenan, J. M., Olson, R. K., & Pennington, B. F. (2021). How specific are learning disabilities? *Journal of Learning Disabilities*, 22219420982981.

Plomin, P., DeFries, J. C., Knopik, V. S., & Neiderhiser, J. M. (2013). *Behavioral genetics* (6th ed.). Worth.

Purpura, D., Hume, L., Sims, D., & Lonigan, C. (2011). Early literacy and early numeracy: The value of including early literacy skills in the prediction of numeracy development. *Journal of Experimental Child Psychology, 110*, 647–658.

Rabiner, D. L., & Malone, P. S. (2004). The impact of tutoring on early reading achievement for children with and without attention problems. *Journal of Abnormal Child Psychology, 32*, 273–284.

Rhee, S. H., Hewitt, J. K., Corley, R. P., Willcutt, E. G., & Pennington, B. F. (2005). Testing hypotheses regarding the causes of comorbidity: Examining the underlying deficits of comorbid disorders. *Journal of Abnormal Psychology, 114*, 346–362.

Semrud-Clikeman, M., Biederman, J., Sprich-Buckminster, S., Lehman, B. K., Faraone, S. V., & Norman, D. (1992). Comorbidity between ADDH and learning disability: A review and report in a clinically referred sample. *Journal of the American Academy of Child and Adolescent Psychiatry, 31*, 439–448.

Sexton, C. C., Gelhorn, H. L., Bell, J. A., & Classi, P. M. (2012). The co-occurrence of reading disorder and ADHD: Epidemiology, treatment, psychosocial impact, and economic burden. *Journal of Learning Disabilities, 45*, 538–564.

Visser, L., Kalmar, J., Linkersdorfer, J., Gorgen, R., Rothe, J., Hasselhorn, M., & Schulte-Korne, G. (2020). Comorbidities between specific learning disorders and psychopathology in elementary school children in Germany. *Frontiers in Psychiatry, 11*, 292.

Wadsworth, S. J., DeFries, J. C., Olson, R. K., & Willcutt, E. G. (2007). Colorado longitudinal twin study of reading disability. *Annals of Dyslexia, 57*, 139–160.

Wadsworth, S. J., DeFries, J. C., Willcutt, E. G., Pennington, B. F., & Olson, R. K. (2015). The Colorado longitudinal twin study of reading difficulties and ADHD: Etiologies of comorbidity and stability. *Journal of Twin Research and Human Genetics, 18*, 755–761.

Wadsworth, S. J., DeFries, J. C., Willcutt, E. G., Pennington, B. F., & Olson, R. K. (2016). Genetic etiologies of comorbidity and stability for reading difficulties and ADHD: A replication study. *Twin Research and Human Genetics, 19*, 647–651.

Wagner, R. K. (1986). Phonological processing abilities and reading: Implications for disabled readers. *Journal of Learning Disabilities, 19*, 623–630.

Wakeman, H. N., Wadsworth, S. J., Olson, R. K., DeFries, J. C., Pennington, B. F., & Willcutt, E. G. (2023). Mathematics difficulties and psychopathology in school-aged children. *Journal of Learning Disabilities, 56*(2), 116–131.

Waschbusch, D. A. (2002). A meta-analytic examination of comorbid hyperactive-impulsive-attention problems and conduct problems. *Psychological Bulletin, 128*, 118–150.

White, J. L., Moffitt, T. E., & Silva, P. A. (1992). Neuropsychological and socio-emotional correlates of specific-arithmetic disability. *Archives of Clinical Neuropsychology, 7*, 1–16.

Willcutt, E. G. (2014). Using behavior genetic methods to understand the etiology of comorbidity. In S. Rhee & A. Ronald (Eds.), *Behavior genetics of psychopathology* (pp. 231–252). Springer.

Willcutt, E. G. (2015). Theories of ADHD. In R. Barkley (Ed.), *Attention deficit hyperactivity disorder: A clinical handbook* (4th ed., pp. 391–404). Guilford Press.

Willcutt, E. G. (2019a). Behavior and molecular genetic approaches to comorbidity. *Current Developmental Disorders Reports, 6*, 31–36.

Willcutt, E. G. (2019b). The etiology of ADHD in adolescents. In S. A. Becker (Ed.), *ADHD in adolescents: Development, assessment, and treatment* (pp. 36–55). Guilford Press.

Willcutt, E. G., Betjemann, R. S., McGrath, L. M., Chhabildas, N. A., Olson, R. K., DeFries, J. C., & Pennington, B. F. (2010). Etiology and neuropsychology of comorbidity between RD and ADHD: The case for multiple-deficit models. *Cortex, 46*, 1345–1361.

Willcutt, E. G., Betjemann, R. S., Pennington, B. F., Olson, R. K., DeFries, J. C., & Wadsworth, S. J. (2007). Longitudinal study of reading disability and attention-deficit/hyperactivity disorder: Implications for education. *Mind, Brain, and Education, 4*, 181–192.

Willcutt, E. G., Betjemann, R. S., Wadsworth, S. J., Samuelsson, S., Corley, R., DeFries, J. C., et al. (2007). Preschool twin study of the relation between attention-deficit/hyperactivity disorder and prereading skills. *Reading and Writing, 20*, 103–125.

Willcutt, E. G., Boada, R., Riddle, M. W., Chhabildas, N., DeFries, J. C., & Pennington, B. F. (2011). Colorado Learning Difficulties Questionnaire: Validation of a parent-report screening measure. *Psychological Assessment, 23*, 778–791.

Willcutt, E. G., Doyle, A. E., Nigg, J. T., Faraone, S. V., & Pennington, B. F. (2005). Validity of the executive function theory of attention-deficit/hyperactivity disorder: A meta-analytic review. *Biological Psychiatry, 57*, 1336–1346.

Willcutt, E. G., McGrath, L. M., Pennington, B. F., Keenan, J. M., DeFries, J. C., Olson, R. K., & Wadsworth, S. J. (2019). Understanding comorbidity between specific learning disabilities. *New Directions in Child and Adolescent Development, 165*, 91–109.

Willcutt, E. G., Nigg, J. T., Pennington, B. F., Solanto, M. V., Rohde, L. A., Tannock, R., et al. (2012). Validity of DSM-IV attention-deficit/hyperactivity disorder dimensions and subtypes. *Journal of Abnormal Psychology, 121*, 991–1010.

Willcutt, E. G., & Pennington, B. F. (2000a). Comorbidity of reading disability and attention-deficit/hyperactivity disorder: Differences by gender and subtype. *Journal of Learning Disabilities, 33*, 179–191.

Willcutt, E. G., & Pennington, B. F. (2000b). Psychiatric comorbidity in children and adolescents with reading disability. *Journal of Child Psychology and Psychiatry, 41*, 1039–1048.

Willcutt, E. G., Pennington, B. F., Duncan, L., Smith, S. D., Keenan, J. M., Wadsworth, S. J.,

& DeFries, J. C. (2010). Understanding the complex etiology of developmental disorders: Behavioral and molecular genetic approaches. *Journal of Developmental and Behavioral Pediatrics, 31*, 533–544.

Willcutt, E. G., Petrill, S. A., Wu, S., Boada, R., DeFries, J. C., Olson, R. K., & Pennington, B. F. (2013). Implications of comorbidity between reading and math disability: Neuropsychological and functional impairment. *Journal of Learning Disabilities, 46*, 500–516.

Willcutt, E. G., Sonuga-Barke, E. J. S., Nigg, J. T., & Sergeant, J. A. (2008). Recent developments in neuropsychological models of childhood disorders. *Advances in Biological Psychiatry, 24*, 195–226.

Woodcock, R. W., McGrew, K. S., & Mather, N. (2001). *Woodcock–Johnson III Tests of Achievement.* Riverside.

World Health Organization. (1992). *The ICD-10 classification of mental and behavioural disorders: Clinical descriptions and diagnostic guidelines.* Author.

Yoshimasu, K., Barbaresi, W. J., Colligan, R. C., Killian, J. M., Voigt, R. G., Weaver, A. L., & Katusic, S. K. (2011). Written-language disorder among children with and without ADHD in a population-based birth cohort. *Pediatrics, 128*, e605–e612.

PART II

INSTRUCTIONAL INTERVENTIONS

The eight chapters in Part II are focused on literacy, mathematics, and interventions in other content areas. In Chapter 11, "Effective Instruction and Intervention for Word-Level Reading for Students with and at Risk for Learning Disabilities," Al Otaiba, Russell Freudenthal, and Zaru first explore theoretical frameworks that explain how proficient reading develops, such as the Simple View of Reading (SVR) and Ehri's multiple-phase developmental trajectory. These frameworks show the interplay between decoding, phonemic awareness, and linguistic comprehension in reading proficiency. The authors also review findings from various studies and meta-analyses, revealing the effectiveness of early, explicit, and systematic reading interventions. These interventions often combine code-focused skills, like phonemic awareness and phonics, with meaning-focused skills, like vocabulary and comprehension. The authors also note the positive impact of writing and spelling instruction on reading skills.

In discussing implications for research and practice, the authors highlight the importance of early, intensive interventions, the benefit of multicomponent approaches, and the need for ongoing, robust interventions, especially for students with persistent difficulties. In conclusion, the authors assert that while prevention and early intervention are more effective, ongoing support is essential to sustain gains in reading proficiency. They call for more research–school partnerships to scale evidence-based approaches and integrate them into multi-tiered systems of support (MTSS) and special education.

In Chapter 12, "Reading Comprehension Instruction and Students with Learning Disabilities in the 21st Century," Wanzek, Sargent, and Fluhler explore the significance of reading comprehension, a critical skill for academic success and lifelong learning. Despite the importance of reading comprehension, national assessments show that only a small percentage of students with disabilities reach proficiency, highlighting a pressing need for targeted interventions.

The authors synthesize research examining reading comprehension interventions for students with learning disabilities (LD) over the last 20 years. They find a limited number of studies that have investigated reading comprehension intervention with a sample of students with LD. These studies document positive outcomes associated with teaching students with LD to organize key information in texts and for instruction in strategies for accessing the key content in texts.

Beyond intervention effectiveness, the authors examine the methodological limitations of existing research and areas requiring further study. They highlight gaps in knowledge regarding the generalization of skills, the impact of interventions on overall academic performance, and the need for more experimental studies. They conclude that research has primarily relied on researcher-developed assessments rather than standardized measures, making it difficult to gauge real-world applicability.

In Chapter 13, "Direct and Extended Vocabulary Instruction and Intervention for Students with Learning Disabilities," Coyne and Loftus-Rattan explore the critical role of vocabulary knowledge in reading comprehension and academic success. Given that many students with LD struggle with vocabulary development and do not acquire new words as effectively through incidental learning, the authors describe the need for direct, intentional vocabulary instruction to help bridge this gap. They review research indicating that explicit vocabulary instruction, which includes defining words in student-friendly terms, providing meaningful contexts, and offering interactive learning opportunities, is effective in improving vocabulary knowledge.

The authors also discuss the importance of intensifying vocabulary instruction for students at risk for reading difficulties through structured interventions, such as small-group instruction within an MTSS framework. Research findings suggest that supplemental Tier 2 vocabulary interventions can accelerate learning and help at-risk students reach vocabulary levels comparable to their peers. Additionally, strategies like oral language activities, extended vocabulary discussions, and continuous review of learned words further enhance comprehension and retention. While direct vocabulary instruction has demonstrated effectiveness, the chapter calls for further research into long-term, sustained vocabulary interventions and alternative instructional approaches that integrate broader language development skills.

Chapter 14 directs our attention to mathematics. In "Interventions to Address the Needs of Students with Mathematics Learning Disabilities," Fuchs, Seethaler, Fuchs, and Espinas focus on the importance of effective intervention for students with MD, given the strong link between mathematics achievement and long-term quality of life. The authors highlight three foundational mathematical domains—arithmetic, word problem solving, and fractions—where structured intervention is particularly crucial. *Scientifically Structured Mathematics Intervention* (SSMI) is introduced as an evidence-based approach designed to compensate for cognitive and linguistic difficulties experienced by students with MD. SSMI is organized around principles for structuring mathematical content, introducing new material, and optimizing practice to improve mathematical understanding and fluency.

The authors then review their validated interventions in each of the three domains: *Galaxy Math* for arithmetic, *Pirate Math* for word problems, and *Super Solvers* for fractions. These interventions emphasize schema-based instruction, explicit modeling, scaffolded learning, cumulative review, and practice strategies aligned with cognitive science. Research findings demonstrate their effectiveness in improving students' mathematical proficiency, though challenges remain in maintaining long-term gains. The authors conclude by emphasizing the need for sustained research on identifying students who require extended support and exploring cost-effective strategies, such as multi-year interventions or booster sessions, to ensure long-term success in mathematics for students with MD.

In Chapter 15, "Writing and Students with Learning Disabilities," Graham and Harris explore the historical origins and evolving purposes of writing and emphasize its critical role in communication, education, and personal expression. Writing challenges faced by students with LD include their tendency to rely on content generation with minimal planning or revision, limited self-regulation strategies, and difficulties with text transcription, sentence construction, and genre knowledge. Research has consistently shown that students with LD produce shorter, less coherent, and lower-quality writing compared to their typically developing peers. Additionally, many students with LD overestimate their writing abilities, which can hinder their motivation and self-regulation.

The authors review various approaches to assessing writing difficulties, including norm-referenced assessments, Response to Intervention models, and curriculum-based measurements—highlighting the need for comprehensive evaluation methods. Effective instructional practices are discussed, with a focus on *Self-Regulated Strategy Development* (SRSD), which has been extensively researched and proven to improve writing outcomes for students with LD. The authors underscore the importance of high-quality teacher preparation in writing instruction, both in preservice programs and through professional development, while also identifying critical research gaps. They recommend that future studies focus on longitudinal writing development, effective teaching practices, and intervention models that support students with LD across different educational settings and throughout their lifespans.

In Chapter 16, "Social Studies and History Instruction for Students with Learning Disabilities," De La Paz, Wissinger, and Otarola document the importance of history education for all students and discuss strategies used by historians that can inform classroom instruction. The authors also present the challenges that students, particularly novices, face when engaging in historical inquiry and the instructional difficulties that educators encounter when teaching historical knowledge and thinking.

The authors review research on interventions designed to support students with language and learning barriers, including cognitive strategies like note-taking, summarization, questioning, and comprehension monitoring. Additionally, the authors discuss strategies that promote higher-level historical reasoning skills, showing that such instructional approaches can benefit students across different learning levels. Finally, the authors emphasize the need for further research on social studies instruction for students with LD, particularly regarding cognitive and linguistic challenges in disciplinary literacy. The authors call for more studies to better understand how students with LD develop historical reasoning skills and to refine teaching strategies that support diverse learning needs.

In Chapter 17, "Science Education for Students with Learning Disabilities," van Garderen, Romine, Abdelnaby, Smith, and Juergensen commend the decades of work conducted by Mastropieri and Scruggs and highlight research demonstrating the effectiveness of instructional strategies like mnemonics, inquiry-based learning, and peer tutoring. Despite this body of evidence, national data show students with LD continue to lag significantly behind their peers in science achievement. The authors posit that one reason for this gap may be the limited implementation of evidence-based teaching practices in general education classrooms. Additionally, teacher preparation programs may not adequately equip educators with the skills needed to support students with LD in science learning.

The authors also explore the shift in science education toward three-dimensional learning, as outlined in the *Next Generation Science Standards* (NGSS). This framework integrates science and engineering practices with core disciplinary ideas and cross-cutting concepts, focusing on inquiry and argumentation rather than rote memorization. The authors discuss their research program, *Linking Science & Literacy for All Learners* (LS&L4AL), which supports middle school teachers in using multimodal science, technology, engineering, and mathematics (STEM) text sets to help students, including those with LD, engage with complex scientific texts and construct evidence-based arguments. Findings from their studies suggest that these strategies can improve scientific literacy for all students, with particularly strong gains for those with disabilities. Despite these promising approaches, challenges remain in fully integrating students with LD into rigorous science instruction. Many students will need support with the complexities of scientific argumentation due to deficits in working memory, reading comprehension, and writing skills. The authors call for further research into how best to adapt science practices for students with LD, ensuring that they can engage meaningfully with disciplinary knowledge while developing essential literacy and reasoning skills.

In Chapter 18, "Key Practices for Preventing and Ameliorating Reading Disabilities among English Learners," Capin, Andress, and Vaughn explore the challenges and strengths of English learners (ELs) with reading disabilities (RD) and highlights the role of bilingualism and socio-contextual factors in their literacy development. While ELs possess valuable linguistic and cultural knowledge, they often face limited opportunities for academic engagement due to systemic inequities, such as underfunded schools and socioeconomic disadvantages. The authors emphasize ELs' untapped potential, particularly those with RD, who can make significant gains with appropriate instructional support.

Research indicates that ELs and their monolingual peers share similar sources of reading difficulties, with word reading playing a crucial role in early literacy and linguistic comprehension becoming more significant in later grades. The authors discuss the role of MTSS in providing structured, evidence-based instruction across three tiers, ensuring early intervention, ongoing progress monitoring, and intensive support when needed. Effective MTSS implementation requires high-quality Tier 1 instruction, culturally responsive interventions, and professional development for educators to ensure ELs receive appropriate support in both literacy and language development.

To improve literacy outcomes for ELs, the authors advocate for structured cooperative learning, explicit vocabulary instruction, and content-area literacy strategies, particularly in the secondary grades. Evidence-based interventions like *Promoting Adolescents' Comprehension of Text* (PACT) and CREATE have shown promise in enhancing ELs' reading comprehension and academic success. The authors recommend prioritizing early intervention, integrating academic language instruction, and designing literacy instruction as if all students are ELs, ensuring that strategies benefit both ELs and their monolingual peers.

CHAPTER 11

Effective Instruction and Intervention for Word-Level Reading for Students with and at Risk for Learning Disabilities

Stephanie Al Otaiba, Dayna Russell Freudenthal, and Mai W. Zaru

Teaching all children to comprehend what they read remains a societal challenge, as only about a third of children in the United States can read proficiently by fourth grade. Furthermore, 17% and 74% of students with disabilities were performing at a basic or below-basic level, respectively. Not even a third of children can read proficiently (31%) by fourth grade, according to the 2024 National Assessment of Educational Progress (NAEP) reading assessment (National Center for Education Statistics, 2025). Practically speaking, reading below basic means that while these fourth graders may recognize some familiar high-frequency monosyllabic words, they struggle to decode multisyllabic words, particularly those that are less common (Hiebert, 2022). A variety of factors can make it challenging for young children to learn to read, such as general language abilities, phonemic awareness, letter knowledge, letter–sound recognition, and exposure to print. The ultimate goal of word-reading instruction (and intervention) is to help children comprehend a variety of texts and content-area genres so they are able to learn from what they are reading.

Purpose of This Chapter

The purpose of this chapter is to describe evidence to inform effective instruction and interventions designed to improve word-level reading, particularly for students with or at risk for reading difficulties. We incorporate research on word-reading instruction and intervention that increases in intensity for multi-tiered systems of support (MTSS) or in response to intervention (RTI) approaches. We acknowledge this may be a somewhat narrow focus, but another chapter in this *Handbook* describes comprehension instruction and intervention. Readers will also learn more about dyslexia specifically and assessment broadly in subsequent chapters, so we will not discuss predictors, identification, or diagnosis in depth. A thorough discussion of the neurological processes of how proficient reading develops is also beyond the scope of this chapter, and certainly beyond our expertise, but we refer readers to Adams (2011), Pugh et al. (2013), and Seidenberg (2017) for more in-depth explanations.

First, we begin by describing theoretical frameworks that explain how proficient reading develops. Second, we synthesize research on word-reading instruction and intervention, including findings from a recent review of reviews summarizing the effects of studies conducted through 2020 and other recent related meta-analyses. Third, we describe findings from individual studies conducted within the context of RTI and MTSS that positively impacted word-reading performance of students with or at risk for reading difficulties. Understanding their response to instruction and intervention is important because earlier intervention has been shown to have a stronger impact than later remediation; therefore, accelerating word-reading growth for students who have not benefited from generally effective interventions requires more robust interventions (e.g., Al Otaiba & Fuchs, 2006; Torgesen, 2000; Lam & McMaster, 2014). This challenge led Miciak and Fletcher (2020) to caution that "persistent lack of adequate response to quality instruction is a marker of disability and educational need" (p. 22). Finally, we discuss implications for research and practice and describe some limitations and directions for future research.

Theoretical Framework to Inform Reading Development, Instruction, and Intervention

As we mentioned previously, the ultimate goal of learning to read words is to comprehend and learn from reading. A variety of theories of reading explain relations between word reading and comprehension. For example, the Simple View of Reading (SVR) (Gough & Tunmer, 1986) explained skilled reading as the product of two sets of skills: those that are *code-focused* (decoding and phonemic awareness) and those that are *meaning-focused* (linguistic skills and listening comprehension). Scarborough (2001) extended the SVR and developed an iconic image of a rope to show these two sets of skills as individual strands in the rope and how these strands become more tightly interwoven and more automatic and strategic across time. Although decoding and phonemic awareness are directly pertinent to this chapter, language comprehension skills are also relevant since they support skilled and fluent reading (e.g., background knowledge, vocabulary, language structures of syntax and morphology, verbal reasoning, and literacy knowledge). The SVR suggested that if either set of code- or meaning-focused skills is lacking, comprehension would suffer, which implied four types of readers: good readers (with strong decoding and linguistic skills) and poor comprehenders (with adequate decoding ability) and the two types that are most relevant to our chapter, poor decoders with good linguistic skills and garden-variety poor readers who lack adequate decoding and linguistic skills. Converging findings from studies have confirmed that decoding and linguistic comprehension predict reading comprehension in diverse populations and languages (e.g., Catts et al., 2015; García & Cain, 2014). However, researchers found that the relative importance of decoding and linguistic comprehension shifted over time, with linguistic comprehension playing an increasing role in later stages of reading development. We acknowledge that the SVR can also be expanded to include other factors related to reading risk, such as resilience and protective factors that could influence word-reading development indirectly, including social and emotional skills, growth mindset towards intelligence and learning, attributions, and motivation (e.g., Catts & Petscher, 2022).

Another enduring theory of how word reading develops that guided our chapter was developed by Ehri (1987, 2020), whose multiple-phase developmental trajectory explains how individuals use their knowledge about *grapheme–phoneme* correspondences with increasing efficiency to decode and spell words. (See also Spear-Swerling and Sterling [1996], who described where and how struggling readers get stuck in their development.) At first, within the *pre-alphabetic* phase, young children have little understanding of the connections between *phonemes*, the sounds' spoken language, and letters or combinations of letters (*graphemes*). A struggling reader in the pre-alphabetic phase may be limited to recognizing words they have memorized and guessing based on context; they have no ability to decode (Ehri & McCormick, 1998). Then, within the *partial-alphabetic* phase, most school-age children begin to understand the workings of letters and sounds, particularly within short, familiar words. These early skills start a progression from understanding a broader *phonological awareness* or sensitivity to sound structures within spoken words (including syllables or onsets). It is crucial to develop *phonemic awareness*, recognizing spoken words as a sequence of phonemes (e.g., Adams, 1990; Brady, 2020). Struggling readers in this phase experience challenges in decoding unfamiliar words. They often attend to the beginning and end of a word only and are likely to misread a new word as a known word because of partial resemblance, as in the words "sack" and "slack." However, they may also begin to recognize words that are very frequent within text (e.g., the, have, and were).

As readers progress to the *fully alphabetic* phase, they can decode familiar and unfamiliar words. Skilled readers can blend sounds to read words and segment words to spell words automatically. In fact, Ehri (2000) described reading and spelling as two sides of a coin. Struggling readers remain slow and laborious. In the final phase, the *consolidated alphabetic* phase, students can quickly and accurately read and spell a variety of words, including multisyllabic words. Over time, proficient readers apply their knowledge to reading novel words (termed the *self-teaching hypothesis*, Share, 1995). They recognize *morphemes*, which are small units of meaning within words. Morphemes include root words, inflectional endings, or suffixes (e.g., the *-es* at the end of suffix*es*, making it plural), prefixes (e.g., the *re-* in *re*view), and derivational affixes (e.g., the *-ful* at the end of hand*ful*). The act of pronouncing the word enhances memory for simple vocabulary words (Rosenthal & Ehri, 2008) and supports grapho-syllabic analysis to pronounce more complex vocabulary, including multisyllabic words (e.g., Bhattacharya & Ehri, 2004). Conversely, struggling readers who have developed inefficient or incomplete word-reading strategies may have their progress impeded as they encounter more complex texts and genres of texts that include unfamiliar words and lengthier, complex multisyllabic words.

Through explicit instruction and the opportunity to build their experience reading known words within connected text, proficient readers have learned what letter sequences are allowed in English and have implicitly and/or explicitly learned how frequently and consistently phonemes are represented by graphemes. Goswami (2005) pointed out that individuals can use a combination of 600 letter–sound patterns and 400 phonological rimes to decode the most frequent 3,000 words in English, even though the relationships between graphemes and phonemes vary in regularity. For example, the spelling of the long *I* in "bike" is more frequent than in "sigh" (e.g., Apel et al., 2006). Proficient readers begin to recognize that not all grapheme–phoneme correspondences (especially vowels within multisyllabic words) are regular or consistent (e.g., Kearns et al., 2016; Venezky, 1999). Proficient readers also use their morphological awareness because roughly 60–80% of words in texts have derived words with multiple syllables (Nagy & Anderson, 1984). Bowers, Kirby, and Deacon (2010) have suggested that phonological, orthographic, and semantic features of multisyllabic words are supported through morphological or morphemic analysis. In other words, understanding that long words can be divided into meaningful parts (i.e., root or base words, prefixes, and suffixes) may be more efficient for reading a long word than analyzing each individual phoneme (e.g., Bhattacharya, 2020; Kearns, 2020). Conversely, struggling readers may devote relatively more effort to decoding; have difficulty analogizing familiar to unfamiliar words, recognizing parts of words they may know; and labor to apply knowledge of less common letter sequences (especially vowel patterns) and morphemes, particularly when trying to read multisyllabic words.

Effective Reading Instruction and Intervention: Big Picture Findings from a Recent Review of Reviews and Other Recent Meta-Analyses and Syntheses

Our intent in writing this chapter was to provide an overview of effective word-reading instruction and intervention rather than an exhaustive and systematic review of all research. So, we begin by synthesizing the major findings about the effects of reading interventions for students who have reading difficulties from a recent review of reviews of studies conducted over the past decade (Al Otaiba et al., 2023). We also integrate findings from other salient recent syntheses and meta-analyses (not part of this review), including a recent synthesis about irregular word reading (Colenbrander et al., 2020), a meta-analysis discussing longer-term intervention effects of reading interventions for struggling readers PreK–grade 6 (Suggate, 2016), and a meta-analysis about longer-term reading interventions for adolescents (Daniel et al., 2021). At a policy level, this past decade represents a time frame when most states promoted RTI for reading or broader MTSS that incorporate additional supports for behavior, social–emotional learning, motivation, mindset, and mental health. RTI and MTSS approaches have varied, and states have not provided consistent guidance for school implementation (e.g., Berkeley et al., 2020). Also, across this time frame, many states passed dyslexia legislation, with requirements such as teacher training, dyslexia screening, and dyslexia-specific interventions (cf. Petscher et al., 2020; Youman & Mather, 2018).

Although Al Otaiba et al.'s (2023) review of reviews focused primarily on studies that were conducted in the elementary grades, some of the meta-analyses also included studies with older students in middle and high school. Within the primary grades, the majority of the early literacy interventions were preventative in nature (i.e., relatively more studies were conducted in kindergarten and first grade), and most targeted beginning code-focused, foundational reading skills, provided in small groups or one-to-one. Findings provided causal evidence for the efficacy of these interventions; small to moderate effects were reported on standardized measures of code-focused skills (*ES* = 0.41 to 0.62), and slightly smaller effects were reported on measures of meaning-focused comprehension skills (*ES* = 0.32 to 0.36). It was noteworthy that only one meta-analysis specifically examined the impact of studies of Tier 3 interventions provided to students who had not responded to previous intervention (Austin et al., 2017). For example, Austin et al. found only three studies that assigned inadequate responders to a more intensive treatment versus a BAU control condition, and the effects on standardized measures of word reading were large to moderate for word attack (*d* = 0.40 to 1.77), letter–word identification (*d* = 0.44 to 0.90), and comprehension (*d* = .07 to 0.42). Although their meta-analysis reported positive effects on reading, the number of studies was small, and students in Tier 3 did not catch up to stronger readers, comprised of either typical groups who never needed Tier 2 or students who had received prior intervention and had responded adequately. Another meta-analysis focused solely on interventions that provided the type of *multi-sensory* components required by some states' dyslexia-specific legislation (Stevens et al., 2021). Their findings revealed no significant differences between treatment and control conditions on either code- or meaning-focused skills. However, they did report small and potentially meaningful effect sizes of 0.32, favoring students who received intervention on the foundational skills of phonological awareness, phonics, fluency, and spelling. Both Austin et al. (2017) and Stevens et al. (2021) cautioned that replication was needed with more rigorous research designs.

Three meta-analyses in the review of reviews focused on the effects of reading interventions for struggling students in upper elementary, middle, and high school (Flynn et al., 2012; Scammacca et al., 2015; Wanzek et al., 2013). In the fourth meta-analysis, Donegan and Wanzek (2021) selected studies only in upper elementary. These meta-analyses also provided causal evidence for the efficacy of explicit and systematic reading interventions across these grades for students with or at risk for reading disabilities. Average mean effect sizes on code-focused skills ranged from (*ES* = 0.09 to 0.43), and slightly larger effects were reported on meaning-focused measures of comprehension skills (*ES* = 0.10 to 0.73). Notably, Flynn et al. (2012) reported the strongest effect sizes for foundational skills such as word identification 0.42 and decoding 0.43. Furthermore, this was the only synthesis focused exclusively on older students with reading disabilities (conceptualized as those falling below the 25th percentile on a norm-referenced reading measure), while the other syntheses were focused more broadly on struggling readers. Wanzek et al. (2013) found small, positive effects for extensive interventions involving 75 or more sessions on reading outcomes. Moderation analyses conducted by Donegan and Wanzek revealed stronger effects for multicomponent interventions and for small groups of 1–2 students.

Although writing is not our focus for this chapter, students with word-reading difficulties commonly also struggle to spell, so it was noteworthy that the review of reviews reported positive effects of writing and spelling instruction on code-focused measures of phonological awareness and word reading (ES ranging for phonological awareness of 0.51 and for word reading from 0.39–0.62) derived from three meta-analyses spanning PreK–high school (Graham et al., 2018; Graham & Hebert, 2011; Graham & Santangelo, 2014). Graham (2020) noted that writing and reading have shared knowledge because they draw on similar systems. These findings support that writing and spelling instruction transfer to reading, which has implications for reading interventions. Moderator analyses suggested that the effects of writing instruction on reading outcomes were stronger when reading and spelling were equally targeted, but more research is needed to inform what type of spelling and writing activities are most beneficial for students with reading difficulties.

Other Recent Syntheses and Meta-Analyses Relevant to This Chapter

In their recent synthesis of the research on teaching irregular words, Colenbrander et al. (2020) noted some debate about how researchers and practitioners have defined *irregular* words. They suggested that regularity could be thought of as a continuum from words that are completely regular in terms of grapheme–phoneme correspondence (e.g., *map*) to words with one irregular correspondence (e.g., *mind*) and words with many irregular correspondences (e.g., *aisle*). For this chapter, we follow their convention of considering a word *regular* only if it can be decoded using the most common pronunciation. Thus, the word "map" would be regular, but not "were" or "was." Colenbrander and colleagues also acknowledged debate among researchers and practitioners regarding how to teach irregular words. They synthesized several studies that have examined different approaches to teaching irregular words (e.g., Shapiro & Solity, 2016), which led them to conclude that there was "no evidence that teaching some irregular sight words alongside regular grapheme-phoneme correspondences is harmful for children or results in 'unlearning' of existing grapheme-phoneme correspondences" (Colenbrander et al., p 98).

It is important to note the phrase "alongside." They highlighted a study that found combining a limited number of sight words with explicit and systematic phonics instruction was beneficial for students with poor phonological awareness (Shapiro & Solity, 2016).

Another issue raised by Colenbrander et al.'s synthesis (2020) was that the term *sight word instruction* meant different methods to researchers and practitioners—including flash cards with or without pictures, practice text, hearing or visualizing the word, or spelling the word. Colenbrander et al. suggested that, to date, many promising sight word approaches have been incorporated within multi-multi-componentomponent interventions and that individual components and combinations may need to be tested in smaller studies. They also noted that because English orthography is related to morphology and etymology, morphological interventions have improved reading and spelling (e.g., Goodwin & Ahn, 2013). Thus, in addition to grapheme–phoneme instruction, some sight word (or word part) instruction, flexible decoding, and morphology instruction may also support reading abilities. They recommended that the optimal forms of instruction may depend on individual differences in age, exposure, reading ability, and the amount and type of instructional resources and time available. They cautioned that future research was needed to determine how many exposures a student required to achieve mastery.

Suggate (2016) conducted a meta-analysis that examined the long-term effects of reading interventions (PreK–grade 6), including phonemic awareness, phonics, fluency, and comprehension components. He categorized participants as "normal," "at risk," "low," or "reading/learning disabled." He was particularly interested in learning whether the intervention components might be associated with more robust effects and to differential transfer to other components over time. Across the studies, the overall mean weighted effect size was $d^w = 0.37$, which declined at follow-up to $d^w = 0.22$. Some findings from his moderation analyses inform this chapter. First, grade did not moderate short-term effects, and there was a trend in studies with younger students demonstrating declining scores, which switched at grade 3 as older students showed increased effects (from $d^w = 0.35$ to 0.43). Second, phonics and purely phonemic awareness interventions were similarly effective ($d^w = 0.43$ and $d = 0.29$, respectively). However, at follow-up, Suggate reported an advantage for phonemic awareness versus phonics ($d^w = 0.36$ and $d^w = 0.07$); comprehension had the largest effects at follow-up ($d^w = 0.47$). Third, he reported that phonemic awareness and comprehension components were associated with transfer to other components, but phonics and fluency components did not transfer. He also noted that students who were struggling had greater retention of intervention effects at follow-up than the normal readers did.

Another recent meta-analysis that examined the effects of reading interventions with older students also considered longer-term effects; Daniel et al. (2021) described findings from 10 reading intervention studies involving adolescent students in grades 6–12 (struggling readers, students with LD or dyslexia). The researchers reported overall large effect sizes across all reading measures of g^w

= 0.78 at immediate posttest, but these declined to g^w = 0.27 at follow-up after approximately 21 weeks. They cautioned that these effect sizes may be inflated by a high number of researcher-developed measures, and no studies occurred in grades 11 or 12.

To briefly summarize, across these meta-analyses and syntheses, it appeared that it was possible to "move the needle" or to substantially impact word reading by providing interventions that delivered explicit and systematic instruction that included grapheme–phoneme correspondences, a mix of decoding and sight word instruction, and reading practice in connected text. Although not our primary focus, writing and spelling instruction also yielded positive effects. After upper elementary, students benefited more from multicomponent interventions that provided meaning-focused intervention components, including vocabulary and comprehension. In the next section of the chapter, we review more recent individual studies with the intent to understand what moved the needle within MTSS approaches, which may inform how to prevent and remediate systematic word-reading interventions, accelerate response, and ensure that intervention gains do not wash out over time.

What Moves the Needle? Effects of MTSS Approaches on Word Reading

Can Struggling Readers Benefit from Early Reading Interventions in Primary and Upper Elementary Grades?

We are mindful that the promising findings we just synthesized contrast sharply with the null to negative effects of a widely cited RTI program evaluation study by Balu et al. (2015), who studied the effects of school-implemented RTI approaches delivered in grades 1–3. These schools reported implementing key RTI components such as screening, progress monitoring, and providing tiered instruction. However, these schools did not receive support from researchers, and their existing programs and processes were not observed, so it was not clear from this study what could be achieved with more support or guidance or when researchers implemented the instruction. Next, we summarize a few of the themes about what can move the needle to improve word reading within research-supported RTI/MTSS initiatives serving students at risk for or with reading difficulties and disabilities. These approaches spanned a continuum of standardized and individualized interventions, with the latter including data-based decision making to select appropriate programs based on student needs and/or data to adjust pacing and grouping (cf. Russell-Freudenthal et al., 2023).

A first theme that emerged was that *providing schools with system supports, such as additional training, resources, and infrastructure to support MTSS, led to stronger reading growth for struggling students.* For example, Fien et al. (2021) explicitly tested the effect of supported MTSS versus unsupported MTSS. The "unsupported" schools were already implementing MTSS and agreed that teachers would implement a strong Tier 1 core reading program daily, conduct universal screening, and provide Tier 2 to struggling students (in the 10th to 30th percentile range). In the supported MTSS condition (Enhanced Core Reading Instruction, ECRI), researchers provided schools with PD, ongoing coaching, materials to enhance systematic and explicit instruction for their core reading, aligned teaching routines for Tier 1 and Tier 2 (focusing on foundational word-reading skills), and teacher training to use data-based decision-making protocols. In the ECRI schools, trained first-grade teachers implemented Tier 1 and Tier 2 for struggling students (also in the 10th to the 30th percentile range). Struggling students in the ECRI schools outperformed those in unsupported RTI schools on phonemic decoding, word identification, and word attack, with small to moderate effects (g = 0.25 to 0.48). Nevertheless, Fien et al. cautioned that some struggling readers would require ongoing, more intensive supports.

Another theme identified was related to *cost-effectiveness*. Foorman et al. (2018) reported positive findings regardless of whether the Tier 2 intervention materials selected to enhance their core reading were aligned with and provided by the Tier 1 core curriculum or were stand-alone supplemental evidence-based programs. They concluded that it may be more cost-effective for schools to utilize commercially available materials aligned to the core rather than adding on additional materials and training. Students in grades K–2 improved their reading performance after receiving daily Tier 1 plus small-group Tier 2 delivered by researcher-trained interventionists throughout the school year. On average, students improved from below the 10th percentile in reading to the 20th percentile, and kindergarteners had the largest gains in word reading, thus supporting early intervention.

A theme derived was that *it may be more cost-effective and efficient to immediately deliver intensive interventions to students with the weakest skills*. Solari et al. (2018) trained first-grade classroom teachers to implement Tier 1 and Tier 2 in two conditions (PD-only or PD + Coaching conditions) and compared the effects of their instruction on students to the effects of teachers on student outcomes in a BAU condition. The intervention included phonemic awareness, phonics, fluent text reading, and comprehension, and it was provided to roughly five struggling readers per classroom. There were no differences between treatment conditions on any measures, but treatment students outperformed students in BAU classrooms on word reading, fluency, and comprehension (with effect sizes ranging from g = 0.41 to 0.72). The effects were stronger for those with the weakest initial skills, but these students had very poor word reading even after intervention and may have benefited from more intensive Tier 3. Moreover, on average, the teachers only completed 66% of the intended number of lessons, suggesting additional support or coaching may have been needed.

Related to the *theme of delivering intensive intervention immediately*, findings from two studies indicated it was more powerful to intervene immediately with struggling first graders than to wait within a typical RTI approach (Al Otaiba, Connor, et al., 2014; Al Otaiba, Kim, et al., 2014). The researchers collaborated with district staff to select interventions for Tier 2 and 3 aligned with the existing Tier 1 core reading program. In one school, only about 16% of students received free and reduced-price lunch (FAPRL); the remaining five schools served a more diverse population, and more received FARPL (42.8% to 89.9%). However, less than 3% of students had limited English proficiency. Students were randomly assigned within classrooms (*n* = 34) to one of two RTI conditions. These RTI interventions were identical and differed only in when students began interventions. In the *Typical RTI* condition, students began in Tier 1 and moved up a tier if they did not respond at the end of 8 weeks. In the *Dynamic RTI* condition, students were immediately assigned to Tier 2 or Tier 3 based on their teacher's nomination of risk and screening scores (*z* scores below the 40th percentile on four brief assessments of letter–sound fluency, word-identification fluency, and sight word- and phonemic-decoding fluency). Classroom teachers received training in a one-day workshop from researchers about RTI and the importance of individualizing instruction by forming small groups. Researchers also provided teachers with ongoing weekly coaching support for Tier 1. Trained research staff provided the Tier 2 and 3 interventions. At both Tier 2 and 3, the meaning-focused aspect of intervention increased in difficulty every 8 weeks: (1) a dialogic read-aloud, (2) student-reading decodable books, and (3) student-reading connected text with a written re-tell using sequencing. Tier 2 incorporated code-focused activities from the core and student-centered activities from the Florida Center for Reading Research (*www.fcrr.org*). Tier 2 was provided to groups of 4–7 students twice a week. Tier 3 was more intensive, with smaller groups of 1–3 students four times a week; the code-focused portion of the intervention used *Early Intervention in Reading* (Mathes et al., 1999). Positive behavior supports were also provided as needed.

Results indicated that, on average, students in the *Dynamic RTI* condition had stronger reading performance (*d* = 0.36) than those in the *Typical* condition. Students who received Tier 2 or Tier 3 immediately demonstrated an advantage, with growth trajectories indicating this benefit accumulated over the year. At the end of the study, overall, 95% of students achieved grade-level basic reading skills; specifically, among struggling students, 83% achieved standard scores at or above 90. Researchers classified students into three groups: (1) those in Tier 1, who had never required intervention (NR), (2) those who were easy to remediate and exited intervention (ER), and (3) students who needed sustained remediation (SR). At the end of second grade, the proportion of students with word-reading standard scores below 90 was low (NR = 1.5%; ER = 3.2%; and SR = 8.7%), and this percentage remained low at the end of third grade (NR = 1.1%; ER = 0%; and SR = 7.9%). However, Al Otaiba, Kim, et al. (2014) cautioned that attrition had occurred and warned that larger proportions of the SR students remained dysfluent or poor comprehenders at the end of grades 2 and 3; relatively more performed below a standard score of 90 on timed measures of word reading (28.6% and 42.1%, respectively, at the end of grades 2 and 3), oral reading fluency (28.6% and 29.4%, respectively), and passage comprehension (36.5% and 24.5%, respectively). Their findings corroborated prior research that early intervention can support most students in achieving (and sustaining) grade-level word-reading skills, but it is harder to promote fluency and comprehension.

Another study related to *the theme of providing early intensive intervention* had even larger effects; Lovett et al. (2017) recruited students in grades 1–3 who scored below a standardized reading score of 85. Their research team implemented the multicomponent intervention that combined decoding and comprehension strategies of the *PHAST Reading Program* (*Phonological and Strategy Training*) (Lovett et al., 2000) and the fluency, orthography, vocabulary, syntax, and morphology activities of *Retrieval, Automaticity, Vocabulary, Engagement-Orthography (RAVE-O)* (Wolf et al., 2000). Notably, researchers explicitly trained students in small groups (1:4) to use a progression of decoding strategies beginning with Sounding Out (letter–sound, blending, and decoding with practice in connected text), to Rhyming (keywords with high-frequency spelling patterns), to Peeling Off (affixes), to Vowel Alert (flexible use of vowel patterns and alerting if a pronunciation is incorrect), and, finally, to I Spy (recognizing parts of words). In addition, PHAST incorporated training for motivation and attribution and provided students with a game plan. Students in the treatment condition outperformed students receiving BAU instruction with moderate to large effects on code-focused measures (d = 0.57 to d = 1.39) and on meaning-focused measures (d = 0.63 to d = 0.90). Importantly, at posttest, significantly more treatment students attained standardized reading scores above 90 in word identification, word attack, and passage comprehension. The importance of earlier intervention was apparent; students were tested through fourth grade, and significantly stronger reading performance continued for students who had received intervention in grade 1 than in grade 2. Future research is needed to replicate these effects with school staff implementing and English language learners who did not participate in this study.

Findings from one further study conducted by Savage et al. (2018) related to *the theme of providing early intervention* emphasized *the promise of teaching students to be flexible decoders*. Savage et al. used a quasi-experimental study to compare the effects of two theoretically different treatments on reading and spelling achievement for first graders whose word reading was below the 30th percentile on a standardized measure. These students had not responded to initial literacy instruction, even though observations of their core reading included research-validated programs that incorporated phonics. In January, both small-group interventions replaced part of core instruction and were provided by trained research assistants. The first intervention was derived from prior research regarding flexible decoding or a "set-for-variability" (e.g., Kearns et al., 2016; Steacy et al., 2016; Venezky, 1999). Their Direct Mapping and Set-for-Variability (DMSfV) intervention provided training in (1) direct mapping of grapheme–phoneme correspondence, including multiple-vowel pronunciations, (2) teaching strategies for being flexible (and self-correcting erroneous pronunciations) while decoding vowels with variable digraph pronunciations (e.g., mouth vs. shoulder), (3) shared reading of text with these patterns, and (4) individualization of practice to ensure mastery. They compared the DMSfV to another explicit and systematic instruction program they developed that also included training on grapheme–phonemes, word reading, and text reading, but without DMSfV components. Although students demonstrated gains in both conditions, the effects were significantly stronger for students in the DMSfV condition on standardized measures (word reading, sight word reading, oral reading fluency, and spelling) with small to moderate effect sizes at posttest (d = 0.08 to 0.41). Most effects decreased at the delayed posttest (d = 0.18 to 0.30), but word attack effects increased (from d = 0.08 to 0.18).

A final theme in this section of studies was that it *was not too late to intervene with struggling readers in upper elementary, but effects were smaller.* This set of studies also included elements of mindset or motivation training. For example, a recent study conducted in upper elementary by Wanzek et al. (2020) used an RCT to directly compare the effect of a word-reading intervention only, to a word-reading intervention plus the Brainology™ growth mindset training, and to BAU. Teachers nominated fourth-grade participants who were struggling readers and qualified for the study if they scored below the 30th percentile on a word-reading test. The research interventionists were trained to implement *Lindamood Phoneme Sequencing Program* (LiPS) (Lindamood & Lindamood, 2010) and provide intervention to small groups of 3–5 students during the school year. Other interventionists were trained to implement Brainology™, and they provided intervention twice a week for the standard 24 sessions. Students in both treatment conditions performed similarly and outperformed the BAU students, albeit with small effects, on measures of nonword reading (d = 0.29 to 0.35), phonological processing (d = 0.20 to 0.28), and comprehension (ES = 0.19 to 0.23). There were no differences across conditions in a survey of students' mindset.

As examples of more targeted recent studies that demonstrated positive effects of explicit multisyllabic instruction, we describe findings from two RCT studies conducted by Toste and colleagues (2017, 2019). Multisyllabic words represent a significant challenge in upper elementary and throughout high school (e.g., Bhattacharya, 2020; Kearns, 2020), particularly given the complexity of how syllables are combined and how prefixes and suffixes connect to root words. After grade 2, the majority of words that students encounter in texts are derived words, and across the grades, they increasingly contain Greek or Latin-bound roots (e.g., Crosson & McKeown, 2016). Toste and her team evaluated the effects of an explicit multisyllabic intervention that included blending, segmenting, reading, and spelling of multisyllabic words and a repeated reading component that allowed students to practice word-reading skills in connected text relative to a BAU control condition. Students received explicit and systematic instruction for reading vowel patterns, learning affixes, and using structural analysis of words. Their studies also tested the value of adding attribution and motivation training by testing the effects of reading-only versus reading plus attribution and motivation. The students were nominated by teachers as struggling readers in both RCT studies. The first study included students in grades 3–4, and they qualified for the study if they had word reading below the 37th percentile. The second study included older students in grades 4–5 with more impaired word reading below the 25th percentile. The older students also learned goal planning in addition to motivation and attribution. Research staff delivered interventions in small groups of 23 students, and Study 1 spanned three 40-minute sessions for 8 weeks, whereas Study 2 included four sessions per week for 10 weeks. In both studies, the effects were similar for the two versions of the intervention, so the conditions were combined. The third- and fourth-grade students in the intervention significantly outperformed controls on sight word efficiency (g = 0.73), and although not significant, the trend was for effect sizes favored the intervention condition for timed decoding (g = 0.31), untimed decoding (g = 0.30), word attack (g = 0.30), and letter–word identification (g = 0.29). Students in the interventions also scored higher than the BAU students on a measure of reading attribution, indicating they were more likely to attribute their failure or success to internal effort or strategy use than to external factors such as luck or teacher assistance. Similarly, the fourth and fifth graders in either intervention condition outperformed BAU students on standardized measures of decoding (ranging from g = 0.17 to 0.43), spelling (g = 0.25), and with larger effects on the proximal multisyllabic word measure (0.90). However, they did not show stronger performance on a reading self-concept measure, but the researchers noted they had switched assessments in this study.

Can Struggling Readers Experience Remediation in Middle and High School?

To answer the question of whether word-reading instruction should remain an active ingredient for interventions with older struggling readers in middle and high school, we highlight some *themes about the findings* of the impact of multi-multi-componentomponent interventions from a few teams of researchers. We caution that compared to the number of studies conducted with younger students, there are far fewer studies with older students who struggle with word reading, and the older the student, the fewer the studies. Struggling older readers may experience difficulties for various reasons; some may have had poor early reading instruction lacking sufficient explicit instruction in skills necessary for proficient reading, while others might have had good instruction but continue to struggle with one or multiple components. The body of research related to adolescent struggling readers points to five skill areas necessary for skilled reading in older readers: word study, fluency, vocabulary, comprehension, and motivation (e.g., Kamil et al., 2008).

A theme that continues with older students is the *time and intensity required to achieve significant effects on the reading of students who have struggled for years*. In one of the earliest large-scale, longitudinal studies of reading intervention for secondary students delivered within the RTI framework, Vaughn and colleagues conducted a 3-year, multi-gated, randomized trial within large urban school settings to evaluate the efficacy of increasingly intensive tiers of instruction for middle school struggling readers (Vaughn et al., 2010, 2011, 2012). In Year 1, at-risk, struggling sixth-grade readers were included if they scored below the cutoff on a statewide reading test. Researchers randomly assigned them to researcher-provided Tier 2 intervention or a comparison BAU condition; their reading growth was also compared to typical readers. Students assigned to the treatment condition in Year 1 were the only participants eligible for the treatment condition(s) in subsequent years, and students in the BAU condition in Year 1 remained eligible only for the BAU in the following years of the study.

For Year 1, students in the Tier 2 treatment condition were placed in homogeneous groups of 10–15 students and received daily intensive intervention implemented by trained tutors coached by the research team. The intervention entailed a three-phase approach. Phase 1 emphasized word study and fluency. Advanced strategies for decoding multisyllabic words were explicitly addressed using REWARDS Intermediate (Archer et al., 2005) to systematically teach students flexible decoding strategies to read long words. In Phase 2, vocabulary and comprehension instruction was prioritized using content-focused expository text and novels, but word study skills were also practiced daily. Phase 3 included word study and vocabulary instruction, but interventionists used researcher-developed units to apply fluency and comprehension strategies to social studies and science expository texts and narrative texts. The BAU comparison students received school-provided reading instruction or intervention, and the typical reading students received no additional reading instruction. Results favored the Tier 2 experimental condition compared to the BAU with significant outcomes and small effect sizes on standardized measures of word attack (d = 0.15) and spelling (d = 0.22). However, the average reading performance of students in Tier 2 was nearly a standard deviation lower than typically performing peers at posttest (d = -0.94). While the raw data for intervention students showed increased proficiency, the researchers concluded that expecting significant growth after a single yearlong intervention in medium-sized groups with little flexibility for students who have struggled with reading for many years may not have been reasonable.

As per their study design, students identified as minimal responders were eligible to receive an additional year of intervention with increased intensity; so in Year 2, Vaughn and her team (2011) examined the efficacy of two different approaches to Tier 3 instruction for those students relative to those who remained in the BAU condition. Students eligible for treatment were randomly assigned to a standard protocol intervention condition or an individualized approach condition and placed in smaller groups of 4–5 students. The interventions were delivered by researcher-hired and trained teachers across the school year during an elective period. The standardized condition utilized the three-phase intervention similar to the prior year. In the individualized condition, teachers used testing and assessment data to develop protocols to meet students' individual needs. Scores on measures related to reading components dictated the makeup of each lesson, advancement and pacing were based on student mastery, and guidelines were provided for instructional time. Word study was flexible but primarily utilized the *Wilson Reading System's* (1996) explicit, intensive word study program along with a research-based scope and sequence of comprehension strategy instruction with narrative and expository text. Teachers made decisions to adjust instruction based on biweekly CBMs. There were significant differences between the two treatment conditions and BAU on comprehension (g = .56). No significant differences were reported between the three conditions on decoding, spelling, and fluency measures, but there was a trend for effects that favored the treatment conditions on standard scores of timed and untimed decoding (g = 0.14 to 0.45), timed and word reading (g = 0.24 to 0.44), and spelling (g = 0.31 to 0.36). The findings in this study did not support the researchers' hypothesis that students in the individualized condition would outperform students in the standardized treatment.

In Year 3 of the longitudinal study, Vaughn and colleagues (2012) examined the effects of an intensive, individualized intervention for students who had not adequately responded to intervention in the 2 prior years. For this study, the researchers hired two teachers with master's degrees in education and extensive experience teaching students with significant reading disabilities. (As a reminder, treatment participants were members of the original treatment conditions in grades 6 and 7, and comparison BAU students were those who had not received the researcher intervention.) The intervention, deemed *Tier 4* by the research team, was an individualized intervention implemented daily in even smaller groups of 2–4 students. Teachers were allowed some flexibility to address student needs but followed a sequential scope and sequence and lessons from an explicit, intense word study program (*Wilson Reading System*, 1996) targeting reading and spelling of mono- and multisyllabic words. Researchers supported teachers in using data to assess student mastery and plan ongoing interventions. The motivational component utilized goal setting, evaluation conferences, motivational text selections, and positive calls home. Results revealed that eighth-grade students in the treatment condition significantly outperformed their peers in the BAU condition on standardized measures of word reading (ES = 0.49) and comprehension (ES = 1.20). The authors noted an important implication: older students with significant reading needs benefited most from intensive instruction provided by expert teachers. Although they still did not close the gap with their typically performing peers, the evidence suggested remediation allowed them to continue to grow, while BAU students (those receiving only school-provided supports and not this intensive intervention) exhibited substantial declines in reading achievement and fell further behind. We note the time, intensity, and expertise required to impact the reading outcomes of secondary students who have been perpetually poor responders in the past.

An example of a study focusing on the *theme of improving adolescent reading skills by fostering reading motivation*, Kim et al. (2017) used an RCT to examine the impact of a new approach, strategic adolescent reading intervention (STARI), on the reading outcomes of adolescent struggling readers who might be reluctant to read and experience low reading motivation. The authors sought to design a framework to promote reading growth by embedding instruction of basic reading skills within challenging content that students can connect to while fostering motivation by supporting self-efficacy, collaboration, and reading engagement. Participants were students in grades 6–8 who had scored below the proficient level on a state literacy assessment and were randomly assigned to the STARI or BAU condition. Students received the intervention during an elective or whole-school intervention period 3–5 days per week across the school year. The intervention was constructed in thematic units addressing complex topics of high interest related to students' social and cultural experiences, with numerous opportunities for students to express their views in discussions and debate. Teachers used researcher-made workbooks for individual and collaborative decoding, fluency, and comprehension practice within engaging and relevant text, along with novels, nonfiction books, and daily lessons for each unit. Students practiced words taught through decoding instruction and morphological analysis in fluency passages with partners, and partner discussion activities emphasizing differing perspectives were part of the fluency cycle. Students in the STARI condition significantly outperformed their peers on measures of word recognition ($d = 0.20$) and morphological awareness ($d = 0.18$). Generally, other outcomes, though not significant, revealed a positive trend suggesting improvement in skills required for reading comprehension. Authors reported a statistically significant mediating effect of engagement on word recognition ($d = 0.35$), morphological awareness ($d = 0.18$), and reading comprehension ($d = 0.35$).

The next study also reinforces the theme that *although it is harder to improve reading performance for older students, it is possible.* Lovett and colleagues (Lovett et al., 2020) conducted a large RCT to test the immediate and 1-year follow-up effects of two PHAST intervention conditions (compared to a special education control condition) provided across the school year in middle school settings for struggling readers in grades 6–8 who scored 1 SD below age-based norms on a broad measure of reading achievement. Students were excluded if they had IQ scores below 75, had English as a second language, or had other sensory impairments or serious mental health issues. Both PHAST conditions were implemented by researcher-hired and trained staff and included the key PHAST decoding and word-identification strategies we described in their elementary study, with some adaptations, such as selecting age-appropriate reading materials. In the PHAST plus Comprehension condition, students were also trained to use and practice metacognitive strategies. In the PHAST plus Fluency condition, the emphasis was on building fluent use of the PHAST strategies across different levels of text, ranging from word lists to connected text. All PHAST conditions included motivation-building aspects to foster self-efficacy, motivation, and attribution of success to effort. The control condition comprised a variety of remedial programs provided by special education teachers in the school. There were no significant differences in performance across the two PHAST conditions, so these groups were combined for the analyses. Lovett et al. (2020) noted that students in the control condition did demonstrate growth on all 16 outcomes. Students in the PHAST conditions demonstrated significantly greater performance than students in the BAU Special Education condition on 8 of 16 outcome measures. Specifically, there were moderate to large effects on standardized measures of word reading ($g = 0.78$ for nonword decoding, 0.56 for word identification) and smaller effects on reading comprehension ($g = 0.36$). Further, students in the PHAST group exhibited a stronger sense of reading competence ($g = 0.61$). A year later at follow-up, PHAST students continued to grow on measures of word identification, sight word-reading efficiency, reading fluency, spelling, text reading accuracy, and oral and reading comprehension; however, they reported a decrease in their sense of competence.

Continuing with the theme of improving reading performance in older students, the next study *illustrated the positive effects of multicomponent reading intervention for older struggling readers in high school.* This study was another large quasi-experimental study conducted by Lovett and colleagues (Lovett et al., 2012). They recruited students in grades 8–9 who lacked basic decoding skills; these students scored below a standard score of 85 on three out of four standardized reading tests of word identification, word attack, or passage comprehension. (On average, the students' reading performance was between 1.5 and 2 SD below age-based standard scores.) Nearly half of the sample (45.6%) were English language learners (ELLs). Lovett et al. (2012) combined three intervention tracks for this multicomponent intervention. The first track was their PHAST reading program that was modified for older students by including relevant vocabulary and multisyllabic words and texts drawn from content-area texts. The next track emphasized text structure strategies. The third track included comprehension strategy instruction they called PACES (an acronym for the strategies taught: Predicting, Activating Prior Knowledge, Clarifying, Evaluating through Questioning, and Summarizing). This track utilized engaging, age-appropriate short stories and texts. The program emphasized metacognitive strategies, attribution retraining, and multiple examples for practice and generalization. In contrast to their prior studies, in which researchers delivered interventions, classroom teachers (English or special education resource room teachers) were trained by the team over 8–10 days, and researchers mentored teachers throughout the project. Teachers taught the program to small groups of 5–10 students as a regular credit-bearing course for one semester. Lovett et al. reported small to moderate effects on standardized word-reading measures (d = 0.45 for Word Attack, d = 0.15 Word Identification, and d = 0.34 for Passage Comprehension); larger effects were found on the proximal measures of letter cluster–sound combinations and multisyllabic words (d = 1.91 and 0.57, respectively). Within their sample, relatively younger students ended with higher standard scores on Word Identification and Passage Comprehension. Students who participated in treatment also received a 1-year follow-up test, and researchers observed decelerating trends on all measures except Passage Comprehension. Generally, students with higher initial vocabulary benefited more at follow-up across most measures. Lovett and colleagues concluded that their study indicated it is not too late to train word-reading skills, noting that high school struggling readers did show a modest narrowing of the gap in standard scores after one semester of PHAST PACES. Further, students were able to master letter–sound clusters and decode multisyllabic words.

Discussion

Our purpose for writing this chapter was to describe an evidence base for effective instruction and intervention for students with word-level reading difficulties. We began by providing a theoretical framework for how reading develops that explained how and why students may struggle to master word-level reading, and that provided a context for intervention components. Then we synthesized findings from a recent review of reviews and other recent meta-analyses and syntheses.

We also summarized findings from recent individual studies to highlight themes about successful RTI and MTSS approaches that have supported word-reading performance. When possible, we reported implications about student response to interventions given that a "persistent lack of adequate response to quality instruction is a marker of disability and educational need" (Miciak & Fletcher, 2021, p. 22).

Major Implications for Practice

Several major implications about improving word reading for struggling readers emerged from our review of meta-analyses and syntheses of studies conducted in the past decade; during this time frame, states have encouraged MTSS implementation as well as supports for students with dyslexia. First, the magnitude of effects was *generally* larger for early intervention than remedial intervention (but this varied at follow-up). Second, the magnitude of effects was *generally* larger for word reading than fluency and comprehension (within the primary grades, but not upper grades). Third, the most common *active delivery ingredient* was explicit and systematic instruction across code- and meaning-focused skills. Fourth, within the primary grades, moderator analyses indicated effects were relatively consistent for primary-grade students regardless of student risk status, intervention type, interventionist training, grade level, or hours of intervention. Within the upper elementary studies, Donegan and Wanzek's (2021) moderator analyses suggested effects were stronger when interventions included multicomponents and were conducted in the smallest groups (1–2). Finally, relatively limited intervention work has been synthesized for adolescents with word-reading difficulties, but converging evidence underscored the persistent nature of reading difficulties.

Other implications for practice that could inform MTSS implementation emerged from the corpus of individual studies conducted in elementary through high school, demonstrating what could move the needle in improving word reading. There were small to moderate effects on struggling word reading when researchers provided schools with additional training, resources, and infrastructure to support data-based decision making within Tier 1 and Tier 2; struggling students benefited more than in schools that implemented MTSS on their own. If schools have the resources to do so, it could be more cost-effective and efficient to immediately provide struggling readers with the weakest initial skills (Tier 3-like intensive intervention) rather than waiting to evaluate response to Tier 2. There also appeared to be emerging support for teaching a variety of decoding strategies to promote flexible word-reading skills. Some of the strongest effects were found when researchers implemented intervention, so it will be important to test these with school staff implementing. It was not too late to intervene with struggling readers in upper elementary in terms of training their single and multisyllabic word reading. There were mixed findings about the effect of mindset, motivation, or attributional components to complement interventions, with relatively strong effects in studies that embedded this training. By middle and high school, it took considerable time, intensity, and teacher expertise to move the needle on word reading for struggling students who appeared stuck in earlier phases of reading development. Finally, it is also worth noting that a similar intervention program (Lovett's PHAST) was robust across grade levels, when modified to be age-appropriate and when woven with additional intervention components.

Some Limitations and Directions for Future Research

As we mentioned, our intent in writing this chapter was not to provide an exhaustive and systematic review of all studies on reading instruction and intervention. Further, we acknowledge that our perspective on *effective*, *evidence-based*, and the *science of reading* within this chapter was informed by experimental and quasi-experimental research studies (e.g., National Early Literacy Panel, 2008; National Reading Panel, 2000; Petscher et al., 2020). This perspective was consistent with the *Every Student Succeeds Act* (ESSA, 2015) and the recommendations for judging the level of evidence by the What Works Clearinghouse. However, the reality in many schools has been that instruction relied less on research evidence and more on traditional teaching practices (e.g., Castles et al., 2018; Seidenberg et al., 2020) or on reading instructional curriculum or interventions that have not been validated through experimental research (e.g., Petscher et al., 2020). Future work using mixed methods and qualitative findings within traditional practices could also provide another perspective on what works.

Another limitation of our chapter was the quality and quantity of studies for students with persistent word-reading difficulties; we echo Austin et al. (2017) caution that there was a relatively limited corpus of research examining effects of Tier 3 interventions for students who had not benefited from prior instruction and intervention and would likely require sustained intensive interventions. In addition, as was noted by Stevens et al. (2021), the field could benefit from larger-scale and more rigorous studies of dyslexia-specific interventions in light of changes in legislation to mandate specific approaches and certain teacher training perspectives. Future larger-scale studies and meta-analyses are needed to understand how to scale up research to help more children read proficiently by attending to understudied moderators or individual differences in response that may or may not be related to students' lived experiences that may relate to resilience, including gender, ethnicity, race, language, or socioeconomic status of their home.

Future research is also needed to help resolve some ongoing debate in the field about how to address the specifics of reading instruction and intervention. As former classroom teachers, we were mindful that while controversy and debate can be healthy within the research community, they can confuse practice and policy, and our intent was not to contribute to confusion. In our role as researchers and teacher educators, many beginning and experienced teachers have asked us questions, such as, "Should students be taught to master phonological sensitivity? Is phonemic awareness enough? Should phonemic awareness *only* be taught with letters? How quickly should I introduce letters and grapheme–phoneme correspondence? Should I continue to teach the most common sight words while also focusing on decoding? When and how should I train students about phonetic rules and syllabication, along with teaching them to be flexible when applying these rules? When and how should multisyllabic irregular words be taught? Should teaching word reading still be a focus of interventions for older students? What is an optimal balance between decodable texts that support practicing words and patterns that are known versus challenging stretch text that is above an independent reading level?" Therefore, when possible, we reported where there appears to be consensus about what works as we understand it today, and we also acknowledge differing viewpoints and caution that research is evolving and that ongoing replication is needed, particularly as the counterfactual or BAU conditions shift.

Future research can further inform and refine instructional design to address such questions about optimizing reading instruction and intervention. We conclude with two examples of such studies for illustrative purposes. The first study, conducted by Vadasy and Sanders (2020), was intended to understand whether it was more promising to provide a slower or faster pace of grapheme–phoneme training and if it was beneficial to introduce units that varied in size (*single* letter-only vs. *mixed* two letters). Their findings suggested that faster rates of instruction had an impact on measures of letter–sound (d = 0.84), letter–sound writing (d = 0.59), and word reading (d = 0.30). Kindergarteners in the mixed condition made greater gains across measures (median d = 0.86). In the second example, across three very brief studies, Gonzalez-Frey and Ehri (2021) compared two methods of decoding instruction to support the transition from the partial to the full alphabetic phase. Participating kindergarten students had not yet learned to decode, but they had mastered the particular letter sounds targeted for instruction. These included five consonants with continuous sounds (f, l, m, n, and s), five consonants with stop sounds (b, d, k, p, and t), and three short vowels (a, i, and o). The two methods contrasted training students to sound out the CVC nonwords using (1) *connected phonation* without pausing between sounds (e.g., mmmmaaaaaffff) or (2) *segmented phonation* with a pause between sounds and then blending them together (nnnn - iiii - ffff). The first author trained students individually for a 20-minute session. In the first two studies, students had already been trained to pause between sounds through their core program, and if these students were assigned to the connected phonation condition, they continued to pause despite training. Therefore, for their third study, the researchers included only students with no prior decoding instruction. They also tested a larger number of students with a greater variety of pretests to determine whether students could blend and segment or if they knew any high-frequency sight words. The students in the connected condition learned to decode in significantly fewer attempts than those in the segmented condition. They also performed significantly better on a transfer test for reading CVC words with stop sounds. Students' ability to read sight words, but not their phonemic awareness, predicted their performance on the transfer task.

To conclude, the evidence for the efficacy of systematic and explicit word-reading instruction and intervention continues to accumulate. Prevention and early intervention may be more effective, but follow-up studies indicate that without ongoing support, the effects may fade, particularly over summers when students receive no instruction. Our review suggests that if schools could use these interventions at the intended intensity, it is possible for more students to achieve grade-level word reading. Future research is also needed to confirm which approach works longer term and for whom, in addition to replication with larger samples and follow-up testing, before translating these findings into practice. We do not yet have evidence about how to move students reading at a basic or below-basic level to a proficient level to ensure they can read for comprehension and learn from what they are reading. More robust interventions are needed for those who need sustained interventions to further test promising components that could promote resilience, such as motivation, attribution, goal setting, and flexible decoding. We also note that this corpus of research has had relatively more attention in the elementary grades than in middle or high school grades, and studies in these grade levels indicate it is very challenging to accelerate reading without ongoing intervention. An important next step is to encourage additional research–school partnerships to scale the evidence about what works and help schools use this evidence within MTSS and within special education.

ACKNOWLEDGMENTS

The research reported here was supported by the Institute of Education Sciences, U.S. Department of Education, through Grant R305A200397 to Southern Methodist University. The opinions expressed are those of the authors and do not represent views of the Institute or the U.S. Department of Education.

REFERENCES

Adams, M. J. (1990). *Beginning to read: Thinking and learning about print.* MIT Press.

Adams, M. J. (2011). The relation between alphabetic basics, word recognition, and reading. In S. J. Samuels & A. E. Farstrup (Eds.), *What research has to say about reading instruction* (pp. 4–24). International Reading Association.

Al Otaiba, S., Connor, C. M., Folsom, J. S., Wanzek, J., Greulich, L., Schatschneider, C., & Wagner, R. K. (2014). To wait in Tier 1 or intervene immediately: A randomized experiment examining first-grade response to intervention in reading. *Exceptional Children, 81*(1), 11–27.

Al Otaiba, S., & Fuchs, D. (2006). Who are the young children for whom best practices in reading are ineffective? An experimental and longitudinal study. *Journal of Learning Disabilities, 39*(5), 414–431.

Al Otaiba, S., Kim, Y. S., Wanzek, J., Petscher, Y., & Wagner, R. K. (2014). Long-term effects of first-grade multitier intervention. *Journal of Research on Educational Effectiveness, 7*(3), 250–267.

Al Otaiba, S., McMaster, K., Wanzek, J., & Zaru, M. W. (2023). What we know and need to know about literacy interventions for elementary students with reading difficulties and disabilities, including dyslexia. *Reading Research Quarterly, 58*(2), 313–332.

Apel, K., Wolter, J. A., & Masterson, J. J. (2006). Effects of phonotactic and orthotactic probabilities during fast mapping on 5-year-olds' learning to spell. *Developmental Neuropsychology, 29*(1), 21–42.

Archer, A. L., Gleason, M. M., & Vachon, V. (2005). *REWARDS secondary.* Sopris West.

Austin, C. R., Vaughn, S., & McClelland, A. M. (2017). Intensive reading interventions for inadequate responders in grades K–3: A synthesis. *Learning Disability Quarterly, 40*(4), 191–210.

Balu, R., Zhu, P., Doolittle, F., Schiller, E., Jenkins, J., & Gersten, R. (2015). *Evaluation of response to intervention practices for elementary school reading* (NCEE 2016-4000). National Center for Education Evaluation and Regional Assistance.

Berkeley, S., Scanlon, D., Bailey, T. R., Sutton, J. C., & Sacco, D. M. (2020). A snapshot of RTI implementation a decade later: New picture, same story. *Journal of Learning Disabilities, 53*(5), 332–342.

Bhattacharya, A. (2020). Syllabic versus morphemic analyses: Teaching multisyllabic word reading to older struggling readers. *Journal of Adolescent & Adult Literacy, 63*(5), 491–497.

Bhattacharya, A., & Ehri, L. C. (2004). Graphosyllabic analysis helps adolescent struggling readers read and spell words. *Journal of Learning Disabilities, 37*(4), 331–348.

Bowers, P. N., Kirby, J. R., & Deacon, S. H. (2010). The effects of morphological instruction on literacy skills: A systematic review of the literature. *Review of Educational Research, 80*(2), 144–179.

Brady, S. (2020). *A 2020 perspective on research findings on alphabetics (phoneme awareness and phonics): Implications for instruction.* Reading League. *www.thereadingleague.org/journal*

Castles, A., Rastle, K., & Nation, K. (2018). Ending the reading wars: Reading acquisition from novice to expert. *Psychological Science in the Public Interest, 19*(1), 5–51.

Catts, H. W., Herrera, S., Nielsen, D. C., & Bridges, M. S. (2015). Early prediction of reading comprehension within the simple view framework. *Reading and Writing, 28*(9), 1407–1425.

Catts, H. W., & Petscher, Y. (2022). A cumulative risk and resilience model of dyslexia. *Journal of Learning Disabilities, 53*(3), 171–174.

Colenbrander, D., Wang, H. C., Arrow, T., & Castles, A. (2020). Teaching irregular words: What we know, what we don't know, and where we can go from here. *The Educational and Developmental Psychologist, 37*(2), 97–104.

Crosson, A. C., & McKeown, M. G. (2016). Middle school learners' use of Latin roots to infer the meaning of unfamiliar words. *Cognition and Instruction, 34*(2), 148–171.

Daniel, J., Capin, P., & Steinle, P. (2021). A synthesis of the sustainability of remedial reading intervention effects for struggling adolescent readers. *Journal of Learning Disabilities, 54*(3), 170–186.

Donegan, R. E., & Wanzek, J. (2021). Effects of reading interventions implemented for upper elementary struggling readers: A look at recent research. *Reading and Writing, 34*(8), 1943–1977.

Ehri, L. C. (1987). Learning to read and spell words. *Journal of Reading Behavior, 19*(1), 5–31.

Ehri, L. C. (2000). Learning to read and learning to spell: Two sides of a coin. *Topics in Language Disorders, 20*(3), 19–36.

Ehri, L. C. (2020). The science of learning to read words: A case for systematic phonics instruction. *Reading Research Quarterly, 55*, S45–S60.

Ehri, L. C., & McCormick, S. (1998). Phases of word learning: Implications for instruction with delayed and disabled readers. *Reading & Writing Quarterly: Overcoming Learning Difficulties, 14*(2), 135–163.

Every Student Succeeds Act. Title 20 § 6301 to 7981 (2015). *www.gpo.gov/fdsys/pkg/BILLS-114s1177enr/pdf/BILLS-114s1177enr.pdf*

Fien, H., Nelson, N. J., Smolkowski, K., Kosty, D., Pilger, M., Baker, S. K., & Smith, J. L. M. (2021). A conceptual replication study of the Enhanced Core Reading Instruction MTSS-reading model. *Exceptional Children, 87*(3), 265–288.

Flynn, L. J., Zheng, X., & Swanson, H. L. (2012). Instructing struggling older readers: A selective meta-analysis of intervention research. *Learning Disabilities Research & Practice, 27*(1), 21–32.

Foorman, B. R., Herrera, S., & Dombek, J. (2018). The relative impact of aligning Tier 2 intervention materials with classroom core reading materials in grades K–2. *The Elementary School Journal, 118*(3), 477–504.

García, J. R., & Cain, K. (2014). Decoding and reading comprehension: A meta-analysis to identify which reader and assessment characteristics influence the strength of the relationship in English. *Review of Educational Research, 84*(1), 74–111.

Gonzalez-Frey, S. M., & Ehri, L. C. (2020). Connected phonation is more effective than segmented phonation for teaching beginning readers to decode unfamiliar words. *Scientific Studies of Reading, 25*(3), 272–285.

Goodwin, A. P., & Ahn, S. (2013). A meta-analysis of morphological interventions in English: Effects on literacy outcomes for school-age children. *Scientific Studies of Reading, 17*(4), 257–285.

Goswami, U. (2005). Synthetic phonics and learning to read: A cross-language perspective. *Educational Psychology in Practice, 21*(4), 273–282.

Gough, P. B., & Tunmer, W. E. (1986). Decoding, reading, and reading disability. *Remedial and Special Education, 7*(1), 6–10.

Graham, S. (2020). The sciences of reading and writing must become more fully integrated. *Reading Research Quarterly, 55*, S35–S44.

Graham, S., & Hebert, M. (2011). Writing to read: A meta-analysis of the impact of writing and writing instruction on reading. *Harvard Educational Review, 81*(4), 710–744.

Graham, S., Liu, X., Bartlett, B., Ng, C., Harris, K. R., Aitken, A., & Talukdar, J. (2018). Reading for writing: A meta-analysis of the impact of reading interventions on writing. *Review of Educational Research, 88*(2), 243–284.

Graham, S., & Santangelo, T. (2014). Does spelling instruction make students better spellers, readers, and writers? A meta-analytic review. *Reading and Writing, 27*(9), 1703–1743.

Hiebert, E. H. (2022). When students perform at the below basic level on the NAEP: What does it mean and what can educators do? *The Reading Teacher, 75*(5), 631–639.

Kamil, M. L., Borman, G. D., Dole, J., Kral, C. C., Salinger, T., & Torgesen, J. (2008). *Improving adolescent literacy: Effective classroom and intervention practices. IES practice guide* (NCEE 2008-4027). National Center for Education Evaluation and Regional Assistance.

Kearns, D. M. (2020). Does English have useful syllable division patterns? *Reading Research Quarterly, 55*, S145–S160.

Kearns, D. M., Rogers, H. J., Koriakin, T., & Al Ghanem, R. (2016). Semantic and phonological ability to adjust recoding: A unique correlate of word reading skill? *Scientific Studies of Reading, 20(6*), 455–470.

Kim, J. S., Hemphill, L., Troyer, M., Thomson, J. M., Jones, S. M., LaRusso, M. D., & Donovan, S. (2017). Engaging struggling adolescent readers to improve reading skills. *Reading Research Quarterly, 52*(3), 357–382.

Lam, E. A., & McMaster, K. L. (2014). Predictors of responsiveness to early literacy intervention: A 10-year update. *Learning Disability Quarterly, 37*(3), 134–147.

Lindamood, P. C., & Lindamood, P. D. (2011). *The Lindamood phoneme sequencing program for reading, spelling, and speech.* PRO-ED.

Lovett, M. W., Frijters, J. C., Steinbach, K. A., Sevcik, R. A., & Morris, R. D. (2020). Effective intervention for adolescents with reading disabilities: Combining reading and motivational remediation to improve outcomes. *Journal of Educational Psychology, 113*(4), 656.

Lovett, M. W., Frijters, J. C., Wolf, M., Steinbach, K. A., Sevcik, R. A., & Morris, R. D. (2017). Early intervention for children at risk for reading disabilities: The impact of grade at intervention and individual differences on intervention outcomes. *Journal of Educational Psychology, 109*(7), 889.

Lovett, M. W., Lacerenza, L., De Palma, M., & Frijters, J. C. (2012). Evaluating the efficacy of remediation for struggling readers in high school. *Journal of Learning Disabilities, 45*(2), 151–169.

Lovett, M. W., Steinbach, K. A., & Frijters, J. C. (2000). Remediating the core deficits of developmental reading disability: A double-deficit perspective. *Journal of Learning Disabilities, 33*(4), 334–358.

Mathes, P. G., Torgesen, J. K., Wahl, M., Menchetti, J. C., & Grek, M. L. (1999). *Proactive beginning reading: Intensive small group instruction for struggling readers.* Southern Methodist University.

Miciak, J., & Fletcher, J. M. (2021). The critical role of instructional response for identifying dyslexia and other learning disabilities. *Journal of Learning Disabilities, 53*(5), 343–353.

Nagy, W. E., & Anderson, R. C. (1984). How many words are there in printed school English? *Reading Research Quarterly, 19*(3), 304–330.

National Center for Education Statistics. (2025). *Nation's report card. National Assessment of Educational Progress.*

National Early Literacy Panel. (2008). *Developing early literacy: Report of the National Early Literacy Panel.* National Institute for Literacy. *www.nifl.gov/earlychildhood/NELP/NELPreport.html*

National Institute of Child Health and Human Development. (2000). *Report of the National Reading Panel. Teaching children to read: An evidence-based assessment of the scientific research literature on reading and its implications for reading instruction* (NIH Pub. No. 00–4769). U.S. Government Printing Office.

Petscher, Y., Cabell, S. Q., Catts, H. W., Compton, D. L., Foorman, B. R., Hart, S. A., & Wagner, R. K. (2020). How the science of reading informs 21st-century education. *Reading Research Quarterly, 55*, S267–S282.

Pugh, K. R., Landi, N., Preston, J. L., Mencl, W. E., Austin, A. C., & Sibley, D. (2013). The relationship between phonological and auditory processing and brain organization in beginning readers. *Brain and Language, 125*(2), 173–183.

Rosenthal, J., & Ehri, L. C. (2008). The mnemonic value of orthography for vocabulary learning. *Journal of Educational Psychology, 100*(1), 175.

Russell-Freudenthal, D., Zaru, M. W., & Al Otaiba, S. (2023). Early literacy, response to intervention, and multi-tiered systems of supports. In S. Cabell, S. Newman, & N. Patton Terry (Eds.), *Handbook on the science of early literacy* (pp. 43–59). Guilford Press.

Savage, R., Georgiou, G., Parrila, R., & Maiorino, K. (2018). Preventative reading interventions teaching direct mapping of graphemes in texts and set-for-variability aid at-risk learners. *Scientific Studies of Reading, 22*(3), 225–247.

Scammacca, N. K., Roberts, G., Vaughn, S., & Stuebing, K. K. (2015). A meta-analysis of interventions for struggling readers in grades 4–12: 1980–2011. *Journal of Learning Disabilities, 48*(4), 369–390.

Scarborough, H. S. (2001). Connecting early language and literacy to later reading (dis) abilities: Evidence, theory, and practice. In S. Neuman & D. Dickinson (Eds.), *Handbook of early literacy research* (pp. 97–110). Guilford Press.

Seidenberg, M. (2017). *Language at the speed of sight: How we read, why so many can't, and what can be done about it.* Basic Books.

Seidenberg, M., Cooper Borkenhagen, M., & Kearns, D. M. (2020). Lost in translation? Challenges in connecting reading science and educational practice. *Reading Research Quarterly, 55*, S119–S130.

Shapiro, L. R., & Solity, J. (2016). Differing effects of two synthetic phonics programmes on early reading development. *British Journal of Educational Psychology, 86*(2), 182–203.

Share, D. L. (1995). Phonological recoding and self-teaching: Sine qua non of reading acquisition. *Cognition, 55*(2), 151–218.

Solari, E. J., Grimm, R. P., McIntyre, N. S., & Denton, C. A. (2018). Reading comprehension development in at-risk vs. not at-risk first grade readers: The differential roles of listening comprehension, decoding, and fluency. *Learning and Individual Differences, 65*, 195–206.

Spear-Swerling, L., & Sternberg, R. J. (1996). *Off track: When poor readers become learning disabled.* Westview.

Steacy, L. M., Elleman, A. M., Lovett, M. W., & Compton, D. L. (2016). Exploring differential effects across two decoding treatments on item-level transfer in children with significant word reading difficulties: A new approach for testing intervention elements. *Scientific Studies of Reading, 20*(4), 283–295.

Stevens, E. A., Austin, C., Moore, C., Scammacca, N., Boucher, A. N., & Vaughn, S. (2021). Current state of the evidence: Examining the effects of Orton-Gillingham reading interventions for students with or at risk for word-level reading disabilities. *Exceptional Children, 87*(4), 397–417.

Suggate, S. P. (2016). A meta-analysis of the long-term effects of phonemic awareness, phonics, fluency, and reading comprehension interventions. *Journal of Learning Disabilities, 49*(1), 77–96.

Torgesen, J. K. (2000). Individual differences in response to early interventions in reading: The lingering problem of treatment resisters. *Learning Disabilities Research & Practice, 15*(1), 55–64.

Toste, J. R., Capin, P., Vaughn, S., Roberts, G. J., & Kearns, D. M. (2017). Multisyllabic word-reading instruction with and without motivational beliefs training for struggling readers in the upper elementary grades: A pilot investigation. *The Elementary School Journal, 117*(4), 593–615.

Toste, J. R., Capin, P., Williams, K. J., Cho, E., & Vaughn, S. (2019). Replication of an experimental study investigating the efficacy of a multisyllabic word reading intervention with and without motivational beliefs training for struggling readers. *Journal of Learning Disabilities, 52*(1), 45–58.

Vadasy, P. F., & Sanders, E. A. (2021). Introducing grapheme-phoneme correspondences (GPCs): Exploring rate and complexity in phonics instruction for kindergarteners with limited literacy skills. *Reading and Writing, 34*, 109–138.

Vaughn, S., Cirino, P. T., Wanzek, J., Wexler, J., Fletcher, J. M., & Denton, C. A. (2010). Response to intervention for middle school students with reading difficulties: Effects of a primary and secondary intervention. *School Psychology Review, 39*(1), 3–21.

Vaughn, S., Wexler, J., Leroux, A., Roberts, G., Denton, C., Barth, A., & Fletcher, J. (2012). Effects of intensive reading intervention for eighth-grade Students with persistently inadequate Response to Intervention. *Journal of Learning Disabilities, 45*(6), 515–525.

Vaughn, S., Wexler, J., Roberts, G., Barth, A. E., Cirino, P. T., & Romain, M. (2011). Effects of individualized and standardized interventions on middle school students with reading disabilities. *Exceptional Children, 77*(4), 391–407.

Venezky, R. L. (1999). *The American way of spelling: The structure and origins of American English orthography.* Guilford Press.

Wanzek, J., Al Otaiba, S., Schatschneider, C., Donegan, R. E., Rivas, B., Jones, F., & Petscher, Y. (2020). Intensive intervention for upper elementary students with severe reading comprehension difficulties. *Journal of Research on Educational Effectiveness, 13*(3), 408–429.

Wanzek, J., Vaughn, S., Scammacca, N. K., Metz, K., Murray, C. S., Roberts, G., & Danielson, L. (2013). Extensive reading interventions for students with reading difficulties after grade 3. *Review of Educational Research, 83*(2), 163–195.

Wilson, B. A. (1996). *Wilson Reading System.* PRO-ED.

Wolf, M., Miller, L., & Donnelly, K. (2000). Retrieval, automaticity, vocabulary elaboration, orthography (RAVE-O): A comprehensive, fluency-based reading intervention program. *Journal of Learning Disabilities, 33*(4), 375–386.

Youman, M., & Mather, N. (2018). Dyslexia laws in the USA: A 2018 update. *Perspectives on Language and Literacy, 44*(2), 37–41.

CHAPTER 12

Reading Comprehension Instruction and Students with Learning Disabilities in the 21st Century

Jeanne Wanzek, Katherine Sargent, and Sally K. Fluhler

Reading comprehension is a vital skill; it has been argued that reading comprehension is the most important skill students learn in school (Mastropieri & Scruggs, 1997). The ability to comprehend written text is not only necessary for learning throughout school years but is also a key skill for finding information throughout life (Vacca et al., 2011). The focus of interventions for students with learning disabilities (LD) is to help students improve their ability to read and understand text. Some reading interventions emphasize required foundational skills for accessing print. For example, the intervention may focus solely on phonemic awareness, fluency, decoding, and other necessary foundational skills. The purpose of these interventions is to ultimately improve access to and understanding of text, or reading comprehension. However, reading comprehension results not only from the ability to decode print fluently but also to extract meaning from the text being read (Klingner et al., 2015; RAND, 2002). This requires coordinating multiple interrelated sources of information to derive meaning from what is being read (Oslund et al., 2016; Perfetti et al., 2005).

Reading Comprehension

One theory of reading, the Simple View of Reading (SVR), posits that reading comprehension is the direct product of an individual's ability to decode words and their ability to understand the meaning of those words, often referred to as linguistic, or listening comprehension (Gough et al., 1986; Hoover & Gough, 1990).

The SVR holds that both decoding and listening comprehension are necessary but insufficient in isolation for reading comprehension. The SVR model explains roughly 60% of the variance in reading comprehension (Quinn & Wagner, 2018). The contributions of the components change over time, however. In first grade, the SVR accounts for 60% of total variance for reading comprehension, with 43% of that variance due to decoding and 36% of the variance due to listening comprehension (Foorman et al., 2018). In seventh grade, the SVR model accounts for only 53% of the total variance in reading comprehension. Decoding accounts for 25% of that variance, with listening comprehension accounting for 46%. By tenth grade, SVR accounts for 61% of total variance, with decoding accounting for 19% of the variance and listening comprehension accounting for 42% (Foorman et al., 2018).

A second theory, the Direct and Inferential Mediational Model (DIME), offers a more complex vision of reading comprehension. In the DIME model, reading comprehension is seen as a result of the relationship between five different areas: background knowledge, inferences, reading comprehension strategies, vocabulary, and word reading (Cromley & Azevedo, 2007). In order to comprehend text, students must not only be able to read and understand the words but also engage in metacognition. This requires students to self-monitor their understanding, make predictions and inferences, as well as be aware of text structure (Cain & Oakhill, 2006). All of these reading practices must be applied simultaneously to effectively comprehend text, especially as texts become more complex throughout the school years. When examining ninth-grade students, the DIME model was found to account for 66% of the variance in reading comprehension. Background knowledge (.34) and reading vocabulary (.41) made the largest contribution to this variance, with inference (.19), strategies (.13), and word reading (.15) making smaller but still significant contributions (Cromley & Azevedo, 2007).

Reading Comprehension and Students with LD

Despite the incredible importance of reading comprehension in both school and life, many students with LD struggle in their ability to read and comprehend text (Mastropieri et al., 2003). Indeed, reading is the most prevalent subtype of LD (Horowitz et al., 2017). Additionally, evidence indicates that we have not been successful in teaching students with disabilities to successfully comprehend text. When examining the most recent National Association of Education Progress results, only 12% of fourth graders, 9% of eighth graders, and 13% of twelfth graders with disabilities scored at or above the proficient level, indicating that these students are not demonstrating competency in the area of reading (National Center for Education Statistics, 2019).

While some of these students' struggles in reading may be the result of deficits in basic reading skills, such as decoding and fluency, difficulties with reading comprehension are also paramount (Klingner et al., 2015; Biancarosa & Snow, 2006). Students with LD may have difficulty monitoring their comprehension, including the ability to successfully apply the strategies good readers use to monitor their comprehension (Swanson et al., 1999). In order for these students to become successful and competent readers, they will need specialized instruction, specifically in reading comprehension.

Reading Comprehension Intervention Research

Previous research has examined the effectiveness of interventions addressing the reading comprehension of students with LD. In 2001, Gersten et al. (2001) conducted a review of interventions targeting reading comprehension for school-age students with LD. They found that strategy instruction interventions (e.g., using advanced organizers, summarizing each paragraph of a story while reading, and using self-questioning), targeting both narrative and expository texts, consistently improved reading comprehension for students with disabilities. They also found that teaching story-grammar elements was particularly effective for narrative text, while expository text required the use of multiple comprehension strategies being used at the same time. Over the last 20 years, additional research in the area of reading comprehension for students with LD has been conducted. A few research syntheses have begun to look at this body of research.

In 2012, Kim et al. conducted a synthesis of critical factors in interventions to improve reading comprehension for students with LD. The interventions in the included research implemented various components of instruction that might affect students' reading comprehension. They identified five critical factors related to reading comprehension instruction: instructional methods (e.g., instructional modifications or strategy instruction), self-monitoring, components of reading incorporated, fidelity of instruction, and instructional group size. They found that strategy instruction was shown to positively impact reading outcomes (*ES* = 0.48–5.23). They also found that self-monitoring was an effective tool, especially when combined with instruction in strategies like main idea strategy instruction (*ES* = 2.26). In addition, instruction that focused solely on comprehension (*ES* = 0.58–1.33) and instruction that addressed other areas of reading (*ES* = 0.07–1.78) were both beneficial. Vocabulary instruction was a particularly helpful addition to reading comprehension instruction (*ES* = 1.53), though the effects were based only on researcher-developed measures. This study provides key guidance to educators on reading comprehension from the first decade of the 21st century, though the identified effects are not specific only to reading comprehension instruction.

Solis et al. (2012) conducted a synthesis focusing specifically on reading comprehension interventions for middle school students with LD. They organized interventions into four categories: summarization-main idea, summarization-main idea with self-monitoring, multiple strategies, and other treatments. Some studies were included in more than one category. Of the 14 studies identified for this synthesis, 7 focused on summarizing or identifying the main idea. With the exception of one measure in one study, these interventions were effective with a range of effect sizes (*ES* = 0.56–6.66). One study, Mastropieri et al. (1996), emphasized reflecting on text meaning beyond summarizing the main idea and simple fact recall. The emphasis in the comparison condition was to recall facts.

The authors found no effects on a measure of fact recall (*ES* = 0.05), but they did find effects when examining students' ability to recall and explain the text as a whole (*ES* = 0.89). Self-monitoring, in addition to summarizing strategies, was examined in seven studies (two of these studies were also included in the summarizing or identifying main idea analysis). These interventions with self-monitoring were also found to be effective with small to large effect sizes (*ES* = 0.33–2.25). Only two studies were identified as examining multiple-strategy interventions (interventions that use three or more reading strategies). Results for these interventions were mixed (*ES* = -0.35–1.42). Specifically, in one study (Klingner & Vaughn, 1996), the results were mixed depending on how students were grouped, with those in peer tutoring groups outperforming those in cooperative groups on researcher-designed measures of comprehension, but those in cooperative groups outperforming those in peer tutoring groups on standardized measures of reading comprehension.

The goal of the present synthesis is to examine the effects of reading comprehension interventions for students with LD over the last 20 years. Specifically, we seek to answer the following questions:

1. What are the effects of reading comprehension interventions for students with LD in the 21st century?
2. What characteristics of the interventions are related to student outcomes?

Identifying Research on Reading Comprehension Interventions for Students with LD

We conducted a comprehensive search of the literature published in the 21st century to identify reading comprehension intervention studies for students with LD. We searched PsycINFO and ERIC from 2000–2020, utilizing terms related to reading comprehension interventions (*reading or comp**) in combination with search terms intended to target students with LD (*learning disab*, or reading disab*, or dyslex* or LD*). The search yielded a total of 8,609 abstracts for screening. We screened the abstracts and, when necessary, the full article to find the studies that met the following criteria:

1. The study was reported in a peer-reviewed journal and printed in English.
2. The participants included students with LD or reading disabilities (e.g., dyslexia); studies with additional participants were included if disaggregated data were provided for the students with LD or reading disabilities.
3. The participants were enrolled in grades K–12 inclusive (ages 5–18), or data were disaggregated for these students.
4. Interventions targeted reading comprehension in English and were not a part of the general education instruction provided to all students.
5. Interventions were provided as part of school programming (i.e., not including home, clinic, or camp programs).

6. Experimental, quasi-experimental, and single-subject designs provided a treatment and a comparison to determine the experimental effect. Single-group, AB single case, and case studies were excluded.
7. Dependent variables address reading outcomes in phonological awareness, phonics (including spelling) and word recognition, reading fluency, oral language/vocabulary, and/or comprehension.

A total of 13 studies met all inclusion criteria (see Table 12.1). Two studies were experimental studies; 11 studies were single case.

TABLE 12.1. Features of the Interventions

Study	*N*	Grade	Frequency (days/week; session min)	Duration (in weeks)	Group size	Implementer
Alturki (2017)	4 LD	6	NR 90 min	NR	2	Researcher
Alves et al. (2015)	3 LD	3/5	2x/week 30 min	5	2–3	Researcher
Ciullo et al. (2015)	7 LD	4–5	5x/week 45 min	6	1	Hired interventionist
Crabtree et al. (2010)	3 LD	12	3x/week 15–30 min	NR	1	Researcher
Firat et al. (2019)	3 LD	6	2x/week 90 min	8	1	Researcher
Fore et al. (2007)	4 LD	11	3x/week 30 min	6	9	Researcher
Fritschmann et al. (2007)	7 LD	9	NR 60–75 min	NR	4	Researcher
Jozwik et al. (2019)	4 LD	5	5x/week 32 min	NR	6	Researcher
Rouse et al. (2014)	2 LD	5	2–3x/week 30 min	NR	1	Researcher
Stagliano & Boon (2009)	3 LD	4	1x/week 15–30 min	8	1	Researcher
Stetter et al. (2011)	6 LD	9	5x/week NR	NR	3	Researcher
Taylor et al. (2002)	5 LD	3–6	NR NR	NR	1	Teacher
Wilder & Williams (2001)	91 LD	6–8	3x/week 45 min	NR	7–11	Teacher

Note. LD = learning disability; NR = not reported.

Coding of Articles

A coding sheet and tables were utilized to organize relevant information about each study. Data were collected on (1) participants (e.g., disability type and grade), (2) research design and methodology, (3) description of experimental and control conditions, (4) measures, and (5) results. There were two independent, experienced coders for each article. Any discrepancies were discussed until consensus was reached. For the two experimental studies, Hedges' *g* effect sizes were calculated using the means and standard deviations and *n*'s for each group.

Research Findings on Comprehension Instruction for Students with LD

We located only two experimental or quasi-experimental studies examining reading comprehension interventions in English for students with LD in the past 20 years. Both studies were conducted at the middle school level, and all included data to calculate effect sizes. In addition, we located 11 single-case studies; all but one of these studies used a multiple-probe across participants design. One study used an alternating treatments design. These single-case studies examined elementary (k = 6), middle (k = 1), and high school (k = 4). All of the studies measured outcomes on researcher-developed comprehension measures, most commonly comprehension questions about a passage. A summary of key characteristics of these studies is provided in Table 12.2 and discussed in the following sections for students in elementary, middle, and high school.

Elementary Grade Findings

Three single-case studies examined the effects of teaching students to identify story structure and complete story maps with their reading to identify the main story elements. All three studies noted improved comprehension for the students when the story map intervention was in place. Stagliano and Boon (2009) examined story mapping with third- and fourth-grade students with LD in a multiple-probe across participants design (24 sessions total). Training on the story map occurred for 3 days (15- to 30-minute sessions) before the student entered the intervention phase, when they had 20-minute sessions where students read an informational passage and completed a story map independently before answering comprehension questions about the passage. All three students demonstrated an immediate level change only at the time of intervention that was maintained throughout intervention and maintenance phases, suggesting positive effects for the story mapping intervention on students' reading comprehension scores.

Alves et al. (2015) also demonstrated overall positive results for a similar story mapping intervention, but the results were not as consistent as the Stagliano and Boon (2009) results. Three participants with LD in third or fifth grade participated in 8–10 sessions of intervention. Each student demonstrated a jump in

TABLE 12.2. Summary of Study Findings

Study/intervention	Measures	Findings		
Alturki (2017) • *T (Story Mapping):* Elements of story and story-mapping strategy taught. Guided practice for each of the elements while reading the nonfiction story aloud. Students completed story maps independently after reading the story. • *C (Comparison):* Students read the nonfiction story aloud until the story was completed.	Comprehension Test	$ES = 1.33$		
Alves et al. (2015) • *T (Story Grammar Instruction):* Researcher read a story aloud, provided instruction on story grammar elements, and filled out story map.	Comprehension Quiz	Baseline 0–80%		Intervention 50–100%
Ciullo et al. (2015) • *T (Graphic Organizer):* After reading a social studies passage, interventionist presented a graphic organizer summarizing information about the big idea question, people or groups of people, vocabulary, events, and how it changed America and people's lives. Students explained the main events and ideas of the graphic organizer, "teaching" the interventionist.	Social Studies Quiz Social Studies Test	Baseline/Pretest $M = 24.7–51\%$ $M = 26–83\%$		Intervention/Posttest $M = 57–84\%$ $M = 56.6–81\%$
Crabtree et al. (2010) • *T (Self-Monitoring of Story Elements):* Researcher trained students on how short fiction stories are structured, looking for information on main characters, what the story was about, and resolutions of conflicts. Students read a one-page fiction story with three stopping points for reflection.	Immediate recall of story facts Comprehension Quiz	Baseline 5–25% 0–60%	Intervention 52–65% 60–100%	Maint. 65–74% 80–100%
Firat et al. (2019) • *T (Think Before Reading, While Reading, After Reading [TWA] Strategy):* Researcher taught nine comprehension strategies taught with self-regulation strategies for use before, during, and after reading expository texts.	Text questions Generalization text Narrative Expository	Baseline 5.66–6.33 40–70% 25–37.5%		After intervention 11–14 60–80% 50–62.5%

Fore et al. (2007) • *T (Story Mapping):* Researcher provided direct instruction on how to construct a story map after reading a story. Students filled out information on the title; characters; setting; events in beginning, middle, and end of the story; and the main idea of the text.	Reading Comprehension Questions	*Baseline* *M* = 37.2–78.94%	*Intervention* *M* = 80–88.25%	*Posttest* *M* = 84.4–90%
Fritschmann et al. (2007) • *T (Inference Strategy Instruction):* Researcher taught students a strategy for reading text and answering multiple-choice questions about the text.	Comprehension Questions	Baseline ~20–60%	Intervention ~60–100%	Maint. ~75–90%
Jozwik et al. (2019) • *T (Self-Regulated Strategy Development):* Researcher provided instruction on how to monitor for text meaning using the TRACK strategy (think, react, ask, connect, and keep track of my thinking) while reading texts.	Strategy Use Comprehension Question	Baseline Median = 1.0–2.0 20–50%	Intervention Median = 3.0–3.5 75–85%	Maint. Median = 3.0
Rouse et al. (2014) • *T (Self-Questioning Strategy with Prompt Fading):* Researcher taught students to answer embedded questions while reading texts; then the embedded questions were systematically faded and replaced with a blank line for students to write a self-generated question and answer. Finally, fading continued to a stop sign in the reading to remind students to stop and ask questions.	Comprehension Quiz	Baseline 26–31% EQ 73%	SQ 73–84% Fade Q 66–81%	Maint. 88–100% General 56–81%
Stagliano & Boon (2009) • *T (Story Mapping):* Researcher reviewed and explicitly taught five story elements, explaining the purpose of using the story map while reading. Students filled in story maps while reading expository texts.	Comprehension Questions	*Baseline* *M* = 6.67–26.67%	*Intervention* *M* = 85–92%	*Maint* *M* = 86.67%

(continued)

TABLE 12.2. *(continued)*

Study/intervention	Measures	Findings		
Stetter et al. (2011) • *T (Computer Assisted Story Mapping):* Researcher modeled story mapping on the computer while students followed on computers. Then students independently mapped stories with computer prompts.	Comprehension Quiz	Baseline M = 8.60–12.80	Intervention M = 7.16–12.40	
Taylor et al. (2002) • *T1 (Story Mapping):* Teacher taught students to complete a story map using a think-aloud. Students filled in story maps while reading texts. • *T2 (Self-Questioning):* Teacher taught students to ask themselves 10 story-element questions at stopping points while reading text. Students had a card with the questions and audio-recorded their answers.	Comprehension Test	Baseline M = 4.28–7.28	Story Mapping M = 7.82–9.0	SQ M = 8.73–9.19
Wilder & Williams (2001) • *T (Theme Identification Program):* Teacher provided instruction about the definition of themes and the story topic. During and after reading, the teacher embedded questions and held a discussion about the main points/outcomes to derive the theme. • *C (Story Comprehension Program):* Traditional comprehension instruction emphasizing vocabulary and plot.	*Near Transfer* Concept of Theme Theme Concepts Theme Identification Theme Application *Far Transfer* Theme Identification Theme Identification Theme Application	 ES = 3.52 ES = 1.66 ES = 5.87 ES = .170 ES = 1.20 ES = 1.44 ES = 0.49		

Note. T = treatment; C = comparison/control; GORT-3 = Gray Oral Reading Tests–3; *ES* = effect size; Maint. = maintenance; EQ = embedded questions; SQ = self-questioning; Q = questioning.

comprehension scores when the intervention was in place; however, two of the students did have an increasing trend in their baseline data prior to intervention. All of the students demonstrated consistently high scores on the comprehension test of the passages when the story map intervention was in place. The posttest given 2 days after intervention ended remained high for two of the three students, but there were noticeable drops in scores at maintenance 2 weeks following intervention.

Taylor et al. (2002) examined story mapping compared to self-questioning in an alternating treatments design. The self-questioning treatment consisted of oral questions/responses about story elements. Thus, both treatments taught the story structure of passages, with only one treatment including the graphic organizer for mapping. Students participated in five 40-minute training sessions for each treatment. Students reached a high level of success completing story maps and answering questions accurately (81.9%–92.8% story map accuracy and 88.2%–94.6% self-questioning accuracy). Student comprehension of passages was similar across both conditions but significantly different than no intervention. Thus, differences between the conditions were largely between the use of the graphic organizer or only oral responding to questions on story structure elements. Overall, the three studies suggested upper elementary students could learn to use a story map with relatively brief training (3–5 days) and improve their comprehension of narrative text.

Ciullo et al. (2015) also examined a graphic organizer intervention, but with informational text rather than stories. A multiple-probe across participants design was conducted with fourth and fifth graders. The graphic organizer intervention covered the main ideas of social studies text. The teacher largely completed the graphic organizer for the student, though once every 3 days there were two boxes left blank for the student to complete. The teacher reviewed the graphic organizer with the student after reading, having the student repeat the information and asking questions about the information. The student then explained the graphic organizer content to the teacher at the end of the session. Student scores on the daily social studies quiz of the content in the reading for the session were consistently higher than baseline, with 97% of the data demonstrating no overlap between baseline and intervention. Mean pre- and posttest scores of the content showed gains in social studies knowledge after the set of intervention sessions across students (5–9 intervention sessions completed). This study demonstrated the graphic organization of content was successful for students reading informational text as well; however, students did not complete the graphic organizers independently, making it difficult for students to generalize this comprehension technique to independent reading.

Two elementary studies approached comprehension intervention with a strategy approach, teaching students step-by-step processes for better comprehending text. Jozwik et al. (2019) worked with four bilingual students with LD in fifth grade, providing seven to ten 32-minute sessions for each participant. The authors implemented self-regulation strategy development (SRSD), specifically the TRACK strategy, in a multiple-probe across participants design. The TRACK strategy consists of students (1) thinking while reading; (2) reacting by changing reading pace or rereading, as well as marking text that is interesting/important/connects or leads to a question; (3) asking relevant questions or marking the text where there is a question; (4) connecting by stating or marking a text connection; and (5) keeping track of thinking, which includes reviewing codes put into the text, answering questions, and positive self-talk about strategy use and text understanding. All four students demonstrated level changes in the TRACK strategy use and in correct comprehension questions answered at the time of intervention that were maintained over time with independent use of the strategy. There were no overlapping data points between baseline and the intervention for any student on either dependent measure.

Rouse et al. (2014) examined a self-questioning strategy with two fifth graders with LD in a multiple baseline across participants design. The self-questioning strategy was taught with prompt fading. First, students answered embedded questions in the text. Then, students were prompted in text to write a self-generated question about the passage and answer it. Then, the prompts for writing were slowly replaced with small stop signs to remind students to stop and ask themselves questions about the text and answer the questions. The intervention was implemented in 30-minute sessions, 2–3 days a week (23–27 intervention sessions). Although one student demonstrated an immediate level change with the introduction of the intervention that was maintained throughout treatment and maintenance, the other students' levels were much more variable and sometimes overlapped with baseline levels. The percentage of nonoverlapping data points was 100% for one student and only 51% for the other student. Thus, the data could not provide evidence of whether the self-questioning strategy with prompt fading was beneficial for multiple students. A training phase for answering the embedded questions stage was described, but there was no training described for helping students identify relevant questions to ask themselves throughout the text. The authors reported that all questions (embedded and self-questions) were literal questions. It is possible that students with LD may need either more explicit instruction in self-questioning or the opportunity to learn other types of questions beyond literal questions to more consistently improve their comprehension of text.

Middle Grade Findings

We located two experimental studies of comprehension interventions for students with LD in the middle grades in the past 20 years (Alturki, 2017; Wilder & Williams, 2001). Alturki (2017) implemented a story mapping intervention similar to the story mapping interventions described for the elementary grades. However, there were several issues with the study that make interpretation of the results difficult. First, the study only included the randomization of four students, and no pretest was given to provide any indication of equivalence of comprehension skills among the students at pretest. In addition, the duration of the intervention was not clear in the manuscript. The study was also unclear regarding whether the comprehension test given at posttest was on a new passage for both study groups or a passage that only the treatment group had worked through story mapping during intervention. Thus, it is difficult to interpret the very high effect size of 1.33 in favor of the treatment group.

Wilder and Williams (2001) examined an intervention to improve the identification of story themes for students with LD in grades 6–8. Classrooms were randomly assigned to the story theme intervention or a story comprehension comparison group. The intervention was implemented three times a week for a total of 12 lessons (45-minute sessions) with seven components included in each lesson: (1) discussion of the purpose of understanding story themes and background for the story in the lesson, (2) teacher reading of the story with comprehension questions, (3) discussion of six organizing story structure questions, (4) identification of a theme in a standard format, (5) application of theme to real-life experiences, (6) a multimodal (role-playing, art, or music) activity exemplifying the theme, and (7) review of the theme questions and developed theme. The comparison group read the same 12 stories but focused on vocabulary and the plot of the story in their discussions. Several researcher-developed near-transfer and far-transfer measures were given to students after the intervention. As would be expected, the highest effect sizes (Hedges' $g = 1.66$ to 5.87) were noted in favor of the treatment group on the near-transfer measures, and the treatment group significantly outperformed the comparison group for each of these near-transfer measures. These measures assessed students' concept of theme, identification of the themes taught in novel stories, and writing a story with the themes taught in the treatment. There were also large effect sizes in favor of the treatment (Hedges' $g = 1.20$ to 1.44) for identification of new themes not taught in the intervention with and without prompts; however, only the new theme identification with prompts was statistically significant. It should be noted that the prompts were the same questions used in the treatment instruction so that they would be more familiar to the students in the treatment group. There were also no statistically significant differences between groups on the measure where students wrote a story with the novel theme applied, though a moderate effect in favor of the treatment group was noted (Hedges' $g = 0.49$). Thus, the story theme instruction significantly improved student scores over the comparison group for the particular themes or with the theme prompts that were taught in the intervention. However, the effect sizes suggest the start of generalization to other themes for the treatment group.

One additional study using a single-case design was conducted at the middle school level. Firat et al. (2019) examined three sixth-grade students with LD in a multiple-probe-across-students design. SRSD was implemented. Specifically, students were taught the TWA strategy (Think before, While, and After reading) 2 days a week for 8 weeks in sessions that lasted 35 minutes to 2 hours, depending on the stage of the strategy. The TWA strategy includes teaching the student to (1) think about the author's purpose, (2) consider what the student knows and wants to know when reading, (3) link knowledge in the passage while reading and reread to understand, (4) identify main ideas, (5) summarize the information, and

(6) consider what the student has learned. All three students in the study showed improvement over baseline when in the intervention and postintervention, though the level increases for one student were minimal. Increases from pretest to posttest on the comprehension test for a generalization passage ranged from 5.34 to 7.67 points. Comprehension levels stayed similar at 3 and 6 weeks postintervention, signifying retention of the gains.

High School Findings

Four single-case design studies have been conducted in the last 20 years at the high school level. There were no experimental or quasi-experimental studies located for this grade level in the past 20 years. Three of the studies examined a story mapping procedure similar to the studies exploring story mapping at the elementary and middle school levels. One study examined inference strategy instruction.

Fore et al. (2007) examined a story mapping procedure with four eleventh-grade students. A multiple-probe-across-participants design was implemented to examine improvement in reading comprehension of a grade-level literature textbook. Students were provided intervention in 30-minute sessions, 3 days a week, for 36 sessions. Although all students had mean comprehension scores above 80% consistently in instruction and at posttest, the overall data across students did not show that these increases occurred only at the time of introduction of the intervention. Therefore, it was not possible to know that the comprehension scores of the students were due specifically to the story mapping intervention.

Crabtree et al. (2010) worked with three 12th-grade students to implement a story map intervention where students stopped at points during the reading to record the characters, setting, plot, problems/conflicts, and story ending. A multiple baseline across participants design was used to examine the effects of the story map intervention. In contrast to Fore et al. (2007), all three students demonstrated higher immediate recall and quiz scores on the story when the story mapping was in place. There were few overlapping points with baseline scores. Scores in maintenance (continued story mapping with fading of prompts) were also above baseline, with one student maintaining or continuing to gain after intervention was completed.

Stetter et al. (2011) examined nine students in ninth grade with LD. A computer-assisted story mapping intervention was implemented in a multiple baseline across participants design with replication. Students received two sessions of training where the researcher defined and clarified story elements and worked together with the student to complete a story map. Then, students independently read passages and completed story maps with computer prompts for the remaining sessions. Across six participants, there were few level or trend differences between baseline, intervention, and maintenance phases. Thus, the computer-assisted story map procedure did not seem to improve students' reading comprehension.

Fritschmann et al. (2007) also worked with seven ninth graders with LD in a multiple baseline across participants design. The authors examined an inferencing strategy intervention to use when reading a text with multiple-choice comprehension questions. The students were taught five steps: (1) preview text and questions, (2) activate background knowledge related to the topic or questions, underline key words in the questions, and mark the type of question, (3) find clues in the text that relate to the key words in the questions and formulate tentative answers, (4) look for additional clues to support tentative answers, and (5) go back to each question and be sure the answer is selected. Students were taught a mnemonic to remember the strategy steps. As a part of the process, students were taught to classify inferential questions into purpose, main idea/summarization, prediction, or clarification questions. All but one student with LD showed a clear level change in scores from baseline to intervention. Most students showed consistent or increasing scores on multiple-choice comprehension questions during intervention. After the intervention, students were asked to read a passage and answer comprehension questions on their own. Scores were generally similar to the intervention scores for each student. Overall, the inference strategy instruction seemed to improve students' ability to answer multiple-choice questions. The intervention was limited to reading text with multiple-choice questions provided, a context that is typically provided in some reading comprehension assessments. This was the only study that examined an inferencing intervention for students with LD.

What Do We Know? What Do We Need to Know?

There have been a limited number of studies (k = 13) specifically examining reading comprehension instruction conducted with full samples of students with LD in the past 20 years. It is promising that studies were found at the elementary, middle, and high school levels. There are more studies examining multicomponent interventions, for which reading comprehension is one component, for students with LD that were not included in this review due to the inability to determine the specific effects of the comprehension instruction. In our search, we also noted how common it is to conduct studies with mixed samples of students with LD and reading difficulties (who may be at risk for identification with LD). These mixed samples can be an artifact of the continued difficulty of accurately defining and identifying students with LD (Fletcher et al., 2019). Mixed samples of students who have similar reading traits (e.g., scoring below a specific percentile level on reading comprehension measure) often allow researchers to conduct larger studies that may generalize to more students. However, some students with reading difficulties, particularly in the higher percentile ranks, may not be representative of the difficulties that students with LD face in reading. Thus, from the most recent research with students with LD, we can identify some key instructional implications for reading comprehension, but additional research focusing on this population of students continues to be needed.

Our review provides support for teaching students to organize key information in the text. Story mapping, for example, has been examined at elementary, middle, and high school with generally positive outcomes, though a computer-assisted version of story mapping did not result in strong outcomes for students. Story mapping includes a text structure element, teaching students to identify the key structural elements of a narrative text, as well as a graphic organizer element where the elements are recorded. A single case study comparing story structure with the mapping (graphic organizer) and to a condition with story questions that only included discussion of the story structure without the graphic organizer demonstrated similar gains for the participants (Taylor et al., 2002). Similarly, a middle school study found positive effects for organizing the text around story themes, which also included identifying story structure elements and extending them to develop story themes but did not include a graphic organizer (Wilder & Williams, 2001). Students improved comprehension of stories with similar themes after intervention over students who solely discussed vocabulary and story plot. At the high school level, another single case study examining the use of a story map intervention also found positive effects on comprehension of the material (Crabtree et al., 2010). Thus, students with LD at varying grade levels seem to benefit from instruction in ways to organize key elements of a text, with the bulk of the research attending to narrative text and story structures.

The findings of our review continue to demonstrate the positive effects of strategy instruction, specifically SRSD, on reading comprehension outcomes for students with LD. One study did also provide strategy instruction for inference making with positive outcomes (Fritschmann et al., 2007). Different comprehension strategies at the elementary and middle school levels were studied. Key elements of these strategies included a step-by-step process for accessing key content in the text (including a mnemonic to remember the steps), explicit instruction on remembering and implementing each of the steps, and slow release of the process to student independence.

Gersten et al. (2001) identified similar instructional implications in their review at the beginning of this century. In contrast, the Solis et al. (2012) review of reading comprehension interventions for middle school students with LD located studies published largely before 2000, and the majority of these interventions examined summarization or main idea, areas that were not the focus of intervention in the more recent research reviewed in this chapter. The current research reviewed provides further examination of the strategy instruction and story-grammar interventions noted in the Gersten et al. review. However, we did not note any novel types or categories of reading comprehension interventions for students with LD in the research published thus far in the 21st century.

The studies we reviewed addressed the linguistic comprehension aspect of the SVR (Gough et al., 1986). More specifically, the studies largely addressed the comprehension strategies' contribution to reading comprehension (Cromley & Azevedo, 2007). Although some studies incorporated quick elements related to accessing background knowledge as a part of the instructional model, we found only one study addressing inferencing for students with LD. Inferencing ability has been noted as a crucial ability to understand text in studies of younger and older readers

(Ahmed et al., 2016; Barth et al., 2015; Cain et al., 2001; Cromley & Azevedo, 2007). This may be one area in need of intervention research for students with LD. Although outside the scope of this review on reading comprehension interventions, Cromley and Azevedo noted the high levels of variance in reading comprehension accounted for by background knowledge and vocabulary. Research on instructional strategies to successfully build student knowledge and language, including academic language, in multiple areas continues to be needed for students with LD (Cabell & Hwang, 2020; Schleppegrell, 2012).

The studies we reviewed included measures that were either highly aligned with the intervention or near-transfer measures. Near-transfer assessments can provide important information related to the specific effects of the targeted instruction practice, which is important for identifying the agents of change within an intervention that can be applied in practice or as a part of multiple-component interventions. The positive findings noted earlier need to be interpreted within this highly aligned context. The studies we reviewed provided no information on the extent to which interventions improved general reading comprehension beyond these more targeted measures, also an important area of measurement of the effects of intervention in assisting students, to accelerate learning toward grade-level expectations. In addition, few of the studies reported on the technical adequacy of the highly aligned or near-transfer measures, making the reliability of the results difficult to ascertain. The measurement aspects of evaluating the efficacy of reading comprehension interventions continue to be an area in need of further research (Clemens & Fuchs, 2022). The measures from the current review provide substantial information on what students learned specific to the subskill being addressed. It is also important to understand the type and duration of reading comprehension instruction required to accelerate the overall reading comprehension of students with LD. The lack of information available in the research on this practical matter requires additional attention.

Summary

Student abilities in linguistic comprehension, inferencing, and comprehension strategies, as well their background knowledge, contribute to a student's overall reading comprehension. We examined the most recent research on interventions in the area of reading comprehension for students with LD to identify effective instructional practices and areas for additional research. We noted limited studies of reading comprehension interventions, specifically with samples of students with LD over the past 20 years. Instruction to help students organize key ideas within text and strategy instruction was found to have positive effects on intervention-aligned or near-transfer reading comprehension measures. The corpus of studies was limited in experimental studies, effects on far-transfer or overall reading comprehension measures, and interventions addressing students' inferencing or comprehension of informational texts.

ACKNOWLEDGMENTS

The research reported here was supported by the Institute of Education Sciences, U.S. Department of Education, through Grants R324A190072 and R324A210021. The opinions expressed are those of the authors and do not represent the views of the Institute or the U.S. Department of Education.

REFERENCES

Ahmed, Y., Francis, D. J., York, M., Fletcher, J. M., Barnes, M., & Kulesz, P. (2016). Validation of the Direct and Inferential Mediation (DIME) model of reading comprehension in grades 7 through 12. *Contemporary Educational Psychology, 44–45*, 68–82.

Alturki, N. (2017). The effectiveness of using group story-mapping strategy to improve reading comprehension of students with learning disabilities. *Educational Research and Reviews, 12* (18), 915–926.

Alves, K. D., Kennedy, M. J., Brown, T. S., & Solis, M. (2015). Story grammar instruction with third and fifth grade students with learning disabilities and other struggling readers. *Learning Disabilities: A Contemporary Journal, 13* (1), 74–93.

Barth, A. E., Barnes, M. Francis, D., Vaughn, S., & York, M. (2015). Inferential processing among adequate and struggling adolescent comprehenders and relations to reading comprehension. *Reading and Writing, 28*, 587–609.

Biancarosa, C., & Snow, C. E. (2006). *Reading next—A vision for action and research in middle and high school literacy: A report to Carnegie Corporation of New York* (2nd ed.). Alliance for Excellent Education.

Cabell, S. Q., & Hwang, H. J. (2020). Building content knowledge to boost comprehension in the primary grades. *Reading Research Quarterly, 55*, S99–S107.

Cain, K., & Oakhill, J. (2006). Profiles of children with specific reading comprehension difficulties. *British Journal of Educational Psychology, 76* (4), 683–696.

Cain, K., Oakhill, J. V., Barnes, M. A., & Bryant, P. E. (2001). Comprehension skill, inference-making ability, and their relation to knowledge. *Memory & Cognition, 29*, 850–859.

Ciullo, S., Falcomata, T., & Vaughn, S. (2015). Teaching social studies to upper elementary students with learning disabilities: Graphic organizers and explicit instruction. *Learning Disability Quarterly, 38* (1), 15–26.

Clemens, N. H., & Fuchs, D. (2022). Commercially developed tests of reading comprehension: Gold standard or fool's gold? *Reading Research Quarterly, 57*, 385–397.

Crabtree, T., Alber-Morgan, S. R., & Konrad, M. (2010). The effects of self-monitoring of story elements on the reading comprehension of high school seniors with learning disabilities. *Education & Treatment of Children, 33* (2), 187–203.

Cromley, J. G., & Azevedo, R. (2007). Testing and refining the Direct and Inferential Mediation model of reading comprehension. *Journal of Educational Psychology, 99*, 311–325.

Firat, T. (2019). Effects of the TWA strategy instruction on reading comprehension of students with learning disabilities. *Educational Research Quarterly, 43* (2), 24–54.

Fletcher, J. M., Lyon, G. R., Fuchs, L. S., & Barnes, M. A. (2019). *Learning disabilities from identification to intervention* (2nd ed.). Guilford Press.

Foorman, B. R., Petscher, Y., & Herrera, S. (2018). Unique and common effects of decoding and language factors in predicting reading comprehension in grades 1–10. *Learning and Individual Differences, 63*, 12–23.

Fore, C., Sceiwe, K., Burke, M. D., & Boon, R. T. (2007). Teaching a story mapping procedure to high school students with specific learning disabilities to improve reading comprehension skills. *Learning Disabilities: A Multidisciplinary Journal, 14* (4), 233–244.

Fritschmann, N. S., Deshler, D. D., & Schumaker, J. B. (2007). The effects of instruction in an inference strategy on the reading comprehension skills of adolescents with disabilities. *Learning Disability Quarterly, 30*, 245–262.

Gersten, R., Fuchs, L. S., Williams, J. P., & Baker, S. (2001). Teaching reading comprehension strategies to students with learning disabilities: A review of research. *Review of Educational Research, 71*, 279–320.

Gough, P. B., & Tunmer, W. E. (1986). Decoding, reading, and reading disability. *Remedial and Special Education, 7*, 6–10.

Hoover, W. A., & Gough, P. B. (1990). The Simple View of Reading. *Reading and Writing: An Interdisciplinary Journal, 2*, 127–160.

Horowitz, S. H., Rawe, J., & Whittaker, M. C. (2017). *The state of learning disabilities: Understanding the 1 in 5*. National Center for Learning Disabilities.

Jozwik, S. L., Cuenca-Carlino, Y., Mustian, A. L., & Douglas, K. H. (2019). Evaluating a self-regulated strategy development reading-comprehension intervention for emerging bilingual students with learning disabilities. *Preventing School Failure, 63* (2), 121–132.

Kim, W., Linan-Thompson, S., & Misquitta, R. (2012). Critical factors in reading comprehension instruction for students with learning disabilities: A research synthesis. *Learning Disabilities Research & Practice, 27*, 66–78.

Klingner, J. K., Vaughn, S., & Boardman, A. (2015). *Teaching reading comprehension to students with learning difficulties* (2nd ed.). Guilford Press.

Mastropieri, M. A., & Scruggs, T. E. (1997). Best practices in promoting reading comprehension in students with learning disabilities: 1976 to 1996. *Remedial and Special Education, 18*, 197–213.

Mastropieri, M. A., Scruggs, T. E., & Graetz, J. E. (2003). Reading comprehension instruction for secondary students: Challenges for struggling students and teachers. *Learning Disability Quarterly, 26*, 103–116.

Mastropieri, M. A., Scruggs, T. E., Hamilton, S. L., Wolfe, S., Whedon, C., & Canevaro, A. (1996). Promoting thinking skills of students with learning disabilities: Effects on recall and comprehension of expository prose. *Exceptionality, 6* (1), 1–11.

National Center for Education Statistics (2019). *The nation's report card: Reading 2019* . Institute of Education Sciences, U.S. Department of Education.

Oslund, E. L., Clemens, N. H., Simmons, D. C., Smith, S. L., & Simmons, L. E. (2016). How vocabulary knowledge of middle-school students from low socioeconomic backgrounds influences comprehension processes and outcomes. *Learning and Individual Differences, 45*, 159–165.

Perfetti, C. A., Landi, N., & Oakhill, J. (2005). The acquisition of reading comprehension skill. In M. J. Snowling & C. Hulme (Eds.), *The science of reading: A handbook* (pp. 227–247). Blackwell.

Quinn, J. M., & Wagner, R. K. (2018). Using meta-analytic structural equation modeling to study developmental change in relations between language and literacy. *Child Development, 89*, 1956–1969.

RAND Reading Study Group. (2002). *Reading for understanding: Toward an R & D program in reading comprehension.*

Rouse, C. A., Alber-Morgan, S. R., Cullen, J. M., & Sawyer, M. (2014). Using prompt fading to teach self-questioning to fifth graders with LD: Effects on reading comprehension. *Learning Disabilities Research & Practice, 29* (3), 117–125.

Schleppegrell, M. J. (2012). Academic language in teaching and learning: Introduction to the special issue. *Elementary School Journal, 112*, 409–418.

Solis, M., Ciullo, S., Vaughn, S., Pyle, N., Hassaram, B., & Leroux, A. (2012). Reading comprehension interventions for middle school students with learning disabilities: A synthesis of 30 years of research. *Journal of Learning Disabilities, 45*, 327–340.

Stagliano, C., & Boon, R. T. (2009). The effects of a story-mapping procedure to improve the comprehension skills of expository text passages for elementary students with learning disabilities. *Learning Disabilities: A Contemporary Journal, 7* (2), 35–58.

Stetter, M. E., & Hughes, M. T. (2011). Computer assisted instruction to promote comprehension in students with learning disabilities. *International Journal of Special Education, 26* (1), 88–100.

Swanson, H. L., Hoskyn, M., & Lee, C. (1999). *Interventions for students with learning disabilities: A meta-analysis of treatment outcomes* . Guilford Press.

Taylor, L. K., Alber, S. R., & Walker, D. W. (2002). The comparative effects of a modified self-questioning strategy and story mapping on the reading comprehension of elementary students with learning disabilities. *Journal of Behavioral Education, 11* (2), 69–87.

Vacca, R. T., Vacca, J. L., & Mraz, M. (2011). *Content-area reading* (10th ed.). Pearson.

Wilder, A. A., & Williams, J. P. (2001). Students with severe learning disabilities can learn higher order comprehension skills. *Journal of Educational Psychology, 93* (2), 268–278.

CHAPTER 13

Direct and Extended Vocabulary Instruction and Intervention for Students with Learning Disabilities

Michael D. Coyne and Susan M. Loftus-Rattan

Vocabulary knowledge is understanding what words mean. When we listen or read, our knowledge of the meanings of words enables us to fully understand or comprehend what we are hearing or reading. When we speak or write, knowledge of word meanings allows us to express ourselves in precise and nuanced ways. Students with broad, rich, and extended knowledge of words and their meanings are not only better readers, they are also better prepared to understand and use language across all academic and social contexts. Many students with learning disabilities, especially those with language and reading disabilities, have less developed vocabulary knowledge than their peers without disabilities and are less likely to develop vocabulary knowledge through typical school practices. The purpose of this chapter is to describe effective practices for teaching the meanings of important academic vocabulary to students with, or at risk for, learning disabilities, as well as implementation strategies for maximizing the intensity of vocabulary instruction with the goal of decreasing the differences in vocabulary knowledge among students.

The Role of Vocabulary Knowledge in Overall Reading Ability

Students' vocabulary knowledge is strongly associated with their overall reading ability (e.g., Elleman et al., 2009; Ouellette, 2006) and is one of the strongest predictors of reading comprehension (Cunningham & Stanovich, 1997; Sénéchal et al., 2006). Researchers and practitioners have long recognized the importance of vocabulary knowledge and teaching vocabulary. For example, in their seminal report, the National Reading Panel (2000) identified vocabulary as one of five "big ideas" in reading instruction. Education standards, policy reports, and practice guides continue to emphasize teaching vocabulary as a top priority for teachers and schools (e.g., Common Core State Standards; National Governors Association, 2010; What Works Clearing House Practice Guides [Foorman et al., 2016]).

The Simple View of Reading (Gough & Tunmer, 1986; Nation, 2019), an influential model of reading comprehension, provides a helpful conceptual framework for understanding the role of vocabulary knowledge in overall reading. According to the Simple View, there are two underlying processes that contribute to successful reading: students' ability to decode words and text and students' ability to understand the words and text once they have been decoded. In other words, students use code-based skills, such as knowledge of letter-sound correspondences and decoding, to read words and then draw on their vocabulary and content knowledge to comprehend, or make sense of the words and text that they have read.

Supporting Vocabulary Development Through Oral Language

There are two important implications of the Simple View of Reading for understanding the role of vocabulary in reading. First, both processes in the Simple View, decoding and understanding, are necessary for reading success; either by itself is insufficient. Vocabulary knowledge therefore is central to overall reading. Even if a student has perfect word-reading ability, she will have no comprehension if she does not understand the meanings of the words she is reading. Second, the Simple View suggests that when students decode words and text, they are essentially turning written language back into oral language. They then use the same language processes they use when understanding speech to comprehend what they read. Therefore, according to the Simple View, oral language abilities directly contribute to reading comprehension. In other words, the development of students' oral vocabulary knowledge is central to their ability to understand what they read.

The importance of supporting vocabulary development through oral language activities, separate from text reading, is particularly important for students with learning disabilities who may be experiencing significant difficulties with decoding. These students will most likely not be able to access sophisticated academic vocabulary in the texts that they are reading to support their word-reading skills (e.g., decodable texts). However, because these students' language abilities are often more highly developed than their reading abilities, vocabulary instruction through oral language activities for these students can include a focus on more sophisticated academic vocabulary than instruction constrained by text at their instructional level. Therefore, teaching vocabulary through oral language activities, exposing students to sophisticated academic vocabulary through reading text aloud, and engaging in rich interactive discussions are primary and important ways that students with reading disabilities learn new vocabulary.

Profiles of Students with Reading Difficulties

The Simple View of Reading also helps us understand different profiles of students experiencing reading difficulties and those with specific learning disabilities in reading (Catts et al., 2005). Given the two processes that contribute to successful reading comprehension, decoding and understanding what has been decoded, students with reading disabilities may have difficulties with one or both of these processes. Some students' reading disabilities are primarily associated with decoding processes. This profile is often referred to as dyslexia (Tunmer & Greaney, 2010). Other students' reading disabilities are primarily related to processes associated with understanding language or text once it has been decoded. These students' reading difficulties are related to vocabulary, content knowledge, and listening comprehension. This profile is often referred to as a specific comprehension difficulty (Catts et al., 2006). Finally, some students with reading disabilities are characterized by difficulties with both decoding and understanding.

The profile associated with dyslexia has received a great deal of recent attention, and there have been important efforts to make effective and systematic phonics instruction accessible to these students. However, evidence suggests that a significant number of students with learning disabilities in reading have specific comprehension difficulties and that a majority of students with reading disabilities are characterized by difficulties with both decoding and understanding. A distinguishing characteristic of students with these reading profiles is less developed vocabulary knowledge. Therefore, an important focus of instruction and intervention for many, if not most, students with reading disabilities should be on supporting vocabulary learning.

The Association Between Vocabulary and Comprehension

There are a number of mechanisms that help explain the association between vocabulary knowledge and reading comprehension and overall reading ability (Anderson & Freebody, 1981). Perhaps the most straightforward of these is the instrumentalist hypothesis (Spencer et al., 2017; Stahl, 1991). The instrumentalist hypothesis posits that a student's comprehension of a sentence of oral or written language is dependent on that student's knowledge of the meanings of the individual words in the sentence. For example, in the sentence "The book Maria was reading was hilarious; she couldn't help but chortle out loud," a student would need to know what hilarious means to comprehend the meaning of the sentence. Additionally, depth of understanding of individual words facilitates a more nuanced and complete understanding of a sentence. A student who understands that when something is hilarious, it is not just funny but extremely funny will more fully comprehend the sentence.

The instrumentalist hypothesis also suggests a mechanism for how deep knowledge of key vocabulary can facilitate incidental learning of other words that co-occur in the same sentence. For instance, in the previous example, if a student knows that "hilarious" means "extremely funny," that provides important contextual information for understanding the meaning of the word "chortle" in the same sentence (e.g., if you are reading something that is extremely funny, you might laugh, or chortle, out loud). Therefore, according to the instrumentalist hypothesis, breadth of vocabulary knowledge and a deep understanding of individual words can theoretically have a generative effect on further vocabulary learning through incidental learning of unknown, or less known, vocabulary that co-occur in sentences or text with known words.

The instrumentalist hypothesis has important implications for supporting vocabulary development and teaching vocabulary to students with reading disabilities and those experiencing reading difficulties (Coyne et al., 2015). Because knowledge of individual words directly supports comprehension of sentences that include those words, teaching the meanings of target vocabulary should theoretically improve local comprehension of sentences or passages that contain taught vocabulary. Moreover, because knowledge of the meanings of key words can accelerate incidental learning of other unknown words that are heard or read in conjunction with known vocabulary, an approach to vocabulary instruction that includes both teaching the meanings of individual words but also provides students with opportunities to develop deep and flexible understanding of those words could lead to incremental accumulation of breadth of overall general vocabulary knowledge.

Rich and Extended Vocabulary Instruction

There is a substantial evidence base that supports the efficacy of directly teaching the meanings of academic vocabulary (Beck et al., 2013; Coyne et al., 2022; Foorman et al., 2016; Marulis & Neuman, 2010). Increasing evidence across studies suggests that direct and extended vocabulary instruction has a positive and meaningful impact on the vocabulary learning of elementary-grade students, particularly words targeted for instruction (e.g., Beck & McKeown, 2007; Goldstein et al., 2016; Justice et al., 2005; Lonigan & Phillips, 2016; Nelson et al., 2011; Silverman, 2007). Convergent evidence also supports the effects of direct vocabulary instruction on the word learning of students with reading and language disabilities and at risk for experiencing reading difficulties (Jitendra et al., 2004; Marulis & Neuman, 2013).

Over the past 15 years, our team has been engaged in research evaluating the effects of direct and extended vocabulary instruction and intervention for young students at risk for experiencing language and literacy difficulties and disabilities. Across studies, we found that an instructional approach that directly teaches the meanings of important academic vocabulary through extended and interactive activities produced greater breadth and depth of word learning than approaches that were less explicit, less interactive, and more incidental (e.g., Coyne et al., 2007, 2009). We also found that direct and extended vocabulary instruction is effective in both whole-class (Coyne et al., 2010) and small-group formats (Loftus et al., 2010).

In our most recent program of research (Coyne et al., 2022), we evaluated the effects of direct and extended vocabulary instruction delivered as a small-group intervention that supplemented classroom vocabulary instruction. Participants included kindergarten students who were identified as at risk for language and reading difficulties and disabilities with scores on a standardized measure of overall vocabulary knowledge below the 30th percentile (i.e., Peabody Picture Vocabulary Test [PPVT]). The average score of participating students was at the 13th percentile. School-based interventionists provided 30 minutes of small-group vocabulary instruction four times per week between November and May. We found large effects of vocabulary instruction on the word learning of at-risk students randomly assigned to the intervention compared to at-risk students who only received classroom vocabulary instruction on measures of receptive and expressive target word knowledge, with Hedges' g effect sizes of 1.14 and 1.05. We also found effects of the vocabulary intervention on a measure of listening comprehension of passages that included taught vocabulary ($g = .47$). We found similar effects in a closely aligned replication study (Coyne et al., 2019), further supporting the efficacy of our approach to direct and extended vocabulary instruction. Finally, we followed participants in the kindergarten study through the end of second grade and continued to find statistically significant effects of our intervention, suggesting that the academic word learning that students experience through direct and explicit instruction is durable and sustained over time (Coyne et al., 2022).

Features of Direct and Extended Vocabulary Instruction

Our approach to direct and extended vocabulary instruction was informed by the work of Isabel Beck and Margaret McKeown (Beck et al., 2013) and includes the following features: (1) selecting academic vocabulary to teach that are representative of the type of decontextualized language found in texts and that is common across content areas (Foorman et al., 2016), (2) developing clear and understandable definitions of words selected for instruction, (3) introducing target academic vocabulary to students in supportive and meaningful contexts, (4) teaching word meanings through explicit instruction, (5) providing students with extended learning opportunities that enable them to interact with academic vocabulary in engaging activities that promote deep processing, (6) providing students with immediate and specific feedback that reinforces their correct use of target vocabulary and corrects errors, and (7) reviewing target vocabulary over time by continuing to discuss words in different meaningful contexts and encouraging students to read widely.

Choosing Vocabulary to Teach

There are various approaches to selecting specific vocabulary words for direct instruction. One approach is to examine the frequency of words that are found in grade-level materials and to choose academic vocabulary that students will likely encounter in their reading or other classwork (Foorman et al., 2016). For example, the Academic Word List (Coxhead, 2000) and the Academic Vocabulary List (Gardner & Davies, 2014) identify academic vocabulary ranked by frequency along with related word forms. Another approach is to examine words that students typically learn at different grade levels and choose words to teach that are either at students' grade level or slightly above. One resource that has compiled grade-specific vocabulary is a word list that contains 5,000 root words that are likely to be known by students in kindergarten through sixth grade (Biemiller, 2009). These approaches to selecting vocabulary are geared toward determining a scope and sequence of words that can be taught at each particular grade level.

In our research, we selected words to teach based on a framework developed by Beck and colleagues (2013) that involves a tiered classification system based on word difficulty and utility. In their framework, Tier 1 words are common words that most students will know before entering school or through nonacademic oral language interactions (e.g., pencil, cat, and tree). Tier 3 words have narrow and often highly specific meanings related to particular areas of study and are better suited to be taught in content-area instruction such as science, social studies, or geography (e.g., nucleus, constellation, and latitude). Tier 2 words are unlikely to be known by students but represent known concepts, can be described in simple terms, and will likely be useful for students to know across content areas. These are words that students will see in their reading, hear in classroom discussions, or use in academic writing and discourse. These Tier 2 words (e.g., fortunate, solitude, and investigate) are a good fit for direct vocabulary instruction. This framework for word selection works well across grade levels and settings and allows teachers to identify words for instruction that are student-specific and already being encountered in books and other class materials.

Developing Clear and Understandable Definitions

The goal of vocabulary instruction is to teach word meanings to students in a way that will allow them to develop both receptive and expressive knowledge of each new word. An important component of this process involves selecting or developing definitions to use when teaching new word meanings. Standard dictionary definitions are often complex and difficult for students to understand. Learners' dictionaries can be helpful when thinking about student-friendly definitions but still may describe words in a way that is too complex for some students. Therefore, teachers should ensure that definitions used when introducing new words are simple, clear, and easy to understand. Students will have opportunities to refine their understanding of words as they continue to encounter them in various contexts over time, but during initial learning, students benefit from unambiguous, student-friendly definitions.

For example, the word *soar* is defined by Merriam-Webster as "to fly aloft or about." This meaning of the word *soar* also suggests flying high in the air and floating on air currents. Additionally, there is an alternate definition that relates to a quick rise in something, such as prices that are soaring. Including all of this information to students who are learning the word *soar* for the first time and who do not have any prior knowledge can be confusing. Instead, introducing the word *soar* with a meaning of "to fly" is a way to convey the central idea of the definition in a manner that is simple to understand. Over time and multiple exposures, students will be able to add nuance to their understanding of *soar* by building on this initial definition.

Providing Both Definitions and Context

Vocabulary instruction that relies solely on providing definitions for unknown words is unlikely to result in a rich understanding of word meanings. When students only learn definitions unconnected from examples, they are likely to rely upon memorization instead of processing word meanings at a deeper level. In order to support deeper processing, it is important to teach definitions in meaningful contexts. Introducing definitions in meaningful and authentic contexts helps students gain a full understanding of how words are used across different sentences and passages. A natural place to find useful contexts is in books. Selecting words for instruction that students will encounter while reading or listening to a text can provide a powerful learning opportunity to show examples of how new words are used in contexts that are meaningful and easy for the students to understand (Wasik et al., 2016). Another approach is to create one or more sentences that contain the new vocabulary word. For example, a sentence that could be used to teach the meaning of the word soar is, "Look at that bird soaring high in the sky." The supportive contextual information in the sentence can help students understand the word's meaning and how it is typically used in language or text. Finally, the use of pictures can also provide context that illustrates words' meanings. For example, showing students pictures of different things that soar in the air, such as birds, planes, and kites, can help to solidify their understanding of the word meaning. Using pictures to provide meaningful contexts to better understand definitions of new vocabulary is a particularly beneficial strategy for students with less developed word-reading skills.

Teaching Through Explicit Instruction

There are two main ways in which students learn new word meanings. One way is through incidental exposure or encountering words in written or spoken language (i.e., books or conversation). When words are encountered multiple times in supportive contexts, students gradually develop incremental knowledge of the meaning of these words. Incidental exposure accounts for many of the words in a student's vocabulary (Nagy & Herman, 1987); however, students with, or at risk for, language and reading disabilities are often less likely to learn from incidental exposure. First, in order to learn new word meanings, students must encounter them in their daily experiences. Students with learning disabilities are less likely to read widely because of word-reading difficulties and, therefore, have less exposure to sophisticated academic vocabulary. Second, the ability to infer a word's meaning relies on strong background knowledge and an understanding of the context surrounding the unknown word.

The second way that students learn new word meanings is through explicit instruction. Although it is not possible to teach the meanings of all words directly, introducing essential academic vocabulary through explicit instruction optimizes the likelihood that all students will learn important words and their meanings (Archer & Hughes, 2010; Coyne & Koriakin, 2017). Teaching vocabulary through explicit instruction means that teachers introduce new words and their meanings directly and do not assume that students will be able to guess or infer what words mean. Explicit instruction involves providing definitions using clear and consistent language and modeling how words are used in different contexts by carefully selecting or developing examples that illustrate a word's meaning. When a new word is introduced using explicit instruction, a teacher indicates that the word is new to the class, pronounces the word clearly, provides a student-friendly definition, and models using the word in context.

Providing Extended Instruction

The introduction of new vocabulary words through explicit instruction that involves providing a student-friendly definition and using the word in context can be referred to as embedded instruction (Coyne et al., 2009). One benefit of embedded instruction is that it is quick and relatively easy to implement. This allows teachers to introduce a large number of new word meanings, contributing to students' overall breadth of vocabulary knowledge. However, this approach alone may not result in a rich, full understanding of new words. Students' knowledge of individual vocabulary words develops over time on a continuum from no knowledge to varying levels of partial knowledge to more complete and full knowledge (Nagy & Scott, 2000).

In order to ensure that students develop more complete and nuanced knowledge of important academic vocabulary, direct instruction can also include more extended activities that go beyond providing a definition and initial context. Extended vocabulary instruction includes interactive activities that allow students to process the words deeply. These activities may involve asking students to create a sentence using the word (e.g., "Tell me about a time when you constructed something"), asking questions about the word that require a knowledge of the word's meaning in order to respond correctly (e.g., "What is an example of something you like to consume?"), asking students to identify examples and non-examples of the word (e.g., Does this picture show something that is hollow?), or having students categorize words and discuss how the new words are similar or dissimilar to other known words (e.g., "Which of our new words can we put together out of the following: immense, timid, and miniature? Why do immense and miniature go together?"). Studies have shown that extended instruction leads to greater depth of word learning than incidental exposure or embedded instruction (Coyne et al., 2009; Loftus-Rattan et al., 2016). It is important to consider, however, that extended instruction requires more time in both preparation of materials and implementation of instruction. Therefore, it may be beneficial to implement a combination of embedded and extended instruction in order to provide opportunities for students to increase both breadth and depth of vocabulary knowledge.

Providing Feedback

As described in the previous section, direct and extended vocabulary instruction involves active student engagement and participation. Student responses during interactive vocabulary activities allow teachers to get a sense of students' understanding and provide corrective feedback. Providing immediate, corrective feedback is an important part of explicit vocabulary instruction. Immediate feedback allows for any misunderstanding to be corrected quickly. An effective strategy for error correction involves providing the correct answer for the student and then allowing the student to have another chance to respond in order to practice the skill or demonstrate knowledge (Gersten et al., 2009). For example, if a student provided an incorrect response to the question, "Is a playscape delicate?" the teacher could reply with the following feedback, "A playscape is not delicate because it cannot be easily broken. Let's try again. Is a playscape delicate?" Feedback can also be used to elicit more comprehensive responses that require students to think deeply about the word meanings and use more extended language. For example, feedback such as, "That's right! Why does this picture show an example of an experiment?" can prompt students to use extended language and engage with new words beyond just giving yes or no responses.

Reviewing Vocabulary

The goal of direct and extended vocabulary instruction is to provide an opportunity for students to develop extended word knowledge that is durable over time and that becomes part of their permanent vocabularies. Students need multiple and ongoing exposures to words in supportive contexts in order to maintain word knowledge after initial instruction (Nagy & Scott, 2000). There is evidence that both embedded review (i.e., providing brief definitions of previously taught words as they are encountered in new situations) and extended review (i.e., leading students in activities related to previously introduced words) result in increased maintenance of word knowledge compared to words that were not reviewed at all (Zipoli et al., 2010). One strategy to review words that align with an embedded approach is to create a vocabulary word wall in the classroom. This allows students to see the words they have learned, and teachers can refer to the words on the wall and provide a brief definition when they come up in class discussions or reading materials. An example of a more extended approach to review is to create a review cycle for previously taught words and include one review activity at the end of each vocabulary lesson to ensure that students are encountering these words multiple times.

Differential Effects of Vocabulary Instruction

Converging evidence supports the efficacy of direct and extended vocabulary instruction for enabling students to develop rich knowledge of important academic vocabulary and to better comprehend text that includes that vocabulary. This research suggests that vocabulary instruction benefits all students. There is also evidence, however, that instruction may not be equally beneficial for all students and that some students respond differentially to vocabulary instruction. For example, students with greater overall vocabulary knowledge respond more strongly to classroom vocabulary instruction than their peers with less vocabulary knowledge (Austin et al., 2021). These students are often those who are at risk for language and reading difficulties and disabilities. In our own research, we found that overall receptive vocabulary measured at the beginning of the school year by the PPVT was highly predictive of target word learning during vocabulary instruction and moderated the impact of our intervention (e.g., Coyne et al., 2019).

This differential response to classroom vocabulary instruction can be explained by the Matthew effect. The Matthew effect was first used to characterize vocabulary development by Keith Stanovich (1986), based on the adage in the book of Matthew that pronounces that "the rich get richer while the poor get poorer." According to the Matthew effect, individual differences in vocabulary knowledge influence students' ability to learn new vocabulary, and this differential learning only increases the gap in vocabulary knowledge among students. For example, students at risk for language and reading difficulties and disabilities often have fewer early experiences with language and literacy or are less able to learn from those experiences. This can result in less developed vocabulary knowledge, which then impacts their ability to leverage existing knowledge to acquire new vocabulary during learning opportunities in school and during wide independent reading. This reciprocal causal relationship results in a cycle in which students with more developed vocabularies continue to outpace their peers with less developed vocabularies, resulting in widening differences in vocabulary knowledge over time.

Although the Matthew effect is most often used to describe natural vocabulary development, it can also be used to better understand students' response to typical classroom vocabulary instruction. In other words, although classroom vocabulary instruction benefits all students, students who already possess larger vocabularies will be better able to leverage their existing knowledge to learn more words during instruction, learn them better, and learn them faster than students with less developed vocabulary. Therefore, even effective direct and extended classroom vocabulary instruction may not be enough to accelerate the word learning of students at risk for language and reading difficulties and disabilities to levels comparable to their not-at-risk peers. In fact, according to the Matthew effect, relying on only whole-class, or Tier 1, approaches to vocabulary instruction may contribute to the widening of the opportunity gap among students.

Intensifying Vocabulary Instruction

Accelerating the vocabulary learning of students with, or at risk for, language and reading disabilities requires intensifying instruction. There are a number of ways that schools and teachers can intensify instruction for students experiencing learning difficulties (Fuchs et al., 2017). Some of these include providing instruction in smaller groups, increasing the amount of instruction, using instructional materials that support effective teaching, leveraging staff with high levels of training and expertise to deliver instruction, adjusting the scope and sequence or rate of introduction of content, and incorporating behavior and engagement strategies into instruction (Lemons et al., 2014).

Multi-tiered systems of support (MTSS), also known as RTI, offer schools and teachers a comprehensive schoolwide framework for intensifying instruction for students based on their academic and behavioral needs (Chard et al., 2008; Gersten et al., 2009; McIntosh & Goodman, 2016). In MTSS, all students receive consistent, high-quality classroom instruction, and those students who are identified as at risk based on universal screening measures take part in supplemental interventions. Interventions are typically delivered to small groups by trained interventionists using evidence-based programs and materials. Student learning during intervention is assessed using progress monitoring measures, and intervention is intensified or adjusted based on student response. Although there is growing evidence base supporting the effects of supplemental interventions for increasing students' code-based skills (e.g., phonemic awareness and phonics) implemented within MTSS frameworks, there is less research on the impact of supporting vocabulary learning within a tiered model.

In our most recent program of research described earlier in the chapter (Coyne et al., 2022), we were able to evaluate whether intensifying direct and extended vocabulary instruction within an MTSS framework accelerated vocabulary learning for kindergarten students at risk for language and reading difficulties and disabilities. We conceptualized our small-group vocabulary instruction as a Tier 2 intervention designed to align with, and supplement, classroom Tier 1 classroom vocabulary instruction. The small-group intervention intensified vocabulary instruction for at-risk students by increasing instructional time or dosage (providing 30 minutes of daily vocabulary intervention in addition to 30 minutes of classroom vocabulary instruction), incorporating review and reteaching of vocabulary introduced during classroom Tier 1 instruction, providing intervention in small groups of two to four students, using carefully designed and highly specified instructional materials, and providing training and ongoing coaching to interventionists.

We found that kindergarten students at risk for language and reading difficulties and disabilities who received Tier 2 intervention in addition to Tier 1 classroom vocabulary instruction experienced accelerated vocabulary learning compared to their at-risk peers who only received Tier 1 instruction. (These findings are described earlier in the chapter.) In addition, we found that at-risk students who received Tier 2 intervention displayed similar, or greater, target word learning as their not-at-risk peers who received Tier 1 classroom vocabulary instruction. These results suggest that Tier 2 vocabulary intervention that aligns with and supplements classroom Tier 1 vocabulary instruction can accelerate the learning of at-risk students to levels comparable to their typically achieving peers. In other words, intensifying vocabulary instruction by providing supplemental Tier 2 intervention within an MTSS framework was able to substantially decrease vocabulary learning differences among students, and at least for words targeted for instruction, counteract Matthew effects in vocabulary learning.

Summary

Possessing deep and flexible knowledge of words and their meanings allows students to fully understand what they read and hear. Many students with, and at risk for, language and reading disabilities have less developed vocabulary knowledge and are less likely to build vocabulary knowledge from incidental learning opportunities. Therefore, these students benefit from a direct and intentional approach to vocabulary instruction and intervention. Converging evidence supports the efficacy of direct and extended vocabulary instruction, especially for teaching the meaning of key academic vocabulary. Directly teaching vocabulary is effective during both reading instruction and during oral language activities (e.g., read-alouds and interactive discussions), which are particularly important for students experiencing reading difficulties.

Direct and extended vocabulary instruction includes (1) selecting important academic vocabulary to teach directly, (2) providing student-friendly definitions of target vocabulary, (3) introducing vocabulary in supportive and meaningful contexts, (4) explicitly teaching word meanings, (5) providing extended instruction that maximizes opportunities for students to interact with new vocabulary, (6) providing immediate corrective feedback, and (7) reviewing taught vocabulary across the school day and over time. Because students with language and reading disabilities may need additional support beyond core Tier 1 vocabulary instruction, small-group intervention can supplement core instruction to intensify support for these students.

Supplemental intervention delivered within an MTSS framework can maximize student engagement, increase learning opportunities, and support extended language use.

Finally, although there is an important role for targeted direct and extended vocabulary intervention for students with, and at risk for, language and reading learning disabilities, additional research could broaden our ability to support these students' language and vocabulary needs. For example, researchers could investigate the effects of sustained vocabulary instruction and intervention over multiple years, along with aligned and coordinated support for general language development. In addition, researchers could consider additional approaches to vocabulary instruction that may have more generative and indirect effects on vocabulary learning and comprehension, like those that focus on other language skills such as morphological, syntactic, or metalinguistic awareness (Nagy, 2007; Gottardo et al., 2018; Spencer et al., 2017).

REFERENCES

Anderson, R. C., & Freebody, P. (1981). Vocabulary knowledge. In J. T. Guthrie (Ed.), *Comprehension and teaching: Research reviews* (pp. 77–117). International Reading Association.

Archer, A. L., & Hughes, C. A. (2010). *Explicit instruction: Effective and efficient teaching.* Guilford Press.

Austin, C. R., Filderman, M. J., & Coyne, M. D. (2021). *Can early vocabulary instruction and intervention combat the Matthew effect?* [Manuscript submitted for publication]

Beck, I. L., & McKeown, M. G. (2007). Increasing young low-income children's oral vocabulary repertoires through rich and focused instruction. *The Elementary School Journal, 107*(3), 251–271.

Beck, I. L., McKeown, M. G., & Kucan, L. (2013). *Bringing words to life: Robust vocabulary instruction* (2nd ed.). Guilford Press.

Biemiller, A. (2009). *Words worth teaching: Closing the vocabulary gap.* SRA/McGraw-Hill.

Catts, H. W., Adlof, S., & Ellis-Weismer, S. (2006). Language deficits in poor comprehenders: A case for the Simple View of Reading. *Journal of Speech, Language, and Hearing Research, 49,* 278–293.

Catts, H. W., Hogan, T. P., & Adlof, S. M. (2005). Developmental changes in reading and reading disabilities. In H. W. Catts & A. G. Kamhi (Eds.), *The connections between language and reading disabilities* (pp. 38–51). Psychology Press.

Chard, D. J., Harn, B. A., Sugai, G., Horner, R. H., Simmons, D. C., & Kame'enui, E. J. (2008). Core features of multi-tiered systems of reading and behavioral support. In C. R. Greenwood, T. R. Kratochwill, & M. Clements (Eds.), *Schoolwide prevention models: Lessons learned in elementary schools* (pp. 31–58). Guilford Press.

Coxhead, A. (2000). A new Academic Word List. *TESOL Quarterly, 34,* 213–238.

Coyne, M. D., & Koriakin, T. A. (2017). What do beginning special educators need to know about implementing intensive reading interventions for students with disabilities? *Teaching Exceptional Children, 49,* 239–248.

Coyne, M. D., McCoach, D. B., & Kapp, S. (2007). Vocabulary intervention for kindergarten students: Comparing extended instruction with embedded instruction and incidental exposure. *Learning Disabilities Quarterly, 30,* 74–88.

Coyne, M. D., McCoach, D. B., Loftus, S., Zipoli, J. R., & Kapp, S. (2009). Direct vocabulary instruction in kindergarten: Teaching for breadth versus depth. *Elementary School Journal, 110*(1), 1–18.

Coyne, M. D., McCoach, D. B., Loftus, S., Zipoli, R., Ruby, M., Crevecoeur, Y., & Kapp, S. (2010). Direct & extended vocabulary instruction in kindergarten: Investigating transfer effects. *Journal of Research on Educational Effectiveness, 3,* 93–120.

Coyne, M. D., McCoach, D. B., Ware, S., Austin, C., Loftus, S., & Baker, D. (2019). Racing against the vocabulary gap: Matthew effects in early vocabulary instruction and intervention. *Exceptional Children, 85,* 163–179.

Coyne, M. D., McCoach, D. B., Ware, S., Loftus-Rattan, S., Baker, D., Santoro, L., & Oldham, A. (2022). Supporting vocabulary development within a multi-tiered system of support: Evaluating the efficacy of supplementary kindergarten vocabulary intervention. *Journal of Educational Psychology, 114*(6), 1225–1241.

Coyne, M. D., Neugebauer, S., Ware, S., McCoach, D. B., & Madura, J. (2015). Vocabulary and its role in early comprehension development. In A. DeBruin, S. Gear, & A. Van Kleek (Eds.), *Pre-reader comprehension: An essential building block to becoming a successful reader* (pp. 19–34). Brookes.

Cunningham, A. E., & Stanovich, K. E. (1997). Early reading acquisition and its relation to reading experience and ability 10 years later. *Developmental Psychology, 33,* 934–945.

Elleman, A. M., Lindo, E. J., Morphy, P., & Compton, D. (2009). The impact of vocabulary instruction on passage-level comprehension of school-age children: A meta-analysis. *Journal of Research on Educational Effectiveness, 2,* 1–44.

Foorman, B., Beyler, N., Borradaile, K., Coyne, M., Denton, C. A., Dimino, J., & Wissel, S. (2016). *Foundational skills to support reading for understanding in kindergarten through 3rd grade* (NCEE 2016-4008). National Center for Education Evaluation and Regional Assistance, Institute of Education Sciences, U.S. Department of Education.

Fuchs, L. S., Fuchs, D., & Malone, A. S. (2017). The taxonomy of intervention intensity. *Teaching Exceptional Children, 50*(1), 35–43.

Gardner, D., & Davies, M. (2014). A new Academic Vocabulary List. *Applied Linguistics, 35,* 305–327.

Gersten, R., Compton, D., Connor, C. M., Dimino, J., Santoro, L., Linan-Thompson, S., & Tilly, W. D. (2009). *Assisting students struggling with reading: Response to intervention and multi-tier intervention for reading in the primary grades. A practice guide* (NCEE 2009–4045). Institute of Education Sciences, U.S. Department of Education.

Goldstein, H., Kelley, E., Greenwood, C., McCune, L., Carta, J., Atwater, J., et al. (2016). Embedded instruction improves vocabulary learning during automated storybook reading among high-risk preschoolers. *Journal of Speech, Language, and Hearing Research, 59*(3), 484–500.

Gottardo, A., Mirza, A., Koh, P. W., Ferreira, A., & Javier, C. (2018). Unpacking listening comprehension: The role of vocabulary, morphological awareness, and syntactic knowledge in reading comprehension. *Reading and Writing, 31*(8), 1741–1764.

Gough, P. B., & Tunmer, W. E. (1986). Decoding, reading, and reading disability. *Remedial and special education, 7*(1), 6–10.

Jitendra, A. K., Edwards, L. L., Sacks, G., & Jacobson, L. A. (2004). What research says about vocabulary instruction for students with learning disabilities. *Exceptional Children, 70*(3), 299–322.

Justice, L., Meier, J., & Walpole, S. (2005). Learning new words from storybooks: An efficacy study with at-risk kindergartners. *Language, Speech, and Hearing Services in Schools, 36*, 17–32.

Lemons, C. J., Kearns, D. M., & Davidson, K. A. (2014). Data-based individualization in reading: Intensifying interventions for students with significant reading disabilities. *Teaching Exceptional Children, 46*(4), 20–29.

Loftus, S. M., Coyne, M. D., McCoach, D. B., Zipoli, R., & Pullen, P. C. (2010). Effects of a supplemental vocabulary intervention on the word knowledge of kindergarten students at risk for language and literacy difficulties. *Learning Disabilities Research & Practice, 25*(3), 124–136.

Loftus-Rattan, S. M., Mitchell, A. M., & Coyne, M. D. (2016). Direct vocabulary instruction in preschool: A comparison of extended instruction, embedded instruction, and incidental exposure. *The Elementary School Journal, 116*(3), 391–410.

Lonigan, C. J., & Phillips, B. M. (2016). Response to instruction in preschool: Results of two randomized studies with children at significant risk of reading difficulties. *Journal of Educational Psychology, 108*(1), 114.

Marulis, L. M., & Neuman, S. B. (2010). The effects of vocabulary intervention on young children's word learning: A meta-analysis. *Review of Educational Research, 80*(3), 300–335.

Marulis, L. M., & Neuman, S. (2013). How vocabulary interventions affect young children at risk: A meta-analytic review. *Journal of Research on Educational Effectiveness, 6*(3), 223–262.

McIntosh, K., & Goodman, S. (2016). *Integrated multi-tiered systems of support: Blending RTI and PBIS*. Guilford Press.

Nagy, W., & Scott, J. (2000). Vocabulary processes. M. L. Kamil, P. B. Mosenthal, P. D. Pearson, & R. Barr (Eds.), *Handbook of reading research* (Vol. 3, pp. 269–284). Erlbaum.

Nagy, W. E. (2007). Metalinguistic awareness and the vocabulary-comprehension connection. In R. K. Wagner, A. E. Muse, & K. R. Tannenbaum (Eds.), *Vocabulary acquisition: Implications for reading comprehension* (pp. 52–77). Guilford Press.

Nagy, W. E., & Herman, P. A. (1987). Breadth and depth of vocabulary knowledge: Implications for acquisition and instruction. In M. G. McKeown & M. E. Curtis (Eds.), *The nature of vocabulary acquisition* (pp. 19–36). Erlbaum.

Nation, K. (2019). Children's reading difficulties, language, and reflections on the Simple View of Reading. *Australian Journal of Learning Difficulties, 24*(1), 47–73.

National Governors Association. (2010). *Common core state standards.*

National Reading Panel. (2000). *Report of the National Reading Panel: Teaching children to read: An evidence-based assessment of the scientific research literature on reading and its implications for reading instruction: Reports of the subgroups.* National Institute of Child Health and Human Development, National Institutes of Health.

Nelson, J. R., Vadasy, P. F., & Sanders, E. A. (2011). Efficacy of a Tier 2 supplemental root word vocabulary and decoding intervention with kindergarten Spanish-speaking English learners. *Journal of Literacy Research, 43*(2), 184–211.

Ouelette, G. P. (2006). What's meaning got to do with it: The role of vocabulary in word reading and word comprehension. *Journal of Educational Psychology, 98*, 554–566.

Sénéchal, M., Ouellette, G., & Rodney, D. (2006). The misunderstood giant: On the predictive role of vocabulary to reading. In S. B. Neuman & D. Dickinson (Eds.) *Handbook of early literacy* (Vol. 2, pp. 173–182). Guilford Press.

Silverman, R. (2007). A comparison of three methods of vocabulary instruction during read-alouds in kindergarten. *The Elementary School Journal, 108*(2), 97–113.

Spencer, M., Quinn, J. M., & Wagner, R. K. (2017). Vocabulary, morphology, and reading comprehension. In K. Cain, D. L. Compton, & R. K. Parrila, R. K. (Eds.), *Theories of reading development* (pp. 239–256). John Benjamins.

Stahl, S.A. (1991). Beyond the instrumentalist hypothesis: Some relationships between word meanings and comprehension. In P. Schwanenflugel (Ed.), *The psychology of word meanings* (pp. 157–178). Erlbaum.

Stanovich, K. E. (1986). Matthew effects in reading: Some consequences of individual differences in the acquisition of literacy. *Reading Research Quarterly, 21*, 360–406.

Tunmer, W., & Greaney, K. (2010). Defining dyslexia. *Journal of Learning Disabilities, 43*(3), 229–243.

Wasik, B. A., Hindman, A. H., & Snell, E. K. (2016). Book reading and vocabulary development: A systematic review. *Early Childhood Research Quarterly, 37*, 39–57.

Zipoli, R., Coyne, M. D., & McCoach, D. B. (2010). Enhancing vocabulary intervention for kindergarten students: Strategic integration of semantically related and embedded word review. *Remedial and Special Education, 32*(2), 131–143.

CHAPTER 14

Intervention to Address the Needs of Students with Mathematics Learning Disabilities

Lynn S. Fuchs, Pamela M. Seethaler, Douglas Fuchs, and Daniel Espinas

Mathematics achievement is a strong predictor of quality of life, financial security, and life expectancy (Every Child a Chance Trust, 2009), and developmental trajectories in mathematics are established early and remain stable over time (Duncan et al., 2007). Mathematics learning disabilities (MLD) are about as prevalent as reading learning disabilities, with estimates ranging from 5.9 to 13.8% depending on the definition (Fletcher et al., 2018). Thus, schools need to act early to ensure children receive quality mathematics classroom instruction and, when needed, early services to prevent unnecessary MLD. Yet, research conducted over the past two decades demonstrates that early prevention is not effective for all students (Fuchs, Fuchs, et al., 2013). For example, Fuchs et al. (2005) showed that although a first-grade mathematics prevention program was highly efficacious at reducing MLD prevalence, 3–6% of students did not respond adequately (varying definitions of inadequate response were used). Thus, efficacious intervention is needed even when supplemental early prevention has been provided.

The focus of this chapter is scientifically structured intervention for students with MLD. Our emphasis is on the elementary grades, when identification of MLD often occurs and where much of the research on scientifically structured mathematics intervention has been conducted (Fletcher et al., 2018). We address three topics, selected because they represent major curricular strands at these grades and because they are foundational for success with more advanced mathematics learning: arithmetic, word problems, and fractions. We begin by providing background information on each aspect of mathematical cognition, a topic discussed in greater detail in Jordan et al. (this volume), and by describing the learning principles that constitute scientifically structured mathematics intervention. Then, for each topic, we feature a scientifically structured mathematics intervention to illustrate how these principles are applied; explain the activities constituting that intervention; describe the results of a randomized controlled trial testing that intervention's effects; and outline an additional study conducted by a different research team. Finally, salient issues are identified concerning scientifically structured mathematics intervention, with implications for future research.

The Importance of Arithmetic, Word-Problem Solving, and Fractions

Arithmetic

Arithmetic refers to simple computation problems (e.g., 3 + 8 = 11; 14 – 6 = 8) that are not solved by applying algorithms. Sometimes arithmetic problems are referred to as *basic facts*. Arithmetic problems pervade mathematics. Research shows that fluency with arithmetic is a pathway to success with third-grade algorithmic calculations and word-problem solving (Fuchs, Gilbert, et al., 2016) and remains a significant predictor of more advanced mathematics before and after students complete their Algebra I course in eighth or ninth grade (Cirino et al., 2022). Consensus exists that arithmetic is an essential form of mathematical knowledge (Kilpatrick et al., 2001).

To answer arithmetic problems, mathematically competent individuals, including children and adults, use a mix of strategies. This includes counting, decomposition, and automatic retrieval of answers from memory. To develop such skill during the primary grades, children require a reservoir of number knowledge. This includes understanding strong associations between number names and the quantities they represent and between number words and Arabic numerals. It also includes an understanding of addition and subtraction concepts and number line concepts. Many but not all children enter kindergarten with such knowledge (Duncan et al., 2007).

With a reservoir of number knowledge, children gradually develop efficiency with counting strategies to solve arithmetic problems. They first count two sets (e.g., 4 + 6) in their entirety (1, 2, 3, 4, 5, 6, 7, 8, 9, 10); then they learn to count on from the first addend (5, 6, 7, 8, 9, 10); then they learn to count on from the larger addend (7, 8, 9, 10). As their knowledge deepens about how numbers are decomposed into constituent sets, they come to understand arithmetic principles (e.g., cardinality, commutativity, and subtraction as the inverse of addition) and develop more sophisticated decomposition strategies for deriving answers (e.g., [4 + 4 = 8] + 2 = 10). As increasingly efficient counting and decomposition strategies facilitate consistent and quick pairing of problems with correct answers, associations are established in long-term memory, and students gradually favor memory-based retrieval of answers (Geary et al., 1987).

Many students with MLD are delayed in number knowledge development, and some do not respond adequately to early classroom instruction designed to solidify such understanding. Students with MLD also experience greater difficulty with counting, persist with immature backup strategies, and fail to make the shift to memory-based retrieval of answers (Geary et al., 1987). When children with MLD do retrieve answers from memory, they commit more errors, and their retrieval speeds are less systematic than younger, typically developing children (Ostad, 1997). Difficulty with automatic retrieval of arithmetic facts is a consistent finding in the MLD literature (e.g., Cirino et al., 2007; Geary et al., 2007).

Arithmetic is incorporated into the curriculum at kindergarten through second grade, although many general educators do not explicitly build arithmetic fluency (Miller & Hudson, 2007). Even so, typically developing students achieve considerable arithmetic fluency by third grade (Cirino et al., 2007). For this reason, early prevention services are important. When students still manifest difficulty in third grade, a pressing need exists for intervention, given the importance of arithmetic fluency within the more advanced topics introduced in later grades.

Word-Problem Solving

Word-problem solving (WPS) requires students to process text to build a mathematics problem model. They must identify and ignore irrelevant information, locate and determine how relevant quantities interact to create a problem model, construct a number sentence with a missing quantity to represent that problem model, and apply correct procedures to solve for the missing quantity. Perhaps due to its simultaneous demands on text processing and mathematics concepts and procedures, WPS is among the best school-age predictors of employment and wages in adulthood (Every Child a Chance Trust, 2009). Because WPS represents a major emphasis in almost every strand of the mathematics curriculum from kindergarten through high school, WPS difficulty also limits school success (Fletcher et al., 2018).

Yet WPS can be a persistent deficit even when computation skill is intact (Swanson & Beebe-Frankenberger, 2004), and the cognitive processes involved in WPS differ from and are more numerous than those underlying computation skill (Fuchs, Gilbert, et al., 2016). WPS thus appears to represent a distinct form of mathematical cognition. Even so, classroom teachers often neglect WPS instructionally by assuming WPS competence will naturally follow computational skill (Daroczy et al., 2015). When teachers do explicitly teach WPS, they often encourage superficial, error-prone strategies, such as using key words to determine operations (Powell & Fuchs, 2018).

WPS difficulty may, therefore, be harder to address than arithmetic difficulty, and WPS difficulty needs to be addressed for students with MLD with intervention specifically focused on WPS. This need is illustrated in a first-grade prevention study (Fuchs, Geary, et al., 2013) in which the main foci were number knowledge and arithmetic; word problems were included only to build number understanding and contextualize arithmetic problems. Findings demonstrated substantially stronger effects on arithmetic than on WPS, and arithmetic performance gaps with classmates decreased over the course of intervention while WPS performance gaps grew dramatically because WPS strategies were not taught.

Fractions

An important goal in the mathematics curriculum is to ensure that students consolidate whole-number and rational-number principles into a single numerical framework (Siegler et al., 2011). This is important for success with algebra and other forms of advanced mathematics learning (Booth et al., 2014). Unfortunately, this transition is challenging for many learners (Durkin & Rittle-Johnson, 2015; Siegler et al., 2011) due to confusion between whole- and rational-number principles and widespread application of whole-number strategies to rational-number concepts and procedures. This phenomenon is known as *whole-number bias* (Ni & Zhou, 2005). Despite widespread difficulty, rational numbers are differentially problematic for students who struggle in the primary grades with whole-number learning. Namkung et al. (2018) reported that students with below-grade-level whole-number skill in the primary grades are 32 times more likely to struggle with fractions than classmates with adequate whole-number knowledge.

Within College- and Career Readiness Standards (CCRS), the focus on fractions begins in third grade and remains strong through middle school. Understanding of fractions includes part-whole ideas (e.g., how many equal parts of whole number and how many items within set of items) and understanding of fraction magnitude (i.e., identifying fraction equivalencies, comparing and ordering fractions, and placing fractions on the number line). The National Mathematics Advisory Panel (2008) hypothesized that a focus on fraction magnitude instruction is more central than part-whole understanding for success with fractions and for advanced mathematics learning.

Intervention research supports this hypothesis. For example, Fuchs et al. (2014) found that improvement in fraction magnitude understanding, but not improvement in part-whole understanding of fractions, mediated (helped explain) intervention effects on fourth-grade students' fraction concepts and on addition and subtraction procedures. This suggests the need for a strong focus on fraction magnitude within intervention.

Scientifically Structured Mathematics Intervention

Studies have established predictive links between students' domain-general cognitive and linguistic resources and trajectories of mathematics development (Fuchs, Geary, et al., 2016). For example, reasoning (e.g., Fuchs, Gilbert, et al., 2016), working memory (e.g., Jordan et al., 2013), and language comprehension (e.g., Jordan et al., 2013) appear important for mathematics success. Because students with MLD often experience limitations in such cognitive and linguistic resources, *Scientifically Structured Mathematics Intervention* (SSMI) (Fuchs & Powell, 2021) is designed to compensate for such resources by relying on 11 principles. We organize SSMI's 11 principles within three phases of intervention design: structuring the mathematics content to be learned, structuring the introduction of new content, and structuring practice (see Table 14.1 for a summary).

TABLE 14.1. Eleven Principles of Scientifically Structured Mathematics Intervention

Structuring the mathematics content to be learned

1. Teach students to understand mathematics within problem types.

Structuring the introduction of new content

2. Introduce new problem types with worked examples.
3. Teach efficient solution strategies.
4. Provide explanations in simple, direct language.

Structuring practice

5. Structure practice so it is distributed.
6. Structure practice so that previously taught content is systematically reviewed.
7. Provide interleaved problem sets.
8. Provide support for correct performance as needed.
9. Structure practice so it supports students' self-analysis and self-explanations.
10. Provide corrective feedback immediately after students complete practice.
11. Incorporate practice activities designed to build fluency.

Structuring the Mathematics Content to Be Learned

The first SSMI principle concerns how mathematics content is conceptualized and organized in intervention. Based on schema theory (Sweller, 1994), structured MLD intervention *teaches students to understand mathematics within problem types* (categories or schemas). Arithmetic, for example, can be conceptualized and organized in terms of four problem types. The Small Step problem type (+/-0, +/-1, +2/-2) is best conceptualized and solved by counting up or down on a paper number line and then a mental number line. With the Doubles problem type (e.g., 2 + 2 = 4, 3 + 3 = 6, . . .), answers are committed to memory by practicing a doubles chant. The Number Set Parts and Families problem type (sets 5–18) is addressed instructionally with real and virtual representations, emphasizing the commutativity principle, subtraction as the inverse of addition, and efficient counting-on strategies to provide the basis for understanding, accuracy, and fluency.

The Small Step, Doubles, and Number Set Parts and Families problem types are invoked within the 2-Step problem type. For example, the answer to 4 + 5 can be derived by decomposing 5 into (4 + 1) and then retrieving the answer to the Doubles problem (4 + 4 = 8) from long-term memory and solving the Small Step problem (8 + 1 = 9) via the mental number line. The answer to the problem 11 – 5 can be derived by decomposing 11 into (10 + 1) and then retrieving the answer to the Doubles problem (10 – 5 = 5) from long-term memory and solving the Small Step problem (5 + 1 = 6) via the mental number line.

Some learners gradually discover schema without formal instruction on problem types as they note and assimilate similarities and differences among problems. Students with MLD, however, require structured instruction to build such understanding and competence. Framing a mathematics domain (e.g., arithmetic) in terms of problem types (or schemas) structures instruction and supports student learning.

Structuring the Introduction of New Content

The next three principles concern structuring the introduction of new content. Based on cognitive load theory (Cooper & Sweller, 1987), MLD intervention *introduces new problem types with worked examples* (Renkl, 2002). This includes modeling a solution strategy for the problem type using the worked example while explaining each step and why each step makes sense. Students gradually assume responsibility for explaining and working solutions as they develop competence with the concepts and procedures underpinning that problem type.

Also based on cognitive load theory, the next principle is that the *solution strategies taught within MLD intervention are efficient.* Efficiency means the solution strategy produces accurate solutions in as few steps as possible while capturing the essential ideas representing that problem type. A related principle, based on the well-established association between language and mathematics (Catts et al., 2005), underscores *the need for intervention to frame explanations for MLD learners in simple, direct language.* This includes using an active voice and vivid words while capturing essential ideas without cluttering explanations with irrelevant information or tangential commentary.

Structuring Practice

The final set of seven principles that guide MLD intervention concerns the structuring of review and practice. Cognitive science demonstrates superior learning (1) when *practice is distributed* rather than massed (Benjamin & Tullis, 2010); (2) when practice systematically includes *cumulative review of previously taught content* such that multiple problem types are included on practice sheets (Rohrer et al., 2015); (3) when *problem sets are interleaved* such that problems are mixed rather than blocked by problem type (Fuchs, Malone, et al., 2021); (4) when *support for correct performance is available* when needed (Sweller, 1988), which includes help cards that provide a problem-solving "map" to make thought processes transparent (Fuchs, Wang, et al., 2021); (5) when *self-analysis and self-explaining of work* occurs (Chi et al., 1989), for example, when students restate the gist of word problems in their own words or check the reasonableness of answers; and (6) when *corrective feedback is promptly provided* (Hattie & Timperley, 2007).

A final principle, again based on cognitive load theory (Sweller, 1994), is *the need to incorporate practice activities designed to build fluency.* Transfer of acquired concepts and skills to automatic processing is essential for integrating foundational knowledge and skills within more complex mathematics. The benefits of speeded practice, with immediate correction of errors, have been experimentally demonstrated for students with MLD (Fuchs, Geary, et al., 2013).

Arithmetic, Word-Problem, and Fractions Intervention That Incorporate These Eleven Principles

For each topic, we feature a validated intervention as a means of illustrating the application of SSMI principles, outline the activities that constitute the intervention, summarize a study testing that intervention effects, and briefly describe one additional prior study conducted by a different MLD research team.

Arithmetic

Galaxy Math is a validated arithmetic intervention at first grade. (See Fuchs, Geary, et al. [2013] for a fuller description of the Galaxy Math program.) Contact *https://frg.vkcsites.org/what-are-interventions/math_intervention_manuals* for Galaxy Math manuals for grades 1–3.

In terms of *structuring content to be learned*, Galaxy Math begins by building students' basic number knowledge (see earlier description). This provides a foundation for Galaxy Math's conceptually rooted focus on arithmetic, centered on the four previously discussed arithmetic problem types: the Small Step problem type, the Doubles problem type, the Number Set Parts and Families problem type, and the 2-Step problem type.

Galaxy Math includes five units. In Unit 1 (Lessons 1–18), instruction focuses on number knowledge. This includes understanding and mapping magnitudes to number words and Arabic numerals, making magnitude comparisons, sequencing magnitudes on the number line (0 to 20), forward and backward counting with and without the number line, part-whole understanding, cardinality and the successor principle, the identity property of 0, the commutative property of addition, addition and subtraction concepts, and the inverse relation between addition and subtraction.

As part of Unit 1's focus on the number line, counting-on, and addition and subtraction concepts, students learn the Small Step arithmetic problem type and efficient counting strategies for addition and subtraction. These counting strategies are central to Galaxy Math because they produce reliably accurate responses, which is important for developing long-term representations of problem stems with the correct answers and for supporting automatic retrieval of answers (Fuchs, Geary, et al., 2013).

The focus of Unit 2 (Lessons 19–20) is the Doubles problem type. Unit 3 (Lessons 21–52) addresses the Number Set Parts and Families problem type. Number Set 5, for example, includes 0 and 5, 1 and 4, 2 and 3; for parts 2 and 3 or 3 and 2, the family includes $2 + 3 = 5$, $3 + 2 = 5$, $5 - 3 = 2$, and $5 - 2 = 3$. Unit 4 (Lessons 53–66) focuses on tens concepts. A small number of students who advance quickly through many lessons also complete the Unit 5 review (Lessons 67–74). In these ways, across units, instruction focuses on the types of number knowledge required in the progression toward arithmetic competence. Instruction incorporates manipulatives and number lines: 0–19 in Units 1–3 and 0–100 in Units 4–5. Across units, tutors and students generate stories to represent addition and subtraction concepts and problems.

In terms of *structuring the introduction of new content*, each form of conceptual knowledge, each arithmetic problem type, and each number set begins with the tutor explaining and modeling worked examples representing the idea behind each problem type. Responsibility for explaining and executing strategies is gradually transferred to students. For example, when introducing counting-on for addition, the tutor initially explains the conceptual basis for the counting-on strategy using a problem (e.g., 3 + 4) by bringing the two parts represented with blocks together into a total and by showing how the solution to the problem is represented while counting up the number line.

Then the tutor models the "counting-in" strategy using fingers. The tutor holds up 3 fingers on one hand to represent the smaller addend and closes the other fist to "hold" the larger addend while gently tapping the closed fist against the other hand and saying the larger addend, 4. Then the tutor counts up the smaller addend, 5 (putting one finger down into the fist), 6 (putting another finger down), and 7 (putting the last finger down). The last number counted is the answer. This is repeated for multiple problems, as the student gradually assumes responsibility for parts of the explanation and demonstration, eventually executing the strategy independently, without reference to blocks or the number line. A similar process is used for subtraction, for which students learn to "count up." For 5 – 2 = 3, they count the difference between the numbers, saying 2 with a closed fist; then they count 3 (hold up a finger), 4 (hold up a finger), and 5 (hold up a finger). The number of raised fingers is the answer.

Galaxy Math *structures practice* in line with SSMI's principles. Take, for example, the Meet or Beat Your Score (MOBYS) practice activity. It incorporates *distributed practice* (the MOBYS activity occurs for 5 minutes each session), with *cumulative review* of previously taught content and *interleaved problem sets* (after the first six lessons, in which flash cards are limited to the Small Step problem type, MOBYS problems are sampled from the entire set of arithmetic problems, across all four problem types every session). *Support for correct performance and self-analysis* is provided in three ways. First, students are taught to "know the answer right off the bat" (retrieve from memory) if confident; otherwise, use the taught counting strategies. Second, students answer each presented problem correctly because, as soon as an error occurs, the tutor requires the student to use the taught counting strategy to produce the correct response. To discourage guessing or careless application of counting strategies, seconds elapse as students execute the counting strategy as many times as needed to produce the correct answer. In this way, careful but quick responses increase the number of correct responses. Third, children have a chance to meet or beat each day's first score, and that day's higher score is graphed. MOBYS is also designed to *promote fluency*.

Galaxy Math's other practice activities occur in the final 5 minutes of each lesson. In Lessons 1–4, practice focuses on number identification and magnitude comparisons. Beginning in Lesson 5, practice is devoted to building facility with arithmetic problems, first with ± 0, 1, and 2 and then with number sets 5 to 12.

Fuchs, Geary, et al. (2013) conducted a randomized controlled trial evaluating Galaxy Math's efficacy while isolating the effects of the speeded-practice

MOBYS activity. First-grade students with or at risk for MLD (N = 591) were randomly assigned to three conditions: a control group condition and to one of the two Galaxy Math tutoring conditions: with MOBYS practice or with non-speeded practice in which students played space-themed games designed to correspond to the content addressed in the first segment of that lesson. Intervention lasted 16 weeks with 30-minute sessions per week. Students in both Galaxy Math conditions significantly outperformed the control group. On a test of arithmetic (sums/minuends between 5 and 12), the effect size (*ES*) was large for Galaxy Math with MOBYS (speeded practice) versus control (0.87), smaller for Galaxy Math with non-speeded game practice (0.38). The effect favoring the speeded condition over the non-speeded condition was also significant and large (*ES* = 0.57). On complex calculations (two-digit addition and subtraction with regrouping), *ES*s were as follows: for Galaxy Math with speeded practice over control, 0.69; for Galaxy Math with non-speeded practice over control, 0.49; and between the two Galaxy Math conditions, 0.21. Given convincingly stronger effects for speeded practice, MOBYS (not games) was incorporated into Galaxy Math. Results provide strong evidence for Galaxy Math's efficacy and specifically support Galaxy Math's MOBYS, which maps onto SSMI's structured practice principles.

Research documents meaningful arithmetic improvement for other interventions that rely on SSMI principles. For example, Bryant and colleagues (2011) randomly assigned first graders to control or an intervention focused on conceptual, strategic, and procedural knowledge of whole numbers and operations. Introduction of new content was structured via modeling with gradual transition to students and immediate corrective feedback. Practice was structured to review previously taught material and build fluency. Intervention students significantly outperformed control students on arithmetic with *ES*s of 0.44 and 0.55.

Word-Problem Intervention

Pirate Math is a validated intervention for improving WPS. It includes three 30-minute sessions each week for 15 weeks. Because the WPS curriculum changes across grades, Pirate Math requires different programs in grades 1–3. In this chapter, we highlight first-grade Pirate Math to illustrate the application of SSMI's instructional principles. For a full description of first-grade Pirate Math and the randomized controlled trial, see Fuchs, Seethaler, et al. (2021). For Pirate Math manuals, contact the first author or go to *https://frg.vkcsites.org/what-are-interventions/math_intervention_manuals.*

In terms of *structuring the content to be learned*, Pirate Math teaches students to understand word problems as belonging to problem types. At the primary grades, Pirate Math addresses three word-problem types: the Combine problem type (referred to as Total problems), the Compare problem type (referred to as Difference problems), and the Change problem type.

Pirate Math begins with an introductory unit focused on skills that are foundational to WPS at first grade (e.g., addition and subtraction concepts; efficient counting strategies to find missing quantities in number sentences). The first WPS unit addresses Total problems, in which parts are combined into a whole (e.g., Jalisa has 2 footballs. She also has 3 soccer balls. How many balls does Jalisa have?). The second WPS unit addresses Difference problems, in which quantities are compared to find a difference (e.g., Sasha has 5 balls. Her cousin Phillipe has 8 balls. How many fewer balls does Sasha have?). The third WPS unit covers Change problems, in which an event causes a starting amount to increase or decrease to a new, ending amount (e.g., Avi had 8 tennis balls. Then he lost 3 balls in the park. How many balls does Avi have left?). The final word-problem unit is review. Pirate Math teaches students to understand and identify word problems as belonging to these problem types. Then, Pirate Math teaches students to use solution strategies with some features that universally apply across problem types but with some features specific to the problem type.

With respect to *structuring the introduction of new content*, each word-problem unit begins by teaching the mathematical structure of that unit's problem type. This involves role-playing the problem type's mathematical event using an intact number story and concrete representations. Teachers use the intact story to connect the mathematical structure with (1) a visual schematic; (2) a hand gesture used across lessons to quickly remind students of that problem type's structure; and (3) a problem type number sentence: P1 + P2 = T (Part 1 plus Part 2 equals Total) or P1 + P2 + P3 = T; B – s = D (bigger quantity minus smaller quantity equals difference); and St +/- C = E (for change increase, start number plus change number equals end number; for change decrease, start number minus change number equals end number).

While teaching the mathematical structure of a problem type, Pirate Math instruction relies on explicit, clear, and direct language to frame explanations and to introduce and review problem-specific math language. For example, although Difference word problems involve comparison of quantities to find the difference between them, many students with MLD do not comprehend the meaning of *compare*, *difference*, and *more* or *fewer than*: terms that must be understood to develop the Difference schema. Thus, the early lessons in that unit explicitly teach students the meanings of important words in clear, precise language using concrete objects, hand gestures, and symbols. Students use the same vocabulary and precise language when restating the problem narrative and checking for reasonableness of answers.

Teachers next introduce a word problem (with a missing quantity), with the same cover story used to introduce the problem type. The word problem is role-played with concrete representations and represented with the word-problem type's schematic, hand gesture, and number sentence. Other word problems are discussed.

Teachers then introduce strategies designed to help students process and solve word problems. Students learn to RUN through problems: R̲ead and restate the gist of the problem in their own words; U̲nderline the word(s) telling what the question is asking them to find (this becomes the answer's label); and N̲ame the problem type. Students write T, D, or C next to the problem to help them remember the identified problem type; then they write the problem type's number sentence. Next, they reread the problem as they identify which quantities belong in which slots of the number sentence, cross out irrelevant numbers, and represent the unknown quantity with an x.

For example, consider this Total problem: There are 8 boys playing soccer. Six girls are on the swings, and 3 girls are on the slides. How many girls are playing outside? Students read and listen to the problem as they follow on paper; restate the word problem in their own words; underline *girls*; identify the problem as Total and write T and the Total number sentence (P1 + P2 = T); reread the problem while crossing out 8 and replacing 6 for P1, 3 for P2, and × for T in the number sentence; solve 6 + 3 = x; and then check the reasonableness of the number answer and check their label (9 *girls*). In each word-problem unit, students also learn how to think about irrelevant information; learn to comprehend challenging word-problem language; and learn to find relevant information in charts and tables.

Solution strategies are shown on posters used by tutors to guide students in translating the text narrative into a number sentence that represents the word-problem structure. Students then use the Pirate Math counting strategy or memory-based retrieval (taught in the introductory unit) to solve for the missing quantity in the number sentence. Training posters are gradually faded and revisited as needed. The structure for initial instruction, solution strategies, and transfer features across the three word-problem types is similar to support integrated thinking across the problem types. The main distinction among the problem types, in terms of the solution strategy, is the selection of the problem-type number sentence.

Pirate Math follows the principles of cognitive science for *structuring practice*. Students have distributed, cumulative, and interleaved practice with each type during each lesson. Three problems are solved in each lesson, always a mix of problem types, which are ordered within lessons in varying ways. Students, therefore, have ongoing practice in distinguishing among problem types. Students engage in self-analysis while working by restating the gist of the word problem and checking the reasonableness of their answers. They rely on the training posters (i.e., help cards) as needed, and tutors provide immediate corrective feedback throughout the lesson.

Pirate Math also relies on speeded practice with immediate corrective feedback in multiple ways. First, during the start of the lesson, students practice counting strategies and memory-based fact retrieval using MOBYS, which (as described earlier) adheres to SSMI practice principles in a timed format. Later in the lesson, students have a short amount of time to sort word-problem flash cards into piles that represent the three word-problem types, with corrective feedback from the teacher. The last segment of each lesson is a timed problem set, including number sentences and a word problem. Thus, the three activities comprising each lesson are MOBYS, the word-problem lesson where structured introduction and review of content occurs, and independent practice. Throughout each lesson, students earn points for on-task behavior and correct performance.

Pirate Math was designed initially as a 1:1 intervention at third grade. Given its efficacy, analogous programs were developed at first and second grade, in formats that allowed for whole-class, small-group, and individual delivery. One or more randomized controlled trial of each adaptation isolated specific effects. Most recently, Fuchs, Seethaler, et al. (2021) isolated the added value of language comprehension instruction at first grade. Children (*n* = 391) were randomly assigned to four conditions: Pirate Math with embedded language comprehension instruction, the same Pirate Math intervention without the language component, Galaxy Math (number knowledge and arithmetic intervention), and control. In the WPS outcome, both versions of Pirate Math produced superior performance over Galaxy Math and over the control group. In WPS, the *ES* favoring Pirate Math with language instruction over control was 1.75; favoring Pirate Math without language instruction over control, 1.08; but favoring Galaxy Math over control, only 0.09. Because WPS was significantly stronger for Pirate Math with embedded language comprehension instruction versus without embedded language comprehension instruction, we incorporated language comprehension instruction as a standard feature of Pirate Math. (In arithmetic, both Pirate Math and the Galaxy Math conditions all produced significantly stronger outcomes than the control group, with ESs ranging between 0.59 and 0.79.)

Schema-based intervention, structured on principles derived from cognitive science, is an important and major approach in the research literature for developing WPS for students with MLD. In another recent study, Powell et al. (2021) isolated the contribution of pre-algebra reasoning instruction on the same three problem types. Third graders (*n* = 304) were randomly assigned to a control group or to one of two WPS conditions, with and without embedded pre-algebra instruction. In the WPS outcome, results favored both intervention groups over control, without significant effects between the Pirate Math conditions: *ES* = 2.66 for Pirate Math with embedded pre-algebra instruction versus control and 2.44 for Pirate Math without embedded pre-algebra instruction versus control. Even so, the effect between Pirate Math conditions was significant on the study's measure of relational understanding of the equal sign, and only in the Pirate Math with pre-algebra instruction did such understanding mediate the effects between Pirate Math and control group. Thus, although effects between the Pirate Math conditions were comparable on WPS, a focus on pre-algebra offered additional advantage.

Fractions

Super Solvers is a validated intervention for grades 4 and 5 focused on fraction magnitude understanding, word problems, and calculations. It includes three 40-minute sessions each week for 13 weeks. In this chapter, we address Super Solver's magnitude understanding component. For a full description of Super Solvers in grades 4 and 5 and the randomized controlled trial testing its effects, see Fuchs, Malone, et al. (2021); for grade 3, see Fuchs, Wang, et al. (2021); and for the word-problem component, see Malone et al. (2019). For *Super Solvers* manuals, contact the first author or go to *https://frg.vkcsites.org/what-are-interventions/math_intervention_manuals3*.

In terms of *structuring the content to be learned*, early Super Solvers lessons focus on the meaning of the numerator and denominator, as students learn conceptual strategies to compare fractions with the same numerator or the same denominator. For comparisons involving fractions with the same denominator (same size parts), they learn to focus on the numerators to decide which fraction has more parts. For comparisons involving fractions with the same numerator (same number of parts), they learn to focus on the denominators to decide which fraction has bigger parts. Conceptual comparing strategies are supported with fraction tiles and representational images.

With this understanding in place, fraction magnitude complexity gradually increases, with the following problem types: comparing two fractions with unlike denominators, ordering three fractions, and placing fractions on number lines (first 0–1 and then 0–2 number lines). For the last three problem types, the conceptual and strategic focus is benchmarking. For comparing fractions with unlike denominators, for example, they first label each fraction as L1 (less than 1), =1 (equal to 1), or G1 (greater than 1). If both fractions are L1, they benchmark to 1/2, labeling each fraction as L1/2, =1/2, or G1/2. If two fractions are L1/2 or G1/2, they find an equivalent fraction with the same numerator or same denominator using multiplication and then compare based on the same denominator problem types. Students convert G1 fractions to mixed numbers: comparing whole numbers and then labeling fractions as just outlined. They apply benchmarking strategies in a similar way for ordering (three) fractions and number line problems, but with adjustments to address the demands of each problem type. These strategies are represented on a Compare Card, which guides students as they process fraction magnitude in terms of the problem types. The card is gradually faded and invoked as needed to support thinking and solutions. The structure of the three main fraction magnitude problem types (comparing, ordering, and number line placement) is designed to support integrated thinking and strategies across the problem types while adjustments differentiate among the problem types.

In terms of *structuring the introduction of new content*, each problem type begins with worked examples, as the tutor models and explains the solution strategy to equip students with the most efficient strategy for each problem type and highlight conceptual thinking. Responsibility for applying and explaining the strategy is gradually transferred to students.

The *structure of practice* begins with students taking turns modeling the solution strategy for the current problem type to each other, with tutor feedback to support thinking. At the end of each lesson, students independently complete a problem set consistent with principles of distributed practice, cumulative review of previously taught content, and interleaved presentation of problem types. The Compare Card is used as needed to support thinking and performance. Students conduct checking routines to evaluate their own work; tutors provide corrective feedback when independent practice ends. Other practice activities are designed to build fluency with subskills embedded within strategies. For example, students complete speeded games in which they name fractions equivalent to 1/2 or identify fraction magnitude relative to 1 and 1/2.

Super Solvers activities are implemented in the following order: *Brain Boost* is designed to promote self-regulated learning and a growth mindset. Students discuss an episode from a comic series focused on how brain power can grow with hard work, how to train the brain to boost learning, and how mistakes help us learn. The emphases are perseverance through challenging tasks, setting SMART (specific, measurable, achievable, realistic, time-bound) goals, and directing one's own learning. Tutors extend these ideas in other lesson activities.

Multi-Minute focuses on multiplication facts due to their necessity for finding fraction equivalencies and reducing fractions. Early lessons focus on skip counting. Later lessons involve a 1-minute practice activity in which students take turns answering multiplication facts. To discourage guessing, students stop for each error to skip count the answer while time elapses. The students' goal is to beat the previous session's score.

Fraction Action focuses on magnitude understanding, as already described. *Calculations Quest* addresses fraction addition, subtraction, multiplication, and division problem types. Tutors introduce each problem type with worked examples to model and explain the efficient solution, gradually transferring responsibility to students with the aid of a Calculation Quest Card. The final activity, *Power Practice*, is independent practice. Super Solvers also includes a *behavior management system* to promote on-task behavior and perseverance through difficult tasks.

Fuchs, Malone, et al. (2021) tested the effects of Super Solvers fraction magnitude and calculations intervention in grades 4–5. (For efficacy of the WPS component, see Malone et al. [2019]; for efficacy of Super Solvers in grade 3, see Fuchs, Wang, et al. [2021]). In the 2021 study for grades 4–5, students with MLD (pretest scores < the 21st percentile) were randomized to three conditions: a control group that received the standard school program; fraction magnitude and calculations intervention (FRAX) with blocked instruction; or FRAX with interleaved calculations instruction. At posttest, effects between FRAX (combined across conditions) versus control were significant and large: ESs ranged from 0.77 on equivalencies to 2.14 on calculations, with comparable effects between the FRAX conditions.

One year after intervention ended, ESs between intervention versus control on fraction magnitude measures had decreased but still demonstrated meaningful impact: 0.39 on ordering, 0.54 on equivalencies, 0.49 on number line estimation, and 1.07 on calculations. On calculations, where effects between the two FRAX conditions had been expected, there was not a significant posttest difference. Yet a posttest *ES* of 0.28 favoring interleaved over blocked instruction increased over time, such that 1-year follow-up effects on calculations were significantly and dramatically stronger for the interleaved over the blocked condition (*ES* = 0.82). This is consistent with cognitive science, which indicates that the effects of interleaved instruction increase over time (e.g., Zigler & Stern, 2014, 2016) as students consolidate the knowledge gained by distinguishing among problem features to identify appropriate solution strategies.

Super Solvers was designed to address the curricular shift in fractions instruction over the past decade, largely due to national reform centered on challenging CCRS. Increased curricular depth on fractions in third grade results in students entering fourth grade with stronger fraction knowledge, even as CCRS refocused the fourth- and fifth-grade curriculum on fraction magnitude understanding and solidified conceptual focus within fraction calculations.

Results from Fuchs, Malone, et al. (2021) in fourth and fifth grades, as well as from Fuchs, Wang, et al. (2021) in third grade, indicate that Super Solvers, an intervention aligned with this curricular shift, addresses the needs of MLD students. Earlier efficacy trials involving fraction intervention (see Ennis & Losinski's [2019] meta-analysis) reported similarly strong *ES*s.

Beyond the two Fuchs et al. studies (Fuchs, Malone, et al., 2021; Fuchs, Wang, et al., 2021), we identified one randomized controlled trial testing the effects of CCRS-aligned fraction magnitude and calculations intervention against a control group also receiving CCRS representative instruction. Jayanthi et al. (2021) intervention, which was conducted in fifth grade, relied on the cognitive science principles incorporated in the Fuchs et al. (Fuchs, Malone, et al., 2021; Fuchs, Wang, et al., 2021) studies, with an innovative method for supporting student explanations. Based on 186 students, approximately half of whom were randomized to receive intervention, significant effects favored intervention over control. *ES*s ranged from 0.66 to 1.08, similar to those reported in the Fuchs et al. (Fuchs, Malone, et al., 2021; Fuchs, Wang, et al., 2021) studies. Study participation in Jaynanthi et al. (2021) was, however, limited to students whose pretest math performance ranged between the 15th and 37th percentile. This precludes conclusions for the most challenged learners. Further, Jayanthi et al. (2021) did not report long-term effects, a point we return to in the next section.

Issues Within Intervention to Address the Needs of Students with MLD

Over the past three decades, the number of randomized controlled trials centered on interventions for improving the mathematics performance of students with MLD has increased substantially. At the same time, the quality of study designs, analytical methods for evaluating effects, and reliance on research-supported instructional principles have improved. Important issues for addressing the needs of students with MLD do, however, remain. In this section, we describe critical issues that warrant systematic inquiry in the decade to come.

The first involves ensuring that intervention effects for students with MLD are sustained and support success with more advanced mathematics. Achieving this goal first necessitates the assessment of follow-up effects in randomized controlled trials. This represents an increasing trend in the literature (e.g., Clarke et al., 2016; Fuchs, Malone et al., 2021; Powell et al., 2021). Yet, as follow-up studies demonstrate, intervention effects usually fade over time. Given the severe needs of the MLD population, along with the mathematics curriculum's ever-increasing complexity and substantive shifts in focus, it is not surprising that a single intervention conducted in a single year, even an intervention that addresses foundational as well as CCRS-infused grade-level topics, fails to inoculate students from further difficulty.

For this reason, research is needed to expand beyond estimating effects at 6 months, 1 year, or even multiple years after intervention ends (Clarke et al., 2016; Fuchs, Malone, et al., 2021; Powell et al., 2021) and beyond technical issues in modeling expected long-term effects (e.g., Bailey et al., 2020). The follow-up research agenda also needs to incorporate a strong focus on identifying pretest and end-of-intervention child-level variables that differentiate students who do and do not require additional intervention.

An initial step in this direction was reported by Bailey et al. (2020), who demonstrated predictive utility for classifying students who did and did not perform adequately in the years following first-grade number knowledge and arithmetic intervention. Students with weaker posttest arithmetic skill, representing weaker response to intervention, were less likely to meet criteria for average or better math achievement at the end of third grade. The other significant predictors involved start-of-first-grade letter knowledge and word reading. This is in line with prior work showing a relation between early literacy skill and later mathematics achievement (Chu et al., 2016; Göbel et al., 2014). Research shows that students who experience concurrent math and reading difficulty suffer worse outcomes in each area than peers with difficulty in one domain (Cirino et al., 2015). This type of follow-up work holds promise for identifying which students require sustained intervention.

Beyond identifying students who require sustained intervention, follow-up research needs to experimentally evaluate methods for improving maintenance of effects over time. Studies might, for example, contrast the efficacy and cost-effectiveness of typical practice (without follow-up support) against various forms of support with varying costs: multi-year intervention versus post-intervention booster sessions versus in-class forms of differentiation. Additionally, identifying child-level moderators of alternative strategies may permit productive personalized post-intervention planning.

Summary

Given the importance of mathematics achievement for quality of life, financial security, and life expectancy (Every Child a Chance Trust, 2009), along with the prevalence of MLD (Fletcher et al., 2018), efficacious intervention is needed to ensure satisfactory mathematics achievement trajectories and outcomes for this population of learners. Scientifically structured intervention, which incorporates principles from cognitive science for structuring the mathematics content to be learned, for structuring the introduction of new content, and for structuring practice, provides a framework for designing efficacious interventions. As illustrated in this chapter, the application of these principles can substantially improve the learning outcomes of students with MLD on three critical mathematics topics that are foundational for advanced mathematics learning: arithmetic, word problems, and fractions. Future work, focused on methods to identify students who are in need of follow-up support and focused on effective and efficient procedures for designing that support, is critical and necessary to address the needs of students with MLD.

REFERENCES

Bailey, D. H., Fuchs, L. S., Gilbert, J. K., Geary, D. C., & Fuchs, D. (2020). Prevention: Necessary but insufficient? A two-year follow-up of effective first-grade mathematics intervention. *Child Development, 91*(2), 382–400.

Benjamin, A. S., & Tullis, J. (2010). What makes distributed practice effective? *Cognitive Psychology, 61*(3), 228–247.

Booth, J. L., Newton, K. J., & Twiss-Garrity, L. K. (2014). The impact of fraction magnitude knowledge on algebra performance and learning. *Journal of Experimental Child Psychology, 118*, 110–118.

Bryant, D. P., Bryant, B. R., Roberts, G., Vaughn, S., Pfannenstiel, K. H., & Porterfield, J. (2011). Early numeracy intervention program for first-grade students with mathematics difficulties. *Exceptional Children, 78*(1), 7–23.

Catts, H. W., Hogan, T. P., & Adolf, S. M. (2005). Developmental changes in reading and reading disabilities. In H. W. Catts & A. G. Kamhi (Eds.), *The connections between language and reading disabilities* (pp. 25–40). Erlbaum.

Chi, M. T. H., Bassok, M., Lewis, M. W., Reimann, P., & Glaser, R. (1989). Self-explanations: How students study and use examples in learning to solve problems. *Cognitive Science, 13*(2), 145–182.

Chi, M. T. H., Feltovich, P. J., & Glaser, R. (1981). Categorization and representation of physics problems by expert and novices. *Cognitive Science, 5*, 1221–152.

Chu, F. W., vanMarle, K., & Geary, D. C. (2016) Predicting children's reading and mathematics achievement from early quantitative knowledge and domain-general cognitive abilities. *Frontiers in Cognitive Psychology, 7*, 775.

Cirino, P. T., Ewing-Cobbs, L., Barnes, M., Fuchs, L. S., & Fletcher, J. M. (2007). Cognitive arithmetic differences in learning disability groups and the role of behavioral inattention. *Learning Disabilities Research and Practice, 22*(1), 25–35.

Cirino, P. T., Fuchs, L. S., Elias, J. T., Powell, S. R., & Schumacher, R. F. (2015). Cognitive and mathematical profiles for different forms of learning difficulties. *Journal of Learning Disabilities, 48*(2), 156–175.

Cirino, P. T., Tolar, T., & Fuchs, L. S. (2022). Domain general and specific contributions to algebra: A sequenced longitudinal path model. *Contemporary Educational Psychology, 68*, 102026.

Clarke, B., Doabler, C., Smolkowski, K., Nelson, E. K., Fien, H., & Baker, S. K. (2016). Testing the immediate and long-term efficacy of a Tier 2 kindergarten mathematics intervention. *Journal of Research on Educational Effectiveness, 9*(4), 607–634.

Cooper, G., & Sweller, J. (1987). Effects of schema acquisition and rule automation on mathematical problem solving transfer. *Journal of Educational Psychology, 79*(4), 347–362.

Daroczy, G., Wolska, M., Meurers, W. D., & Nuerk, H.-C. (2015). Word problems: A review of linguistic and numerical factors contributing to their difficulty. *Frontiers in Psychology, 6*, 348.

Duncan, G. J., Dowsett, C. J., Classens, A., Magnuson, K., Huston, A., & Klebanov, P. (2007). School readiness and later achievement. *Developmental Psychology, 43*(6), 1428–1446.

Durkin, K., & Rittle-Johnson, B. (2015). Diagnosing misconceptions: Revealing changing decimal fraction knowledge. *Learning and Instruction, 37*, 21–29.

Ennis, R. P., & Losinski, M. (2019). Intervention to improve fraction skills for students with disabilities: A meta-analysis. *Exceptional Children, 85*(3), 367–386.

Every Child a Chance Trust. (2009). *The long-term costs of numeracy difficulties. www.everychildachancetrust.org/counts/index.cfm*

Fletcher, J. M., Lyon, G. R., Fuchs, L. S., & Barnes, M. A. (2018). *Learning disabilities: From identification to intervention* (2nd ed.). Guilford Press.

Fuchs, L. S., Compton, D. L., Fuchs, D., Paulsen, K., Bryant, J. D., & Hamlett, C. L. (2005). The prevention, identification, and cognitive determinants of math difficulty. *Journal of Educational Psychology, 97*(3), 493–513.

Fuchs, L. S., Fuchs, D., & Compton, D. L. (2013). Intervention effects for students with comorbid forms of learning disability: Understanding the needs of nonresponders. *Journal of Learning Disabilities, 46*(6), 534–548.

Fuchs, L. S., Geary, D. C., Compton, D. L., Fuchs, D., Schatschneider, C., & Hamlett, C. L. (2013). Effects of first-grade number knowledge tutoring with contrasting forms of practice. *Journal of Educational Psychology, 105*(1), 58–77.

Fuchs, L. S., Geary, D. C., Fuchs, D., Compton, D. L., & Hamlett, C. L. (2016). Pathways to third-grade calculation versus word-reading competence: Are they more alike or different? *Child Development, 87*(2), 558–567.

Fuchs, L. S., Gilbert, J. K., Powell, S. R., Cirino, P. T., Fuchs, D., & Hamlett, C. L. (2016). The role of cognitive processes, foundational math skill, and calculation accuracy and fluency in word-problem solving versus pre-algebraic knowledge. *Developmental Psychology, 52*(12), 2085–2098.

Fuchs, L. S., Malone, A. S., Preacher, K. J., Cho, E., & Fuchs, D. (2021). *Next-generation fraction intervention for students with intensive mathematics and the long-term advantage of interleaved instruction* [Manuscript submitted for publication].

Fuchs, L. S., & Powell, S. R. (2021). *A model of scientifically structured mathematics intervention to improve student outcomes* [Manuscript submitted for publication].

Fuchs, L. S., Schumacher, R. F., Sterba, S. K., Long, J., Namkung, J., & Malone, A. S. (2014). Does working memory moderate the effects of fraction intervention? An aptitude-treatment interaction. *Journal of Educational Psychology, 106*(2), 499–514.

Fuchs, L. S., Seethaler, P. M., Sterba, S. Y., Craddock, C., Fuchs, D., & Compton, D. L. (2021). Closing the word-problem achievement gap in first grade: Schema-based word-problem intervention with embedded language comprehension instruction. *Journal of Educational Psychology, 113*(1), 86–103.

Fuchs, L. S., Wang, A., Y., Preacher, K. J., Malone, A. S., Fuchs, D., & Pachmayr, R. (2021). Addressing challenging mathematics standards with at-risk learners: A randomized controlled trial on the effects of fractions intervention at third grade. *Exceptional Children, 87*(2), 163–182.

Geary, D. C., Hoard, M. K., Byrd-Craven, J., Nugent, L., & Numtee, C. (2007). Cognitive mechanisms underlying achievement deficits in children with mathematics learning disability. *Child Development, 78*(4), 1343–1359.

Geary, D. C., Widaman, K. F., Little, T. D., & Cormier, P. (1987). Cognitive addition: Comparison of learning disabled and academically normal elementary school children. *Cognitive Development, 2*(3), 249–269.

Göbel, S. M., Watson, S. E., Lervåg, A., and Hulme, C. (2014). Children's arithmetic development: It is number knowledge, not the approximate number sense, that counts. *Psychological Science, 25*(3), 789–798.

Hattie, J., & Timperley, H. (2007). The power of feedback. *Review of Educational Research, 77*(1), 81–112.

Jayanthi, M., Gersten, R., Schumacher, R. F., Dimino, J., Smolkowski, K., & Spallone, S. (2021). Improving struggling fifth-grade students' understanding of fractions: A randomized controlled trial of an intervention that stresses both concepts and procedures. *Exceptional Children*. Advanced online publication.

Jordan, N. C., Hansen, N., Fuchs, L. S., Siegler, R. S., Gersten, R., & Micklos, D. (2013). Developmental predictors of fraction concepts and procedures. *Journal of Experimental Child Psychology, 116*(1), 45–58.

Kilpatrick, J., Swafford, J., & Findell, B. (Eds.) (2001). *Adding it up: Helping children learn mathematics*. National Academy Press.

Malone, A. S., Fuchs, L. S., Sterba, S. K., Fuchs, D., & Foreman-Murray, L. (2019). Does an integrated focus on fractions and decimals improve at-risk students' rational number magnitude performance? *Contemporary Educational Psychology*, *59*, 101782.

Miller, S. P., & Hudson, P. J. (2007). Using evidence-based practices to build mathematics competence related to conceptual, procedural, and declarative knowledge. *Learning Disabilities Research and Practice, 22*(1), 47–57.

Namkung, J. M., Fuchs, L. S., & Koziol, N. (2018). Does initial learning about the meaning of fractions present similar challenges for students with and without adequate whole-number skill? *Learning and Individual Differences, 61*, 151–157.

National Mathematics Advisory Panel (2008). *Foundations for success: Final report of the National Mathematics Advisory Panel.* U.S. Department of Education.

Ni, Y., & Zhou, Y. D. (2005). Teaching and learning fraction and rational numbers: The origins and implications of whole number bias. *Educational Psychologist, 40*(1), 27–52.

Ostad, S. A. (1997). Developmental differences in addition strategies: A comparison of mathematically disabled and mathematically normal children. *British Journal of Educational Psychology, 67*(3), 345–357.

Powell, S. R., Berry, K. A., Fall, A.-M., Roberts, G., Barnes, M. A., & Fuchs, L. S. (2021). Does word-problem performance maintain? Follow-up one year after implementation of a word-problem intervention. *Journal of Research on Educational Effectiveness.* Advanced online publication.

Powell, S. R., & Fuchs, L. S. (2018). Effective word-problem instruction: Using schemas to facilitate mathematical reasoning. *TEACHING Exceptional Children, 51*(1), 31–42.

Renkl, A. (2002). Learning from worked examples: Instructional explanations supplement self-explanations. *Learning and Instruction, 12*(5), 529–556.

Rohrer, D., Dedrick, R. F., & Burgess, K. (2015). The benefit of interleaved mathematics practice is not limited to superficially similar kinds of problems. *Psychonomic Bulletin Review, 21*(5), 1323–1330.

Siegler, R. S., Thompson, C. A., & Schneider, M. (2011). An integrated theory of whole number and fractions development. *Cognitive Psychology, 62*, 273–296.

Swanson, H. L., & Beebe-Frankenberger, M. (2004). The relationship between working memory and mathematical problem solving in children at risk and not at risk for serious math difficulties. *Journal of Educational Psychology, 96*(3), 471–491.

Sweller, J. (1988). Cognitive load during problem solving: Effects on learning. *Cognitive Science, 12*(2), 257–285.

Sweller, J. (1994). Cognitive load theory, learning difficulty, and instructional design. *Learning and Instruction, 4*(4), 296–312.

Zigler, E., & Stern, E. (2014). Delayed benefits of learning elementary algebraic transformations through contrasted comparisons. *Learning and Instruction, 33*, 131–146.

Zigler, E., & Stern, E. (2016). Consistent advantages of contrasted comparisons: Algebra learning under direct instruction. *Learning and Instruction, 41*, 41–51.

CHAPTER 15

Writing and Students with Learning Disabilities

Steve Graham and Karen R. Harris

Every story starts somewhere. With writing, the story started in three different locations: Mesopotamia around 3200 BCE, China around 1250 BCE, and Mesoamerica around 250 CE (Schmandt-Besserat & Erard, 2008). The earliest known uses of writing in these three locations included recording the number of commodities on a clay tablet, inscribing symbols on cow bones or turtle shells to pose a question to an oracle, and creating glyphs on stone to show calendar calculations or the actions of kings. The invention of the alphabet occurred somewhere around 1700 BCE, possibly in Lebanon. All alphabets evolved from this initial endeavor (Healey, 1990).

Since these early applications of writing, purposes for writing have undergone an incredible transformation to accomplish a variety of human goals. This includes communicating, recording and sharing information, informing and persuading others, chronicling one's own and others' personal experiences, thinking about topics, learning new information and ideas, creating imaginary worlds, entertaining others, exploring the meaning of events, and healing psychological and physiological wounds (Graham, 2018a; Harris et al., 2023). Writing, however, is not acquired naturally, easily, or effortlessly (Harris & Graham, 2016). While some knowledge about how to write can be gained as a result of writing and reading (e.g., Fitzgerald & Shanahan, 2000), engaging in these activities alone is not enough for most children to learn how to write effectively. This is especially true for students who experience difficulty learning to write and/or read, such as students with learning disabilities (LD) (As a result, students who do not learn to write well are at a distinct disadvantage educationally, occupationally, and socially. This is particularly true for students with LD, who experience Graham, Harris, et al., 2016; Harris et al., 2019).

Today, writing is an essential tool at school, work, and home (Graham, Harris, et al., 2016). The scientific study of writing has occurred for slightly over

100 years, with a considerably shorter time period focused on students with LD. Further, we do not yet have the body of research necessary to adequately describe typical writing development, which hampers research on students with LD and their typically achieving peers.

In this chapter, we review what is currently known about writing and school-age students with LD and their peers, drawing on scientific research from multiple disciplines, including special education, educational psychology, English, and educational sciences. Research on the writing of students with LD supports conclusions about how they write and how to teach them to write. Even so, much is still unknown, and we note where additional research is needed. We begin by considering the writing of students with LD and how assessment is used to identify these students' writing difficulties and to inform instruction. The final sections of this chapter focus on evidence-based writing practices for preservice teacher preparation and professional development in writing for students, including those with LD.

The Writing of Students with LD

Research on the writing characteristics of students with LD generally addresses three areas of investigation. The first includes studies examining the writing or writing processes of students with LD. A second area compares students with LD to their typically developing peers on one or more writing attributes. Experimental manipulations designed to identify factors that contribute to the writing difficulties of students with LD are the focus of the third area. Drawing on these areas of investigation, we consider how students with LD write, how their writing compares to that of other students, and which factors contribute to writing difficulties among students with LD.

How Students with LD Write

The approach to writing that students with LD most often employ, especially when they are younger, involves little in the way of planning, thinking, and reflecting (Harris & Graham, 2013; Thomas et al., 1987). Instead, these students rely heavily on one composing process: generation of writing content. With this approach, students compose by creating or drawing from memory a relevant idea, writing it down, and using each preceding phrase or sentence to stimulate the next idea. Little effort is made to evaluate or rework these ideas or to consider the constraints imposed by the topic, the needs of the audience, or the organization of text. The resulting composition is generally a list of topic-related ideas rather than a coherent discussion or examination of the topic. This approach to writing functions much like an automated and forward-moving content generation program (McCutchen, 1988). Although this may be a useful approach for some writing tasks, it is not particularly effective for many school-related writing demands, such as writing an essay, report, narrative, or story.

Content generation dominates the planning and composing process for most students with LD and is a relatively unproductive approach. One of the most striking characteristics of these students' writing is that there is so little of it. Their papers are inordinately short, containing little elaboration or detail (Myklebust, 1973; Newcomer & Barenbaum, 1991).

Self-Regulation of Writing

The two aspects of self-regulation in writing with students with LD, where we can draw reasonably strong conclusions involving planning before writing and revising, involves monitoring and evaluation (Wong et al., 1989). Students with LD typically do little or no planning before starting to write (FitzPatrick & McKeown, 2021; Garcia & Fidalgo, 2008), even when asked to plan in advance. For example, MacArthur and Graham (1987) prompted fifth- and sixth-grade students with LD to plan before writing. These students averaged less than 1 minute of advanced planning time, whether they were writing papers by hand, typing their compositions on a word processor, or dictating them to an adult.

Students with LD also demonstrate a restricted approach to revising text. They focus their revising efforts mainly on making word substitutions, correcting mechanical errors, and producing a neater product (MacArthur et al., 1991). Less than 20% of the revisions made by these students appreciably change what they write; the majority of their revisions involve minor changes to the surface-level features of text (MacArthur & Graham, 1987; MacArthur et al., 1991). Over 70% of these changes are attempts to correct capitalization, punctuation, spelling, format, and other mechanical errors. The changes made are generally ineffective, as the only thing that typically improves across drafts is the legibility of handwriting.

One possible reason why the planning, drafting, and revising of students with LD are so limited is that they have trouble managing the processes underlying each of these activities (Graham, Harris, et al., 2016; Harris et al., 2009, 2011, 2018). Support for this hypothesis was found in two separate experiments involving revising (De La Paz et al., 1998; Graham, 1997). Revising for students with LD improved when they received support designed to ensure that separate elements of the revising process were coordinated and occurred in a regular way.

In the first study (Graham, 1997), fifth- and sixth-grade students with LD executed a revising routine where they evaluated each sentence written, explained their evaluation, selected a tactic for revising the sentence (if one was needed), and executed the revision. Revising one sentence at a time, the child first selected one of seven possible evaluations written on separate index cards. Three of the evaluations were written from the writer's perspective (e.g., "This is not what I wanted to say.") and three from the reader's perspective (e.g., "People may not understand this part."). The seventh evaluative statement was, "This is good." Once they selected an evaluation, they explained how it applied. Next, they selected a tactic for revising the sentence, drawing upon five possible directives; again, each was written on a separate index card. The directives were "Leave it the same," "Say more," "Leave this part out," "Change the wording," and "Cross out and say it a different way." Students then executed the change. This routine reduced the executive burden involved in revising by signaling movement from one element of revising to the next and limiting the number of decisions students made. The participating students indicated that the procedure made the process of revising easier. There was also an improvement in the quality of their revisions and the type of text that they changed, resulting in more revisions involving larger units of text, such as phrases and t-units.

Even more impressive results were obtained in the second study (De La Paz et al., 1998). Eighth-grade students with LD used a similar routine that involved making two passes through their composition. The first pass focused on more global concerns (e.g., "Part of the essay is not in the right order."), whereas the second pass concentrated on local concerns primarily situated at the sentence level (e.g., "This one doesn't sound right.") Students indicated that the executive routine made revising easier. It also prompted more, better, and lengthier revisions substantive enough to improve the overall quality of their text.

Skills

Even when students with LD receive support in regulating planning, revising, or other strategic processes, they may still experience problems because they do not possess the skills for carrying out these processes. In the two revising studies reviewed earlier (Graham, 1997; De La Paz et al., 1998), there were many instances where students failed to make a constructive evaluation. Some students lacked the skills and knowledge needed to adequately evaluate their text. For instance, one student told us he deleted three sentences that were central to understanding his story (a negative change) because "people won't care about that part."

There were also instances in these two revising studies where revisions were ineffective because students did not have the skills needed to carry out the intended change. To illustrate, one child wrote a persuasive essay to support her claim that boys and girls should be educated together because they can give each other advice. She identified the sentence, "But sometimes you need a girl's more than you do a boy's," as not a complete idea and decided to add information. Instead of adding the word *advice* after the word *girl*, she added a sentence, "And sometimes you don't have advice to give," which did not address the problem.

Difficulties with basic text transcription skills are marked among students with LD. They routinely misspell words, write letters so they are difficult to read, and ignore or misplace capitalization and punctuation. Many produce letters slowly, at almost half the rate of their more fluent peers (Søvik et al., 1987). These problems not only make their papers more difficult to read but also undermine the writing process in at least three ways (Graham, Hebert, et al., 2016). One, having to switch attention to mechanical concerns while writing, such as how to spell a word, may cause them to lose ideas or plans held in working memory. Two, possible writing content may be lost because children's writing (or typing) is not fast enough to keep up with their thoughts, and ideas are lost before they can be transcribed onto paper. Finally, opportunities for thinking about writing ideas and making written output fit intentions are reduced when children's attention is occupied with mechanical concerns. These students also experience difficulties with sentence construction (Saddler & Graham, 2005), which is likely to have similar effects.

Knowledge

For many students with LD, their knowledge about writing—its genres, devices, and conventions—is limited (Montague et al. 1990; Saddler & Graham, 2007). For example, they are often unfamiliar with the basic parts of a story. In a recent interview with a third-grade child with LD, for example, he started off on the right track but quickly veered into questionable territory. When asked to tell a friend what to include in a story, he indicated, "I would tell him main character, a subject, predicate, and main idea." These students' incomplete knowledge is further noticeable in their stories as they often omit basic elements such as the location, problem, or ending (Foxworth et al., 2017; Lin et al., 2007). Lack of genre knowledge is also evident in their writing to inform, persuade, and argue (Harris & Graham, 2018).

Gaps in what students with LD know are not limited to genre knowledge and other aspects of the written product but extend to knowledge about how to write. When compared with their regularly achieving peers, for instance, students with LD are less knowledgeable about the processes involved in organizing and categorizing writing ideas as well as evaluating and revising text (Englert et al., 1989; Harris et al., 2009, 2011, 2018). Equally important to writing is knowledge about the writing topic (Olinghouse et al., 2015). Even when these students possess knowledge about a topic, other factors, such as we have discussed here, may interfere.

Self-Efficacy, Attitudes, and Motivation

Students with LD or writing difficulties, particularly young students, are often overconfident about their capabilities, making measurement of variables such as self-efficacy, attitudes, and motivation difficult. In addition, disparate conceptualizations of what each means and how each can be measured also lead to difficulties in writing research (c.f. Ekholm et al., 2018; Harris et al., 2015; Sawyer et al., 1992). For example, Sawyer et al. (1992) found high self-assessments of self-efficacy for writing among fifth- and sixth-grade students with LD at pretest, despite low performance in writing, and noted a body of research that indicates students with LD frequently make overly positive self-evaluations and reviewed articles regarding this challenge in younger students as well. When Graham et al. (1993) assessed the self-efficacy of 10- to 14-year-old students with LD, for example, they were just as positive about their writing capabilities as their peers who were better writers, favorably rating their ability to write reports, stories, and book reports. They were also positive about their abilities to get and organize ideas for writing, transcribe ideas into sentences, sustain their writing effort, and correct mistakes. Although a positive judgment about one's capabilities may promote persistence, there are downsides as well. Children who overestimate their capabilities may fail to allocate needed resources and effort to writing tasks and may be unable to evaluate their writing adequately.

Surprisingly little is known about attitudes toward writing among students with LD and their relationship to motivation (Graham et al., 2007). When students in the Graham et al. (1993) study were asked to indicate their agreement or disagreement with six attitude questions (e.g., "Writing is a waste of time."), the students with LD were generally positive about writing. Their responses stand in contrast to anecdotal and clinical reports where students with LD commonly indicate they dislike and avoid writing (Berninger et al., 1997). Self-efficacy for writing and attitudes about writing are both believed to impact motivation, as are a number of other factors (e.g., effort, persistence, and time-on-task). All of these constructs need far more research among students with LD and present thorny issues in construct validity.

How the Writing of Students with LD Compares to the Writing of Other Students

Four meta-analyses are reviewed here. In all four of these meta-analyses, comparisons were made to writers in the same grade who were not identified with the specific disability examined. Graham et al. (2017) conducted a meta-analysis examining the writing of students with LD. Meta-analyses focusing on the writing of students with ADHD (Graham, Fishman, et al., 2016), speech and language difficulties (Graham et al., 2020), and reading difficulties (Graham et al., 2021) have also been conducted.

Graham et al. (2017) located 53 studies that compared the writing of school-age students with LD with their same-age peers. On every aspect of writing in every study, students with LD had lower scores than their same-grade counterparts. Spelling was particularly problematic for students with LD, as they scored 1.5 standard deviations below their typically developing peers. The overall quality of their text, how well it was organized, the richness of ideas presented, the voice projected, and the mastery of writing conventions were also problematic. Students with LD scored 1 standard deviation or more below their peers on these measures. Students with LD scored one-half a standard deviation to close to a full standard deviation below same-age peers without LD on vocabulary writing measures, amount written, inclusion of pertinent genre elements in their writing, knowledge of writing, sentence fluency, handwriting, and grammar. Scores on motivation measures were almost one-half of a standard deviation lower than their peers. Many, although not all, students with LD find virtually every aspect of writing challenging.

When the writing of students with LD is compared to the writing of students with other disabilities in the other three meta-analyses, students with LD almost always have lower writing scores than students with identified reading difficulties, ADHD, and speech and hearing difficulties. The only exceptions involved lower scores for grammar and vocabulary for students with identified reading difficulties and lower scores for grammar for students with speech and hearing difficulties.

While some caution must be exercised in interpreting these findings (e.g., students with LD were not directly compared to students with other disabilities, and it was not possible to make comparisons between these students on all aspects of writing), the effect sizes in these studies reinforce just how difficult writing is for students with LD.

Research examining how and what students with LD write, however, is limited and less frequent now than in the past (Graham et al., 2017). Some areas, like students' knowledge about writing, self-regulation of the writing process, and motivation, are particularly in need of further research. Hopefully, researchers interested in students with LD will address these aspects of writing further, as they can help provide guidance to the field on what to assess and teach.

Assessing Writing

Numerous issues and approaches are relevant in assessing writing among students with disabilities. Here, we address approaches to determining if a student has an LD in writing and the roles of summative and formative assessments in writing.

Identification of LD in Writing

Multiple approaches have been implemented to determine if a student has an LD in writing (Pullen, 2017). One common approach is the discrepancy model, where one or more tests of writing may be administered to students to determine how their writing abilities compare to a normative sample of students at the same age or grade. A basic concern with this method of identification involves how students' writing is sampled. Norm-referenced writing tests available today assess a very limited range of writing genres, skills, and processes. In many assessments for writing difficulties or LD in writing, only a single norm-referenced writing test is given, and this test assesses just one writing genre (Harris, Lane, Graham, et al., 2012), most commonly narrative writing (Calfee & Wilson, 2004). Such an assessment also assumes that a single measure of writing provides a reliable measure of a student's ability to write in multiple genres. This is not a valid presumption. Nor is it safe to assume that a single sample of writing provides an adequate indication of how a student writes in the genre assessed. As a study by Graham, Hebert, et al. (2016) demonstrated, multiple samples of writing are needed to obtain a reliable estimate of the writing performance of students at risk for or with LD. Thus, when assessing if a student has an LD in writing using the discrepancy approach, it is necessary to assess multiple forms of writing, multiple writing skills and processes, and multiple assessments in each genre.

A second common approach to identifying if a student has an LD in writing is the response-to-intervention (RTI) approach. In this case, identification is based on students' lack of adequate responsiveness to targeted and intensive Tier 2 writing instruction. This approach may involve using curriculum-based measures (CBM) of writing to judge students' responsiveness. When this is the case, CBM measures are administered frequently (e.g., once a week) to monitor the success of the Tier 2 instruction. These measures are typically efficient (e.g., 3- to 5-minute samples of writing are collected), reliable, and relatively easy to score (Dockrell et al., 2018). Unfortunately, these assessments may not be sensitive to the effects of instruction delivered over a week, a relatively short period of time. Further, most available writing CBM measures focus on narrative writing, younger students, and easily countable indices of productivity and accuracy (e.g., number of words written, correct word sequences, and correct spelling). These short CBM measures may not adequately assess writing quality or writing processes (Dockrell et al., 2018; Ritchey & Coker, 2013; McMaster & Espin, 2007). Further, reliance on these measures may inadvertently narrow the focus of Tier 2 instruction, as practitioners may tailor the Tier 2 instruction provided to the aspects included in the CBM measure administered. While progress is being made, the utility of CBM measures for writing remains limited across ages, genres, and differing populations. The use of additional assessments in writing is frequently advised (Dockrell et al., 2018).

If students are to be provided special education services for writing, additional research is needed to refine existing identification procedures and develop new ones. How writing is assessed is not only a serious concern for identification of students with LD, but a problem for formative assessment of writing as well.

Summative and Formative Writing Assessment

Writing assessments can serve summative and formative functions (Graham, 2018b). Summative assessments, which can range from norm-referenced to teacher-designed assessments, are designed to determine a student's current writing attainment and are typically used to determine growth and mastery. They can also be used for some formative purposes to inform instruction. Formative assessments involve reliable and valid evidence collected to design or adjust instruction based on students' writing strengths and needs (Lane, 2010).

Students with LD are likely to participate in a variety of summative writing assessments. This includes writing tests or assessments to determine if they met IEP goals as well as standardized tests administered by a school district or state to monitor student growth and evaluate teachers and schools. The value of high-stakes summative assessments, such as state assessments, has been hotly debated (Graham et al., 2011). One possible value of these tests is that teachers may come to view writing as an important skill to teach to students with LD. This must be tempered by the fact that these tests may be less accurate than advertised.

There are many different forms of formative/performance assessment in writing, including writing portfolios, student self-assessment, writing rubrics, teacher feedback, peer assessment, teacher professional judgment, and computer feedback (Calfee & Wilson, 2004; Graham, 2018b; Lane, 2010; McMaster & Espin, 2007). A meta-analysis by Graham, Hebert, et al. (2015) provided support for using teacher, student, and peer assessments in writing, but this applied to students in general and not students with LD specifically. While we expect such procedures would enhance the writing of students with LD, research is needed to determine if this is the case and how such assessment procedures can best be applied to this population of students.

Test accommodations have been used as a means to provide a more accurate picture of the writing of students with LD on high-stakes assessments. Accommodations can include extended testing time, different modes of writing (e.g., speech-to-text synthesis), and taking the test in a different setting. An example of a successful test accommodation was illustrated by MacArthur and Cavalier (2004), who found that changing the response mode from writing by hand to speech-to-text synthesis enhanced the writing of students with LD, but not the writing of their peers. Despite the widespread availability of test accommodations, there is little research on their effectiveness. This needs to be rectified if they are to be used effectively.

Teaching Writing

Students with LD spend most of their school day in the regular classroom (U.S. Department of Education, 2015). The writing and other instruction they receive there is often referred to as Tier 1 instruction. They may also receive writing instruction or support from a special or general education teacher in the regular classroom or from a special educator in another setting (e.g., resource room). This instruction may be provided in small groups or individually and may involve the regular and special education working or teaching together. For example, Harris et al. (2015) found that following intensive professional development, second-grade general education teachers implemented Tier 2 self-regulated strategy development (SRSD) writing instruction (described later in this chapter) with small groups of at-risk writers with high fidelity. Students made large gains in writing outcomes, and motivation for writing improved.

A basic assumption is that all students, including students with LD, are less likely to experience writing difficulties if the Tier 1 instruction they receive is evidence-based. While both survey and observational studies provide evidence that some teachers provide evidence-based instruction at Tier 1, this is generally not the case (Graham, 2019), although general education teachers report they make a variety of instructional adaptations for writing for students with disabilities (Troia & Graham, 2017). The overall findings from these investigations are that students in elementary and secondary classrooms receive little writing instruction and spend very little time writing. While teachers do report use of evidence-based writing practices, they use these procedures infrequently.

The poor quality of Tier 1 writing instruction might be alleviated somewhat if students with LD received effective writing instruction from their special education teachers. The little evidence available suggests this is not likely. We located only one study, quite dated now, that examined this proposition. Christenson et al. (1989) found that special and regular education teachers provided very little writing instruction to students with LD. If we assume that the available evidence is an accurate portrayal of the writing instruction students with LD receive, these findings are particularly unfortunate, as researchers have identified a variety of evidence-based practices for teaching writing to all students (Tier 1) and to students with LD specifically. We examine these practices next.

Evidence-Based Practices for Tier 1 Writing Instruction

A number of meta-analyses have been conducted to identify effective writing practices in the general education classroom. In two chapters (Graham & Harris, 2018; Graham, Harris, et al., 2016), we drew this work together along with meta-analyses conducted by other researchers to present meta-analyses that included studies from all of these sources. The studies included in this new meta-analysis were true and quasi-experiments and covered grades 1 to 12. In addition, we included a meta-analysis of single-case design studies (Rogers & Graham, 2008) and a meta-synthesis of qualitative studies that examined how highly effective literacy teachers have taught writing (Graham, Harris, et al., 2015).

Table 15.1 presents writing practices that have been demonstrated to be effective in improving writing in the inclusive classroom. In all but two cases, effect sizes presented are for writing quality. The only exceptions are writing about classroom content material or material read. The outcomes for these types of writing were content learned and reading comprehension.

As seen in Table 15.1, an important element of a strong Tier 1 writing program is to ensure that students write. This includes using writing as a tool to support students' learning of content material and to better understand material read. As students write, the quality of what they write can be improved by providing them various supports, including establishing goals for writing; participating in activities to generate and organize possible writing content; encouraging students to work together as they write; providing structure where students are expected to plan; drafting and revising what they write; sharing model text that students can emulate; and providing students with digital tools to support their writing. Support can also be provided by providing students with feedback, which can come from the teacher, peers, or computer programs. Just as importantly, students need to be taught basic writing foundational skills, such as genre knowledge, strategies for planning and revising, transcription skills (spelling, handwriting, and typing), sentence formation, procedures for regulating the writing process, as well as grammar and vocabulary skills. Fostering motivation, creativity, and the use of imagery can further enhance the quality of what students write.

Single-case studies (Rogers & Graham, 2008) also found that many of the practices in Table 15.1 were effective, and qualitative studies of exceptional teachers found that they applied most of these practices (Graham, Harris, et al., 2015). More research is needed, however, to identify other effective writing practices and to determine how and for whom evidence-based writing practices can best be implemented.

Evidence-Based Practices Specifically for Students with LD

Two meta-analyses have provided evidence on writing practices that are effective specifically with students with LD. These practices were tested with true- and quasi-experimental designs (Gillespie & Graham, 2014) and single-case designs (Rogers & Graham, 2008). These writing practices, presented in the following list,

TABLE 15.1. Effect Sizes for Evidence-Based Writing Practices

Writing interventions (Graham & Harris, 2018)	Number of studies	Effect size	*p*-value
Ensure that students write			
• Increase how much students write	9	0.24	<.038
• Write about information presented in class	31	0.29	<.001
• Write about information read (research-designed tests)	55	0.50	<.001
• Write about information read (norm-referenced tests)	11	0.37	<.001
Support students as they write			
• Implement a process approach to writing	33	0.34	<.001
• Provide word processors for writing	39	0.44	<.001
• Provide word processing programs for writing that included additional writing supports	4	1.46	<.001
• Have students collaboratively plan, draft, and/or revise their papers	8	0.74	.001
• Set specific goals for students' writing	9	0.80	<.001
• Use prewriting activities that help students gather and organize writing information	13	0.55	<.001
• Engage students in inquiry activities to gather, organize, and think about information for their writing	6	0.37	.025
• Provide students with model text to analyze and emulate	7	0.30	<.001
Teach writing explicitly			
• Teach planning, drafting, and revising strategies	42	1.26	<.001
• General strategy instruction	14	0.56	<.001
• SRSD (self-regulated strategy development)	28	1.59	<.001
• Add self-regulation (e.g., goal setting and self-assessment) procedures to strategy instruction	6	0.50	.003
• Implement procedures to enhance motivation	3	1.0	.001
• Teach student to use imagery or be more creative	4	0.76	<.001
• Teach sentence construction skills through sentence combining	5	0.50	<.001
• Teach grammar skills	10	−0.17	.36
• Teach transcription skills (spelling, handwriting, and typing)	8	0.55	.02
• Teach vocabulary skills for writing	3	0.78	.003
Conduct formative assessment			
• Teacher or other adult provides students with feedback about their writing	7	0.87	<.001
• Teach peers to provide each other with feedback about their writing	10	0.77	<.001
• Teach students to self-assess their own writing	13	0.51	<.001
• Use a computer program to provide students with feedback on their writing	5	0.34	.036

overlap somewhat with evidence-based practices for regular classroom instruction. A primary difference between many of the studies testing the effectiveness of a writing practice with students with LD and students generally involved intensity. In many of the studies conducted with students with LD, but not all of them, instruction was administered individually or in small groups and for a more sustained period of time. Most of the studies conducted with students in general, but not all of them, were conducted with the whole class. There was one notable exception, however. Studies testing the process approach, regardless of type of student, almost always involved the whole class.

Evidence-based writing practices that were effective *with students with LD* included:

- Apply a process approach to writing where students write for extended periods of time, engaging in cycles of planning, drafting, revising, and editing.
- Teach strategies for planning, drafting, revising, and editing text as well as self-regulating the writing process. The SRSD model of writing instruction is especially effective; description of SRSD components and characteristics follows.
- Teach strategies for constructing different types of paragraphs.
- Encourage students to use prewriting strategies to help them generate and organize their writing ideas.
- Teach students how to monitor their writing by recording their writing productivity or on-task behavior.
- Provide extra handwriting and spelling instruction.
- Teach grammar skills through modeling and guided practice.
- Teach students to write more complex sentences through sentence combining or by teaching sentence-writing formulas.
- Provide students with elaborated goals for what they are to do when writing.
- Make word processing the primary mode of writing for students with LD.

While the field of LD has come a long way in identifying writing practices effective with students with LD, the evidence base is relatively slim for most practices (a notable exception is strategy instruction). More attention is needed to identify a broader array of effective practices, especially ones that can be applied by special education teachers in inclusive and other settings.

Self-Regulated Strategy Development Instruction for Students with LD

Given the manifold demands of writing reviewed here, SRSD is a complex, multicomponent instructional approach that supports differentiation across students based on strengths and needs. SRSD is the most researched approach to writing instruction for students with LD (FitzPatrick & McKeown, 2021). SRSD instruction is not scripted (Harris et al., 2015), includes formative and summative assessment, and incorporates both writing strategies for planning and revising, as well as instruction in and support for development of the four cornerstones of self-regulation: goal setting, self-instruction/self-talk, self-assessment (self-monitoring and self-evaluation), and self-reinforcement. Knowledge, attitudes and beliefs about writing, self-efficacy for writing, and motivation are directly addressed and supported in SRSD; skills should be addressed in tandem with SRSD instruction (Harris & Graham, 2016; Harris et al., 2006, 2023). SRSD instruction includes active, discourse-based, scaffolded, and explicit learning of strategies for genre-specific and general aspects of writing and the writing process, the knowledge (e.g., academic vocabulary, background knowledge, declarative knowledge, procedural knowledge, and conditional knowledge) needed to use these strategies, and strategies for self-regulating writing behavior (e.g., persistence and attention) as well as for memory of what is learned. Students are active collaborators in learning; peer supports and group discussion are integral (Harris et al., 2006, 2018).

Multiple elements of SRSD instruction (e.g., development of attributions for effort, use of powerful strategies and self-monitoring, and celebrating of progress toward goals) help teachers support students in the development of motivation, positive attitudes toward writing, and belief in themselves as capable writers. Multiple procedures that promote long-term maintenance and appropriate generalization are integrated throughout instruction. SRSD instruction takes place across six adaptable and recursive stages that are criterion-based rather than time-based (Develop background knowledge, Discuss it, Model it, Memorize it, Support it, and Independent performance), with gradual release of responsibility for writing to students. SRSD has been deemed an evidence-based practice for students with LD or EBD; the What Works Clearinghouse deemed it evidence-based for inclusive classrooms as well, noting it has the largest evidence base of any approach to writing instruction (Graham et al., 2018). Further, the research base indicates that SRSD has had positive effects on self-regulation, attitudes about writing, motivation, persistence, engagement, knowledge about writing, strategy use, what and how students write, and maintenance and generalization (Graham & Harris, 2018; Graham et al., 2013; Harris & Graham, 2016, 2018; Harris et al., 2019). Much remains to be investigated in SRSD research, however (Harris, 2021; Harris & Graham, 2018; McKeown et al., 2019).

Teacher Preparation in Preservice Programs and in Professional Development

Preservice

As Cochran-Smith and Zeichner (2005) noted, "Teachers are among the most, if not the most, significant factors in children's learning" (p. 1). While factors outside of school play a role in students' writing development, a primary responsibility of schooling is to teach students to write. This requires that teachers are prepared to teach this complex skill. Unfortunately, a majority of teachers in the United States and other countries are not particularly positive about their preparation in this area. In reviewing studies conducted since 2000, Graham (2019) found that general education teachers typically did not believe that their preservice preparation to teach writing was adequate, and many questioned the in-service preparation they received.

We know of only one study examining preparation of special education teachers. Graham et al. (2022) compared special and regular education teachers' beliefs about their preservice preparation to teach writing. All of these teachers taught students with disabilities, including students with LD, and they worked in the same schools. Both groups indicated they were not adequately prepared to teach writing to students with disabilities. Surprisingly, general education teachers believed they were better prepared to teach writing than special education teachers and were more positive about their efforts to learn to teach writing. They also held more positive attitudes about teaching writing and their own capabilities as a writer than special education teachers. Additionally, they were more likely than special educators to indicate that writing developed through effort and process and less likely to think that writing knowledge came from experts. However, more research is needed here, as these beliefs may relate to specific paradigms (e.g., writers' workshop) and data on effectiveness of writing instruction, neither of which was assessed.

It is not unreasonable to expect that specialists would be more knowledgeable and prepared to teach writing to students with LD. Both groups' lack of preparation was due, in part, to a lack of coursework and practicum emphasizing writing instruction in their preservice college programs. Over the past 40 years, we have found that few special education programs require even one course in teaching writing across grades K–12. This must change if we are to provide students with LD, and others, the writing instruction they deserve. This will take a concerted effort on the part of special education and general education faculty members.

Professional Development

Given inadequate preservice preparation in writing for the majority of teachers, effective PD is imperative, yet research on PD for writing has been relatively rare in both general and special education. Harris et al. (2022), however, found 21 studies of professional development for SRSD in writing across the United States, Portugal, and Spain. Six additional studies involved two instructional approaches similar to SRSD in Spain and the Netherlands. The majority of these studies involved practice-based professional development (PBPD) for SRSD. Ball and Cohen (1999) indicated that the focus of practice-based PD is to develop teacher knowledge, understanding, and skills related to an effective educational practice; support is provided once classroom implementation begins. The complex reality of practice and the opportunity to develop important knowledge, skills, and understandings are addressed by (1) collective participation of teachers within the same school with similar needs; (2) basing PD around the characteristics, strengths, and needs of current students; (3) attention to content knowledge needs of teachers, including pedagogical content knowledge; (4) opportunities for active learning and practice of the new methods being learned, including opportunities to see and analyze examples of these methods being used; (5) use of materials and other artifacts during PD that are identical to those to be used in the classroom; and (6) feedback on performance while learning, prior to classroom use, so that understandings and skills critical in implementation are developed. Recent reviews of PD research, however, have neglected to identify and include this research base in writing (McKeown et al., 2019). A detailed description of PBPD for SRSD can be found in McKeown et al. (2019) and Harris, Lane, Driscoll, et al. (2012).

Space precludes a thorough discussion of Harris et al.'s (2022) findings. Notable here is that 12 of the 21 PBPD for SRSD studies took place in inclusive classrooms, studies existed across student SES levels, and the majority of students involved in these studies were Black, White, or Latinx (52%, 41%, and 27%, respectively). Only three studies focused specifically on students with or at risk for EBD; only one study focused specifically on students at risk for LD in writing. Studies that involved inclusive classrooms typically did not have the N required to separate outcomes for students with or at risk for disability in writing. While it is encouraging that a large number of studies were conducted in inclusive classrooms, more research on PD for teachers working specifically with students with LD or other disabilities is clearly needed. Only one study was found that involved both special and general education teachers; only one study was found that focused on special educators. Research on PBPD for this evidence-based writing intervention among special education teachers is clearly needed. As noted previously, special education teachers do not feel particularly well-prepared to teach writing and are not efficacious about their capabilities as writers or to teach this complex skill.

Also notable is that every one of the 27 studies reviewed resulted in one or more significant and meaningful outcomes in student writing, most commonly quality and/or length (multiple other outcomes were investigated as well). A few studies, however, particularly the one mixed-methods study and three single-case design studies, found that not all students improved as expected and that meaningful variability in outcomes existed. The results of studies at the whole class or inclusive classroom level can mask this issue, highlighting the importance of continued SCD and mixed-methods research. Also notable is that in the RCT and quasi-experimental studies, effect sizes were comparable to those achieved in studies where research team members delivered SRSD instruction, contrary to the oft-cited finding that teacher-implemented interventions rarely attain the effect sizes found in researcher-implemented interventions (McKeown et al., 2019). Finally, eight studies included a measure of social validity of SRSD among students; outcomes were high in each study.

The primary teacher outcomes reported were fidelity (reported in 20 of the 27 studies; range = 74%–98%, mean = 90%) and social validity (reported in 11 of 27 studies, high in all). Only one study reported on possible improvements in self-efficacy for teaching writing. A significant problem for research in writing is the lack of teacher-level outcome measures with proven reliability and validity in areas such as genre knowledge, cross-genre characteristics of effective writing, and attitudes and self-efficacy for writing and for teaching writing. A great deal more work is needed here to enhance research on PD in writing. Finally, Harris et al. (2022) found only three studies of reading to learn and writing to inform or persuade. While additional research in SRSD for reading and writing to learn from text has been conducted (c.f. Foxworth & Mason, 2018; Mason et al., 2012), far more research in reading to learn and writing to inform, persuade, or argue is needed, as is research on PD for these approaches.

Conclusion and Suggestions for a Research Agenda

The field of LD has come a long way in the study of writing among students at risk for LD or other disabilities and with students with LD. Here, we have reviewed research on writing among school-age students with LD and their peers and factors that influence how these students write. Practices for assessing writing and identifying LD in writing were examined, as were preservice and in-service teacher development in writing. While much has been accomplished, much remains to be studied.

We would like to provide seven recommendations for future research. One, we need to know more about how writing develops for students with LD and how such development differs from typically developing writers. This requires longitudinal studies of writing comparing students with and without LD. Two, and somewhat similarly, we need to know more about how students with LD write as well as the personal and contextual factors that facilitate and impede their writing. We also need to know more about the processes that students with LD apply while writing, the knowledge they draw on as they write, their beliefs about writing, and how varying contexts interact with these factors and other related skills, such as reading, to shape what they write. Three, research on students with LD and writing is mostly limited to school-age children. We need to take a broader lifespan view of writing, including its use, value, and growth (as well as decline) for people with LD from childhood through adulthood.

Four, our knowledge about how students are taught to write is limited. We currently possess very little information on how these youngsters are taught writing by either general or special education teachers. Observational studies that examine the writing instructional practices of both groups of teachers are sorely needed. Such research can be especially impactful if it is carried out over time and in different settings, examining the associations between observed instructional practices and the writing growth of students with LD. Five, and directly related to teaching writing, is the need for an increased investiture in writing intervention research. This includes studies that test and replicate the effectiveness of new (and old) writing practices for students with LD in Tier 1, 2, and 3 settings.

Our sixth recommendation is not aimed solely at research. The preparation of preservice special education teachers to teach writing, and that of general educators, is inadequate. We need special and general education faculty to advocate for effective coursework in teaching writing and for collaboration in writing development. In addition, we need research that accompanies such teacher preparation, identifying what is working, where we still are not doing enough, and how we can improve teacher preparation in this critical area.

Finally, our seventh recommendation focuses on further research in SRSD and in PD for SRSD. SRSD research on writing for students with LD needs to expand in new directions. For example, we lack research on text structures other than opinion/persuasive writing, narrative writing, and informative writing. Text structures common in reading, such as compare and contrast, cause and effect, and problem and solution, need to be addressed separately and in tandem with the three genres focused on now. In addition, research on SRSD needs to expand to include young children (ages 5–6), high school students, and adults with LD. The role of family, and family supports, in developing as a writer has been neglected. Longitudinal research on outcomes of SRSD instruction across grades is nonexistent yet badly needed. The effectiveness of incorporating SRSD within a larger writing program, perhaps including aspects of writers' as well as transcription, sentence construction, and vocabulary, needs to be examined (Harris & Graham, 2018). Research on integrating SRSD instruction in the classroom with online intelligent tutors or other web-based approaches for all students in inclusive classrooms, as well as students receiving special education services, is needed. Finally, the emergent body of research on PD for teachers working with students with LD and other disabilities needs to be sustained and expanded to help guide our work with practicing special educators and their peers.

Even though there is still much to learn, the growth and increasing attention devoted to writing research for students with and without LD in the last several decades is encouraging. We look forward to following writing research for students with LD and their peers in the years to come.

REFERENCES

Ball, D. L., & Cohen, D. K. (1999). Developing practice, developing practitioners: Toward a practice-based theory of professional education. In L. Darling-Hammond & G. Sykes (Eds.), *Teaching as a learning profession: Handbook for policy and practice* (pp. 3–31). Jossey-Bass.

Berninger, V., Vaughn, K., Abbott, R., Abbott, S., Rogan, L., Brooks, A., et al. (1997). Treatment of handwriting problems in beginning writers: Transfer from handwriting to composition. *Journal of Educational Psychology, 89*, 652–666.

Calfee, R., & Wilson, K. (2004). A classroom-based writing assessment framework. In C. Stone, E. Silliman, B. Ehran, & K. Apel (Eds.), *Handbook of language and literacy: Development and disorders* (pp. 583–599). Guilford Press.

Christenson, S., Thurlow, M., Ysseldyke, J., & McVicar, R. (1989). Written language instruction for students with mild handicaps: Is there enough quantity to ensure quality? *Learning Disability Quarterly, 12*, 219–222.

Cochran-Smith, M., & Zeichner, K. (Eds.) (2005). *Studying teacher education: The report of the AERA Panel on research and teacher education*. American Educational Research Association.

De La Paz, S., Swanson, P., & Graham, S. (1998). The contribution of executive control to the revising of students with writing and learning difficulties. *Journal of Educational Psychology, 90*, 448–460.

Dockrell, J., Connelly, V., Walter, K., & Critten, S. (2018). The role of curriculum based measures in assessing writing products. In B. Miller, P. McCardle, & V. Connelly (Eds.), *Writing development in struggling learners: Understanding the needs of writers across the life course* (Studies in Writing, Vol. 35, pp. 182–215). Brill.

Ekholm, E., Zumbrunn, S., & DeBusk-Lane, M. (2018). Clarifying an elusive construct: A systematic review of writing attitudes. *Educational Psychology Review, 30*, 827–856.

Englert, C., Raphael, T., Anderson, L., Gregg, S., & Anthony, H. (1989). Exposition: Reading, writing, and metacognitive knowledge of learning disabled students. *Learning Disabilities Research, 5*, 5–24.

Fitzgerald, J., & Shanahan, T. (2000). Reading and writing relations and their development. *Educational Psychologist, 35*, 39–50.

FitzPatrick, E., & McKeown, D. (2021). Writing from multiple source texts: SRSD for fifth grade learners in inclusive settings. *Learning Disabilities Research & Practice, 36*(3), 188–200.

Foxworth, L., & Mason, L. H. (2018). Writing to learn instruction that works. In R. Fidalgo, K. R. Harris, & Braaksma, M. (Eds.), *Design principles for teaching effective writing: Theoretical and empirical grounded principles* (pp. 119–151). Brill.

Foxworth, L., Mason, L. H., & Hughes, C. (2017). Improving narrative writing skills. *Exceptionality, 25*, 217–234.

Garcia, J.-N., & Fidalgo, R. (2008). Orchestration of writing processes and writing products: A comparison of sixth-grade students with and without learning disabilities. *Learning Disabilities: A Contemporary Journal, 6*, 77–98.

Gillespie, A., & Graham, S. (2014). A meta-analysis of writing interventions for students with learning disabilities. *Exceptional Children, 80*, 454–473.

Graham, S. (1997). Executive control in the revising of students with learning and writing difficulties. *Journal of Educational Psychology, 89*, 223–234.

Graham, S. (2018a). A writer(s) within community model of writing. In C. Bazerman, V. Berninger, D. Brandt, S. Graham, J. Langer, S. Murphy, et al. (Eds.), *The lifespan development of writing* (pp. 271–325). National Council of Teachers of English.

Graham, S. (2018b). Instructional feedback in writing. In A. Lipnevich & J. Smith (Eds.), *The Cambridge handbook of instructional feedback* (Cambridge Handbooks in Psychology, pp. 145–168). Cambridge University Press.

Graham, S. (2019). Changing how writing is taught. *Review of Research in Education, 43*, 277–303.

Graham, S., Aitken, A., Hebert, M., Santangelo, T., Camping, A., Harris, K. R., et al. (2021). Do children with reading difficulties experience writing difficulties? A meta-analysis. *Journal of Educational Psychology, 113*(8), 1481–1506.

Graham, S., Berninger, V., & Fan, W. (2007). The structural relationship between writing attitude and writing achievement in young children. *Contemporary Educational Psychology, 32*, 516–536.

Graham, S., Bollinger, A., Booth Olson, C., D'Aoust, C., MacArthur, C., McCutchen, D., & Olinghouse, N. (2018). *Teaching elementary school students to be effective writers: A practice guide (NCEE 2012-4058), Revised.* National Center for Education Evaluation and Regional Assistance, Institute of Education Sciences, U.S. Department of Education.

Graham, S., Collins, A., & Ciullo, S. (2022). Special and general education teachers' beliefs about writing and writing instruction. *Journal of Learning Disabilities, 56*(3), 163–179.

Graham, S., Collins, A., & Rigby-Wills, H. (2017). A meta-analysis examining the writing characteristics of students with learning disabilities and normally achieving peers. *Exceptional Children, 83*, 199–218.

Graham, S., Fishman, E., Reid, R., Hebert, M. (2016). Writing characteristics of students with ADHD and their normally achieving peers. *Learning Disabilities Research & Practice, 31*, 75–89.

Graham, S., & Harris, K. R. (2018). Evidence-based writing practices: A meta-analysis of existing meta-analyses. In R. Fidalgo, K. R. Harris, & M. Braaksma (Eds.), *Design principles for teaching effective writing: Theoretical and empirical grounded principles* (pp. 13–37). Brill.

Graham, S., & Harris, K. R. (2020). Writing and students with learning disabilities. In A. Martin, R. Sperling, & K. Newton (Eds.), *Handbook of educational psychology and students with special needs* (p. 509). Routledge.

Graham, S., Harris, K. R., & Chambers, A. (2016). Evidence-based practice and writing instruction. In C. MacArthur, S. Graham, & J. Fitzgerald (Eds.), *Handbook of writing research* (Vol. 2, pp. 211–226). Guilford Press.

Graham, S., Harris, K. R., & McKeown, D. (2013). The writing of students with LD and a meta-analysis of SRSD writing intervention studies: Redux. In L. Swanson, K. R. Harris, & S. Graham (Eds.), *Handbook of learning disabilities* (2nd ed., pp. 405–438). Guilford Press.

Graham, S., Harris, K. R., & Santangelo, T. (2015). Research-based writing practices and the Common Core: Meta-analysis and meta-synthesis. *Elementary School Journal, 115*, 498–522.

Graham, S., Hebert, M., Fishman, E., Ray, A., & Gillespie-Rouse, A. (2020). Do children classified with specific language impairment experience writing difficulties? A meta-analysis. *Journal of Learning Disabilities, 53*, 292–310.

Graham, S., Hebert, M., & Harris, K. R. (2011). Throw 'em out or make 'em better? High-stakes writing assessments. *Focus on Exceptional Children, 44*, 1–12.

Graham, S., Hebert, M., & Harris, K. R. (2015). Formative assessment and writing: A meta-analysis. *Elementary School Journal, 115*, 524–547.

Graham, S., Hebert, M., Sandbank, M., & Harris, K. R. (2016). Credibly assessing the writing achievement of young struggling writers: Application of generalizability theory. *Learning Disability Quarterly, 39*, 72–82.

Graham, S., Schwartz, S., & MacArthur, C. (1993). Knowledge of writing and the composing process, attitude toward writing, and selfefficacy for students with and without learning disabilities. *Journal of Learning Disabilities, 26*, 237–249.

Harris, K. R. (2021). SRSD instructional research for students with or at-risk for LD across the content areas: History and reflections. *Learning Disabilities Research and Practice, (36)*, (3), 235–241.

Harris, K. R., & Graham, S. (2013). "An adjective is a word hanging down from a noun": Learning to write and students with learning disabilities. *Annals of Dyslexia, 63*, 65–79.

Harris, K. R., & Graham, S. (2016). Self-regulated strategy development in writing: Policy implications of an evidence-based practice. *Policy Insights from Behavioral and Brain Sciences, 3*, 77–84.

Harris, K. R., & Graham, S. (2018). Self-regulated strategy development: Theoretical bases, critical instructional elements, and future research. In R. Fidalgo, K. R. Harris, & Braaksma, M. (Eds.), *Design principles for teaching effective writing: Theoretical and empirical grounded principles* (pp. 119–151). Brill.

Harris, K. R., Graham, S., & Adkins, M. (2015). Practice-based professional development and self-regulated strategy development for Tier 2, at-risk writers in second grade. *Contemporary Educational Psychology, 40*, 5–16.

Harris, K. R., Graham, S., Brindle, M., & Sandmel, K. (2009). Metacognition and children's writing. In D. Hacker, J. Dunlosky, & A. Graesser (Eds.), *Handbook of metacognition in education* (pp. 131–153). Erlbaum.

Harris, K. R., Graham, S., MacArthur, C., Reid, R., & Mason, L. (2011). Self-regulated learning processes and children's writing. In B. Zimmerman & D. H. Schunk (Eds.), *Handbook of self-regulation of learning and performance* (pp. 187–202). Routledge.

Harris, K. R., Graham, S., & Mason, L. (2006). Improving the writing, knowledge, and motivation of struggling young writers: Effects of self-regulated strategy development with and without peer support. *American Educational Research Journal, 43*(2), 295–340.

Harris, K. R., Graham, S., Mason, L., McKeown, D., & Olinghouse, N. (2018). Self-regulated strategy development in writing: A classroom example of developing executive function processes and future directions. In L. Meltzer (Ed.), *Executive functioning in education: From theory to practice* (2nd ed., pp. 326–356). Guilford Press.

Harris, K. R., Kim, Y-S., Yim, S., Camping, A., & Graham, S. (2023). Yes, they can: An RCT of Tier 2 SRSD plus transcription and oral language skills for writing to inform using source text at 1st and 2nd grades. *Contemporary Educational Psychology, 73*, 102150.

Harris, K. R., Lane, K., Driscoll, S., Graham, S., Wilson, K., Sandmel, K., Brindle, M., & Schatschneider, C. (2012). Teacher-implemented class-wide writing intervention using Self-Regulated Strategy Development for students with and without behavior concerns. *Elementary School Journal, 113*, 160–191.

Harris, K. R., Lane, K. L., Graham, S., Driscoll, S., Sandmel, K., Brindle, M., & Schatschneider, C. (2012). Practice-based professional development for self-regulated strategies development in writing: A randomized controlled study. *Journal of Teacher Education, 63*(2), 103–119.

Harris, K. R., McKeown, D., & Camping, A. (2022). *Practice-based professional development for scaling up writing interventions: Lessons learned and challenges remaining* [Manuscript submitted for publication].

Harris, K. R., Ray, A. Graham, S., & Houston, J. (2019). Answering the challenge: SRSD instruction for close reading of text to write to persuade with 4th and 5th grade students experiencing writing difficulties. *Reading and Writing: An Interdisciplinary Journal, 32*, 1345–1357.

Healey, J. (1990). *The early alphabet.* University of California Press.

Lane, S. (2010). *Performance assessment: The state of the art* (SCOPE Student Performance Assessment Series). Stanford University, Stanford Center for Opportunity Policy in Education.

Lin, S. C., Monroe, B. W., & Troia, G. A. (2007). Development of writing knowledge in grades 2–8: A comparison of typically developing writers and their struggling peers. *Reading & Writing Quarterly: Overcoming Learning Difficulties, 23*, 207–230.

MacArthur, C., & Cavalier, A. (2004). Dictation and speech recognition technology as test accommodation. *Exceptional Children, 71*, 43–58.

MacArthur, C., & Graham, S. (1987). Learning disabled students' composing with three methods: Handwriting, dictation, and word processing. *Journal of Special Education, 21*, 22–42.

MacArthur, C. A., Graham, S., & Fitzgerald, J. (Eds.). (2016). *Handbook of writing research.* Guilford Press.

MacArthur, C., Graham, S., & Schwartz, S. (1991). Knowledge of revision and revising behavior among students with learning disabilities. *Learning Disability Quarterly, 14*, 61–74.

Mason, L. H., Reid, R., & Hagaman, J. (2012). *Building comprehension in adolescents: Powerful strategies for improving reading and writing in content areas.* Brookes.

McCutchen, D. (1988). "Functional automaticity" in children's writing: A problem of metacognitive control. *Written Communication, 5*, 306–324.

McKeown, D., Brindle, M., Harris, K. R., Sandmel, K., Steinbrecher, T. D., Graham, S., et al. (2019). Teachers' voices: Perceptions of effective professional development and classwide implementation of self-regulated strategy development in writing. *American Educational Research Journal, 56*, 753–791.

McMaster, K., & Espin, C. (2007). Technical features of curriculum-based measurement in writing: A literature review. *Journal of Special Education, 41*, 68–84.

Montague, M., Maddux, C. D., & Dereshiwsky, M. I. (1990). Story grammar and comprehension and production of narrative prose by students with learning disabilities. *Journal of Learning Disabilities, 23*, 190–197.

Myklebust, H. R. (1973). *Development and disorders of written language: Studies of normal and exceptional children* (Vol. 2). Grune & Stratton.

Newcomer, P., & Barenbaum, E. (1991). Written composing ability of children with learning disabilities: A review of literature from 1980 to 1990. *Journal of Learning Disabilities, 24*, 578–593.

Olinghouse, N., Graham, S., & Gillespie, A. (2015). The relationship of discourse and topic knowledge to writing performance. *Journal of Educational Psychology, 107*, 391–406.

Pullen, P., Lane, H., Ashworth, K., & Lovelace, S. (2017). Specific learning disabilities. In J. M. Kauffman, D. P. Hallahan, & P. C. Pullen (Eds.), *Handbook of special education* (2nd ed., pp. 286–299). Routledge.

Ritchey, K. D., & Coker, D. L. (2013). An investigation of the validity and utility of two curriculum-based measurement writing tasks. *Reading & Writing Quarterly, 29*(1), 89–119.

Rogers, L., & Graham, S. (2008). A meta-analysis of single subject design writing intervention research. *Journal of Educational Psychology, 100*, 879–906.

Saddler, B., & Graham, S. (2005). The effects of peerassisted sentence combining instruction on the writing performance of more and less skilled young writers. *Journal of Educational Psychology, 97*, 43–54.

Saddler, B., & Graham, S. (2007). The relationship between writing knowledge and writing performance among more and less skilled writers. *Reading and Writing Quarterly, 23*, 231–247.

Sawyer, R. J., Graham, S., & Harris, K. R. (1992). Direct teaching, strategy instruction, and strategy instruction with explicit selfregulation: Effects on learning disabled students' composition skills and selfefficacy. *Journal of Educational Psychology, 84*, 340–352.

Schmandt-Besserat & Erard, M. (2008). Origins and forms of writing. In C. Bazerman (Ed.), *Handbook of research on writing* (pp. 7–22). Routledge.

Søvik, N., Arntzen, O., & Thygesen, R. (1987). Writing characteristics of "normal," dyslexic and dysgraphic children. *Journal of Human Movement Studies, 31*, 171–187.

Swedlow, J. (1999). The power of writing. *National Geographic, 196*, 110–132.

Thomas, C., Englert, C., & Gregg, S. (1987). An analysis of errors and strategies in the expository writing of learning disabled students. *Remedial and Special Education, 8*, 21–30.

Troia, G., & Graham, S. (2017). Use and acceptability of adaptations to classroom writing instruction and assessment practices for students with disabilities: A survey of grade 3–8 teachers. *Learning Disabilities Research & Practice, 32*, 257–269.

U.S. Department of Education. (2015). *37th annual report to congress on the implementation of the Individuals with Disabilities Education Act.* Office of Special Education and Rehabilitation Services, Office of Special Education Programs.

Wong, B. Y. L., Wong, R., & Blenkinsop, J. (1989). Cognitive and metacognitive aspects of learning disabled adolescents' composing problems. *Learning Disability Quarterly, 12*, 300–322.

CHAPTER 16

Social Studies and History Instruction for Students with Learning Disabilities

Susan De La Paz, Daniel R. Wissinger, and Josue Otarola

This chapter reviews recent exemplary research on social studies and history instruction for students with learning disabilities (LD). Society has changed significantly since the second edition of this *Handbook* in 2014, with national and worldwide challenges including the COVID-19 pandemic, nationwide calls for reckoning on racism and police violence following George Floyd's murder in 2020, and the rise of false or misleading *disinformation* spread intentionally for profit, harm, or political or ideological purposes (Freelon & Wells, 2020). Issues such as school safety, critical race theory, and how to respond to over 600 Americans attacking the U. S. Capital in response to the transfer of presidency from Donald Trump to Joe Biden in 2021 were once viewed as contentious issues but are now polarized topics, and many people believe that what now counts as evidence of truth claims is hard to agree upon (Ferretti et al., 2023). We believe social studies and history education are, therefore, of vital importance.

In this chapter, we discuss theoretical underpinnings for teaching social studies and history to students with LD. Next, we highlight exemplary strategies from the research literature that can be used by teachers to facilitate the development of generic cognitive strategies, such as note taking and summarizing a text passage, questioning, monitoring comprehension, or prewriting strategies. We then describe exemplary cognitive strategies interventions that align with recommendations for promoting more sophisticated conceptual knowledge and epistemic ways of reasoning with historical information. We end with calls for researchers to focus on understudied topics in social studies and for research that explores how cognitive, linguistic, and social challenges impact the participation of students with LD in these subjects.

Social studies and history education can be understood through comparisons in subject matter goals and in activities that take place in schools. At the elementary level, the National Council for the Social Studies (NCSS) defines social studies as an interdisciplinary study of history, geography, economics, and government/civics and is defined through disciplinary, cross-disciplinary, and interdisciplinary subjects at higher levels. Secondary disciplines and courses include history (e.g., United States, world, and African American), geography, economics, government and citizenship, social sciences (e.g., anthropology, LGBTQ+ studies, psychology, and religious studies), ethnic studies, human rights and social justice, financial literacy, and contemporary issues (e.g., current events and the study of social studies topics in current contexts). It is through studying these topics that students gain a sense of our collective past; by learning about people, places, problems, solutions, and the outcomes of those solutions, students prepare for a lifelong practice of civil discourse and civic engagement in their communities.

The NCSS curriculum standards, civic mission, and the College, Career, and Civic Life (C3) Framework all emphasize the importance of meeting the needs of diverse students and providing meaningful and powerful teaching and learning opportunities that are scaffolded and engaging (Minarik & Lintner, 2024). The C3 Framework further stresses the importance of inquiry activities in which students have the opportunity to develop their own questions; apply disciplinary concepts; gather sources and use evidence; and work collaboratively to develop conclusions and take action. These make clear that ambitious expectations for learning apply equally to students who find school to be challenging. Unfortunately, the field lacks adequate understanding of how to support students with LD because researchers and educators often under-report findings for academically diverse students.

National Assessment of Educational Progress (NAEP) reports also consistently indicate the need for improved outcomes for students with and without disabilities. In 2022, the average U.S. history score for eighth-grade students in the nation was 5 points lower compared to 2018. Only 13% of the eighth graders demonstrated proficient knowledge of U.S. history and historical thinking skills (in comparison, the average scores for students with disabilities were at the basic level); in addition, the percentage of students who performed below the basic level on the 2022 Civics Assessment increased by 3%. Also in 2022, a mere 6% of eighth-grade students with disabilities performed at or above proficient, and these results were not significantly different from previous civics assessments (NCES, 2022).

Students, teachers, and administrators answered survey questions about educational experiences both inside and outside the classroom. Results in 2022 indicate that larger percentages of higher-performing students (scoring at or above the 75th percentile) participated in U.S. history-related instructional practices, such as exploring information from multiple sources, as compared to lower-performing students (scoring below the 25th percentile). Significantly more higher-performing students *often*, *always*, or *almost always* investigated causes and effects of important events in U.S. history; analyzed relationships between historical events; and compared and evaluated different points of view, as compared to lower-performing students. Unfortunately, we do not know if these gaps were due to lack of instructional opportunity or whether they were due to challenges associated with having a disability. Because students with LD struggle in multiple areas, we now address linguistic, cognitive, and affective needs that impact their learning in social studies and history.

Academic Challenges and Instructional Considerations

It is not surprising that social studies and history instruction is challenging for students with LD, as these students experience significant barriers to comprehending written texts and producing comprehensible texts (Ferretti & De La Paz, 2011). Poor reading comprehension is ubiquitous among students with a learning disability (Kennedy et al., 2015), and many adolescents with LD have difficulty understanding complex historical events, often due to their low reading abilities (O'Connor et al., 2017). However, in comparison with novices who do not have learning difficulties, students with LD may have comprehension problems that also result from lack of relevant background knowledge, restricted vocabularies, limited text structure or genre knowledge, and restrictions in self-regulatory skills needed to monitor comprehension and repair misunderstandings (De La Paz, 2005; Mastropieri et al., 2003).

Moreover, students with LD routinely experience writing problems. Compared to their normally achieving peers, the essays of students with LD contain more spelling, punctuation, and grammatical errors (Englert et al., 2009). These production problems tax the writer's working memory capacity, thereby limiting the processing resources available for planning, revising, and regulating the writing process (Nokes & De La Paz, 2018). Although limited, the available evidence also suggests that without instruction, students with LD frequently write less than their peers (Bulgren et al., 2011; Okolo et al., 2011). Their writing often lacks critical discursive elements. For example, students with LD are more likely than their peers to fail to consider alternative perspectives (De La Paz & Wissinger, 2017; Wissinger & De La Paz, 2020).

There are many potential underlying reasons for these literacy challenges. Struggling learners often have limitations in being able to consider multiple perspectives (Bouck et al., 2008). Further cognitive and socioemotional delays constrain some students' ability to develop historical empathy (Okolo & Ferretti, 1996). Students with LD have been shown to have limitations in their ability to transform information and differentiate relevant from irrelevant details (Bulgren et al., 2007), have more misconceptions about the processes involved in historical reasoning (Ferretti et al., 2007), and generally know less factual historical content than their peers without disabilities (De La Paz, 2005; Ferretti et al., 2001).

Developmental Challenges

As some researchers have identified strategies historians use, other researchers have considered how students approach historical thinking. Observational research clearly shows that historical reading and writing is challenging for neurotypical novices (De La Paz & Nokes, 2020). For example, Lee and Ashby (2000) observed the unsophisticated strategies used by students. When faced with multiple sources that contain conflicting accounts, the youngest students, lacking any strategies, admitted that they could not know what happened in the past. Older, middle-school-aged students arbitrarily labeled some accounts as deliberate falsifications, agreeing with others. Slightly older students ruled with the majority of the accounts. Rather than creating a synthesized interpretation that relied on the best evidence from multiple documents, they discounted some accounts and accepted others as factual.

And, almost 10 years previously, Wineburg (1991) observed gifted high school students solve historical reading and writing tasks in a now seminal study. They skillfully applied generic reading strategies, such as summarizing, monitoring comprehension, making connections to background knowledge, and rereading. However, the historical thinking strategies they used were as unsophisticated as those Lee and Ashby (2000) observed. For instance, most students sought a nonexistent objective source that lacked bias, being enticed by a textbook account. Wineburg's seminal work also revealed that high school students failed to interrogate sources, primarily because they did not see the texts as written by individuals with specific purposes and intentions—even trusting textbooks as the most reliable source of information.

Students might not only lack sophisticated strategies for formulating a compelling historical argument, such as relying on everyday notions about argumentation (De La Paz et al., 2012), but they might also fail to understand why argumentation is needed in history (Monte-Sano, 2010; Nokes et al., 2007). For example, when writing historical arguments, students often respond to requests to create arguments by first figuring out what they want to say and then using the documents to support their standpoint or looking for a single, objective interpretation (Monte-Sano, 2010). They tend to have difficulty grasping the nature of historical context, often judging past actors and actions by present standards (VanSledright, 2002). Further, without instruction, even advanced students face challenges analyzing and using historical evidence (De La Paz et al., 2022; Monte-Sano, 2010; Wineburg, 1991). In sum, novices have less sophisticated understandings of the cognitive strategies underlying historical reading and writing processes.

Classroom Challenges

Integrating disciplinary literacy into classroom practice is ambitious, and it poses challenges to teachers who are tasked with bringing reading, writing, and content together in an integrated way that fosters disciplinary learning and related literacy development. Increasingly, history classrooms have embraced primary source–based investigation and inquiry (Thacker et al., 2017); however, writing is not a regular part of students' social studies experience in school. When teachers assign reading and writing in secondary history classrooms, the focus typically involves reading comprehension and summary of information (Kiuhara et al., 2009), as well as the use of textbooks as authoritative sources of information (Nokes, 2014).

This set of findings is, however, fragmented and incomplete, as educational researchers and national history assessment data have yet to give precise information about the gaps between students with LD and other novices when considering conceptual foundations, linguistic abilities, and procedural knowledge related to reading and writing in social studies and history. Moreover, we have conflicting reports as to the capability of students with LD to develop more nuanced understandings of history. Some researchers (e.g., Swanson et al., 2014) suggest that cognitive processing difficulties lead students with LD to have difficulty developing deep historical understandings, whereas others (Bouck et al., 2008; De La Paz & Hernández-Ramos, 2013; Ferretti et al., 2001) show that when students are given sustained opportunities to engage in historical inquiry and construct their own interpretations, students with LD are able to reason with primary and secondary sources in ways that are as advanced as their peers who do not have disabilities.

Over the past two decades, extensive reforms in social studies education have changed the way students with LD learn in the classroom. The Common Core State Standards (CCSS) further make clear that students are expected to incorporate literacy skills in the subjects they are learning. For example, students should be able to "construct effective written arguments and convey intricate or multifaceted information" and support their ideas with "relevant evidence" (CCSS, 2010, p. 3). Students must also "identify aspects of text that reveal an author's point of view" (CCSS.ELA-Literacy.RH.6-8.8) as they read and "compare the point of view of two or more authors for how they treat the same topics, including which details they emphasize in their respective accounts" (CCSS.ELA-Literacy.RH.9-10.6). However, referring to "supporting ideas with relevant evidence" and identifying "an author's point of view" without further specification minimizes the role that each subject matter plays (Moje, 2008). This means that teachers must attend to what it means to learn in each subject and consider what counts as knowledge in the discipline(s) that provide a foundation for those subjects, or they will struggle to integrate literacy instruction in those subjects.

Subsequently, Monte-Sano (2010, 2016) and others advocate for reading and writing activities that prioritize historical cognitive strategies, using specialized ways of thinking more common to historians to analyze and use evidence in support of an interpretation. Historical writing,[1] like most other types of academic writing, uses data, warrants, and claims to construct a rational argument; however, the nature of the data and warrants and the way evidence is framed is singular in the manner historians write. Moreover, the study of the past is further complicated by the nature of historical evidence. Most historical evidence, including written records and artifacts, is produced by humans and, as such, is susceptible to human frailties, including biases, imperfect perceptions, and selective recordkeeping (Collingwood, 2005). As a result of the nature of historical evidence, subjective evaluations of significance and causation, and the role of perspective in the

[1]Readers should consult authors such as van Boxtel and van Drie (2018), Monte-Sano (2011), Nokes (2014), Reisman (2012), Seixas (2017), VanSledright (2002), and Wineburg (1991, 2001) for further information on historical reasoning and the nature of historian's writing.

production and analysis of evidence, the narratives that historians construct are interpretive reflections of the past rather than snapshots of reality (Nokes & De La Paz, 2023).

As such, history has its own epistemic norms and practices for constructing historical knowledge (Nokes, 2014; van Boxtel & van Drie, 2018). Fortunately, calls for the integration of disciplinary literacy instruction in subject matter classrooms are consistent with models used in cognitive research and assert that mastery evolves from domain-general declarative knowledge to discipline-specific procedural knowledge (Alexander, 2003).

Alexander's (2003) Model of Domain Learning (MDL) explains how students' knowledge, strategic processing, and interest change over time as they become acclimated to, competent, and finally proficient in a given discipline such as history. Acclimation, the initial stage, signifies the learner has limited domain and topic knowledge, resulting in the need for generic, surface-level strategies (e.g., rereading, comprehension, and paraphrasing) and a concomitant increase in procedural knowledge for analyzing and constructing history (e.g., asking questions, constructing interpretations, and evaluating historical evidence). According to the MDL, academic competence is demonstrated when learners flexibly use surface-level and deep processing strategies during academic problem-solving tasks, such as when reading and writing in social studies and history.

When applied to social studies, topic knowledge (also called *first-order knowledge*) refers to specific, factual knowledge about historical dates, figures, or events. Domain knowledge includes both *first-order knowledge* and *second-order knowledge*, which are characterized as conceptual knowledge about elements of domain thinking, such as cause and using evidence to construct narratives about the past. This model proposes that students' beliefs about knowledge shift after they begin to view domain knowledge as something that can be constructed (i.e., they develop epistemological beliefs). They are then likely to view the domain as more engaging, which facilitates greater interest and the capacity to generalize domain-specific thinking and knowledge to other topics and subjects (Alexander, 2003).

Research on Social Studies and History Instruction for Students with LD

Alexander's (2003) model can be used to organize the literature on social studies literacy. Several meta-analyses highlight the utility of effective interventions for developing students' learning and knowledge in social studies classrooms (Ciullo et al., 2020; Swanson et al., 2014; Wissinger & Ciullo, 2018). While most of the studies have targeted students' topic and domain knowledge, a corpus of more recent studies reveals several promising strategies and forms of instruction that teachers can use to facilitate the use of deep-level strategies and changes in epistemological beliefs.

We begin with interventions in which special education researchers taught students with LD to acquire vocabulary, improve reading comprehension, or produce written summaries of informational text. Research shows that textbooks are still used for at least part of secondary social studies and history instruction (O'Connor et al., 2017); therefore, domain-general cognitive strategies are also needed. Because this body of literature has been summarized elsewhere (e.g., Ciullo et al., 2020; Scruggs et al., 2010; Wissinger & Ciullo, 2018), we do not provide comments about designs or intervention conditions, except when reviewing component analyses, and do not discuss statistical conclusions in depth.

Vocabulary Instruction

Seminal work by Mastropieri, Scruggs, and colleagues showed that one of the most effective ways to teach content-area vocabulary to students with disabilities is through explicit instruction in mnemonic strategies (Scruggs et al., 2010). Mnemonic instruction has been extensively researched with students with LD and found to be a highly effective approach for learning first-order knowledge (names of significant people, events, and dates). However, designing mnemonic vocabulary strategy lessons is time-consuming for teachers. More importantly, because students do not use vocabulary in isolation, researchers have combined mnemonics with note-taking strategies or focused on students working in teams to learn vocabulary and social studies content (Mastropieri et al., 2003).

Bulgren and colleagues investigated the effectiveness of a question-exploration routine (QER) on diverse seventh-grade students' ability to ask and answer inferential questions as they read and studied researcher-developed social studies content (Bulgren et al., 2011). Students used a graphic organizer while learning note-taking strategies, formed main-idea statements to answer critical questions, and learned to relate main ideas to the real world. The results showed that participants with LD had better performance on multiple-choice, matching, and short-answer content test, in comparison to students who were exposed to lecture and discussion. The positive effects of QER instruction extended to high achievers, average achievers, those identified with disabilities, and low achievers. In 2013, Bulgren and colleagues published information on related cognitive routines that facilitate learning.

Kennedy and colleagues used effective multimedia design principles to develop "podcasts" (PowerPoint presentations with embedded video) for teaching social studies information as an alternative to reading passages (Kennedy et al., 2015). Their focus was on teaching word definitions and broader conceptual understanding of words to improve ninth-grade students' vocabulary learning. Outcomes included a 30-item multiple-choice assessment of vocabulary definitions and world history concepts (e.g., imperialism) and an application task that required students to write synonyms, antonyms, and any additional information that they knew about each term. An interesting aspect of this study is that the researchers provided a component analysis of intervention elements, comparing explicit cues (i.e., providing video with explicit definitions of vocabulary and signals as to what is important to understand) with and without mnemonic instruction and, in comparison, to the same information in audio format. Findings indicated that effective design principles (i.e., multimedia materials with redundancy, signaling, images, and video) combined with mnemonic strategies were most effective (*ES* = 0.69) for teaching vocabulary to adolescents with LD in secondary classrooms.

Text Comprehension Instruction

Several meta-analyses and syntheses show large effects for using social studies and history content for teaching reading comprehension strategies to students with LD (e.g., Ciullo et al., 2020). We share two exemplary multicomponent interventions, one developed by Vaughn and colleagues (Vaughn et al., 2013; Swanson et al., 2014), called PACT (Promoting Acceleration of Comprehension and Content through Text) and one by O'Connor and colleagues (2017), referred to as BRIDGES (Building Reading Interventions Designed for General Education Subjects). Eighth-grade students in both studies received explicit instruction in high-frequency academic vocabulary and two to three high-utility words or concepts to understand social studies content, with embedded strategies, for example, for decoding multisyllabic words or answering comprehension questions. Of note, in both studies, students read materials that were designed to help them learn cause–effect relationships (e.g., How did events and ideas cause conflict between Great Britain and the American colonies and lead to the signing of the Declaration of Independence?).

These Tier 1 literacy practices have been shown to be effective for students with LD. Swanson and colleagues (2014) reported on the effectiveness of the PACT intervention with students with and without disabilities, including individuals with LD, other health impairments, language disorder, emotional disturbance, or intellectual disability. In this approach, teachers provided lessons with an overarching question for the instructional unit, such as the one shared previously, with a "motivational springboard" (short video, photo, or map), which is referred to as a *comprehension canopy*. Students learned four to five vocabulary words each day and reviewed previously learned words in subsequent lessons. Students then read and discussed informational texts in small teams. Teachers provided constructive feedback and encouraged students to offer text evidence and justification for answers to the comprehension canopy question. Eighth-grade students with disabilities who were in the PACT condition outperformed comparison peers with disabilities on content knowledge and reading comprehension measures.

In O'Connor and colleagues' (2017) work, teachers taught students with disabilities reading comprehension strategies and a strategy for decoding multisyllabic words as they read expository texts. Teachers followed scripted lesson plans that included: 5 minutes of decoding practice using multisyllabic words pulled from the text; 5 minutes of academic word instruction; and 10–15 minutes of a comprehension strategy (main idea, compare–contrast, and cause–effect relationships) for reading brief history passages taken from textbooks, primary sources, or history websites that were modified to a lower reading level. Outcomes included multiple-choice vocabulary tests and researcher-designed comprehension measures that required students to express their understanding in writing. Students also completed a multiple-choice and short-answer content assessment that was based on the participating teachers' bank of content items. Students in the intervention condition made strong gains in reading and outperformed peers with disabilities in the control condition, but they did not improve on a standardized reading comprehension measure. This was not surprising; there were only three 3-week instructional cycles, with students learning a different comprehension strategy in each.

Integrating Reading and Writing Instruction

Teachers commonly require students to demonstrate content understanding in writing, so it makes sense to provide cognitive strategies instruction in both domains. One form of cognitive strategies instruction, the Self-Regulated Strategy Development (SRSD) (Harris et al., 2011) model, is an evidence-based approach for teaching writing to students with and without disabilities (Ciullo et al., 2020). The SRSD approach to teaching incorporates a process by which students gradually take ownership of learning by (1) moving from teacher modeling to collaborative (group) practice to independent execution of specific academic and self-regulation strategies and (2) fading procedural scaffolds, such as the use of graphics or other prompts that contain strategy steps. In SRSD, instruction takes place over 2 or more weeks, on average, as teachers scaffold students' learning as well as transfer responsibility for independent use of the target strategies (De La Paz, 2005).

Collins et al. (2021) examined the effectiveness of SRSD to improve third-grade students' ability to read and summarize information from social studies texts in expository essays. Teachers provided SRSD strategy instruction using the heuristic, TIDE (*Topic Sentence, Important Details, Explain Details, Ending*), which had been used in a prior study to promote comprehension of science information, to that of social studies. The results indicated that SRSD students included more genre elements in their expository essays and produced essays of higher holistic quality. Students in the SRSD condition also included more elements when writing about an expository topic they remembered learning and outperformed control students on a norm-referenced writing measure. Students did not, however, show a statistically significant positive effect on expository essays written from social studies text on a maintenance probe, nor improve in their performance on a norm-referenced reading comprehension measure. Despite these limitations, the authors' findings suggest that writing can be improved through shared reading and writing strategy instruction.

Summary

Special education researchers have a strong tradition of developing effective interventions to address the cognitive and linguistic challenges students with LD face in acquiring content knowledge through reading and writing in social studies classrooms. NAEP history data indicate these strategies are relevant in the elementary and early middle grades, as students often read and summarize information from textbooks. However, more recent NAEP data indicate the need for instruction in historical thinking skills, such as perspective taking and teaching argumentative writing. Historical writing generally orients students toward history as an interpretive discipline grounded in analysis of evidence rather than one focused on factual recall. Research also tells us that writing essays in history can improve students with LDs' mastery of information (Wissinger & De La Paz, 2016). We, therefore, now move to discuss historical reasoning instruction and the implications of such instruction for students with LD.

Historical Reasoning Instruction

We first acknowledge that despite extensive work highlighting the benefits of discipline-specific strategy instruction (e.g., Moje, 2008; Monte-Sano, 2010, 2011, 2016; Nokes, 2014), we also recognize the view that ambitious disciplinary literacy interventions could frustrate learners or negatively affect domain-general learning (Faggella-Luby et al., 2012). Fortunately, a growing body of research suggests that teachers can nurture struggling learners and students with LD in developing historical thinking strategies and improve the resulting products (e.g., argumentative historical writing) by building background knowledge, teaching skills, and addressing students' understanding of historical inquiry (Reisman, 2012) and writing (De La Paz & Felton, 2010; De La Paz & Wissinger, 2017; Wissinger & De La Paz, 2020).

We now review exemplary studies from this body of research, highlighting instruction developed to teach students historians' cognitive strategies. The majority of the instructional approaches reviewed here are complex, often lengthy, multicomponent interventions, each with more than one heuristic, strategy, or procedural facilitator (e.g., the use of model texts) to teach students more sophisticated historical reasoning. In addition, researchers define the primary focus of their interventions differently. Some study the cognitive frameworks that influence students' conceptual understanding of the processes of historical inquiry. Others attend to cognitive processes (e.g., reading and writing); still others study how class discussions impact student reasoning. We review studies according to the authors' emphasis, theoretical framing, and choice of student learning outcomes.

Historical Discussions and Debates

Classroom discussions help to promote student reasoning. They can enhance text comprehension because sustained interactions allow students to explore topics in greater depth (Swanson et al., 2019). When used during historical inquiry involving primary and secondary sources, discussion helps students to clarify different perspectives and to learn about multiple interpretations (Bouck et al., 2008; Ferretti et al., 2001, 2007). While recognizing benefits to integrating opportunities to discuss documents during project-based and technology-enhanced project-based inquiry (e.g., De La Paz & Hernández-Ramos, 2013; Okolo et al., 2007), research on the use of discussion that focuses on historical reasoning with students with LD remains limited.

In 2017, De La Paz and Wissinger examined whether middle school students with LD could use argumentation schemes proposed by Walton et al. (2008) as heuristics during discussion to learn content and write historical arguments. Though Walton et al.'s argumentative schemes and patterns of human reasoning are used widely by philosophers and those in the legal field, two schemes are consistent with the practices of historians and observed in the writing of advanced secondary students (De La Paz et al., 2012). Therefore we used the *argument from expert opinion* as a model for teaching sourcing, and the *argument from consequences* scheme prompted students to consider causal relationships of historical events. Teachers used critical questions to help students test the strength of their argument or its premises, similar to those by Nokes et al. (2007). Students' historical reasoning was evaluated according to four aspects of historical thinking: *substantiation*, students' ability to use evidence to support a claim; *perspective recognition*, students' acknowledgment of texts as representing a certain point of view; *contextualization*, students' ability to situate their argument within an accurate historic, geographic, and social setting; and *rebuttal*, students' ability to deal rationally with opposing points of view. The results ($\partial\eta^2 = 0.40$) indicated that students in the experimental condition wrote essays that evidenced greater levels of substantiation, perspective recognition, contextualization, and rebuttals than their peers.

Reading and Writing Historically

As noted, historians engage in strategic and purposeful recursive reading and writing processes when engaged in inquiry. They critically analyze the purpose behind texts written by others, simultaneously considering their purposes, plans, and goals for constructing written (or spoken) interpretations that contribute new knowledge (Nokes & De La Paz, 2018). In schools, however, van Boxtel and van Drie (2018) explain that it is "difficult to disentangle historical reading from reading and writing history because historical reasoning ability is largely expressed in the reading and writing of history" (p. 158). Therefore, it also seems productive to teach students historical reading and writing through disciplinary inquiry (Monte-Sano, 2011; Monte-Sano et al., 2017; Reisman, 2012; van Boxtel & van Drie, 2018).

Monte-Sano's (2010) close analysis of advanced high school students' historical reasoning and use of evidence revealed characteristics that distinguished argumentative historical writing from generic argumentation, suggesting that historical arguments require "conceptual understanding, procedural knowledge of historical analysis, an underlying grasp of the topic and discipline, and background content knowledge" (p. 560). Because most novices view history as the past—simply what happened—factual, fixed, and indisputable (Wineburg, 2001), instruction must confront students' misunderstanding that historical writing simply relates what happened (i.e., engaging in knowledge telling) as opposed to interpreting the past events. Assignments in traditional, content-focused history classrooms, such as a short essay on an exam to demonstrate factual recall, further distract students from more authentic types of historical writing. Fortunately, research shows that with instruction and practice, students in elementary school begin to assume an epistemic stance that leads to more mature ways of thinking about the past (Nokes, 2014; VanSledright, 2002; Wissinger et al., 2021).

Making Historical Reasoning Visible

Epistemological issues and the inability to use evidence are not the only barriers to students' engaging in historical writing. The limitations of their working memory may also interfere (Nokes & De La Paz, 2018). Historical writing often involves sifting through multiple, conflicting, overlapping, and/or fragmentary bits of evidence in order to develop and defend an interpretation. Therefore, students with LD need scaffolds such as graphic organizers to facilitate learning. Explicit instruction in cognitive strategies, such as sourcing, corroboration, and contextualization, as well as explicit instruction on second-order concepts (e.g., continuity and change, significance, progress and decline, and perspective taking), will help students develop a better grasp of the discipline. In addition, providing them feedback on their attempts to write arguments grounded with evidence will help students develop more advanced knowledge of historical analysis procedures.

In a series of studies on historical reading and writing instruction, De La Paz and colleagues (De La Paz, 2005; De La Paz & Felton, 2010; De La Paz et al., 2014, 2017, 2022, 2023, 2025; Wissinger & De La Paz, 2020; Wissinger et al., 2021) used a cognitive apprenticeship (Brown et al., 1989; Collins et al., 1991) to embed explicit instruction on writing, argument, and thinking in history classrooms.

Incorporating a cognitive apprenticeship (CA) framework further enhances instruction by embedding literacy practices within disciplinary tasks, connecting reading, writing, and argumentation to historical analysis. Unlike SRSD instruction, which emphasizes analyzing model texts as a means to learn about genre, CA connects reading, writing, and argumentation directly to disciplinary goals. This is particularly effective in teaching conceptual knowledge of history (e.g., metaconcepts like evidence and perspective) and procedural skills for historical analysis. Our CA approach integrates goal setting, teacher feedback, and progress monitoring, aligning with SRSD (Harris, 2021; Harris et al., 2011).

In CA, an expert models thinking processes for learners and gradually shifts responsibility for completing tasks to them. CAs help teachers organize the learning environment and are used to help students see the actions involved in otherwise hidden cognitive processes. In the CA formed by De La Paz and her colleagues, middle and high schoolteachers made visible the heuristics used by experts by (1) explicitly discussing writing and historical reasoning processes; (2) modeling, coaching, and providing scaffolding as novices used general and disciplinary heuristics; (3) gradually releasing responsibility for reading, thinking, and writing to the students as they acquired competence; and (4) providing feedback as students use historical thinking and literacy practices independently.

In their early work with eighth graders, De La Paz et al. (2017) created a series of historical inquiry lessons they labeled "investigations" that gave students with and without LD opportunities to practice historical reading and writing. During these lessons, teachers moved through several stages of instruction, helping students set goals for learning and develop metacognitive strategies. Six investigations were spread across an entire year using different historical controversies. In keeping with the CA model, during the first half of the year, teachers actively taught historical reading and writing heuristics and modeled them by thinking aloud (Collins et al., 1991). During the second half of the year, teachers gradually released responsibility to students who applied the heuristics with decreasing levels of scaffolding. Scaffolding included tools for students to use while reading, planning, and writing and tools for teachers to use for monitoring students' progress (Monte-Sano et al., 2014, 2017).

We now more fully describe the disciplinary scaffolds and explain how they were used in our lessons to help students learn strategies for historical reading, analysis, and argumentative writing: The mnemonic IREAD was developed to guide students' general reading comprehension *and* historical reading, and the "how to write your essay" (H2W) text structure and sample essays were used to guide students' planning and composing in our work with middle and high school students. In addition, we supported teachers' learning through sustained professional development, based on Grossman, Smagorinsky, and Valencia's (1999) approach to appropriating pedagogical tools (see Monte-Sano et al., 2014, 2017, for more information). At the core, using this model, teachers are given both conceptual and practical tools, and they engage in practice with each other, using and adapting tools in ways that are responsive to their learners.

Overview of IREAD

We used IR ("Identify the author's purpose" and "Read each paragraph and ask about the author's main ideas") to prompt students to identify and summarize what the author wrote. One cue for I is to consider what the author would say in response to the historical question. Certainly, the authors of historical texts did not write with the questions we ask in mind; however, this cue supports students' reading comprehension by having them connect the text to the investigative question, providing guidance and purpose as students read.

The next two elements, EA ("Evaluate the author's reliability" and "Assess the influence of context"), prompt students to source and contextualize texts (Wineburg, 1991) so they might begin to regard historical texts as the product of an author with intentions and as situated in a different time and place. We added the final prompt, D ("Determine the quality of the author's facts and examples"), to highlight the idea that authors use evidence to support their own arguments. Evidence in our materials also included information provided by individual historical actors who could be considered to be knowledgeable (i.e., experts) on the given topic.

Together, these prompts encouraged students to analyze and critique the texts rather than amass information about them. IREAD embeds a process of annotation to help struggling students notice specific aspects of texts and track their thinking. In previous work, Monte-Sano observed the annotation process used effectively with advanced students (Monte-Sano, 2010). We prepared IREAD in a foldable version for the eighth-grade students, in which the front flap included questions to prompt students' historical thinking and the inside flap directed students to make specific notations for each step of IREAD or way of thinking (e.g., underline anything that has to do with the setting or context) (Monte-Sano et al., 2014). Later, we switched to virtual materials (Google Docs) that teachers used in Google classrooms.

Overview of H2W

We created a graphic organizer to display particular aspects of an argumentative historical text visually, based in part on prior research that text structure allows readers to identify and remember top-level or central information from text. Explicit signals (e.g., topic statements, summary statements, and key words) cue text structure and the location of expository content. Good readers who detect these cues can remember more ideas when reading expository texts than students who do not search for or identify text structure (De La Paz & Nokes, 2020). Moreover, intervention work on the use of text structure (as introduced by Englert et al., 1991) indicates that providing students with direct instruction on how expository ideas are organized into text structures is a successful scaffold for helping students to write better essays.

We extended this work by creating a disciplinary text structure, representing it in a graphic organizer that included essential components of historical writing *and* general argument, as well as information that signaled how to organize essential components in the composition. We embedded a list of transition words and phrases (e.g., "this point makes sense" and "when all of the facts on both sides are considered") that were shown in relevant categories for historical writing (e.g., evaluating a quote and wrapping things up) based on the success of this type of scaffold in prior work (De La Paz, 2005). H2W reminded students to use evidence they had identified and evaluated through reading and discussion when writing their historical arguments as well as their critique of the evidence. During the 2017 study, we further clarified the writing process by creating an essay planning sheet and a reflection guide that mimicked H2W, reinforcing important aspects of historical *and* general argument writing. And the high school teachers with whom we worked modeled for students how to read and write with digital documents (De La Paz et al., 2023).

Throughout the year, students were taught to manage reading, thinking, and writing with increasing independence as they learned how to analyze primary sources, evaluate evidence, and plan and write arguments. Rather than addressing skills as discrete or decontextualized, De La Paz and her colleagues sought to maintain the complexity of historical writing by situating students' learning in the context of authentic historical inquiry, such as working with conflicting primary sources to investigate a central question. During teacher professional development, the researchers modeled and discussed the differences between simply telling students what to do and forming cognitive apprenticeships. After the researchers modeled instructional methods, teachers practiced and planned how to adapt their teaching for different types of learners and analyzed student work to make instructional decisions.

This work (De La Paz et al., 2017; Monte-Sano et al., 2017) collectively shows that when implemented with reasonable levels of fidelity, even when controlling statistically for students' entry learning characteristics (e.g., reading proficiency), academically and culturally diverse students improve in their ability to write historical arguments. Students in each subgroup (basic readers, students with LD, English learners, and proficient and advanced readers) demonstrated increased levels of *substantiation*, *perspective recognition*, *contextualization*, and *rebuttal* in their written arguments (*ES* = 0.45), although proficient and advanced readers showed greater learning gains than struggling learners. Although our most recent study (De La Paz et al., 2025) is currently in review, our prior work with high school students (De La Paz et al., 2022; *ES* = 0.32–0.44) shows similar positive outcomes for older students. Further, students' general writing ability improved, providing strong support for simultaneously teaching reading and writing strategies. Interviews suggested that many students gained a more sophisticated epistemological approach, though to varying degrees and in ways that correlated with their incoming reading abilities.

Extensions for Younger Students

Recognizing that younger students need additional support, Wissinger et al. (2021, 2020) evaluated the benefits in teaching fourth through sixth graders a historical reading ("I3C") and historical writing strategy ("PROVE IT!"). Because elementary students were presumed to know less about history than secondary learners (VanSledright, 2002), the authors integrated timelines, historical cartoons, and excerpts from newspapers into secondary sources. Digital images, audio, and other video media were integrated into the lessons. Each historical investigation was taught in 5 days, allowing teachers time to provide background information, model, facilitate guided practice, and hold discussions on the qualities of strong writing. I3C prompted students to (1) identify the author's stance, (2) identify 3 ideas supporting the author's stance, and (3) check for limitations in the author's argument. PROVE IT! prompted students to focus on text structure and the skills of historical argumentation, reminding students to (1) provide background information on the historical problem, (2) report their interpretation, (3) offer 3 evidence-based reasons, (4) voice the other side's interpretation, (5) establish a rebuttal, then consider (6) is the argument convincing, and (7) total up what you know by adding a concluding sentence. After controlling for gender, ethnicity, and pretest scores, students in the intervention scored higher in historical writing and overall writing quality (a holistic writing measure) and wrote longer essays after instruction and on maintenance probes. Moreover, students with disabilities benefited to the same degree as students without disabilities, after controlling for students' initial reading proficiency.

Conclusions and Future Directions

All students, including those with LD, multilingual students, and other struggling learners, must learn to grapple with complex historical and political information. Doing so will support their ability to make sense of conflicting and/or politicized information that pervades the media today and to judge for themselves what counts as evidence and truth. Substantial research in the past five decades has demonstrated that students with LD benefit from contextually appropriate cognitive strategies and that students benefit most when strategies are integrated as part of the regular curriculum, using them when needed, and as appropriate for the assigned task.

Collectively, the field has established effective approaches for teaching students with LD vocabulary, text comprehension, and writing strategies for literacy skills that are highlighted in the CCSS. While we did not mention all such approaches in this chapter, studies with students who have LD have included children as young as in the second grade, up through high school students (Ciullo et al., 2020). However, despite calls by Okolo and Ferretti (2014), our understanding about how students' linguistic, cognitive, and social–emotional challenges related to having an LD interacts with historical reasoning tasks remains limited (i.e., those with more severe reading challenges may require greater adaptations to sources, different vocabulary supports, longer or more guidance during practice, etc.).

It is equally important for social studies teachers to have options for providing differentiated instruction for students who are proficient and advanced learners. Interventions should be designed to address both generic and disciplinary skills, with cognitive strategies that are designed to do both. For example, vocabulary instruction might focus on the development of basic knowledge (e.g., historical facts or meaning in context) as well as second-order outcomes (e.g., historical significance and analyzing cause and consequence). Text comprehension strategies might include topics such as significance or explore ways to help students with LD learn how to reason across time periods, historical eras, or geographical locations. These efforts have been shown to help diverse groups of students improve conceptual understanding about the discipline (De La Paz et al., 2017; De La Paz et al., 2025; Wissinger et al., 2021). Interventions that assist proficient and advanced learners are more likely to be seen as acceptable by general education teachers.

Given the number of students with and at risk for LD in elementary and secondary schools (Scruggs et al., 2010), we call on history education colleagues to provide more nuanced information about the degree to which their research promotes learning for all students. According to the National Center for Education Statistics (NCES, 2024), the percentage of multilingual learners (ML) in the U.S. K–12 population was 10.3% in the fall of 2020. Given long-standing gaps in achievement between students who are and are not ML on the history, civics, reading, and writing assessments, it is essential to formally consider the needs of ML, including those with LD, as additional student subgroups. These challenges may cause students to struggle with or be less willing to participate in discourse (Bueso, 2022), particularly if they have not mastered English (Boyd & Rubin,

2002), creating additional instructional challenges. Thus, researchers should design interventions to address the needs of ML students and to report outcomes for subgroups with different cognitive, linguistic, academic, and cultural profiles.

We encourage more researchers to explore the benefits of discussion. Both small- and large-group dialogue provides an opportunity for students to reason with each other, problem solve, and listen to multiple perspectives (Reisman, 2012). De La Paz and Wissinger's work (2016, 2017) provides compelling evidence that younger students, including those with LD, benefit from disciplinary discussions to improve students' historical writing. We encourage more researchers to explore similar goals or to examine the effectiveness of discussions that center on other aspects of the C3 Framework with elementary and middle-level learners.

Teachers need support for this work and for schools to change the way they provide professional development (PD) in ways that are backed by educational research findings. Monte-Sano and colleagues (2014, 2017) have pointed out effective practices for how to support teacher learning using Grossman et al.'s (1999) framework. Core elements involve providing time to practice new approaches and to engage with other teachers about how to adapt the instructional approach while remaining faithful to the core principles. In our federally funded work, we observed teachers using our lessons and provided feedback to the group (often by posing questions related to teaching challenges) during follow-up workshops (spread across the year, about once per month).

We also shared representative samples of student work during PD sessions and elicited teachers' thinking about how to focus instruction based on what was evident in each sample. In our most recent project with high school students (De La Paz et al., 2023, 2025), we provided virtual webinars with lead teachers attending additional 1:1 virtual sessions focused on problem solving, based on questions and feedback from other teachers at each participating school. We encouraged teachers to adapt our materials (adding video, links to Spanish translations on slides, and documents) and used team decision making during the webinar follow-up to decide on the simplest scaffolds and activities to emphasize within and between schools.

It is also important to consider new historical reasoning activities that take into consideration students' lived experiences. One example might be to focus on social and historical problems that are relevant to a local community. In addition, it is critical to inform students about the effects of systemic, structural racism, which affects everyday workers, small business owners, and even sports and entertainment figures (among others). Another issue that is important to address is the increased polarization of politics in America and elsewhere. These issues and many more are seen as the purview of social studies teachers, who are asked to tackle challenging societal issues (see, e.g., *www.socialstudies.org/about/ncss-news*).

When we think of the purposes of social studies and history education, we recognize that an important civic goal is to develop students' capacity to engage with people who have other perspectives, with open-mindedness, tolerance, and a willingness to change one's opinion. The C3 Framework explains that civics education teaches virtues, such as honesty, mutual respect, cooperation, and attentiveness, to multiple perspectives, that citizens should use when they interact with each other on public matters, and that "by the end of grade 8, students [should be able to] apply civic virtues and democratic principles in school and community settings" (NCSS, 2013, p. 33).

A recent study by Bueso (2022) reveals important differences in civics learning opportunities for students with and without disabilities. While her data did not disaggregate outcomes specifically for students with LD, Bueso found statistically significant differences between the civic education experiences provided to SWD and students without disabilities. In particular, SWD were less likely to participate in discussions about controversial issues and the credibility of online information than neurotypical peers, even when controlling for socioeconomic status, race/ethnicity, and gender. Conversely, they were more likely to participate in service learning projects. The author questioned whether "SWD are more likely to be excluded from activities [requiring] cognitive or communicative competence, but not from activities that ask students to lend a helping hand" (p. 78) and highlighted how these differences may impact their future civic engagement.

Ultimately, argumentation, which is at the heart of historical inquiry, is central to citizenship. In its essence, the argumentative process is an ongoing conversation bringing together what multiple voices say in an effort to construct an evidence-based and reasonable interpretation (Graff et al., 2015). To date, we know of no interventions that have explored how to teach students to apply their historical argumentation skills in ways that promote civic engagement. Much work remains to be done on the best ways to prepare young people for 21st-century historical and civic reading, writing, and thinking.

REFERENCES

Alexander, P. A. (2003). The development of expertise: The journey from acclimation to proficiency. *Educational Researcher, 32*, 10–14.

Bouck, E. C., Okolo, C. M., Englert, C. S., & Heutsche, A. (2008). Cognitive apprenticeship into the discipline: Helping students with disabilities think and act like historians. *Learning Disabilities: A Contemporary Journal, 6*(2), 21–40.

Boyd, M. P., & Rubin, D. L. (2002). Elaborated student talk in an elementary ESOL classroom. *Research in the Teaching of English, 36*(4), 495–530.

Brown, J. S., Collins, A., & Duguid, P. (1989). Situated cognition and the culture of learning. *Educational Researcher, 18*(1), 32–42.

Bueso, L. (2022). Civic equity for students with disabilities. *Teachers College Record, 124*(1), 62–86.

Bulgren, J. A., Deshler, D. D., & Lentz, K. (2007). Engaging adolescents with LD in higher concepts using integrated content enhancement routines. *Journal of Learning Disabilities, 40*, 121–133.

Bulgren, J. A., Marquis, J. G., Lenz, B. K., Deshler, D. D., & Schumaker, J. B. (2011). The effectiveness of a question-exploration routine for enhancing the content learning of secondary students. *Journal of Educational Psychology, 103*(3), 578–593.

Ciullo, S., Collins, A., Wissinger, D., McKenna, J., Lo, S., & Osman, D. (2020). Students with learning disabilities in the social studies: A meta-analysis of intervention research. *Exceptional Children, 86*(4), 393–412.

Collingwood, R. G. (2005). *The idea of history.* Oxford University Press.

Collins, A., Brown, J. S., & Holum, A. (1991). Cognitive apprenticeship: Making thinking visible. *American Educator, 15*(3), 6–11, 38–46.

Collins, A., Ciullo, S., Graham, S., Sigafoos, L., Guerra, S., David, M., & Judd, L. (2021). Writing expository essays from social studies texts: A self-regulated strategy development study. *Reading and Writing: An Interdisciplinary Journal, 34*, 1623–1651.

Common Core State Standards Initiative. (2010). *Common core state standards for English language arts & literacy in history/social studies, science, and technical subjects. www.corestandards.org/assets/CCSSI_ELA%20Standards.pdf*

De La Paz, S. (2005). Effects of historical reasoning instruction and writing strategy mastery in culturally and academically diverse middle school classrooms. *Journal of Educational Psychology, 97*, 139–156.

De La Paz, S., & Felton, M. K. (2010). Reading and writing from multiple source documents in history: Effects of strategy instruction with low to average high school writers. *Contemporary Educational Psychology, 35*(3), 174–192.

De La Paz, S., Felton, M., Monte-Sano, C., Croninger, R., Jackson, C., Deogracias, J. S., & Hoffman, B. P. (2014). Developing historical reading and writing with adolescent readers: effects on student learning. *Theory & Research in Social Education, 42*(2), 228–274.

De La Paz, S., Ferretti, R., Wissinger, D., Yee. L., & MacArthur (2012). Adolescents' disciplinary use of evidence, argumentative strategies, and organizational structure in writing about historical controversies, *Written Communication, 29*, 412–454.

De La Paz, S., & Hernández-Ramos, P. (2013). Project-based learning in history: Effects on historical thinking for students with and without learning disabilities. *Journal of Special Education Technology, 28*, 1–14.

De La Paz, S., Monte-Sano, C., Felton, M., Croninger, R., Jackson, C., & Piantedosi, K. W. (2017). A historical writing apprenticeship for adolescents: Integrating disciplinary learning with cognitive strategies. *Reading Research Quarterly, 52*(1), 31–52.

De La Paz, S., & Nokes, J. D. (2020). Strategic processing in history and historical strategy instruction. In D. L. Dinsmore, L. K. Fryer, & M. M. Parkinson (Eds.), *Handbook of strategies and strategic processing* (pp. 195–215). Routledge.

De La Paz, S., Otarola, J., & Butler, C. (2023). Using virtual teacher PD to support implementation of a historical literacy curriculum. *Social Studies Research and Practice, 18*(2), 164–179.

De La Paz, S., Otarola, J., & Wissinger, D. R. (2025). *Teaching academically and linguistically diverse high school students to write historical arguments* [Manuscript submitted for publication].

De La Paz, S., & Wissinger, D. (2017). Improving the historical knowledge and writing of students with or at-risk for LD. *Journal of Learning Disabilities, 50*(6), 658–671.

De La Paz, S., Wissinger, D., Gross, M., & Butler, C. (2022). Strategies that promote historical reasoning and contextualization: A pilot intervention with urban high school students. *Reading and Writing, 35*(2), 353–376.

Englert, C. S., Okolo, C. M., & Mariage, T. V. (2009). Informational writing across the curriculum. In G. Troia (Ed.), *Instruction and assessment for struggling writers: Evidence-based practices* (pp. 132–161). Guilford Press.

Englert, C. S., Raphael, T. E., Anderson, L., Stevens, D. D., & Fear, K. L. (1991). Making writing strategies and self-talk visible: Cognitive strategy instruction in writing in regular and special education classrooms. *American Educational Research Journal, 28*(2), 337–372.

Faggella-Luby, M., Graner, P. S., Deshler, D., & Drew, S. (2012). Building a house on sand. Why disciplinary literacy is not sufficient to replace general strategies for adolescent learners who struggle. *Topics in Language Disorders, 32*, 69–84.

Ferretti, R. P., & De La Paz, S. (2011). On the comprehension and production of written texts: Instructional activities that support content-area literacy. In R. O'Connor & P. Vadasy (Eds.), *Handbook of reading interventions* (pp. 326–355). Guilford Press.

Ferretti, R. P., De La Paz, S., & Mason, L. H. (2023). Perspectives about disciplinary argumentation in the era of post-truth: Introduction to the special issue. *Written Communication, 409*(2), 289–299.

Ferretti, R. P., MacArthur, C. A., & Okolo, C. M. (2001). Teaching for historical understanding in inclusive classrooms. *Learning Disability Quarterly, 24*(1), 59–71.

Ferretti, R., MacArthur, C., Okolo, C. (2007). Students' misconceptions about U.S. westward migration. *Journal of Learning Disabilities, 40*, 145–153.

Freelon, D., & Wells, C. (2020). Disinformation as political communication. *Political Communication, 37*(2), 145–156.

Graff, G., Birkenstein, C., & Durst, R. (2015). *They say, I say: The moves that matter in academic writing*. W. W. Norton & Co.

Grossman, P. L., Smagorinsky, P., & Valencia, S. (1999). Appropriating tools for teaching English: A theoretical framework for research on learning to teach. *American Journal of Education, 108*, 1–29.

Harris, K. R. (2021). SRSD instructional research for students with or at-risk for LD across the content areas: History and reflections. *Learning Disabilities Research & Practice, 36*, 1–7.

Harris, K. R., Graham, S., MacArthur, C., Reid, R., & Mason, L. H. (2011). Self-regulated learning processes and children's writing. In B. J. Zimmerman & D. Schunk (Eds.), *Handbook of self-regulation of learning and performance* (pp. 187–202). Routledge.

Kennedy, M. J., Deshler, D. D., & Lloyd, J. W. (2015). Effects of multimedia vocabulary instruction on adolescents with learning disabilities. *Journal of Learning Disabilities, 48*, 22–38.

Kiuhara, S., Graham, S., & Hawken, L. (2009). Teaching writing to high school students: A national survey. *Journal of Educational Psychology, 101*(1), 136–160.

Lee, P. J., & Ashby, R. A. (2000). Progression in historical understanding among students age 7–14. In P. N. Stearns, P. Seixas, & S. Wineburg (Eds.), *Knowing, teaching, and learning history. National and international perspectives* (pp. 199–222). New York University Press.

Mastropieri, M., Scruggs, T., Spencer, V., & Fontana, J. (2003). Promoting success in high school world history: Peer tutoring versus guided notes. *Learning Disabilities Research & Practice, 18*(1), 52–65.

Minarik, D., & Linter, T. (2024). The social studies classroom. In D. Minarik & T. Lintner (Eds.), *Creating an inclusive social studies classroom for exceptional learners* (pp. 3–16). Information Age.

Moje, E. B. (2008). Foregrounding the disciplines in secondary literacy teaching and learning: A call for change. *Journal of Adolescent and Adult Literacy, 52*, 96–107.

Monte-Sano, C. (2010). Disciplinary literacy in history: An exploration of the historical nature of adolescents' writing. *Journal of Learning Sciences, 19*, 539–568.

Monte-Sano, C. (2011). Beyond reading comprehension and summary: Learning to read and write in history by focusing on evidence, perspective, and interpretation. *Curriculum Inquiry, 41*, 212–249.

Monte-Sano, C. (2016). Argumentation in history classrooms: A key path to understanding the discipline and preparing citizens. *Theory into Practice, 55*(4), 311–319.

Monte-Sano, C., De La Paz, S., & Felton, M. (2014.) *Reading, thinking, and writing about history: Teaching argument writing to diverse learners in the common core classroom, grades 6–12*. Teachers College Press.

Monte-Sano, C., De La Paz, S., Felton, M., Worland, K., Yee, L. S., & Carey, R. L. (2017). Learning to teach disciplinary literacy across diverse eighth-grade history classrooms within a district-university partnership. *Teacher Education Quarterly, 44*(4), 98–124.

National Center for Education Statistics. (2022). *2022 NAEP civics assessment*. U.S. Department of Education, Institute of Education Sciences. *www.nationsreportcard.gov/highlights/civics/2022/*

National Council for the Social Studies. (2013). *The College, Career, and Civic Life (C3)*

Framework for social studies state standards: Guidance for enhancing the rigor of K–12 civics, economics, geography, and history.

Nokes, J. D. (2014). Elementary students' roles and epistemic stances during document-based history lessons. *Theory and Research in Social Education, 42*(3), 375–413.

Nokes, J., & De La Paz, S. (2018). Writing and argumentation in history education. In S. A. Metzger & L. McArthur Harris (Eds.), *International handbook of history teaching and learning* (pp. 551–578). Wiley-Blackwell.

Nokes, J., & De La Paz, S. (2023). Historical argumentation: Watching historians and teaching youth. *Written Communication, 40*(2) 333–372.

Nokes, J. D., Dole, J. A., & Hacker, D. J. (2007). Teaching high school students to use heuristics while reading historical texts. *Journal of Educational Psychology, 99*, 492–504.

O'Connor, R. E., Sanchez, V., Beach, K., & Bocian, K. (2017). Special education teachers integrating reading with eighth grade U.S. history content. *Learning Disabilities Research & Practice, 32*(2), 99–111.

Okolo, C. M., Englert, C. S., Bouck, E. C., Heutsche, A., & Wang, H. (2011). The virtual history museum: Learning American history in diverse eighth grade classrooms. *Remedial and Special Education, 32*, 417–428.

Okolo, C. M., & Ferretti, R. P. (1996). Knowledge acquisition and technology-supported projects in the social studies for students with learning disabilities. *Journal of Special Education Technology, 13*, 91–103.

Okolo, C. M., & Ferretti, R. (2014). History instruction for students with learning disabilities. In L. Swanson, K. Harris, & S. Graham (Eds.), *Handbook of learning disabilities* (2nd ed., pp. 462–486). Guilford Press.

Okolo, C. M., Ferretti, R. P., & MacArthur, C. A. (2007). Talking about history: Discussions in a middle school inclusive classroom. *Journal of Learning Disabilities, 40*(2).

Reisman, A. (2012). Reading like a historian: A document-based history curriculum intervention in urban high schools. *Cognition and Instruction, 30*(1), 86–112.

Scruggs, T., Mastropieri, M. A., Berkeley, S., Graetz, & J. E. (2010). Do special education interventions improve learning of secondary content? A meta-analysis. *Remedial & Special Education, 31*, 437–449.

Seixas, P. (2017). A model of historical thinking. *Educational Philosophy and Theory, 49*, 593–605.

Swanson, E., Hairrell, A., Kent, S., Ciullo, S., Wanzek, J. A., & Vaughn, S. (2014). A synthesis and meta-analysis of reading interventions using social studies content for students with learning disabilities. *Journal of Learning Disabilities, 47*(2), 178–195.

Swanson, E., Stevens, E. A., & Wexler, J. (2019). Engaging students with disabilities in text-based discussions: Guidance for general education social studies classrooms. *Teaching Exceptional Children, 51*(4), 305–312.

Thacker, E. S., Lee, J. K., & Friedman, A. M. (2017). Teaching with the C3 Framework: Surveying teachers' beliefs and practices. *Journal of Social Studies Research, 41*(2), 89–100

van Boxtel, C., & van Drie, C. (2018). Historical reasoning: Definitions and educational applications. In S. A. Metzger & L. McArthur Harris (Eds.), *The Wiley international handbook of history teaching and learning* (pp. 149–176). Wiley.

VanSledright, B. (2002). *In search of America's past: Learning to read history in elementary school.* Teachers College Press.

Vaughn, S., Swanson, E. A., Roberts, G., Wanzek, J., Stillman-Spisak, S., Solis, M., & Simmons, D. (2013). Improving reading comprehension and social studies knowledge in middle school. *Reading Research Quarterly, 48*(1), 77–93.

Walton, D., Reed, C., & Macagno, F. (2008). *Argumentation schemes.* Cambridge University Press.

Wineburg, S. S. (1991). Historical problem solving: A study of the cognitive processes used in the evaluation of documentary and pictorial evidence. *Journal of Educational Psychology, 83*, 73–87.

Wineburg, S. S. (2001). *Historical thinking and other unnatural acts: Charting the future of teaching the past.* Temple University Press.

Wissinger, D. R., & Ciullo, S. (2018). History literacy research for students with or at risk for learning disabilities: A systematic review. *Learning Disabilities Research & Practice, 33*(4), 237–249.

Wissinger, D. R., & De La Paz, S. (2016). Effects of critical discussions on middle school students' written historical arguments. *Journal of Educational Psychology, 108*(1), 43.

Wissinger, D. R., & De La Paz, S. (2020). Effects of discipline-specific strategy instruction on historical writing growth of students with writing difficulties. *Journal of Learning Disabilities, 53*, 199–212.

Wissinger, D. R., De La Paz, S., & Jackson, C. (2021). The effects of historical reading and writing strategy instruction with fourth- through sixth-grade students. *Journal of Educational Psychology, 113*(1), 49–67.

CHAPTER 17

Science Education for Students with Learning Disabilities

Delinda van Garderen, William Romine, Heba Z. Abdelnaby, Cassandra M. Smith, and Rachel L. Juergensen

In the second edition of the *Handbook on Learning Disabilities* (2013), Drs. Scruggs and Mastropieri wrote a chapter on students with learning disabilities (LD) in both science and social studies. In that chapter, they summarized their research that, at that time, represented—and arguably still represents to date—the largest and most comprehensive body of work spanning over 30 years on students with LD in science by one team of researchers. The focus of their research has been on teaching and learning strategies designed to facilitate content learning. Many studies have focused on the use of single strategy types, including text-processing strategies (e.g., main idea and list or order structures), mnemonic strategies (e.g., key word method), elaborative interrogation (e.g., coached elaboration for facts), inquiry, and activity-oriented learning (e.g., construction of a telegraph). Several studies have examined combinations of strategies with classwide peer tutoring. (See summary of studies, Scruggs and Mastropieri [2013].) All the strategies examined in their research have reported positive outcomes for students with LD. Using strategies such as these with students with learning disabilities, as demonstrated by the findings in their studies, can result in improved outcomes for science learning. But to what extent are students with LD in general, beyond those involved in the research studies, improving in science outcomes?

According to the latest test results on the National Assessment of Educational Progress (NAEP) science assessment in 2019 (U.S. Department of Education, 2019), students with disabilities (SWD) continue to significantly lag behind their peers without disabilities. For example, for fourth-grade students, 56% of SWD, as compared to 22% of students without disabilities, were below basic on the NAEP. This gap continues to widen across the grades (eighth grade: 65% of SWD vs. 28% of students without disabilities were below basic; 12th grade: 71% of

SWD vs. 37% of students without disabilities were below basic). Nor has this gap significantly reduced since the NAEP began in 2009. The question then is, despite the availability of evidence-based instructional practices (e.g., strategy instruction) for students with LD in science, why does the gap remain?

One possible reason may simply be that teachers, whether general or special education, are not or are poorly using the available evidence-based instructional practices with their students with LD when teaching science. The research suggests that teacher knowledge and use of evidence-based instructional practices are of concern (Bradley-Black, 2013; Guckert et al., 2016; Jones, 2009). Consequently, implementation fidelity is low, negatively impacting the quality of instruction students receive (Cook & Odom, 2013). Compounding this issue is that teacher preparation programs may not be sufficiently preparing teacher candidates about evidence-based instructional practices and how to use them in their classrooms (Bradley-Black, 2013; Scheeler et al., 2016). And when taught about evidence-based instructional practices, a significant concern is that teacher candidates are not transferring what has been learned to actual teaching settings beyond their training program (Markelz et al., 2017; Scheeler et al., 2016). While lack of improved student outcomes may be attributed to these factors, other factors need to be considered, such as the existing set of evidence-based instructional practices for teaching science that are currently available. We would suggest that they target not science but more domain-general skills (e.g., main idea comprehension of informational text) with an emphasis on recalling content (e.g., mnemonics). And while these evidence-based instructional practices have been demonstrated to work for SWD and they are often essential to the success of learners with disabilities because of their unique learning needs (Cook et al., 2017), how well they match the current teaching conditions needs to be appraised.

The purpose of this chapter is to discuss the current teaching conditions and expectations for science instruction and the implications of these for students with LD. We then share our work and its connections to current expectations. We conclude by discussing implications for research and practice. It is important to note that we are not suggesting that the available research on teaching and learning strategies that target more domain-general skills in science has no value—on the contrary! (We highly recommend reading Scruggs et al. [2013] to see how the domain-specific strategies in science could connect to current standards and expectations for teaching science to SWD.) Rather, we seek to identify ways to improve outcomes in science that not only target domain-general skills but focus on disciplinary knowledge, understanding, and practices in science for students with learning disabilities.

Science Instruction for SWD: State of the Field

The Individuals with Disabilities Education Act (IDEA, 2004) requires SWD, including students with learning disabilities, to have access to the general education curriculum to the fullest extent possible. As such, 75.3% of SWD spend at least 80% of their day in the general education classroom (U.S. Department of Education, 2024). This number has dramatically increased from 66.2% reported in 2013 (U.S. Department of Education, 2009), the year the second edition of the *Handbook for Learning Disabilities* (2nd edition) was published. Therefore, it is safe to assume that for the majority of students with LD, science instruction is taking place within the general education classroom (Kahn & Lewis, 2014).

Content standards for science instruction, or science, technology, engineering, and mathematics (STEM), have evolved considerably over almost three decades. Building on the previous work of *Science for All Americans*, *Benchmarks for Science Literacy* (American Association for the Advancement of Science [AAAS], 1993) and the *National Science Education Standards* of the National Research Council (NRC, 1996), *A Framework for K–12 Science Education* followed (NRC, 2012), from which the Next Generation Science Standards (NGSS) (NGSS Lead States, 2013) were developed and disseminated. While there are no specific science content standards included in the Common Core State Standards (CCSS) (National Governors Association Center for Best Practices, Council of Chief State School Officers, 2010), there are many connections between the NGSS and CCSS, particularly when thinking about the integration of science and literacy.

Three-Dimensional Learning in Science

The NGSS puts heavy emphasis on science engineering practices (SEPs) and focuses on a limited set of crosscutting concepts (CCCs) and disciplinary core ideas (DCIs). Together, the SEPs, CCCs, and DCIs are referred to as three-dimensional learning (NGSS Lead States, 2013). SEPs describe the work scientists engage in as they conduct investigations, build models, and test theories about the world around them, whereas the CCCs apply to all domains of science (e.g., patterns, similarity, and diversity; cause and effect; scale, proportion, and quantity; systems and system models; energy and matter; structure and function; and stability and change). Finally, the DCIs serve to focus science curriculum, instruction, and assessments on four critical aspects of science, including (1) physical sciences, (2) life sciences, (3) earth and space sciences, and (4) engineering, technology, and applications of science. The three-dimensional learning framework is built on the idea that learning content cannot be separated from the practice of science; hence, content and practice should be taught and assessed as a single outcome, as opposed to separate and unrelated outcomes (Krajcik, 2015).

The shift toward three-dimensional learning is quite different from past conceptualizations of science education. As Lee and Stephens (2020) write, "Contemporary views emphasize that students make sense of phenomena and problems in the classroom community (*knowledge-in-use)*, whereas traditional views have focused on learners' mastery of discrete elements of content" (p. 429). Consequently, science instruction is more than learning content; it also requires an emphasis on practices. But as Reiser et al. (2012) note, the practices are not "separate learning goals that define what students should know *about* the processes of science. Instead, the science practices identify the reasoning behind, discourse about, and application of core ideas in science" (p. 8). Important to also note is the shift from focusing on "inquiry" to focusing on "practices," within which inquiry is a part (Bybee, 2011). In the 1990s, the idea of "scientific inquiry" was a central theme within state standards and school science programs (NRC, 1996, 2000). Although changes were seen in science instruction, such as increased attention to inquiry-based learning (e.g., Scruggs et al., 1993), scientific inquiry was not implemented as widely as expected (Bybee, 2011).

The central focus on science instruction within the NGSS is to enable students to be able to explain phenomena and design solutions to problems (National Science Teachers Association, 2018). Effective three-dimensional learning works towards this focus, where an understanding of the DCIs and crosscutting concepts is used along with science and engineering practices. Within three-dimensional learning, students are (1) focused on explaining and making sense of the natural and designed world, (2) using science and engineering practices to develop and apply these explanatory ideas, and (3) asking questions arising from phenomena to build, revisit, and revise ideas over time (Reiser, 2013). In three-dimensional learning, then, knowledge and practice are intertwined in any learning experience in K–12 science education (NRC, 2012). One without the other is insufficient, as each dimension is required to make sense of natural phenomena (Anderson et al., 1998).

Science and Engineering Practices

The *Framework for K–12 Science Education* identified eight science and engineering practices for K–12 classrooms. The practices outlined include (1) asking questions and defining problems; (2) developing and using models; (3) planning and carrying out investigations; (4) analyzing and interpreting data; (5) using mathematics and computational thinking; (6) constructing explanations and designing solutions; (7) engaging in argument from evidence; and (8) obtaining, evaluating, and communicating information.

Building scientific knowledge involves all eight practices. Each practice is interdependent and interrelated. As Reiser et al. (2012) note, the practices serve two very important functions: "The practices involve *doing* the work of building knowledge in science and *understanding* why we build, test, evaluate and refine knowledge as we do" (p. 9). Science practices should be thought of as learning outcomes and instructional strategies (Bybee, 2011).

Research has advanced our knowledge about how students learn science and how science functions, leading to the recognition that scientific inquiry is a form of scientific practice (Bybee, 2011). Practices such as "Asking questions and defining problems," "Planning and carrying out investigations," and "Engaging in argument from evidence" relate directly to inquiry. As Bybee (2011) writes, "When students engage in scientific practices, activities become the basis for learning about experiments, data and evidence, social discourse, models and tools, and mathematics and for developing the ability to evaluate knowledge claims, conduct empirical investigations, and develop explanations" (p. 5). Note, however, although the scientific practices are related and can be used as a part of inquiry, they can also be practiced and utilized individually at a particular time. For example, it is possible to "Analyze and interpret data" without necessarily "Planning and carrying out an investigation."

Summary

The challenge in any research agenda focused on students with LD and science is to connect the two fields, in this case, science education *and* special education. To date, the predominant research that has been carried out has connected science and special education via a focus on using strategies to learn and recall information (e.g., mnemonics; see Scruggs & Mastropieri, 2013). This approach connects well with the research that suggests a core deficit for many SWD is difficulty with working memory (Swanson, 1993; Swanson & Zheng, 2013). However, this work is less connected to current expectations in the field of science education related to three-dimensional learning that not only includes building knowledge of the content but, importantly, using and learning about practices to do science.

The need to focus on practices is important as they have become front and center of both the CCSS and the Next Generation Science Standards (NGSS Lead States, 2013). Taken together, the standards and practices call for all students, including students with LD, to (1) build a strong base of knowledge through content-rich texts; (2) read, write, and speak grounded in evidence; (3) construct viable arguments and critique the reasoning of others; and (4) engage in argument from evidence. In the following section, we describe our research program that is designed to help all learners, including students with LD, develop skills to engage in argumentation in science, namely Claim-Evidence-Reasoning (CER) via complex text.

Our Research Program: Core Components

Our program, *Linking Science, Math & Literacy for All Learners* (LSM&L4AL), formerly known as *Liking Science & Literacy for All Learners* (LS&L4AL), supports sixth- to eighth-grade science, English Language Arts (ELA), and special education teachers as they develop and implement STEM multimodal text sets. The LSM&L4AL program involves a yearlong teacher professional development program. The "core" of professional development occurs during the summer. During the professional development, teachers are introduced to foundational ideas about multimodal STEM text sets and learn or review the NGSS and CCSS practices and life science content for the development of their own multimodal STEM text sets. In addition, teachers learn how to scaffold instruction for their diverse learners. Time is provided to develop and/or refine a multimodal STEM text set that they plan on using with their students. During the academic year, regroup meetings are held where the teachers continue to learn about or share instructional practices designed to help students link science and literacy.

Multimodal STEM Text Set

For the purposes of our program, a multimodal STEM text set comprises a coherent sequence of multimodal "texts" (e.g., printed text, video, and online resources) and activities pertaining to a specific STEM topic or line of inquiry. The line of inquiry of the text set is determined by an anchor text—a rich, complex, grade-level text that reflects the grade-level science and literacy standards. Within the multimodal STEM text set scaffolds–both instructional and content that are based on learner needs—are integrated to support in building the vocabulary and background knowledge required for reading comprehension and practices, which, in our case, is argumentation. (We discuss the importance of argumentation later in this chapter.) The multimodal STEM text set is organized as a series of learning cycles/lessons that are implemented with students.

Learning Cycles/Lessons

Across the learning cycles/lessons of a multimodal STEM text set, teachers strategically select and sequence multimodal texts to scaffold the knowledge and skills students need to engage in the anchor text and construct evidence-based arguments. The texts are multimodal as they may consist of articles, videos, inquiry (hands-on) activities, novels, picture books, infographics, pictures, simulations, poems, audio recordings, and much more; however, each multimodal text serves the purpose of developing students' scientific knowledge and argumentation skills. The teachers purposefully select the multimodal texts to use within their learning cycles/lessons to serve as either a content (designed to build knowledge about the content) or instructional scaffold (designed to support the learner to access [e.g., simpler text] or demonstrate knowledge [e.g., choice of response] of content). For example, Figure 17.1 shows an example of one learning cycle lesson where one teacher used a video, inquiry activity, and picture book to develop students' background knowledge and vocabulary regarding pollination, pollinators, and plants. Teachers also include evidence-based instructional scaffolds (e.g., graphic organizers) to provide students with the individualized support and/or extension required for students to engage in the multimodal STEM text set. Copies of the anchor texts, scaffolds, and example teacher text sets can be found on our website: *https://scienceandliteracy.missouri.edu.*

Anchor Texts Content and Foci

Central to the multimodal STEM text set is the anchor text. An anchor text is a complex, grade-level text grounded in a specific STEM topic or line of inquiry that aligns with the NGSS science standards. To date, the program key personnel and

<table>
<tr><td>Guiding Questions</td><td colspan="2">How are flowers adapted to attract specific pollinators?
What is the relationship between pollinators and plants?</td><td></td></tr>
<tr><td></td><td>Key Idea</td><td>Learning Activities</td><td></td></tr>
<tr><td>Engage</td><td>Pollinators serve an important role in our lives.</td><td>Have snacks on the table or counter at the beginning of class. On the board, have the question "Why do we need pollinators?" or "Why are pollinators important?" After a brief discussion, point to the snacks and ask the class what they think all of these snacks have in common. Pollinators! You could also remove all of the snacks and say, "Without pollinators, none of these snacks exist."
Ask the students the following questions:
"What are your favorite flowers?"<br>"Why do plants have flowers?"</td><td></td></tr>
<tr><td rowspan="3">Explore</td><td rowspan="3">Flowers are in a symbiotic relationship with pollinators.
Flowers are designed to attract specific pollinators.
Pollinators are attracted to specific traits that flowers have.</td><td>Ask the students the following questions before watching the video: Do you think all flowers are trying to attract the same pollinators? Why are there so many types of flowers?</td><td></td></tr>
<tr><td>Watch the video Trading Food for Fertilization. While you watch, write in your journals. What are some facts that you learned from the video? Be prepared to share.</td><td>→ Video to build background knowledge and vocabulary</td></tr>
<tr><td>After the video, allow time for sharing their video facts. Ask them if they would like to add to or modify their answers to the questions: Do you think all flowers are trying to attract the same pollinators? Why are there so many types of flowers?
Pass out the Pollinator Observation Data Sheets from Part One of Flowers Seeking Pollinators. Assign each group a pollinator (there are 6 choices). Briefly explain what this chart is about and how it is organized. Look at the question on the back. Explain to the class that they need to look at which flower or flowers that their pollinator visited the most. Some pollinators clearly visit one flower more than any other. Other pollinators may visit more than one flower. On the paper, list the 3 flower traits that you think attract your pollinator.</td><td>→ Inquiry actvity to build background knowledge and vocabulary</td></tr>
<tr><td>Explain</td><td>Flowers are designed to attract specific pollinators.
Pollinators are attracted to specific traits of flowers.</td><td>Pass out the Constructing Explanations sheet from Part Two of Flowers Seeking Pollinators. Also pass out the Pollinator Profile cards.
Have a student read the directions. Use the Pollinator Profile card and your Datasheet to help you complete this assignment. Using all of the information, what are 3 traits that you think attract your pollinator? Find evidence on your card or data sheet to support your claims.</td><td></td></tr>
</table>

(continued)

FIGURE 17.1. 5E Learning cycle with embedded content scaffolds.

Elaborate	There are many types of flowers and pollinators. Flowers are designed to attract specific pollinators.	Post the following questions on the board: What is the author's purpose? What is something new you learned from this book? How does this book add to what you learned already? What new questions does it raise? Explain that you will be reading a book to them and that they need to answer those questions in their notebooks. Be prepared to share at least one thing from your notes with the class. Show them the front of the book. What do you think the title means? Read the book The Flowers Are Calling by Rita Gray. After reading, have students share from their notes. If students have new questions you can also take a moment to research the answers.	→	Picture book to build background knowledge and vocabulary
Evaluate		Part Three of Flowers Seeking Pollinators "Imaginary Garden." Students will think about the traits that their pollinator looks for in a flower. They will look through several fake flowers and decide which one their pollinator is attracted to the most. Once the group has decided on their flower, they need to create a presentation for the class. The presentation should explain to the class why their pollinator is attracted to that flower. They could create a Keynote, Google Slide show, or Clips App presentation about their pollinator. The presentation could also require them to show two-three other flowers that their pollinator is attracted to. Explain why your pollinator is attracted to each of those flowers. **COLLECT EVIDENCE:** Go back to your Claim, Evidence, and Reasoning worksheet and go the **Lesson 5 Evidence** section. What evidence have you discovered to explain why pollinators are important?		

FIGURE 17.1. *(continued)*

staff, assisted by MU undergraduate and graduate students, have developed three "foundational" grade 6–8 band anchor texts and selected scaffolds that address NGSS and CCSS shared practices, the NGSS crosscutting concepts, and selected NGSS DCIs (Table 17.1). The anchor texts address Earth and human activity, science and engineering, and human and body activity standards. In the *Flight of the Bumblebee,* the anchor was made based on Miller-Struttmann et al. (2017), which investigates the use of acoustics to measure bees' sound waves for monitoring bumblebee behavior and pollination services. The second anchor, *Heat Waves in Missouri,* was developed based on Steinweg and Gutowski (2015) and highlights the increasing heat waves in the St. Louis, Missouri, area and the negative impact on human health and daily activities. *Vaping: Not for the Young at Heart!,* the third anchor text, was inspired by the work of Moheimani et al. (2017) and Middlekauff (2020). It addresses the impact of vaping and vaping fluids on heart rhythms and human health. See Table 17.1 for an overview of the multimodal text sets, anchor text topics, and DCI connections to the NGSS.

TABLE 17.1. Overview of Multimodal STEM Text Sets

Anchor text	"Flight of the Bumblebee: Using Acoustics to Eavesdrop on Bees and Pollination"	"Heat Waves in Missouri—Is It Getting Hotter or Is It Just Me?"	"Vaping: Not for the Young at Heart!"
Foundational text set title	"Flight of the Bumblebee"	"Earth and Human Body Systems"	"Vaping: Not for the Young at Heart!"
Anchoring phenomena	Worldwide, declining bee numbers and species threaten biodiversity, agriculture, and human health. Analyses of bees' sound waves (buzzes) can distinguish between different bee sizes (functional groups), numbers, and pollination activities to help understand and mitigate bee declines.	Earth's warming climate impacts all living species. Recent climate models project more heat waves in the St. Louis area that will increase heat stresses and harm human health and daily activities. Actions can be taken to address climate warming and the harm it causes.	Scientific studies show the nicotine in tobacco and vaping fluids cause altered heart rhythms and premature death, as well as increased risk of COVID-19. Young people are being targeted by advertisements to encourage vaping. How can they distinguish what is true from false?
Pertinent disciplinary core ideas (DCIs)	MS-PS4 Waves and their Applications in Technologies for Information Transfer; MS-LS2 Ecosystems—Interactions, Energy, and Dynamics.	MS-PS3 Energy; MS-ESS2: Earth's Systems; MS-ESS3: Earth and Human Activity; MS-LS1 From Molecules to Organisms: Structures and Processes.	MS-LS1 From Molecules to Organisms: Structures and Processes; MS-PS4 Waves and their Applications in Technologies for Information Transfer.

Engaging Learners in a Complex Text

As previously noted, central to the multimodal STEM text set is the anchor text. The anchor text is a complex scientific text. While definitions of text complexity vary (Amendum et al., 2018), we use Mesmer et al. (2012) distinction that *text complexity* refers to properties (e.g., structure, language conventionality and clarity, and knowledge demands) of a text, regardless of reader or task, while *text difficulty* refers to how easy or hard a text is for readers.

All students must grapple with complexity to learn. Furthermore, national and state standards state that all learners should be able to use grade-band level complex informational text in science (e.g., Next Generation Science Standards [NGSS] and CCSS-ELA-Reading in Science and Technical Subjects [RST]). Litman and Greenleaf (2018) noted that "Reducing the complexity of texts and the effort required of students to make sense of them may similarly compromise student learning . . ." (p. 110). A major concern, however, is that engaging students in grade-level science texts can be an extremely difficult task, and as a result, complex texts are often avoided in science instruction (Amendum et al., 2018; Fisher & Frey, 2014; Shanahan, 2020).

Engaging Learners in Argumentation in Science

A key practice focus within each multimodal STEM text set is to develop students' ability to use argumentation. The ability to make evidence-based claims is central to literate science and responsible citizenship (Sjöström & Eilks, 2018). In the context of science education, this practice leads to asking: What does it mean to engage in argumentation? From the perspective of science, we can think of argumentation as a key scientific practice that involves making a claim, supporting it with evidence, and making a creative but logic-driven case for how the evidence provided supports the claim (NGSS Lead States, 2013). At the forefront, we caution against the misconception that argumentation is about taking sides in a debate. Rather, argumentation should be framed as a dialogue where many perspectives are welcomed and negotiated through evidence. The process of argumentation was formalized by Toulmin (1958), suggesting that an argument in its complete form includes a claim, evidence, and a warrant. This formulation has been contextualized in science education as helping students understand how to both construct their own arguments and evaluate the arguments of others (Osborne et al., 2016).

Toward argument construction, Gotwals and Songer (2010) advanced the CER framework, which gives emphasis to the use of scientific theory and data toward advancing and reasoning around scientific claims. Under the premise that the various processes behind argument construction and evaluation entail different levels of complexity, Berland and McNeill (2010) proposed a learning progression for argumentation that takes into account the complexity of the instruction and tasks that the students are asked to negotiate, the completeness of the argumentation product (e.g., whether or not a claim is supported with evidence), and the fluidity of the argumentation process (e.g., the extent to which students engage in argumentative discourse without prompting from the instructor). Based on the qualitative findings from a study by Berland and McNeill (2010), Toulmin's model was utilized more directly by Osborne et al. (2016) to develop and validate a formal quantitative measure of students' ability to not only make valid arguments but also to critique competing arguments. Using a similar logic with regards to progression of complexity, their progression moves from easier competencies that focus on simply identifying a claim up to the highest levels, where students are asked to evaluate multiple competing arguments and propose alternative explanations (Osborne et al., 2016).

Challenges Students with Learning Disabilities Experience Engaging in Complex Text and Argumentation

Ability to engage in and use complex texts as well as argumentation contributes to students developing scientific literacy. While many students may experience difficulty accessing grade-level complex text (Fisher & Frey, 2014; Shanahan, 2020) and engaging in argumentation (Zohar, 2007), students with LD have been found to have specific challenges related to both.

Four characteristics of complex, expository text have been found to challenge diverse learners (Mason & Hedin, 2011; Sáenz & Fuchs, 2002). First, these texts often use complex structures (e.g., compare–contrast) that can occur at any level within a text (e.g., sentence and paragraph), and sometimes multiple structures appear in a single passage. Many diverse learners find these structures unfamiliar and difficult to understand. Second, concepts and vocabulary are often densely packed so that learners struggle to connect prior knowledge to new learning (Diehl & Reese, 2010). Third, many texts contain high levels of novel and technological vocabulary with few supports for vocabulary development (Fang, 2008). Fourth, many learners lack the background knowledge and comprehension skills necessary to draw inferences that are critical to understanding (Mason & Hedin, 2011).

Based on the available research, many students struggle with different aspects of activities, including writing and scientific argumentation (Sampson & Clark, 2011). Difficulties have been observed in all aspects of argumentation from struggling to make sense of the phenomenon and relying on personal beliefs or past experiences (Kuhn & Reiser, 2005) to generating, justifying, and providing evidence and reasoning for an argument (Kuhn & Reiser, 2005; Sandoval, 2003).

For students with LD, difficulties in argumentation are often further compounded by difficulties in the writing process itself. Students with LD have been observed to experience challenges with planning, writing, editing, and revising their writing due to limitations in working memory, processing, memorizing, and information recall, which are functions of executive functioning and metacognition (Boyle et al., 2016; De La Paz & Levin, 2018; Hebert et al., 2018; Levin et al., 2021). These challenges are further magnified by trouble with foundational writing skills such as spelling, mechanics, and transcription (De La Paz, 1999; De La Paz & Levin, 2018). The goal, then, of our program is to use multimodal STEM text sets as a way to scaffold instruction to support students with LD in engaging in complex text and argumentation. We describe the extent to which we meet that goal next.

Our Research Program: Research Findings

In this section of the chapter, we describe 3 years of iterative development of multimodal STEM text sets and discuss what we have learned about their potential to positively impact SWLD's ability to construct arguments around socio-scientific issues. We describe three studies in turn that have facilitated the initiation and subsistence of the work. The goal of Study 1 (Romine et al., 2022) was to start to understand different models of best practice that teachers used and how this affected students' learning; namely, we wanted to study teachers who model best practice for multimodal STEM text set implementation and how this impacted science and language arts students' argumentation ability. This would be used to inform multimodal STEM text set development in the coming years. Study 2 (Romine et al., 2024) presents a quasi-experimental approach across multiple teachers with diverse practices aligned with our program. Study 2 focused specifically on construct validity of the assessments of argumentation with a focus on potential biases in SWLD as well as differential effects of the intervention of the multimodal STEM text set for students with and without LD. We then proceed to present the most recent data, Study 3, supporting the efficacy of our efforts to positively impact argumentation in SWLD through multimodal STEM text sets. It is important to note that in all studies, we did not focus only on students with LD; all students with an IEP were included. However, given the number of students with LD who are 80% or more in the general education classroom, we suspect a higher number of our students on IEPs were students with LD.

Overview of Studies: Constants Across All Studies

Multimodal STEM Text Selection and Development

In helping students learn science through multimodal STEM text sets, we gave the teachers flexibility in what they asked students to do and how they implemented the materials. The teachers chose the anchor text and connecting standards (i.e., NGSS and CCSS-ELA) to focus on to match their building and/or district scope and sequence requirements. Fidelity to the intervention depended not on doing a specific set of activities but rather doing activities consistent with our programmatic framework. Specifically, we asked that teachers require all students to read an anchor text at some point within the multimodal STEM text set implementation. Given the expectation that students will be at different levels of understanding of the anchor text, both in terms of reading level and disciplinary content, the teachers used supplementary texts, which served to scaffold students toward developing a better comprehension of the anchor text. The teachers were able to choose which supplementary texts they could use to support the phenomena they focused on. In carrying out the activities, we also asked that each teacher focus on CER when asking students to interpret the texts; namely, students were asked to write about what they read and use their content knowledge to negotiate the authors' position with respect to their own position on the issues they read about. Further, students were encouraged to use evidence and data gathered from the readings to support their positions. These activities were to take a duration of approximately 2 weeks and, in most cases, were approximately five instructional sessions. Note, because of COVID-19, teachers used either a face-to-face, online, or hybrid approach for instruction.

Measuring Argumentation

To measure students' argumentation, students completed a scenario-based assessment (SBA). An SBA is a situation that contains a specific scenario along with accompanying quantitative data (e.g., table and graph) that students are to respond to by making a claim and using the accompanying data as evidence to support the claim and explain their reasoning for the claim. In the current study, we utilized Gotwals and Songer's (2010) CER framework in order to develop a learning progression-based measure of argumentation in which argumentation tasks are contextualized with respect to scenarios aligning with current socio-scientific issues (SSIs) (Romine et al., 2024). Data from this study demonstrate that the product of making a claim and the process of writing about the claim are the easiest tasks. Use of discipline-specific vocabulary to support the claim was found to represent moderate complexity. The most difficult competencies included identifying appropriate sources of evidence and using reasoning to explain how the evidence supports the claim. Through multifaceted Rasch analysis, these scenario-based assessments were found to generate reliable measures of CER (r = 0.96), which were transferable across different SSI contexts.

For the current study described in this chapter, the SBA was constructed using the CER framework (Gotwals & Songer, 2010). Each student was given one of two possible scenarios that contained six parallel competencies that measured the ability to make a claim, use evidence, draw upon content-specific vocabulary, reason around evidence, and communicate the argument. Students were scored on each competency on a 4-point scale by at least 2 raters randomly assigned out of a pool of 11 trained raters comprising participating teachers, university faculty, and graduate students. Since inter-rater reliability was found to be moderate, we utilized the multifaceted Rasch model similar to Romine et al. (2024) to provide CER measures that were corrected for differences in rater severity.

Study 1: Pilot Work

Study 1 was a multiple case study of two teachers: one (Ms. Jane) who implemented a multimodal STEM text set in life sciences classes (n = 61) and another (Ms. Laura) who implemented a multimodal STEM text set in ELA classes (n = 129). Both used *Flight of the Bumblebee* as their anchor text around which other supplementary texts and activities were situated, but the disciplinary context differed. Ms. Jane's multimodal STEM text set was designed for use during a unit on ecosystems, and she intentionally included scaffolds that were multimodal to engage her learners. She used an inquiry approach, emphasizing use of the readings to help students construct their own knowledge. Through the processes of journaling and discussion, focus on CER was woven throughout all of Ms. Jane's lessons; for example, in connection with the readings on pollinators she provided for her students, she asked her students to find evidence about their pollinator and flower to support their claims. She took an explicit approach to teaching CER, which included looking at examples of each of the elements of an argument and then asking students to identify each within a scientific article. These served as scaffolds to support them in working with the anchor text.

Ms. Laura also embedded CER throughout the multimodal STEM text set. She implemented this text set in two sections of eighth-grade English, which consisted of a diverse group of students with a variety of needs and abilities. She designed the scaffolds to strengthen students' background knowledge, vocabulary, and literacy skills. CER was integrated into rolling journals, inquiry activities, and class discussions. Students created a claim regarding why bees are important, utilizing their rolling journals for evidence. At the end of the activities, students presented their flowers and explained why their flower is matched to a certain pollinator.

During a fishbowl discussion, students read a text about honeybees and discussed their claims and evidence regarding which bees are important. To scaffold students' use of CER, Ms. Laura provided a mnemonic framework: RACE (Restate and Answer to create a Claim, cite evidence, and Explain how the evidence supports the claim). Overall, the integration of CER throughout the text set provided students with opportunities to practice CER within a science context.

We used both qualitative and quantitative data to better understand the impact of these experiences on Ms. Jane's and Ms. Laura's students. For the quantitative analysis, which consisted of SBAs of CER, we used a double pretest design, where the first pretest of CER was given at least 2 weeks before the intervention started, a second pretest was given at the beginning of the intervention, and a posttest was given after the intervention. A total of 53 students in Ms. Jane's class and 106 students in Ms. Laura's class completed the SBA at all three testings. Scores changed significantly for both teachers ($F_{2,314}$= 48.96, $p < 0.001$, $\eta^2_{partial} = 0.24$), and we found a significant differential effect in this change between the respective teachers' students' scores ($F_{2,314} = 9.32$, $p < 0.001$, $\eta^2_{partial} = 0.056$).

Both teachers indicated in their interviews that their implementations fostered inclusion for students with diverse levels of literacy. For example, Ms. Jane commented that multimodal texts gave her a new way of thinking about differentiated instruction, "*Being able to use different levels of reading material was really helpful. . . . You know, like that we could have it on all these different levels in the same class, and I didn't really know how to make that work until I did this program.*"

In turn, Ms. Laura commented on how offering a variety of texts connected to the anchor text and encouraging students to actively engage with these texts was integral in helping the students starting at lower levels of literacy build the confidence they need to engage in argumentation: "*the confidence that the kids had by being able to build at those lower levels . . . having those text sets at the level that they needed and being able to be the first ones to talk about what they read and have the other kids really listen to them and taking notes on what they said. I think that gave a layer of accountability to it. And also just made them feel like 'I'm the expert here.' . . . And then when they would sit down and then need to take notes on more complex ideas, I think were better able to make sense of them than if they had not had that initial experience of really having to delve into that text that they were given.*"

By studying these two teachers through a mixed-methods approach, we were able to inform our next year's professional development through the understanding of the types of approaches that worked well toward helping all students improve their ability to comprehend, negotiate, and communicate scientific information; namely, both teachers used a supported inquiry-based approach facilitated by access to multiple supplementary texts and scaffolds, and both teachers gave students the opportunity to actively interact with the texts they read through consistent use of journaling and other writing and discussion activities. Hence, these approaches formed a foundation for the next year's professional development.

Study 2: Comparison of Effects between Students With and Without LD

The following year included a cohort of 14 middle school teachers enrolled in the yearlong PD, which was the focus of Study 2 (Romine et al., 2024). Based on the generally positive efficacy findings, especially for students starting with lower levels of literacy, from Ms. Jane's and Ms. Laura's classes in Study 1, we structured the learning experiences to support inclusion by asking each teacher to select one foundational anchor text as their focus for their multimodal STEM text set and to include a variety of scaffolds tied to the anchor text. Using the foundational anchor text along with recommended scaffold texts, the teachers developed their own multimodal STEM text set around that anchor text, which included the standards of focus, the learning objectives, lesson plans/5E learning cycles, resources, and materials for implementation with their students. In reviewing the teachers' multimodal STEM text sets, we confirmed that all teachers included these components.

For our evaluation (Romine et al., 2022), we generated measures using a model that accounts for the difficulty of the particular SBA context and the specific teacher scoring the SBA. Based on a repeated measures ANCOVA procedure described in Romine et al. (2024), we found that being a SWD had a significant effect on students' argumentation scores as they came into instruction with lower levels of argumentation ability than the other students ($F(1,642) = 11.47, p = 0.001, \eta^2_{partial} = 0.02$); however, the differential effect of instruction between SWDs and students without disabilities was non-significant ($F(1,642) = 1.83, p = 0.176, \eta^2_{partial} < 0.01$), meaning there was no significant difference in gains between SWD and students without disabilities in terms of the effect of instruction. Specifically, SWDs started at -2.72 logits (the unit of measure derived from our measurement model) and ended up at -1.27 logits, representing a significant gain of 1.45 logits ($t(72) = 3.23$, $p = 0.002$, Hedges' g effect size = 0.33). Students without disabilities started higher, at -0.44 logits, and ended up at 0.27 logits, representing a gain of 0.71 logits ($t(589) = 4.62, p < 0.001$, Hedges' g effect size = 0.19). It is also noteworthy that the Time × IEP × Teacher three-way interaction is non-significant ($F(9,642) = 0.56, p = 0.832, \eta^2_{partial} = 0.01$); this indicates that there was no statistically significant difference in the effects of individual teachers' implementations between SWLDs and students without disabilities.

The finding in Study 2 that SWLDs made gains in CER that were statistically similar in magnitude, as students without disabilities mirror what we found in the mixed-methods case study design in Study 1. These results offer a strong case for the efficacy of multimodal texts in helping all students improve their science literacy, regardless of where they begin or whether or not they have a disability. Data show that these methods are robust to different teaching styles and school environments. This led us to give the assessments again the following year (Study 3) in order to evaluate the extent to which these findings hold up over time.

Study 3: How do These Findings Translate to Future Implementation?

A total of 502 students nested within 6 teachers participated in the study. Of these students, 308 students in total, including 44 SWD, completed an SBA at both points. Our analysis of the effects of the curricula was done in two steps. In the first step, we simply wanted to take a descriptive look at the gains in CER between the pre- and posttests. We were then interested in the extent to which there were differential effects of the intervention for special education students. This was done using a three-level mixed-effects linear model to account for multiple measures within students who were in turn nested within teachers. Time and Time × IEP status were included as within-subjects effects, and IEP status was included as a between-subjects effect. Random intercepts were allowed at the student and classroom levels, which were modeled with an independent covariance structure. Robust standard errors were used to calculate the statistical significance of Time, IEP, and IEP × Time at the 99% confidence level (two-tailed).

On average, the cohort made positive and significant gains in CER, moving from an average measure of –1.53 logits (SD = 3.63) on the pretest to 0.27 logits (SD = 3.56) on the posttest. This change is statistically significant ($T_{df=307} = 7.64$, $p < 0.001$), and the standardized mean difference (Cohen's d = 0.50) indicates a moderate effect.

Parameter estimates from the three-level mixed-effects model give us a more holistic look at how the effects of the curricula differentially impacted special education students. Although special education students started with significantly lower levels of CER ($b = -3.82$, $SE = 0.44$, $Z = -8.73$, $p < 0.001$), the gains they made as a result of the text sets were significantly larger on average ($b = -1.06$, $SE = 0.36$, $Z = -2.98$, $p = 0.003$). These findings provide compelling evidence to support use of multimodal text to improve key skills related to argumentation and negotiation of SSIs. Given that the CER construct exemplifies many aspects of scientific practice laid out in the NGSS, integration of contemporary texts targeted to a variety of literacy levels may provide a mechanism for closing the achievement gap.

When comparing average pre- and post-measures for students with and without an IEP, we found that both groups made significant gains in their ability to use CER in their written responses (Table 17.2). The data indicate that students on an IEP started lower (pretest = –4.70 logits, SD = 2.68) on average than students who were not on an IEP (pretest = –1.00 logits, SD = 3.50). However, the students on

TABLE 17.2. Student Gains in CER between the Pre- and Posttest

IEP status	*N*	Pre	*SD*	Post	*SD*	Gain	*SD*	Cohen's *d*	*T*-score
IEP	44	–4.70	2.68	–1.76	2.87	2.94	3.44	1.06	5.67*
Non-IEP	264	–1.00	3.50	0.61	3.56	1.61	4.21	0.46	6.20*
All	308	–1.53	3.63	0.27	3.56	1.80	4.13	0.50	7.64*

*Significant gain in CER at alpha = 0.01.

an IEP made larger gains on average (gain = 2.94 logits, *SD* = 3.44, $T_{df=43} = 5.67$, $p < 0.001$) than students without an IEP (gain = 1.61 logits, *SD* = 4.21, $T_{df=263} = 6.20$, $p < 0.001$). The magnitude of the gain for students on an IEP (Cohen's $d = 1.06$) indicates a large effect. It was interesting that the magnitude of the gain for students on IEPs was over two times the magnitude for the other students (Cohen's $d = 0.46$).

Summary

Thus far, our data indicate that linking science and argumentation via multimodal STEM text sets can serve as a mechanism to improve all students' argumentation but, most importantly, for SWD. Further, the students were able to make gains in argumentation regardless of the classroom they attended (special education, science, or ELA) via instruction that connected to science literacy benchmarks, such as those of the NGSS and CCSS. These findings from the research we have carried out so far are promising. Yet there is still more work to do. Although the SWD made gains in argumentation, they remained behind their peers without disabilities, reflective of the concern we raised earlier in the chapter. But the SWD made greater gains than their peers without disabilities, thus working toward eliminating the gap.

Expanding Research in Science Education for Students with LD

The need to use evidence-based instructional strategies with students with LD has been well-established (Therrien et al., 2011). Numerous evidence-based instructional strategies exist for teaching different content, including science. The importance of not only understanding the science content and concepts but also the practices needed to do science should not be overlooked. Yet the extent to which the existing evidence-based instructional strategies in science reflect current science education expectations is limited. In addition to our work, several other researchers have also begun to address this gap with some success.

Doabler et al. (2021) and Maddox et al. (2025) investigated a program, Scientific Explorers (Sci2), which embedded the principles of explicit instruction in a guided inquiry-based design framework. Each lesson in the program connected to second-grade DCI and CCC related to Earth's systems and comprised four key components: activities designed to engage the learner and activate prior knowledge, explicit vocabulary instruction, read-aloud of research-developed expository text, and hands-on and simulation activities. The results from both studies suggest that the Sci2 program shows promise for improving science outcomes for students, including students with or at risk for a learning disability. The improvements are particularly attributed to the vocabulary instruction, suggesting that when SWD are pre-taught vocabulary with repeated exposure and opportunities to use the vocabulary, they are better positioned to engage in exploring phenomena and participate in meaningful discussions.

Several researchers have examined the effectiveness of using a Science Writing Heuristic (SWH) approach to improve students' science learning and critical thinking skills (e.g., Hand et al., 2004; Jang & Hand, 2017). The SWH is used in conjunction with any form, including inquiry-based, of science instruction, where students keep science notebooks and journals to record their experiences. The SWH is designed to enhance science argumentation, where students are expected to generate research questions, make a claim, and provide evidence using the heuristic as a guide. Students are provided with specific questions on a template to answer as they participate in the lesson and activities (e.g., Beginning ideas: What are my questions?), and teachers are provided a template to use to structure their learning experiences. Recently, the SWH has been demonstrated to be effective in science achievement scores on a standardized measure with third- to fifth-grade SWD (Taylor et al., 2018).

Benedek-Wood et al. (2014) investigated a Self-Regulated Strategy Development strategy for quick writing for informative writing with students, including SWD, in middle school science classrooms. Using explicit instruction, students were taught by their teacher the strategy POW-TIDE[2] (topic sentence, important details, elaborations, and ending sentence) to write a complete quick-write response during their science lessons. Performance in organizational writing quality, as well as total number of words written, improved for all students in the intervention, including SWD.

Lee and De La Paz (2021) examined the effect of cognitive apprenticeship with contextualized language instruction on middle school students', including those with learning disabilities, ability to compose scientific explanations. The cognitive apprenticeship approach had distinct instructional phases, including (1) preparing students to learn by defining objectives and building background knowledge through the use of a science experiment; (2) modeling well-written explanations and explaining tools to support writing; (3) supporting students' practice by allowing students to work collaboratively with the supportive tools and learn through discussion; and (4) independent practice where students were given two or more opportunities to practice their writing. Additionally, as part of the intervention, students were provided with language activities on language parts that students may use to communicate scientific ideas. After receiving instruction via the cognitive apprenticeship approach, the students were able to use more details in their scientific explanations. Moreover, the students produced clearer responses that were longer and more complex. Importantly, students maintained these skills 2 weeks after instruction ended.

Each of these studies, like ours, strives to find ways to balance current science education demands with the specific learning needs of students with LD. While the research shows promise for improving science outcomes for SWD, such as those with LD, much more needs to be done. For example, of the research summarized in this chapter, there were limited connections to a few of the DCIs; the only practice, of the many, of focus is argumentation, and none were connected to the high school setting. Compounding these needs are larger challenges for teaching science to students with and without LD that need to be addressed. For example, elementary science instruction is critical for building students' foundational science knowledge, but scientific practice is rarely emphasized in elementary classrooms (Banilower et al., 2018). Further compounding this challenge is that science instruction is often a time frame when SWD are pulled out of the classroom for services, resulting in these students missing crucial learning experiences (Banilower et al., 2018). In middle school and high school, many teachers do not think they are prepared to teach science to SWD (Kahn & Lewis, 2014). Consequently, they do not plan for SWD and often revert to practices that are not best practices and that result in disengaging their students from learning science (Dori, Tal, & Tsaushu, 2003; Maeng & Bell, 2015). But this does not need to be the case. There is evidence that shows it is possible to create a science classroom where all students are given the opportunity to build key science practices, and in doing so, it is possible to close the gap in literacy skills, including argumentation and comprehension of expository text between students with and without LD.

REFERENCES

Amendum, S. J., Conradi, K., & Hiebert, E. (2018). Does text complexity matter in the elementary grades? A research synthesis of text difficulty and elementary students' reading fluency and comprehension. *Educational Psychology Review, 30*(1), 121–151.

American Association for the Advancement of Science. (1993). *Science for all Americans. Benchmarks for science literacy.*

Anderson, A., Druger, M., James, C., & Katz, P. (1998). An NSTA position statement: The national science education standards: A vision for the improvement of science teaching and learning. *Science and Children, 35*(8), 32.

Banilower, E. R., Smith, P. S., Malzahn, K. A., Plumley, C. L., Gordon, E. M., & Hayes, M. L. (2018). *Report of the 2018 NSSME+.* Horizon Research, Inc.

Benedek-Wood, E., Mason, L. H., Wood, P. H., Hoffman, K. E., & McGuire, A. (2014). An experimental examination of quick writing in the middle school science classroom. *Learning Disabilities: A Contemporary Journal, 12*(1), 69–92.

Berland, L. K., & McNeill, K. L. (2010). A learning progression for scientific argumentation: Understanding student work and designing supportive instructional contexts. *Science Education, 94*(5), 765–793.

Boyle, J. R., Rosen, S. M., & Forchelli, G. (2016). Exploring metacognitive strategy use during note-taking for students with learning disabilities. *Education 3–13, 44*(2), 161–180.

Bradley-Black, K. H. (2013). *Teachers and evidence-based practices.* George Mason University.

Bybee, R. W. (2011). Scientific and engineering practices in K–12 classrooms. *Science Teacher, 78*(9), 34–40.

Cook, B. G., & Odom, S. L. (2013). Evidence-based practices and implementation science in special education. *Exceptional Children, 79*(2), 135–144.

Cook, B. G., Simpson-Steele, J., & Cook, L. H. (2017). Using evidence-based practice in teaching students with and at risk for developing disabilities. In J. B. Crockett & S. M. Malley (Eds.), *Handbook of arts education and special education policy, research & practices* (pp. 72–90). Routledge.

De La Paz, S. (1999). Self-regulated strategy instruction in regular education settings: Improving outcomes for students with and without learning disabilities. *Learning Disabilities Research & Practice, 14*(2), 92–106.

De La Paz, S., & Levin, D. M. (2018). Beyond "they cited the text": Middle school students

and teachers' written critiques of scientific conclusions. *Research in Science Education, 48*(6), 1433–1459.
Diehl, V., & Reese, D. D. (2010). Elaborated metaphors support viable inferences about difficult science concepts. *Educational Psychology, 30*(7), 771–791.
Doabler, C. T., Therrien, W. J., Longhi, M. A., Roberts, G., Hess, K. E., Maddox, S. A., & Toprac, P. (2021). Efficacy of a second-grade science program: Increasing science outcomes for all students. *Remedial and Special Education, 42*(3), 140–154.
Dori, Y. J., Tal, R. T., & Tsaushu, M. (2003). Teaching biotechnology through case studies—can we improve higher order thinking skills of nonscience majors? *Science Education, 87*(6), 767–793.
Fang, Z. (2008). Going beyond the fab five: Helping students cope with the unique linguistic challenges of expository reading in intermediate grades. *Journal of Adolescent & Adult Literacy, 51*(6), 476–487.
Fisher, D., & Frey, N. (2014). *Checking for understanding: Formative assessment techniques for your classroom.* ASCD.
Gotwals, A. W., & Songer, N. B. (2010). Reasoning up and down a food chain: Using an assessment framework to investigate students' middle knowledge. *Science Education, 94*(2), 259–281.
Guckert, M., Mastropieri, M. A., & Scruggs, T. E. (2016). Personalizing research: Special educators' awareness of evidence-based practice. *Exceptionality, 24*(2), 63–78.
Hand, B., Wallace, C. W., & Yang, E. M. (2004). Using a Science Writing Heuristic to enhance learning outcomes from laboratory activities in seventh-grade science: Quantitative and qualitative aspects. *International Journal of Science Education, 26*(2), 131–149.
Hebert, M., Bohaty, J., Nelson, J. R., Roehling, J., & Christensen, K. (2018). Taking notes on informational source text using text structures: An intervention for fourth grade students with learning difficulties. *Learning Disabilities: A Multidisciplinary Journal, 23*(2), 34–55.
Individuals with Disabilities Education Improvement Act, 20 U.S.C. § 614 et seq. (2004).
Jang, J. Y., & Hand, B. (2017). Examining the value of a scaffolded critique framework to promote argumentative and explanatory writings within an argument-based inquiry approach. *Research in Science Education, 47*(6), 1213–1231.
Jones, M. L. (2009). A study of novice special educators' views of evidence-based practices. *Teacher Education and Special Education, 32*(2), 101–120.
Kahn, S., & Lewis, A. R. (2014). Survey on teaching science to K–12 SWD: Teacher preparedness and attitudes. *Journal of Science Teacher Education, 25*(8), 885–910.
Krajcik, J. (2015). Three-dimensional instruction. *The Science Teacher, 82*(8), 50–52.
Kuhn, L., & Reiser, B. (2005, April). *Students constructing and defending evidence-based scientific explanations* [Presented paper]. Annual meeting of the National Association for Research in Science Teaching, Dallas, TX.
Lee, O., & Stephens, A. (2020). English learners in STEM subjects: Contemporary views on STEM subjects and language with English learners. *Educational Researcher, 49*(6), 426–432.
Lee, Y., & Paz, S. D. L. (2021). Writing scientific explanations: Effects of a cognitive apprenticeship for students with LD and English learners. *Exceptional Children, 87*(4), 458–475.
Levin, D. M., De La Paz, S., Lee, Y., & Escola, E. N. (2021). Use of cognitive apprenticeship models of instruction to support middle school students' construction and critique of written scientific explanations and arguments. *Learning Disabilities: A Multidisciplinary Journal, 26*(1), 58–72.
Litman, C., & Greenleaf, C. (2018). Argumentation tasks in secondary English language arts, history, and science: Variations in instructional focus and inquiry space. *Reading Research Quarterly, 53*(1), 107–126.
Maddox, S. A., Gersib, J. A., Fall, A.-M., Longhi, M. A., Therrien, W. J., Roberts, G., et

al. (2025). The role of instructional design in the delivery of early science instruction. *Remedial and Special Education*. Advance online publication. *https://doi.org/10.1177/07419325251314119*

Maeng, J. L., & Bell, R. L. (2015). Differentiating science instruction: Secondary science teachers' practices. *International Journal of Science Education, 37*(13), 2065–2090.

Markelz, A., Riden, B., & Scheeler, M. C. (2017). Generalization training in special education teacher preparation: Does it exist? *Teacher Education and Special Education, 40*(3), 179–193.

Mason, L. H., & Hedin, L. R. (2011). Reading science text: Challenges for students with learning disabilities and considerations for teachers. *Learning Disabilities Research & Practice, 26*(4), 214–222.

Mesmer, H. A., Cunningham, J. W., & Hiebert, E. H. (2012). Toward a theoretical model of text complexity for the early grades: Learning from the past, anticipating the future. *Reading Research Quarterly, 47*(3), 235–258.

Middlekauff, H. R. (2020). Cardiovascular impact of electronic-cigarette use. *Trends in Cardiovascular Medicine, 30*(3), 133–140.

Miller-Struttmann, N. E., Heise, D., Schul, J., Geib, J. C., & Galen, C. (2017). Flight of the bumble bee: Buzzes predict pollination services. *PLOS One, 12*(6), e0179273.

Moheimani, R. S., Bhetraratana, M., Yin, F., Peters, K. M., Gornbein, J., Araujo, J. A., & Middlekauff, H. R. (2017). Increased cardiac sympathetic activity and oxidative stress in habitual electronic cigarette users: Implications for cardiovascular risk. *JAMA Cardiology, 2*(3), 278–284.

National Governors Association Center for Best Practices & Council of Chief State School Officers. (2010). *Common core state standards for English language arts & literacy in history, science, and technical subjects.* Authors.

National Research Council. (1996). *National science education standards.* National Academies Press.

National Research Council. (2000). *Inquiry and the national science education standards: A guide for teaching and learning.* National Academies Press.

National Research Council. (2012). *A framework for K–12 science education.* National Academies Press.

National Science Teachers Association. (2018). *NSTA position statement: Transitioning from scientific inquiry to three-dimensional teaching and learning.*

NGSS Lead States. (2013). *Next generation science standards: For states, by states.* National Academy Press.

Osborne, J. F., Henderson, J. B., MacPherson, A., Szu, E., Wild, A., & Yao, S. Y. (2016). The development and validation of a learning progression for argumentation in science. *Journal of Research in Science Teaching, 53*(6), 821–846.

Reiser, B. J. (2013, September). *What professional development strategies are needed for successful implementation of the Next Generation Science Standards* [Paper presentation]. Invitational Research Symposium on Science Assessment, Educational Testing Services.

Reiser, B. J., Berland, L. K., & Kenyon, L. (2012). Engaging students in the scientific practices of explanation and argumentation. *The Science Teacher, 79*(4), 34.

Romine, W., Lannin, A., Palmer, T., van Garderen, D., Juergensen, R., Smith, C., & Folk, W. (2022). Complex multimodal text sets to support science literacy. In P. Short, H. Hensen, & J. R. McConnell (Eds.), *Age of inference: Cultivating a scientific mindset* (pp. 157–182). Information Age.

Romine, W., van Garderen, D., Follk, W., Lannin, A., Juergensen, R., Smith, C., et al. (2024). Science literacy: Using multimodal STEM text sets to help students with learning disabilities get ahead. *Learning Disability Quarterly, 47*(2), 84–96.

Sáenz, L. M., & Fuchs, L. S. (2002). Examining the reading difficulty of secondary students with learning disabilities: Expository versus narrative text. *Remedial and Special Education, 23*(1), 31–41.

Sampson, V., & Clark, D. B. (2011). A comparison of the collaborative scientific argumentation practices of two high and two low performing groups. *Research in Science Education, 41*(1), 63–97.

Sandoval, W. A. (2003). Conceptual and epistemic aspects of students' scientific explanations. *The Journal of the Learning Sciences, 12*(1), 5–51.

Scheeler, M. C., Budin, S., & Markelz, A. (2016). The role of teacher preparation in promoting evidence-based practice in schools. *Learning Disabilities: A Contemporary Journal, 14*(2), 171–187.

Scruggs, T. E., Brigham, F. J., & Mastropieri, M. A. (2013). Common core science standards: Implications for students with learning disabilities. *Learning Disabilities Research and Practice, 28*(1), 49–57.

Scruggs, T. E., & Mastropieri, M. A. (2013). Science and social studies education for students with learning disabilities. In H. L. Swanson, K. R. Harris, & S. Graham (Eds), *Handbook of learning disabilities* (2nd ed., pp. 448–462). Guilford Press.

Scruggs, T. E., Mastropieri, M. A., Bakken, J. P., & Brigham, F. J. (1993). Reading versus doing: The relative effects of textbook-based and inquiry-oriented approaches to science learning in special education classrooms. *The Journal of Special Education, 27*(1), 1–15.

Shanahan, T. (2020). What constitutes a science of reading instruction? *Reading Research Quarterly, 55*, S235–S247

Sjöström, J., & Eilks, I. (2018). Reconsidering different visions of scientific literacy and science education based on the concept of bildung. In Y. Dori, Z. Mevarech, D. Baker (Eds.), *Cognition, metacognition, and culture in STEM education–learning, teaching and assessment* (part of the Innovations in Science Education and Technology book series, vol. 24) (pp. 65–88). Springer.

Steinweg, C., & Gutowski, W. J. (2015). Projected changes in greater St. Louis summer heat stress in NARCCAP simulations. *Weather, Climate, and Society, 7*(2), 159–168.

Swanson, H. L. (1993). Working memory in learning disability subgroups. *Journal of Experimental Child Psychology, 56*(1), 87–114.

Swanson, H. L., & Zheng, X. (2013). Memory difficulties in children and adults with learning disabilities. In H. L Swanson, K. R. Harris, & S. Graham (Eds.), *Handbook of learning disabilities* (2nd ed., pp. 214–238). Guilford Press.

Taylor, J. C., Tseng, C. M., Murillo, A., Therrien, W., & Hand, B. (2018). Using argument-based science inquiry to improve science achievement for SWD in inclusive classrooms. *Journal of Science Education for Students with Disabilities, 21*(1), 1–14.

Therrien, W. J., Taylor, J. C., Hosp, J. L., Kaldenberg, E. R., & Gorsh, J. (2011). Science instruction for students with learning disabilities: A meta–analysis. *Learning Disabilities Research & Practice, 26*(4), 188–203.

Toulmin, S. E. (1958). *The Uses of Argument*. Cambridge University Press.

U.S. Department of Education. (2009). *31st Annual Report to Congress on the Implementation of the Individuals with Disabilities Education Act. https://www2.ed.gov/about/reports/annual/osep/index.html*

U.S. Department of Education. (2019). *2019 NAEP science assessment*. Institute of Education Sciences, National Center for Education Statistics.

U.S. Department of Education. (2024). 45th Annual Report to Congress on the Implementation of the Individuals with Disabilities Education Act. *https://sites.ed.gov/idea/2023-individuals-with-disabilities-education-act-annual-report-to-congress/*

Zohar, A. (2007). Science teacher education and professional development in argumentation. In S. Erduran & M. P. Jiménez-Aleixandre (Eds.), *Argumentation in science education* (pp. 245–268). Springer.

CHAPTER 18

Key Practices for Preventing and Ameliorating Reading Disabilities among English Learners

Philip Capin, Tim T. Andress, and Sharon Vaughn

English learners (ELs) are a heterogeneous population of students with a variety of strengths and needs, including differing degrees of language proficiency in multiple languages, literacy skills, and content-area knowledge. Yet discussions of ELs and their English reading abilities often center upon their deficits and the achievement gap between ELs and their monolingual, English-speaking peers. This is particularly true for ELs identified with reading disabilities (RD), who are the focus of this chapter. It is important to consider the benefits of bilingualism and the sociocontextual factors that influence their development in the United States. Bilingual students possess important linguistic knowledge in their primary language and cultural knowledge, which can provide an advantage to them in their language and literacy development in a second language. Children who are bilingual are better able "to develop and sustain strong ties with their immediate and extended families" and "establish a strong cultural identity" (Espinosa, 2007, p. 2). In the long term, there may also be economic benefits to bilingualism as employers increasingly favor employees who are multilingual, contribute cultural expertise, and work well with others across ethnic and cultural backgrounds (Gándara, 2015).

Unfortunately, relative to their monolingual peers, many ELs experience fewer opportunities to engage with texts and academic experiences in English that contribute to successful academic language and reading proficiency. Spanish-speaking ELs in the United States are more likely than their native English-speaking peers to attend less-resourced, lower-performing schools (Cosentino de Cohen et al., 2005) and have parents with less financial resources and less favorable working hours that limit their time at home with their children (Capps et al., 2005). As others have noted (e.g., Patton Terry, 2020), Spanish-speaking Latinos and other ethnic groups (e.g., Black students) in the United States are also negatively impacted by policies and practices in and outside of schools, such as inequitable laws that couple property taxes with school funding. Thus, we interpret the difference in academic performance between ELs and their monolingual peers as reflective of a disparity in English learning opportunities. When we consider the significant strengths of ELs and their limited opportunities to develop their English language and literacy skills, it becomes clear that ELs have considerable untapped potential. ELs with RD may have the greatest opportunity to improve, as they typically perform well below grade level.

With that as our backdrop, the purpose of this chapter is to address the question: How can we best prevent and ameliorate reading difficulties among ELs? To this end, we describe the promise of multi-tiered systems of support (MTSS) as a framework for providing high-quality instruction and assessment to ELs and evidence-based practices for teaching ELs in the primary grades and beyond. Since the last edition of the *Handbook of Learning Disabilities*, there has been a surge in research examining evidence-based practices for ELs, including those with RD. This is reflected in the systematic reviews and meta-analyses published over the past decade (e.g., Baker et al., 2014; Hall et al., 2017; Richards-Tutor et al., 2016). Although more research is needed to understand what instructional practices are most effective and under what conditions, the available studies provide a strong basis for making evidence-based decisions. We begin this chapter by examining how the sources of reading difficulties are similar and different for ELs with RD relative to their monolingual peers and the implications for instruction. From there, we describe why MTSS is a promising framework for supporting the needs of ELs with or at risk for RD and present evidence-based instructional practices for students in the primary grades (K–3) and the upper elementary grades and beyond (grades 4–12).

Understanding the Sources of Reading Difficulties among ELs with LD

The Simple View of Reading (SVR) (Gough & Tunmer, 1986) provides a helpful starting place for understanding sources of reading difficulties. The SVR posits that reading comprehension is equal to the product of word reading and linguistic comprehension. Across an abundance of studies, results consistently substantiate the SVR as a strong model for understanding individual differences in reading comprehension performance (e.g., Catts et al., 2015). An important finding from this research is that word reading accounts for greater variation in reading comprehension until about age 10 (or grade 4). At this age, for students with average reading development, word reading becomes automatic, and the texts become increasingly more difficult to understand, which results in linguistic comprehension playing a larger role. However, students with disabilities are an exception to this trend. Students with RD continue to show considerable variability in their word-reading skills; thus, word reading accounts for variation in text comprehension into adolescence (e.g., Braze et al., 2007).

The SVR framework has also been used to understand what, if any, differences exist between ELs and their monolingual peers in the sources of reading difficulties. The research conducted with primary-grade students suggests there are no substantial differences between ELs and monolingual children in the degree to which word reading and linguistic comprehension predict reading comprehension performance. For instance, Kieffer and Vukovic (2012) collected cross-sectional data on grade 1 and 2 students and found word reading and linguistic comprehension skills were similarly predictive of reading comprehension across ELs and monolingual speakers. This is consistent with longitudinal research that shows there are no significant differences between language groups in the extent to which the component skills assessed in grades 1 through 3 predict later reading comprehension (Lesaux et al., 2007). We know that ELs, by definition, have limited English language knowledge, but they have similar performance on code-based tasks (e.g., word reading and spelling tasks) (Lesaux et al., 2007). It may be that the linguistic demands required by the reader to successfully understand texts in the primary grades are less complicated, thus explaining the lack of differences between subgroups.

However, it appears that differences in the contributions of the component skills of reading to reading comprehension between ELs and monolingual students begin to emerge as students advance beyond the primary grades (Babayigit, 2012; Droop & Verhoeven, 2003). In perhaps the most relevant study, Cho and colleagues (2019) compared the sources of difficulties among grade 4 ELs and monolingual students with significant reading problems using the SVR. The authors reported that the contribution of linguistic comprehension was greater for ELs than for monolingual students. Additionally, word reading was a greater predictor of reading comprehension for monolingual students than ELs. However, it is important to note that word reading remained a greater predictor of reading comprehension than listening comprehension for both ELs and monolingual students with significant reading difficulties.

Collectively, these findings shed light on the sources of reading difficulties of ELs and the instructional approaches that may be most impactful for ELs with RD. In the primary grades, word reading plays an outsized role in understanding texts, both among ELs and monolingual students. The finding that word reading matters just as much for ELs underscores the importance of establishing word-reading proficiency in the early grades. Studies with older ELs with reading difficulties reveal that word reading still has a large effect on students' reading comprehension, suggesting that instruction may need to target word reading beyond the primary grades. However, these findings should not undermine efforts—early and often—to establish the broader English language facilities of ELs. Research shows that beginning in the upper elementary grades, developing linguistic processes is particularly important for ELs, including those with RD.

MTSS: A Promising Framework for ELs

MTSS provides a promising framework ideally suited to support ELs by establishing the provisions of ongoing screening, progress monitoring to inform instruction, research-based approaches to improving instruction, and approaches to remedy learning difficulties. With a focus on early intervention, using data to monitor progress, and intensive interventions when needed, MTSS has the potential to prevent and ameliorate RD among ELs.

MTSS service delivery systems use tiered levels of instruction that begin in the general education classroom (Tier 1). In many ways, the success of an MTSS system is reliant on classroom instruction in language and literacy that is well-grounded in research and thus is most likely to reduce the number of students with RD. Well-developed and implemented Tier 1 instruction increases accuracy in identifying students with "real" literacy challenges rather than students who have received inadequate or inappropriate Tier 1 instruction. Of particular importance for ELs is the need for both high-quality literacy and language learning from Tier 1 instruction so that they have access to successful literacy as they are co-developing their language. We consider research-based instruction provided within Tier 1 reading instruction as the "secret sauce" that enables all students the opportunity to launch onto a literate path.

MTSS frameworks provide increasingly customized reading interventions to students across three tiers. All students receive Tier 1 instruction, which consists of effective, evidence-based reading instruction. Roughly 15% of students do not make adequate improvement in reading from Tier 1 instruction alone, warranting supplemental instruction in Tier 2. Additionally, 5% of students experience continued reading difficulties when given Tier 1 and 2 supports and require intensive customized intervention. These students are often referred for special education or dyslexia services. These estimates are expected to vary considerably based on factors such as opportunities to learn and language development in English. Developing a systemic MTSS approach to support teachers so that they can meet the needs of ELs with RD requires that all of these pieces (i.e., screening, progress monitoring, core literacy instruction, and interventions) are seamlessly assembled to develop an effective MTSS system.

A considerable amount of evidence suggests that approaches involving effective classroom instruction, early intervention, and ongoing progress monitoring consistent with MTSS are associated with improved outcomes for the majority of students in early reading (e.g., Burns et al., 2007). Though there is less information about the effectiveness of these approaches with ELs (Linan-Thompson et al., 2006), the extant evidence is consistent with findings for English-only students (Fletcher & Vaughn, 2009).

Caveats and Considerations about MTSS for ELs with RD

When considering MTSS approaches for students who are ELs, it is worthwhile to consider the EL program and supports provided for the student as part of their Tier 1 literacy instruction. For example, is the student in a bilingual literacy program (e.g., dual-language program), or what other language instruction or supports are provided? It is also worthwhile to consider how their home language is assessed and monitored and the core literacy programs they have received in previous grades. When implementing MTSS approaches with ELs, a significant challenge is determining students' knowledge and skills in their first language and then understanding their performance in English. For example, there are subgroups of students whose literacy knowledge and skills in their first language (e.g., Spanish) are adequate, but whose literacy skills in their second language (e.g., English) are low. These students have demonstrated the capacity to acquire reading skills and now require instruction so they can apply those skills to the acquisition of English literacy. Other students may have low literacy in both their first language and English because they have not received adequate instruction in either language. Another group of students may demonstrate low literacy skills in both their home language and English even after receiving adequate instruction. Further complicating these issues is when the student's home language is not shared by other students or teachers at their school. This may be made even more complex when there are inadequate print sources in their home language or when their home language does not have a written orthography. We recognize that these caveats and considerations may guide decision making; however, educators may not postpone decision making and interventions for ELs. In most cases, providing the best instructional practices for students in their Tier 1 literacy program and supplementing this with Tier 2 interventions when students are not making adequate progress is the best pathway to success for ELs with RD.

Effectively Implementing MTSS for ELs

Educators may be reluctant to provide screening, assessment, and Tier 2-type interventions to students who are ELs with RD because they perceive they have inadequate resources (e.g., assessments and programs) or knowledge and skills. We recognize the immediate need for research-based assessments, screening resources, and materials and that the immediate provision of best practices for these students is essential. Ways educational leaders can support teachers and other personnel in meeting the needs of ELs with RD include (1) provide ongoing professional development, coaching, and professional groups aimed to improve research-based knowledge and skills; (2) improve knowledge of language development and mechanisms to support language use and acquisition schoolwide; (3) improve knowledge about the family contexts, home language, and cultural background of students to facilitate interpretation of assessments and instructional response; and (4) recognize that students who are ELs, as well as other learners in their classrooms, have more in common as learners than differences and these commonalities require explicit instruction in the same foundational literacy skills.

Universal Screening

Several MTSS models for preventing RD describe screening and identification of literacy problems as the critical first step (Fletcher & Vaughn, 2009). Missing from these models for ELs is consideration of how their language development in English impacts their performance on early literacy screening assessments.

Students who are ELs may perform poorly on screening measures because they have had inadequate exposure to the constructs tested in English, yet, when provided the necessary instruction, demonstrate success. Thus, we recommend that for ELs, educators consider not just students' performance on the screening measures but also their rate of successful learning in the classroom and their language experiences. It is this focus on instructional response within MTSS systems as the method for identifying students who need instructional supports that makes it particularly beneficial for ELs. Assessing students in their native language may also provide useful information about who needs instructional supports, though we recognize this may not always be feasible (Project ELLIPSES et al., 2021). Some reading assessments (e.g., Dynamic Indicators of Basic Early Literacy Skills [DIBELS] have parallel versions in English and another language, such as Spanish.

Most schools across the United States are implementing screening approaches to RD that ostensibly identify children who are at risk for reading failure. Screening is mandated for dyslexia in over 40 states (National Center on Improving Literacy, 2021). There are several critical elements to effective screening: (1) able to be administered and scored easily and quickly (screening measures in early reading ought to require 10 minutes or less per child), (2) demonstrate strong psychometric properties, (3) provide readily usable data that identifies students as either at risk or not at risk, and (4) is developmentally appropriate and can be administered two to three times per year. Identification errors when utilizing brief screeners are inevitable. We think schools should focus on reducing errors that result in not identifying risk when risk is present (false negatives), even if the number of children identified as at risk increases and includes some children without true risk (false positives) because early identification of reading difficulties is crucial. Screeners are not diagnostic and should indicate a need to monitor a child because of the at-risk designation. By treating screening as a recursive, dynamic process, false-positive errors can be corrected over time (Fletcher et al., 2021). The following guidelines may be helpful when screening ELs:

- ELs can be screened on the same early reading indicators as those used for monolingual English students (e.g., phonological awareness and word and text reading) (Gersten et al., 2007); however, it would be ideal to use a screener with evidence of reliability and validity for ELs.
- Incorporate screening measures that tap not only code-based skills (e.g., phonological awareness) but also oral language skills (e.g., vocabulary, listening comprehension).
- Universal screening measures should demonstrate high validity and reliability.
- When screening ELs, consider their performance in both home language and English. Students with high proficiency in early reading skills in their home language(s) and low English proficiency can be considered instructionally different from students with low proficiency in both their home language(s) and English.

- Universal screening and other assessment scores should be interpreted in light of the language(s) of instruction.
- Provide instructional support to ELs with low performance in reading areas even when oral language skills in English are low. Interventions should simultaneously address development of language and literacy skills in English.

Progress Monitoring of ELs with RD

The goal of progress monitoring is to determine whether students are learning the intended goals of instruction (e.g., the phonics elements taught and the words students are expected to read correctly) and whether students are making expected progress toward grade-level expectations. In an MTSS model, progress monitoring aims to determine whether students are acquiring proficiency in the target areas taught and whether they can integrate these target areas to demonstrate reading growth. Thus, progress monitoring is often based on short probes involving timed word or passage reading to determine students' progress so that teachers can make instructional decisions. In many ways, these measures yield information about whether our teaching is effective and what instructional adjustments may be needed. These types of assessments are aimed at improving instruction and determining students' incremental progress, recognizing that for students who are consistently making inadequate progress, either more intensive interventions or different interventions may be warranted.

Within an MTSS framework, this type of progress monitoring data can be useful when instructing ELs in several ways. First, these data can be used to document that students are learning the critical aspects of reading instruction taught (e.g., sight words, phonic elements, and text reading with comprehension). Second, the types of responses students provide can be used to guide instruction, highlighting each student's needs for reteaching and additional practice and those elements that appear to be successfully learned and can be monitored for maintenance. Third, data from these measures can facilitate curriculum decisions (e.g., whether additional or different curricula are needed), grouping decisions (e.g., some students may benefit from a more advanced group; students may benefit from a mini one-on-one lesson to enhance performance), and whether students continue or discontinue an intervention. Consider the following guidelines when providing progress monitoring for ELs with RD:

- Monitor ELs' progress at least as frequently as you monitor the progress of other students.
- Determine whether the research-based practices for Tier 1 and interventions include adequate support for ELs and use progress monitoring data to inform adjustments.
- Do not penalize students for accents or dialectic features when scoring tests.
- Recognize that students' rate of progress in oral reading fluency may decelerate over time as students begin reading texts with many words that may be new to their oral vocabulary.

Implementing MTSS for ELs in the Secondary Grades

Although MTSS was originally designed as a framework for preventing RD among younger students, MTSS is also beneficial for adolescent ELs (Baker et al., 2014; Echevarria et al., 2015). The core components of MTSS remain the same, but there are differences in MTSS implementation for students in the secondary grades. Related to universal screening, secondary schools schedule students into classes prior to the start of the school year, which makes it challenging for schools to administer and use beginning-of-year screening measures to determine instructional schedules. However, research indicates that additional screeners of reading performance may not be needed to identify secondary struggling readers because their challenges are often well-documented (Fuchs et al., 2010; Vaughn & Fletcher, 2012). Secondary school structures also present challenges for using progress monitoring data to move students between instructional tiers on an ongoing basis. Specifically, it is difficult for schools to transition because of scheduling barriers and staffing limitations. Survey data indicate that secondary schools often schedule students with reading difficulties into interventions during separate class periods and keep students in these classes for an entire semester (Savitz et al., 2021). Given these constraints, teachers may need compelling data from multiple sources to make changes to students' schedules. A centralized, online system that enables content-area teachers, intervention staff, and special education staff to input and access assessment results may be helpful. Additionally, a schedule for how often progress monitoring data should be collected and when educators meet to assess progress and adapt instructional plans. Schools that develop a flexible block scheduling approach that enables students to move across instructional tiers may be best positioned to use this data to inform instructional placements (Thomas et al., 2020).

Evidence-Based Instructional Practices for Young ELs with or at Risk for RD

Tier 1 Instruction

All of the elements of MTSS are important; however, Tier 1 instruction is arguably the most important. Teachers who set high but reasonable instructional expectations and provide ongoing instructional support to ensure that these expectations are met, providing EL students a strong base for learning. Fundamental to success for ELs is assuring foundational skills are systematically and explicitly taught, such as phonemic awareness and phonics, with continued emphasis on vocabulary and concept building throughout the instructional process. Reading words accurately and with prosody, as well as reading for meaning and learning, are emphasized through listening comprehension early and then later through reading comprehension. It is also essential that support for literacy is not delayed until English language is adequately developed. Provide supports for language and vocabulary development throughout the day through whole-class supports as well as small-group structures. See Table 18.1 for several suggestions for enhancing Tier 1 literacy instruction in the early grades.

TABLE 18.1. Tier 1 Supports for ELs with Reading Difficulties in the Early Grades

Academic language and vocabulary

- Promote language and key vocabulary use throughout the day. Utilize organized opportunities to turn and talk, as well as oral language, to summarize ideas.
- Develop word and world knowledge throughout all content learning.
- Teach vocabulary, particularly high-utility words related to content areas.
- Give students opportunities to engage in participatory story read-alouds that encourage them to signal when they hear new vocabulary and practice retelling.

Phonemic awareness and phonics

- Provide fun, game-like ways to promote phonological awareness with an emphasis on blending and segmenting sounds within words.
- Teach and practice high-frequency words in phrases, sentences, and texts.
- Teach foundational phonics and word analysis skills explicitly and provide opportunities for practice opportunities over a long period of time.
- Intensify instruction by reducing group size, increasing instructional time, matching instruction with student needs, and frequently tracking progress.

Reading fluency

- Engage students in reading increasing amounts of texts, starting with words and sentences and building to multiple sentences and then to pages of text.
- Develop peer-assisted routines to support reading fluency and comprehension.

Reading comprehension

- Systematically develop students' knowledge within and across content areas to support text comprehension.
- Teach students to monitor their understanding of vocabulary and text comprehension using the "click-and-clunk" strategy (Capin & Vaughn, 2017).
- Teach comprehension strategies that can be applied before, during, and after reading explicitly (see Collaborative Strategic Reading; Klingner et al., 1998).
- Use structured cooperative learning techniques in which each student is assigned a specific role and responsibility that allows each student to develop oral language skills and practice taught comprehension strategies.

Tier 2 and 3 Interventions

Fundamental to a successful MTSS program for ELs is the effective use of supplemental interventions to enhance opportunities for acquiring on-level language and literacy. This requires providing sufficiently intensive reading interventions to ELs demonstrating low reading skills immediately and for as long as needed. Most of the research examining the effects of instruction for school-age ELs has focused on young learners in the primary grades (Ludwig et al., 2019). These meta-analyses reveal that early reading interventions yield significant benefits on reading outcomes for ELs (Ludwig et al., 2019), including ELs with or at risk for RD (Richards-Tutor et al., 2016). A variety of instructional practices have been incorporated into past interventions, with many focused on multiple reading domains, such as phonics, fluency, vocabulary, and comprehension. Members of our author team were involved in two such studies, which can provide a glimpse into what works for ELs in the primary grades.

Vaughn and colleagues conducted a multi-year intervention project involving first-grade ELs with reading difficulties (Vaughn, Linan-Thompson, et al., 2006; Vaughn, Mathes, et al., 2006). Specifically, they conducted two separate student randomized studies, with the second study replicating the first using the same methods. The treatment group instruction supplemented the core reading instruction that was occurring in students' classrooms, and this instruction (and assessments) were provided in the same language as that of the students' core reading instruction (either English or Spanish, as determined by schools). Treatment students were taught in groups of three to five students for approximately 50 minutes a day for about 7 months. To address the multiple needs of ELs with or at risk for RD in the primary grades, the intervention used explicit instructional techniques to target both the development of code-based reading skills (e.g., phonemic awareness and word recognition) and broader oral language skills (e.g., vocabulary and oracy). The instructional components of the English and Spanish intervention were the same, except the Spanish phonics instruction focused on more complex word structures sooner than the English intervention because Spanish is a more transparent orthography. English and Spanish interventionists were trained and received semi-scripted lessons that promoted the use of explicit instruction in language use, multiple opportunities for elaborated responses, and visual aids and story retells to support language understanding.

Table 18.2 presents the instructional strands targeted in the intervention (e.g., phonemic awareness and oral reading fluency) and the effect sizes for both cohorts of the English and Spanish interventions on related measures. Significant differences in favor of treatment were present across multiple reading indicators, regardless of whether the intervention occurred in English or Spanish. These findings

TABLE 18.2. Intervention Strands and Effect Sizes from First-Grade Studies (Vaughn, Linan-Thompson, et al., 2006; Vaughn, Mathes, et al., 2006)

		Effect size (Cohen's *d*)			
Intervention strands	Construct measured	English Cohort 1	English Cohort 2	Spanish Cohort 1	Spanish Cohort 2
Vocabulary and oral language development →	Oral language composite	0.43	−0.17	0.35	0.23
Phonemic awareness and encoding →	Phonemic awareness	1.24	0.38	0.73	0.81
Letter–sound recognition →	Letter-sound identification	1.01	0.36	0.72	0.53
Word recognition →	Word attack	1.09	0.06	0.85	0.45
Repeated connected text reading →	Oral reading fluency	0.16	0.27	0.75	0.28
Comprehension strategies →	Passage comprehension	1.08	06	0.55	0.45

Note. The number of intervention strands targeted shifted over the course of the intervention. The start of each arrow represents the time when intervention strand began. For example, the repeated connected text reading strand started after word recognition, which started after phonemic awareness and encoding. Once an intervention strand (e.g., word recognition) started, it was continued through the rest of the intervention.

highlight the power of explicit and systematic instruction in code-based skills, an emphasis on vocabulary development with repeated practice, and oral language development through routines such as story retells. They are also consistent with other studies with ELs with or at risk for RD in the primary grades that incorporate explicit and systematic instruction to address components of early reading (e.g., Richards-Tutor, 2016).

Evidence-Based Instructional Practices for Older ELs with RD (Grades 4–12)

Tier 1 Instruction

Relative to younger students, less research exists examining the effects of reading instruction for ELs in the upper elementary grades and beyond (e.g., Hall et al., 2019; Richards-Tutor et al., 2016). For example, Hall and colleagues (2017) identified 11 studies examining the effects of whole-class, Tier 1 instructional practices implemented with ELs in grades 4 through 8. Consistent with previous reviews of research (Baker et al., 2014; Shanahan & Beck, 2006), Hall and colleagues identified three common features of interventions that were found to be effective for ELs in the upper elementary and middle school grades. They found that vocabulary instruction that taught students the meaning of target words using explicit instructional techniques and opportunities to use the words across multiple contexts was valuable. Reading comprehension instruction was also present in several studies, and this instruction was associated with improved outcomes in reading comprehension. In each of these studies, treatment instruction engaged students in comprehension instruction (often using reading comprehension strategies) and provided frequent opportunities to read text, apply strategies, and engage in text-based discussions. Hall and colleagues found that interventions that targeted both reading comprehension and vocabulary ($g = .39$) yielded larger gains in comprehension than studies that focused on only vocabulary ($g = .08$). Finally, the authors found empirical support across multiple studies for the use of Spanish language supports during English instruction helped ELs who were learning English as a Second Language.

Hall and colleagues' (2017) findings correspond to the recommendations put forth by the Institute of Education Sciences (IES) panel focused on improving literacy among ELs (Baker et al., 2014). The IES report also underscored the need to support ELs during content-area learning because students are expected to read and understand complex informational texts according to progressive state standards. Baker and colleagues (2014) provide four suggestions related to content-area teaching for ELs: (1) strategically use instructional tools (e.g., short videos) to help students make sense of content, (2) explicitly teach key academic vocabulary, (3) provide daily opportunities for small-group discussions, and (4) integrate writing opportunities.

Members of our research team have played a primary role in the development of two content-area reading programs tailored to meet the needs of ELs in social studies by supporting the development of vocabulary and reading comprehension: Center for Research on the Educational Achievement and Teaching of English

TABLE 18.3. Summary of Findings from Middle School Studies Conducted in Social Studies Classes for ELs

Program	Grade level	Research design	Measures	Effect size
CREATE (Vaughn et al., 2009; Cohort 1)	7	Within-teacher experimental design	Vocabulary	$g = 0.63$ for ELs; $g = 0.49$ for non-ELs
			Comprehension of Social Studies Texts	$g = 0.71$ for ELs; $g = 0.71$ for non-ELs
CREATE (Vaughn et al., 2009; Cohort 2)	7	Within-teacher experimental design	Vocabulary	$g = 0.49$ for ELs; $g = 0.36$ for non-ELs
			Comprehension of Social Studies Texts	$g = 0.83$ for ELs; $g = 0.47$ for non-ELs
CREATE (Reutebuch et al., 2018; Cohort 3)	7	Within-teacher experimental design	Vocabulary	$g = 0.54$ for ELs; $g = 0.55$ for non-ELs
			Comprehension of Social Studies Texts	$g = 0.49$ for ELs; $g = 0.56$ for non-ELs
PACT for ELs (Vaughn et al., 2017)	8	Within-teacher experimental design	Social Studies Knowledge	$g = 0.40$ for total sample[a]
			Comprehension of Social Studies Texts	$g = 0.20$ for total sample
			Generalized Reading Comprehension	$g = 0.12$ for total sample

[a]Vaughn et al. (2017) did not report effect sizes by language group. However, moderation results indicated that the effects of PACT did not vary by EL status on either measure of reading comprehension. On the content knowledge measure, the authors reported a significant three-way interaction between treatment, EL status, and the proportion of ELs in classroom, indicating that the effects of PACT were slightly smaller than non-ELs when the percentage of ELs in classrooms was at or above 12%.

Language Learners (CREATE) intervention (Vaughn et al., 2009) and Promoting Adolescents' Comprehension of Text (PACT) for ELs (Vaughn et al., 2017). Both programs are responsive to the need to develop ELs' literacy and knowledge of academic content in the middle grades and incorporate the key practices for content-area learning identified by Baker et al. (2014). Findings from experimental studies demonstrate the effectiveness of these programs in accelerating reading and social studies outcomes among middle school ELs as well as their monolingual peers (Vaughn et al., 2009; 2017). We present the results from experimental studies with CREATE and PACT in Table 18.3 and provide an overview of the more recently developed instructional program (PACT).

PACT

PACT was initially developed to help all learners in eighth-grade classrooms meet progressive state standards for reading and social studies knowledge. The results from randomized control trials underscored its efficacy in improving social studies knowledge and reading outcomes among all learners (e.g., Vaughn et al., 2015). PACT was further developed to ensure it promoted best practices for teaching ELs.

In particular, three primary enhancements were made: (1) increasing the focus on academic vocabulary by providing students multiple opportunities to interact with key academic vocabulary throughout each instructional unit, (2) integrating structured opportunities for students to use their learned vocabulary and content knowledge during academic discussion and writing, and (3) using additional scaffolds in order to prepare them to engage in academic discourse (e.g., provide visuals and graphic organizers or opportunities to work in pairs or small groups). These practices were interlaced into the five PACT components and found to be effective for ELs (Capin & Vaughn, 2017).

1. *Comprehension Canopy.* The comprehension canopy routine serves as the introduction to the unit and contains a springboard (short video, photo, or map) to help generate motivation and background knowledge and an overarching question that motivates the unit.

2. *Essential Words.* Within each unit, PACT teachers introduce four to five keywords that are likely to be unfamiliar to students and key to the central content in the unit. For each word, teachers introduce the words directly using friendly definitions, pictures, synonyms, examples and non-examples, and a turn-and-talk prompt. In subsequent lessons, the words are reviewed, and students have opportunities to engage with words across literacy activities.

3. *Knowledge Acquisition.* Knowledge acquisition is the primary text-reading activity in PACT. In this activity, text reading occurs with primary and secondary social studies text sources, and classroom discussion is focused on addressing the comprehension canopy, making connections with essential words, and developing content expertise.

4. *Team-based Learning (TBL) Comprehension Check.* A key feature of PACT is TBL, which engages students in collaborative discourse in small teams (four to five students). The TBL comprehension check consists of a 10-question comprehension check focused on vocabulary and content knowledge. To assess individual learning gains, each comprehension check occurs individually before team members confer to complete the comprehension check.

5. *TBL Knowledge Application.* The TBL knowledge application activity serves as a culminating activity that helps students apply the knowledge gained throughout the unit to address a prompt that is related to the comprehension canopy. In response to a short text and a prompt that requires students to address a new perspective or problem, students work in their teams to develop a written product, present their work to the class, and then answer questions from their peers and the teacher related to their presentation.

Tier 2 and 3 Instruction

Earlier, we discussed the findings from Hall and colleagues' (2017) systematic review of classwide approaches for ELs in the middle grades. Although their meta-analysis revealed a moderate effect size across all reading measures (g = .35), it is worth noting the effect size for standardized reading assessments was near zero (g = .01). This may not be entirely surprising given (1) the use of standardized measures is consistently associated with smaller effect sizes (e.g., Scammacca et al., 2015), and (2) many of these effect sizes were calculated based on performance in reading comprehension, which is notoriously difficult to improve among older struggling readers regardless of primary language status (e.g., Catts, 2021). Although the use of evidence-based instructional practices in Tier 1 is critical, these findings suggest these efforts may be unsatisfactory in improving the broad reading achievement of ELs with RD.

To date, empirical reports of reading interventions for ELs with RD beyond the primary grades are relatively sparse. In a review of interventions for ELs with or at risk for RD, Richards-Tutor et al. (2016) identified only four reading comprehension studies conducted with ELs with RD beyond the primary grades and found the effects were "minimal" across the four studies. Taken together, the effects of interventions for ELs in general education settings (Hall et al., 2017) and ELs with RD (Richards-Tutor et al., 2016) on standardized measures appear smaller than studies conducted with all students with RD (e.g., Scammacca et al. [2015] found a small mean effect size [g = .21] on standardized measures of reading for all struggling readers), suggesting there is an important need to develop and test reading comprehension approaches for middle-grade ELs with RD. Why have the few interventions tested for ELs with RD in the middle grades yielded little to no impact on reading comprehension? One explanation is that they may not have adequately focused on ELs' academic language, which is a primary source of their reading comprehension difficulties (e.g., Mancilla-Martinez & Lesaux, 2010; Cho et al., 2019). In a review of interventions for ELs with RD, Richards-Tutor et al. (2016) noted, "none of the studies reviewed included building of academic vocabulary or academic language as an explicit goal," and only two of the studies included any academic language instruction (p. 153).

Several researchers (e.g., Proctor et al., 2019) have suggested that interventions for ELs must address "the constellation of high-utility language skills" that support reading comprehension among ELs (Uccelli et al., 2015, p. 338). A few academic language programs have been carefully crafted to improve the academic language performance of ELs (e.g., ALIAS) (Lesaux et al., 2010; Word Generation; Snow et al., 2009). These programs have shown promise in improving academic language and content knowledge outcomes among ELs in general education settings (Truckenmiller et al., 2019) and may serve as a key instructional component for ELs with RD. Recently, Proctor et al. (2019) developed a small-group, language-focused academic language and reading comprehension intervention for typically developing ELs in the upper elementary grades that informs this project. The intervention focused on multiple aspects of language development by teaching vocabulary knowledge, morphology, and syntax and supporting comprehension discussions about text and writing activities. Study results were encouraging, but it is unclear how these effects will generalize to ELs with RD. Additionally, given research shows ELs with RD beyond the primary grades have difficulties related to word reading (e.g., Cho et al., 2019), it is likely that systematic word-reading instruction may need to be integrated within interventions for some ELs with RD.

Vaughn and colleagues (2019) conducted one such study that merged word-reading instruction with broader reading comprehension and vocabulary instruction for ELs with RD. This study sought to examine the effects of a 2-year intervention for ELs with RD beginning in grade 9. Students randomized to reading intervention received a supplemental reading intervention that front-loaded word-reading instruction for one semester using REWARDS Secondary (Archer et al., 2014) and then primarily focused on developing vocabulary and reading comprehension for the next three semesters. Relative to the control participants, students in the intervention group made significant growth on one standardized measure of reading comprehension (g = .18) and a proximal measure of vocabulary (g = .41), but not on other standardized measures of general reading skills. These findings further underscore the difficulty of ameliorating persistent reading problems of ELs with RD in high school and the need for additional investigations with older ELs with RD. They also accentuate the importance of early interventions that address vulnerabilities to reading difficulties before "achievement gaps become achievement chasms" (Balfanz, 2009, p.6).

Recommendations for Moving the Needle with ELs with RD

Our work understanding the sources of ELs with RD and developing and testing intervention effects for these students with MTSS has led us to a few realizations that may inform further research and practice.

1. *Do not underestimate the importance of developing code-based skills for ELs with RD.* There is compelling research to suggest that ELs are at no greater risk for word-reading difficulties than their monolingual peers (e.g., Lesaux et al., 2007). It is also true that most ELs who struggle to meet grade-level demands in language and literacy have difficulties due to their developing English language proficiency. However, this finding cannot be generalized to ELs with RD. Though more research is needed in this area, our research suggests that students with significant reading difficulties, even those beyond the primary grades, have instructional needs related to word reading that contribute to their inability to effectively understand texts (Capin et al., 2021; Cho et al., 2019). Given this, explicit and systematic code-based instruction will play an important role in preventing and remediating reading difficulties among students with or at risk for RD, even for students in the secondary grades (Vaughn et al., 2019).

2. *It is better to err on the side of providing interventions to ELs at risk for RD than to wait.* It can be difficult to determine whether ELs with underdeveloped reading skills have true reading difficulties or whether their ostensible challenges arise from a lack of opportunity to engage in academic activities in English. Some educators may assume that ELs' reading skills will eventually catch up once their

English language proficiency improves. This reasoning may be why recent research suggests that ELs are underidentified with learning disabilities and speech/language impairments relative to their native English-speaking peers (Morgan et al., 2015). We contend there are two important questions to consider when determining whether to provide an intervention to ELs who are struggling in reading, "Do we want to wait to provide the customized instruction and risk that these students develop significant needs in reading while their reading difficulties are untreated? Or would we rather provide the customized instruction to students at risk for RD knowing that for a few students waiting might have worked?" (Capin et al., 2020, p. 30). Our answers to these questions reflect a proactive approach to providing early, evidence-based interventions and using students' response to instruction as an indicator of whether an EL student has a true reading difficulty (Miciak & Fletcher, 2020).

3. *We should use structured cooperative learning techniques to foster high-quality academic discussions about text.* Providing opportunities for structured discussion is an effective practice for ELs (Dicerbo et al., 2014) because it affords opportunities to integrate foundational language skills (e.g., vocabulary, syntax, and morphology) as well as higher-order cognitive processes (e.g., inference-making) related to oral language in English. These practices can be particularly valuable in the late elementary and secondary grades as the language in schools shifts from conversational to academic English and students are expected to read, understand, and acquire knowledge from informational texts. In our experience, cooperative learning groups work best when groups are heterogeneous and their members are each assigned a specific role (for example, see Collaborative Strategic Reading [Klingner et al., 1998] or PACT [Vaughn et al., 2013]). In our recent work, we have also wondered whether enhancing students' expressive language and listening comprehension through high-quality, text-based discussions may serve as mechanisms for enhancing reading comprehension among struggling readers (Barth et al., 2016). Several studies have found the linguistic processes involved in listening comprehension are malleable (e.g., Gillam et al., 2012), and a few small-scale studies have evaluated the effectiveness of explicitly teaching oral language skills to struggling readers, revealing encouraging results on language and reading measures (Barth et al., 2016; Clarke et al., 2010). This may serve as a rewarding line of future research for ELs with RD, given that developing oral language and listening comprehension are key to their development.

4. *Engage ELs in complex tasks, knowing language development is a product of learning and interaction, not a prerequisite.* Our final recommendation relates to holding high expectations for ELs and ensuring ELs have ample opportunities to engage in complex literacy tasks that will support the development of English language proficiency and build knowledge. Some educators may believe that ELs need a certain threshold of English language proficiency to engage in literacy activities, particularly demanding, content-area literacy tasks. We consider language development a product of learning, not a prerequisite, and advocate for teachers to provide ELs, including those with RD, with language-rich,

intellectually challenging tasks in supportive contexts. PACT is an example of a set of high-quality instructional practices that enables secondary ELs with varying levels of English language and literacy proficiency to develop their academic language and social studies knowledge. Educators who recognize language and content knowledge are inextricably linked and support ELs with RD to effectively engage in demanding disciplinary learning are likely to see the most gains in language, literacy, and content learning.

5. *The best way to improve instruction for ELs and their monolingual peers may be to teach all students as if they are ELs.* Providing high-quality instruction is a strenuous task for teachers even when teachers are provided adequate resources and supports. We know many teachers face many daily challenges, including, but not limited to, inadequate preparation time, large class sizes, lack of training and professional development, insufficient teaching resources, and high turnover among teacher colleagues. Considering these challenges and reports from teachers that it is difficult to understand how and when to differentiate instruction for ELs in classes with ELs and non-ELs (Rubinstein-Avila & Lee, 2014), we wonder whether it is time to flip the script when it comes to instructing ELs. What if we designed all instruction to optimize learning for ELs? We contend that the practices described in the chapter for ELs with or at risk for RD will also benefit their monolingual peers, and this approach may be more feasible for teachers. This aligns with the IES practice guide on ELs, which observed, "Research suggests that effective teaching for English learners also benefits native English speakers" (Baker et al., 2014, p. 46).

Summary

As illustrated in this chapter, there is growing research to draw upon when considering (1) the sources of reading difficulties ELs with RD present, (2) how to develop MTSS systems responsive to the needs of ELs, and (3) instructional practices with evidence for ELs across tiers of instruction. MTSS provides a useful framework for providing assessment and instruction to ELs with RD and can lead to substantial improvements for these students. Yet, there is much rigorous research to be done investigating evidence-based practices for ELs with RD, a growing yet traditionally (and still) understudied population of students. A sustained program of research has the potential to reduce the gap in academic opportunities and performance between ELs and their monolingual peers and improve the lives of English learners.

ACKNOWLEDGMENTS

This work was supported by the Institute of Education Sciences (IES), U.S. Department of Education, through Grant R305C200016, as well as Grant 2P50 HD052117-11 from the Eunice Kennedy Shriver National Institute of Child Health and Human Development

(NICHD), National Institutes of Health (NIH). The content is solely the responsibility of the authors and does not necessarily represent the official views of the IES, NICHD, or NIH.

REFERENCES

Archer, A. L., Gleason, M., Vachon, V., & Archer, A. L. (2014). *REWARDS, reading excellence: Word attack & rate development strategies: Multisyllabic word reading strategies.* Cambium Learning Group Sopris Learning.

Babayigit, S. (2012). The role of oral language skills in reading and listening comprehension of text: A comparison of monolingual (L1) and bilingual (L2) speakers of English language. *Journal of Research in Reading, 37*, 22–47.

Baker, S., Lesaux, N., Jayanthi, M., Dimino, J., Proctor, C. P., Morris, J., & Newman-Gonchar, R. (2014). *Teaching academic content and literacy to English learners in elementary and middle school* (NCEE 2014-4012). What Works Clearinghouse.

Balfanz, R. (2009). *Putting middle grades students on the graduation path: A policy and practice brief.* National Middle School Association.

Barth, A. E., Vaughn, S., Capin, P., Cho, E., Stillman-Spisak, S., Martinez, L., & Kincaid, H. (2016). Effects of a text-processing comprehension intervention on struggling middle school readers. *Topics in Language Disorders, 36*(4), 368.

Braze, D., Tabor, W., Shankweiler, D. P., & Mencl, W. E. (2007). Speaking up for vocabulary: Reading skill differences in young adults. *Journal of Learning Disabilities, 40*(3), 226–243.

Burns, M. K., Griffiths, A., Parson, L. B., Tilly, W. D., & VanDerHayden, A. (2007). *Response to intervention: Research for practice.* National Association of State Directors of Special Education.

Capin, P., Cho, E., Miciak, J., Roberts, G., & Vaughn, S. (2021). Examining the reading and cognitive profiles of students with significant reading comprehension difficulties. *Learning Disability Quarterly, 44*(3), 183–196.

Capin, P., Hall, C., & Vaughn, S. (2020). Evidence-based practices in the treatment of reading disabilities among English learners. *Perspectives on Language and Literacy, 46*, 26–31.

Capin, P., & Vaughn, S. (2017). Improving reading and social studies learning for secondary students with reading disabilities. *Teaching Exceptional Children, 49*(4), 249–261.

Capps, R., Fix, M., Murray, J., Ost, J., Passel, J. S., & Herwantoro, S. (2005). *The new demography of America's schools: Immigration and the No Child Left Behind Act.* Urban Institute. *www.urban.org/sites/default/files/publication/51701/311230-The-New-Demography-of-America-s-Schools.PDF*

Catts, H. W. (2021). Rethinking how we teach and assess reading comprehension. *American Educator, 45*(4), 26–33.

Catts, H. W., Herrera, S., Nielsen, D. C., & Bridges, M. S. (2015). Early prediction of reading comprehension within the simple view framework. *Reading and Writing, 28*(9), 1407–1425.

Cho, E., Capin, P., Roberts, G., Roberts, G. J., & Vaughn, S. (2019). Examining sources and mechanisms of reading comprehension difficulties: Comparing English learners and non-English learners within the simple view of reading. *Journal of Educational Psychology, 111*(6), 982.

Clarke, P. J., Snowling, M. J., Truelove, E., & Hulme, C. (2010). Ameliorating children's reading-comprehension difficulties: A randomized controlled trial. *Psychological Science, 21*(8), 1106–1116.

Cosentino de Cohen, C., Deterding, N., & Clewell, B. C. (2005). *Who's left behind? Immigrant children in high and low LEP schools.* Urban Institute. *www.urban.org/research/publication/whos-left-behind*

DiCerbo, P. A., Anstrom, K. A., Baker, L. L., & Rivera, C. (2014). A review of the literature on teaching academic English to English language learners. *Review of Educational Research, 84*(3), 446–482.

Droop, M., & Verhoeven, L. (2003). Language proficiency and reading ability in first- and second-language learners. *Reading Research Quarterly, 38*(1), 78–103.

Echevarria, J., Richards-Tutor, C., & Vogt, M. (2015). *Response to intervention (RTI) and English learners: Using the SIOP model* (2nd ed.). Pearson.

Espinosa, L. (2007). *Second language acquisition in early childhood. Early childhood education.* Greenwood Publishing Group.

Fletcher, J. M., Francis, D. J., Foorman, B. R., & Schatschneider, C. (2021). Early detection of dyslexia risk: Development of brief, teacher-administered screens. *Learning Disability Quarterly, 44*(3), 145–157.

Fletcher, J., & Vaughn, S. (2009). Response to intervention: Preventing and remediating academic difficulties. *Child Development Perspectives, 3*, 30–37.

Fuchs, L. S., Fuchs, D., & Compton, D. L. (2010). Rethinking response to intervention at middle and high school. *School Psychology Review, 39*(1), 22–28.

Gándara, P. (2015). Is there really a labor market advantage to being bilingual in the U.S.? *ETS Research Report Series, 2015*(2), 1–34.

Gersten, R., Baker, S. K., Shanahan, T., Linan-Thompson, S., Collins, P., & Scarcella, R. (2007). *Effective literacy and English language instruction for English learners in the elementary grades: A practice guide.* National Center for Education Evaluation and Regional Assistance, Institute of Education Sciences, U.S. Department of Education.

Gillam, S. L., Gillam, R. B., & Reece, K. (2012). Language outcomes of contextualized and decontextualized language intervention: Results of an early efficacy study. *Journal of Speech, Language, and Hearing Research, 43*(1), 276–291.

Gough, P., & Tunmer, W. (1986). Decoding, reading, and reading disability. *Remedial and Special Education, 7*(1), 6–10.

Hall, C., Roberts, G. J., Cho, E., McCulley, L. V., Carroll, M., & Vaughn, S. (2017). Reading instruction for English learners in the middle grades: A meta-analysis. *Educational Psychology Review, 29*, 763–794.

Hall, C., Steinle, P. K., & Vaughn, S. (2019). Reading instruction for English learners with learning disabilities: What do we already know, and what do we still need to learn? *New Directions for Child and Adolescent Development, 166*, 145–189.

Kieffer, M. J., & Vukovic, R. K. (2012). Components and context: Exploring sources of reading difficulties for language minority learners and native English speakers in urban schools. *Journal of Learning Disabilities, 45*(5), 433–452.

Klingner, J. K., Vaughn, S., & Schumm, J. S. (1998). Collaborative strategic reading during social studies in heterogeneous fourth-grade classrooms. *Elementary School Journal, 99*(1), 3–22.

Lesaux, N. K., Kieffer, M. J., Faller, S. E., & Kelley, J. G. (2010). The effectiveness and ease of implementation of an academic vocabulary intervention for linguistically diverse students in urban middle schools. *Reading Research Quarterly, 45*(2), 196–228.

Lesaux, N. K., Rupp, A. A., & Siegel, L. S. (2007). Growth in reading skills of children from diverse linguistic backgrounds: Findings from a 5-year longitudinal study. *Journal of Educational Psychology, 99*(4), 821–834.

Linan-Thompson, S., Vaughn, S., Prater, K., & Cirino, P. T. (2006). The response to intervention of English language learners at risk for reading problems. *Journal of Learning Disabilities, 39*(5), 390–398.

Ludwig, C., Guo, K., & Georgiou, G. K. (2019). Are reading interventions for English language learners effective? A meta-analysis. *Journal of Learning Disabilities, 52*(3), 220–231.

Mancilla-Martinez, J., & Lesaux, N. K. (2010). Predictors of reading comprehension for struggling readers: The case of Spanish-speaking language minority learners. *Journal of Educational Psychology, 102*(3), 701.

Miciak, J., & Fletcher, J. M. (2020). The critical role of instructional response for identifying dyslexia and other learning disabilities. *Journal of Learning Disabilities, 53*(5), 343–353.

Morgan, P. L., Farkas, G., Hillemeier, M. M., Mattison, R., Maczuga, S., Li, H., & Cook, M. (2015). Minorities are disproportionately underrepresented in special education: Longitudinal evidence across five disability conditions. *Educational Researcher, 44*(5), 278–292.

National Center on Improving Literacy. (2021). *State of dyslexia. https://improvingliteracy.org*

Patton Terry, N. (2020). Diverse vulnerable learners with reading disabilities: A call to action. *Perspectives on Language and Literacy, 46*(2), 7–9.

Proctor, C. P., Silverman, R. D., Harring, J. R., Jones, R. L., & Hartranft, A. M. (2019). Teaching bilingual learners: Effects of a language-based reading intervention on academic language and reading comprehension in grades 4 and 5. *Reading Research Quarterly, 55*, 95–122.

Project ELLIPSES, Project ELITE^2, & Project LEE. (2021). *Meeting the needs of English learners with and without disabilities: Brief 3, English learners with significant learning difficulties or disabilities: Recommendations for practice.* U.S. Office of Special Education Programs.

Reutebuch, C. K., Vaughn, S., & Martinez, L. R. (2018). Enhancing reading and critical thinking skills for English learners in social studies: Findings from three experimental studies. In D. L. Baker, D. L. Basaraba, & C. Richards-Tutor (Eds.), *Second language acquisition: Methods, perspectives and challenges* (pp. 269–294). Nova Science.

Richards-Tutor, C., Baker, D. L., Gersten, R., Baker, S. K., & Smith J. M. (2016). The effectiveness of reading interventions for English learners: A research synthesis. *Exceptional Children, 89*, 144–169.

Rubinstein-Avila, E., & Lee, E. H. (2014). Secondary teachers and English language learners (ELLs): Attitudes, preparation and implications. *The Clearing House: A Journal of Educational Strategies, Issues and Ideas, 87*(5), 187–191.

Savitz, R. S., Allen, A. A., & Brown, C. (2021). Variations in RTI literacy implementation in grades 6–12: A national study. *Literacy Research and Instruction, 61*(1), 18–40.

Scammacca, N. K., Roberts, G., Vaughn, S., & Stuebing, K. K. (2015). A meta-analysis of interventions for struggling readers in grades 4–12: 1980–2011. *Journal of Learning Disabilities, 48*(4), 369–390.

Shanahan, T., & Beck, I. L. (2006). Effective literacy teaching for English-language learners. In D. L. August & T. Shanahan (Eds.), *Developing literacy in second-language learners: Report of the National Literacy Panel on language-minority children and youth* (pp. 415–488). Erlbaum.

Snow, C. E., Lawrence, J. F., & White, C. (2009). Generating knowledge of academic language among urban middle school students. *Journal of Research on Educational Effectiveness, 2*(4), 325–344.

Thomas, E. R., Conoyer, S. J., & Lembke, E. S. (2020). Districtwide evaluation of RTI implementation: Success, challenges, and self-efficacy. *Learning Disabilities Research & Practice, 35*(3), 118–125.

Truckenmiller, A. J., Park, J., Dabo, A., & Newton, Y. W (2019). Academic language instruction for students in grades 4 through 8: A literature synthesis. *Journal of Research on Educational Effectiveness, 12*(1), 135–159.

Uccelli, P., Galloway, E. P., Barr, C. D., Meneses, A., & Dobbs, C. L. (2015). Beyond vocabulary: Exploring cross-disciplinary academic-language proficiency and its association with reading comprehension. *Reading Research Quarterly, 50*(3), 337–356.

Vaughn, S., & Fletcher, J. M. (2012). Response to intervention with secondary school students with reading difficulties. *Journal of Learning Disabilities, 45*(3), 244–256.

Vaughn, S., Linan-Thompson, S., Mathes, P. G., Cirino, P. T., Carlson, C. D., Pollard-Durodola, S. D., & Francis, D. J. (2006). Effectiveness of Spanish intervention for first-grade English language learners at risk for reading difficulties. *Journal of Learning Disabilities, 39*(1), 56–73.

Vaughn, S., Martinez, L. R., Linan-Thompson, S., Reutebuch, C. K., Carlson, C. D., & Francis, D. J. (2009). Enhancing social studies vocabulary and comprehension for seventh-grade English language learners: Findings from two experimental studies. *Journal of Research on Educational Effectiveness, 2*(4), 297–324.

Vaughn, S., Martinez, L. R., Wanzek, J., Roberts, G., Swanson, E., & Fall, A. M. (2017). Improving content knowledge and comprehension for English language learners: Findings from a randomized control trial. *Journal of Educational Psychology, 109*(1), 22.

Vaughn, S., Martinez, L. R., Williams, K. J., Miciak, J., Fall, A. M., & Roberts, G. (2019). Efficacy of a high school extensive reading intervention for English learners with reading difficulties. *Journal of Educational Psychology, 111*, 373–386.

Vaughn, S., Mathes, P., Linan-Thompson, S., Cirino, P., Carlson, C., Pollard-Durodola, S., & Francis, D. (2006). Effectiveness of an English intervention for first-grade English language learners at risk for reading problems. *The Elementary School Journal, 107*(2), 153–180.

Vaughn, S., Roberts, G., Swanson, E. A., Wanzek, J., Fall, A. M., & Stillman-Spisak, S. J. (2015). Improving middle-school students' knowledge and comprehension in social studies: A replication. *Educational Psychology Review, 27*(1), 31–50.

Vaughn, S., Swanson, E. A., Roberts, G., Wanzek, J., Stillman-Spisak, S. J., Solis, M., & Simmons, D. (2013). Improving reading comprehension and social studies knowledge in middle school. *Reading Research Quarterly, 48*(1), 77–93.

PART III

FUTURE DIRECTIONS IN LEARNING DISABILITIES

This third part of the book collects seven chapters that address recent developments in learning disabilities (LD) identification, assessment, progress monitoring, differentiated instruction, teacher education, and new research perspectives. In Chapter 19, "Recent Trends in Dyslexia Legislation," Odegard, Farris, Middleton, Rimrodt-Frierson, and Washington underscore that while dyslexia, the most common specific learning disability, affects a significant portion of students, its identification and support within public education remain inconsistent. The authors discuss how concern for low literacy levels has stimulated new initiatives. Nearly all U.S. states have enacted dyslexia legislation mandating universal screening, explicit identification criteria, and structured interventions. These laws, largely influenced by parental advocacy, prescribe specific instructional approaches, often aligned with Orton Gillingham-based approaches emphasizing systematic, explicit phonics instruction.

The authors critique the limitations of dyslexia legislation, highlighting inconsistencies in screening implementation, the narrow focus on early grades, and the lack of attention to socioeconomic and environmental factors. Additionally, they call for a broader focus on high-quality instruction for all students rather than a reactive approach that isolates dyslexia from the larger literacy crisis. The authors argue that policies should prioritize widespread access to effective reading instruction, ensuring that struggling readers, regardless of background, receive timely and appropriate support.

A key issue raised in the chapter is the gap between policy mandates and practical implementation in schools. While states require universal screening and structured literacy interventions, many schools lack the resources, trained personnel, and instructional support necessary to carry out these policies effectively. Teachers often receive limited training in evidence-based reading instruction, and intervention programs may be inconsistently applied or fail to reach all students in need. Additionally, disparities in school funding and access to high-quality literacy instruction mean that students from under-resourced communities are disproportionately affected by inadequate reading support. The authors recommend that, for literacy policies to be effective, they must be accompanied by comprehensive teacher training, improved instructional materials, and systemic changes that ensure equitable access to high-quality education for all students.

Chapter 20, "Advances in Assessment to Monitor Progress and Performance," by Burns, Romero, Duesenberg-Marshall, Wan, and Abdelnaby, describes progress monitoring, which has been a critical tool in education for decades, rooted in precision teaching and data-based program modification. The chapter details three primary progress monitoring approaches: curriculum-based measurement (CBM), computer-adapted testing (CAT), and subskill mastery measures (SMM). Each of these methods offers unique advantages, with CBM serving as a widely used tool for tracking progress in reading, mathematics, and writing. CATs, on the other hand, employ item response theory to adjust assessments dynamically to a student's ability level, allowing for more efficient testing. Meanwhile, SMMs provide a more granular view of student learning by focusing on specific subskills, making them particularly useful for monitoring targeted intervention outcomes.

One of the key discussions in the chapter revolves around the psychometric properties of these assessments. Reliability and validity are crucial factors in ensuring that progress monitoring data can be used to make informed instructional decisions. CBM has been extensively researched and found to correlate strongly with standardized achievement tests, making it a valuable predictor of future academic success. Similarly, research on CATs suggests that they provide valid growth estimates when administered regularly, though their use in progress monitoring is not as well established as CBM. SMMs, while less common, are particularly effective in tracking student improvement on narrowly defined academic skills, thereby enhancing the precision of intervention strategies. Additionally, the authors outline best practices for interpreting progress monitoring data, including the use of decision rules to determine whether an intervention is effective or needs modification. Both datapoint and trendline decision rules are discussed, with trendline analysis emerging as the more reliable approach for making high-stakes decisions.

The authors emphasize the importance of integrating multiple data sources—CBM, CATs, and SMMs—to obtain a comprehensive picture of student progress. Examples are provided to illustrate how educators can use these assessments in real-world scenarios, demonstrating how data can inform intervention decisions in both reading and math.

In Chapter 21, "Child × Instruction Interactions: Using Technology to Support Differentiated Instruction," Sanabria and Siegal explore the importance of individualized instruction in special education, particularly for students with language and learning disabilities. However, implementing individualized instruction is challenging due to teacher training gaps, larger class sizes, and resource limitations. The response-to-intervention (RTI) model helps structure instruction, but research emphasizes the need to improve Tier 1 core instruction to prevent students from requiring more intensive interventions.

While many instructional models focus on broad teaching methods, research increasingly supports child-by-instruction (CXI) interactions, which tailor teaching methods to individual student needs. For example, studies show that students benefit from different instructional approaches based on their relative reading skill levels—those with weaker phonemic awareness require more explicit code-focused instruction, while stronger language learners benefit from meaning-focused strategies. Tools like the Assessment to Instruction (A2i) system use student data to personalize instruction, and research demonstrates that small-group, tailored instruction leads to significant literacy gains. The implementation of A2i in classrooms has led to improved reading outcomes, particularly for students who receive individualized instruction over multiple years.

Research using A2i underscores the necessity of moving beyond one-size-fits-all instruction to a more dynamic model that considers individual student differences. The authors contend that leveraging CXI interactions allows educators to better support students' literacy development, ensuring that all learners receive effective, research-based instruction. This approach also informs decisions about additional interventions in multi-tiered systems of support (MTSS). Schools using data-driven instruction can allocate resources more effectively and prevent struggling students from falling behind.

In Chapter 22, "Trends in Research Methods in the Learning Disabilities Field," Cook, Fleming, Therrien, and Wong note that the field has increasingly emphasized evidence-based instruction, leading to the adoption of rigorous research designs such as randomized controlled trials (RCTs) and single-case designs. The growth of systematic reviews and meta-analyses has also helped synthesize findings across studies, improving the reliability of research conclusions. Additionally, the development of research standards by organizations such as the What Works Clearinghouse and the Council for Exceptional Children has enhanced the transparency and validity of LD research. However, despite these advancements, challenges remain in ensuring the credibility, applicability, and impact of research findings in educational practice.

A major challenge is the lack of replication studies, which are essential for confirming the validity and generalizability of intervention effects. Although the frequency of replication studies has increased in recent years, they remain scarce in special education research. Another issue is the reliance on small and non-representative samples, which limits the generalizability of findings and reduces statistical power, making it harder to detect meaningful effects. To address these challenges, researchers are encouraged to adopt systematic replication frameworks, engage in crowdsourcing to increase sample sizes, and use tools like the Generalizer to ensure study results apply to diverse populations. Moreover, questionable research practices (QRPs), such as selective outcome reporting, p-hacking, and hypothesizing after results are known (HARKing), pose additional threats to validity. Strategies like preregistration and registered reports can help mitigate these issues by promoting transparency and accountability in the research process.

Another pressing concern is the gap between research and practice. Many research findings remain inaccessible to educators due to paywalls, complex technical language, and impractical interventions. Implementation science offers solutions by promoting researcher-practitioner collaborations, fostering practice-based evidence, and considering feasibility throughout the research process. Open-access publishing and sharing intervention materials can also help bridge this gap, making evidence-based practices more accessible and usable for educators. Despite the remaining challenges, ongoing efforts to improve research validity through replication, transparency, and better implementation strategies will strengthen the connection between research and educational outcomes. Addressing these issues requires a combination of grassroots initiatives from researchers and top-down changes in policies, funding, and publication standards to ensure that research findings translate into meaningful improvements in education for students with LD.

In Chapter 23, "Beyond Demography: Integrating Mind, Culture, and Equity in LD Research," Ferrell and Artiles begin by examining LD as defined under the Individuals with Disabilities Education Act (IDEA) and the ongoing debates surrounding its classification. One of these is the explicit exclusion of environmental, cultural, and economic factors in diagnosis and identification. The exclusionary clause has been challenged for disregarding the systemic inequalities affecting racialized and multilingual students, contributing to disparities in LD identification. The authors also critique the subjectivity of LD diagnoses, emphasizing that professional judgment plays a significant role, which leads to inconsistencies in classification and overrepresentation of certain student groups. Furthermore, the use of standardized assessments that fail to account for diverse learning backgrounds reinforces inequities, privileging dominant cultural and linguistic norms while marginalizing students from historically underserved communities.

The authors further argue for a cultural perspective on learning, asserting that traditional LD research often isolates learning difficulties from broader sociocultural and institutional contexts. The historical tension between biological and environmental explanations of LD is traced back to early neurological studies and later policy decisions that sought to secure resources for LD students while excluding culturally influenced learning difficulties. The authors advocate for an intersectional and sociocultural approach that recognizes how race, language, and socioeconomic status influence learning experiences. They suggest rethinking LD research and interventions through frameworks that integrate cognitive, emotional, and cultural dimensions, moving beyond rigid diagnostic categories toward a more inclusive understanding of learning diversity. This shift requires acknowledging how systemic barriers—such as restrictive instructional practices, limited access to multilingual education, and deficit-based perspectives—shape students' academic trajectories.

In Chapter 24, "Integrated Multi-Tiered Systems of Support (I-MTSS): New Directions for Supporting Students with or at Risk for Learning Disabilities," Gruner Gandhi, Clemens, Coyne, Goodman, Lane, Lembke, and Simonsen provide a comprehensive discussion of Integrated Multi-Tiered Systems of Support (I-MTSS), outlining its historical evolution, policy framework, benefits, and challenges in implementation, particularly for students with disabilities. The authors highlight how traditional academic and behavioral tiered systems have been treated separately but argue for a cohesive integration of these domains to enhance student outcomes.

The chapter draws from four research projects funded by the Institute of Education Sciences (IES) to explore I-MTSS implementation, fidelity, and impact. These projects focus on aspects such as behavioral support in academic interventions, professional development for educators, and the creation of fidelity rubrics for assessing I-MTSS implementation and evaluating the effects of integrated behavior and reading support at different intervention tiers. The discussion traces the historical shift from a reactive, within-child approach to learning and behavior challenges toward a systemic, proactive model that incorporates academic, social–emotional, and behavioral support. The authors emphasize how I-MTSS frameworks help schools provide targeted interventions based on data-driven decision making and structured tiers of support. Research shows the benefits of I-MTSS include improved academic and behavioral outcomes, increased teacher efficacy, and reduced exclusionary discipline. The authors also acknowledge ongoing challenges, such as siloed implementation, lack of integrated instructional materials, and difficulties in aligning school-level and district-level supports. They call for continued collaboration between researchers and practitioners to refine I-MTSS frameworks.

In Chapter 25, "Understanding and Developing Expert Teachers for Students with Learning Disabilities," the concluding chapter of the *Handbook*, Brownell, Leko, and Benedict emphasize the critical role of knowledgeable and skilled teachers in effectively educating students with LD. Since most of these students spend much of their education in general education classrooms, both general and special education teachers must be equipped to implement high-quality instruction and collaborate in designing interventions that complement the general curriculum.

The authors document the importance of using validated classroom assessments and evidence-based practices (EBPs) to support students' academic and social–emotional development. However, research indicates that teachers often do not implement EBPs with consistency or fidelity, pointing to a persistent research-to-practice gap. To address this issue, scholars have turned to implementation science to investigate the factors influencing teachers' use of EBPs, emphasizing the importance of preservice training, ongoing professional development, and professional coaching.

The authors also discuss the broader contextual factors that impact teaching quality, including school culture, leadership, collaborative opportunities, and access to instructional resources. The authors argue that effective teaching is not solely about mastering EBPs but also requires deep domain knowledge, pedagogical expertise, and an understanding of how students learn specific content. Furthermore, there remains a pressing need for a more integrated approach to teacher preparation, where general and special education teachers learn collaboratively rather than in separate tracks. The authors call for systemic changes in teacher education, advocating for practice-based learning opportunities that emphasize modeling, feedback, and analysis. They conclude by recommending policy and research efforts that focus on creating comprehensive, collaborative systems of teacher development, ensuring that educators are better prepared to support students with LD in diverse classroom settings.

CHAPTER 19

Recent Trends in Dyslexia Legislation

Timothy N. Odegard, Emily A. Farris, Anna E. Middleton,
Sheryl Rimrodt-Frierson, and Julie A. Washington

The scientifically informed knowledge base documenting effective reading instruction in the early grades is well established. The seminal reports reviewing and summarizing the empirical basis for early reading instruction and policy are over 20 years old (i.e., National Institute of Child Health and Human Development [NICHD], 2000). The major elements reviewed in the National Reading Panel (NRP) report were codified into policy (No Child Left Behind; U.S. Department of Education, 2002) and are a central focus of state standards (National Governors Association Center for Best Practices & Council of Chief State School Officers, 2010). In the ensuing decades, empirical study of reading, reading development, and reading disabilities continued, which allowed theoretical models to be refined and elaborated, but the basic science and models remain mostly the same (Garcia & Cain, 2014; Kim, 2017) including the major findings from a National Academy of Education report (Pearson et al., 2020).

Although we have learned much about reading and reading development, research's true potential is its translation into instructional practices in classrooms for the betterment of students' reading outcomes—a potential that has not been realized. Before the global coronavirus pandemic, 30% of fourth-grade students scored below basic on the National Assessment of Educational Progress (NAEP) Reading Literacy test (NAEP, 2019). The First Look report on the 2018 NAEP Special Study of oral reading revealed that the majority of the students who perform below basic on this test lack sufficient foundational skills (White et al., 2021). They struggle with oral reading fluency and word-reading accuracy, and these outcomes disproportionately are observed for Black, Hispanic, and Native American students, students eligible for free/reduced-price lunch, and English language learners. The same pattern was observed in the previous study of oral reading (Daane, 2005; Sabatini et al., 2018).

These outcomes are largely preventable based on what has been learned about the potential for instruction to provide students with a solid foundation to develop advanced literacy skills and abilities (Castles et al., 2018; Foorman et al., 2016). With that said, it is also well documented that learning rates vary from child to child. For example, they do not arrive at school with equivalent language and early literacy knowledge and skills (Hart & Risley, 1995). Also, research on language development and learning disabilities suggests some students struggle to read and spell words accurately even under ideal conditions, and some of these students present as persistently poor responders even when provided with sustained high-quality instruction and intervention (Middleton et al., 2021; Wagner et al., 2020).

Society has a term for struggles with learning to read and spell words—dyslexia. Dyslexia is the most widely studied form of a specific learning disability. It is also the most prevalent. Estimates of its prevalence vary, ranging from 3–5% of the population to as much as 17–20% (Elliott & Grigorenko, 2014; Fletcher et al., 2018). Moreover, it is specified as one cause of a specific learning disability (SLD) that gives rise to academic underachievement in reading and is referenced in the fifth edition of the *Diagnostic and Statistical Manual of Mental Disorders* (DSM-5; American Psychiatric Association, 2013). Yet in 2019, only 5% of public school students in the United States were identified with an SLD and received support through special education (Hussar et al., 2020). These rates are far less than the 31% of public school students who perform below basic when NAEP reading test data are aggregated across 4th, 8th, and 12th grades (NAEP, 2019).

Additionally, the rate at which students struggle with basic reading skills based on NAEP estimates is far greater than the identification rates of dyslexia in public schools in three states: Arkansas, Tennessee, and Texas, where schools are mandated to report the identification rates of dyslexia to their respective state oversight agencies (Odegard et al., 2020; Phillips & Odegard, 2017). These findings point to a discrepancy in public schools between objective measures of reading, the distribution of resources to protected classes of students under federal law, and the identification of students with dyslexia.

Dyslexia Legislation

Within this educational landscape, legislatures in almost every state in the United States have passed laws intended to address the needs of students who struggle to read and spell as a result of dyslexia. Historically, dyslexia initiatives have been led by concerned parents (Fletcher, 2009). The children of these parents were not learning to read in school, and the parents believed that their children were not learning to read despite their potential to do so. As a result, parents advocated for legislation that would identify their children's reading struggles as exceptional and mandate schools to provide specialized forms of reading intervention. Parent advocacy was in direct response to schools not meeting the needs of students. The problem they identified is difficult to dispute. It is a problem that emerging evidence suggests persists today (Odegard et al., 2021). Yet, how we respond to this challenge as a society is a point of disagreement, and dyslexia laws represent one possible response—a response that is reactionary and prescriptive.

Dyslexia laws are reactionary in that they are reacting to an educational system that overwhelmingly does not provide direct instruction in essential skills in the early grades in a way that positively affects students' reading outcomes. This position has some empirical support in light of NAEP data and high-stakes state reading assessments. Moreover, when schools strive to independently implement empirically validated reading instruction, the instructional methods are associated with smaller effects than researcher-implemented interventions (Scammacca et al., 2015). In addition, dyslexia laws are prescriptive. They are written to prescribe (1) what school personnel should look for, (2) how school personnel should look for it, and (3) how they should intervene once they find it.

These are the major components found in dyslexia laws across the country that will be the focus of this chapter. First, the laws uniformly define a condition—dyslexia. Second, they often include a mandate for public schools to screen all students for dyslexia. Laws with screening provisions typically specify the constructs that must be included as part of universal screening for dyslexia and the grades in which this screening must occur. Third, many of these laws mandate that once a student has been identified with dyslexia, they must receive a dyslexia-specific intervention. The laws almost always specify what should be taught to students with dyslexia (i.e., the instructional targets) and the instructional methods used.

Dyslexia Defined

Any discussion of dyslexia as it relates to public policy must grapple with how it is defined. At this point, all states with a dyslexia law include a definition of dyslexia, and 34 states included the definition of dyslexia adopted by the International Dyslexia Association (IDA) or a slightly modified version. To appreciate this definition and its implication for public policy, we must consider the core assumptions built into this definition. Dyslexia has been studied for well over a century, and the collective understanding of it has evolved through scientific inquiry (Fletcher, 2009). Based on the amassed evidence, it has been established that individuals with dyslexia struggle to read and spell words—central characteristics specified in the IDA definition and other definitions (Miciak & Fletcher, 2020). In one widely held view of dyslexia, these deficits are proposed to result from abnormalities in brain development that give rise to difficulties processing the phonological components within spoken words and mapping them to the orthographic structure of a written language (Norton et al., 2015).

However, for most of the 20th century, explanations of dyslexia were not grounded in theories of reading development established through systematic empirical studies of large groups of individuals. It was not until the latter part of the 20th century that a more formal, systematic, empirical approach was adopted to investigate the characteristics of dyslexia and to construct a model for its classification and identification (Vellutino, 1979). These efforts helped establish a variety of well-supported developmental models of reading and a more refined understanding of language function in the brain (Gough & Tunmer, 1986; Perfetti & Stafura, 2014; Vellutino et al., 2007), but before this research was undertaken, a movement started that led to the creation of SLD as a construct, which was codified into law through the IDEA in 1975 (Education for All Handicapped Children Act, 1975; U.S. Department of Education, 2006).

IDEA was established to ensure that all children with disabilities receive a free, appropriate public education that meets their unique needs and prepares them for further education, employment, and independent living. SLD is the largest eligibility category under IDEA, and the most prevalent form of SLD impacts reading (Office of Special Education and Rehabilitative Services, 2017). Thus, we find it essential to highlight SLD and IDEA because the motivation for dyslexia legislation is intertwined with the provision of protection for individuals with disabilities. It is also important to highlight that many of the concepts incorporated into the current definition of SLD were borrowed from initial understandings of dyslexia. As a result, central to the concept of SLD is the notion of exceptionalism. Like dyslexia, the construct of SLD is based on the premise that children labeled as having an SLD struggle to learn due to intrinsic factors. Their learning struggles are not the result of apparent primary sensory system differences (e.g., vision and/or hearing impairments) or lack of instruction due to other factors such as poor attendance or the child not having access to instructional opportunities. Without an obvious set of factors to account for the learning difficulties, the basis of these learning struggles was thought to be neurobiological. Thus, a determination of an SLD is made by exclusion—determining what is not causing the academic underachievement documented for an individual.

Support for the notion that the nexus of academic underachievement is intrinsic and neurobiological was provided by appealing to older concepts, such as minimal brain dysfunction and neurobiological causes offered for dyslexia (Hinshelwood, 1917; McCandliss & Noble, 2003; Orton, 1928; Turkeltaub et al., 2003; Wender, 1975). However, it was not possible when SLD was first conceptualized to demonstrate a neurobiological difference at the individual level to drive identification efforts. Thus, there was and still is a need for guiding principles to operationalize who does and who does not qualify as having an SLD. From this need arose the notion that children with learning disabilities were unified by their "developmental discrepancies in abilities and achievement" (Kirk & Gallagher, 1979, p. 281). This idea came to be conceptualized as "unexpected underachievement" in policies and procedures used to guide the identification and classification of children based on the presence of a learning disability (Education for All Handicapped Children Act, 1975; U.S. Department of Education, 2006).

The unexpected underachievement concept served two functions. It was a proxy for the neurobiological assumption of SLD. It also differentiated those students who were failing to meet their potential to learn—the exceptional from those who were not failing to meet their potential—the unexceptional. Variations of these initial policies and procedures continue to determine how resources are allocated and who receives educational opportunities through special education (U.S. Department of Education, 2004). These procedures are set forth by government agencies and diagnostic manuals (for a discussion of these procedures, see Fletcher et al., 2018). However, who is said to be exceptional and have an SLD is determined just as much by which tests are used (Fletcher & Miciak, 2017).

IDA Definition of Dyslexia

Since the inception of SLD and IDEA, research in dyslexia and other forms of reading disabilities has continued. The current definition of dyslexia adopted by IDA represents the culmination of research efforts at the time of its adoption (Lyon et al., 2003).

> Dyslexia is a specific learning disability that is neurobiological in origin. It is characterized by difficulties with accurate and/or fluent word recognition and by poor spelling and decoding abilities. These difficulties typically result from a deficit in the phonological component of language that is often unexpected in relation to other cognitive abilities and the provision of effective classroom instruction. Secondary consequences may include problems in reading comprehension and reduced reading experience that can impede growth of vocabulary and background knowledge.

By highlighting the characteristics of dyslexia, the IDA definition was a shift toward specificity that was not present in earlier definitions of dyslexia. It characterizes a specific manifestation of a reading disability based on an empirically derived literacy profile. Rather than lumping all aspects of reading into a single category, the definition was written to acknowledge that various breakdowns in the skills that support this ability can result in different manifestations of a reading disability. Specified within the definition are the hallmark deficits characteristic of individuals with dyslexia: deficits in word recognition and spelling. The group who drafted the definition found it warranted and prudent to specify that evidence pointed to a language basis for dyslexia—implicating phonological decoding, a reading skill that supports word recognition, as commonly deficient. It also denotes the role that phonological processing deficits can have in the manifestation of dyslexia. This specificity is grounded in an empirically derived understanding of how reading develops.

Although it broke with earlier definitions by highlighting positive indicators of the condition, the IDA definition maintained the notion of exceptionalism present in previous definitions of dyslexia. Moreover, the language-based deficits that likely give rise to the word-reading and spelling deficits resulting from dyslexia were thought to be brain-based. This aspect of the definition harkens back to why dyslexia emerged historically. It is conceptualized as being neurobiologically based. In the IDA dyslexia definition, exceptionality is indicated in two ways.

An individual with dyslexia fails to acquire proficiency with word recognition and spelling despite the potential to learn, and they demonstrate a lack of response to instruction. Although the definition may not align with current understandings of dyslexia, it is how dyslexia is defined in most states, and this definition informs the screening and intervention provisions specified in state dyslexia laws.

Screening for Dyslexia

At this time, laws in 34 states require schools to universally screen for dyslexia. Gearin et al. (2021) noted tremendous variability in the constructs named and a lack of accompanying definitions in dyslexia laws. However, we can still learn from what is specified in these laws and use it to inform discussions about the implications of screening mandates. Most screening mandates require schools to measure multiple constructs when screening for dyslexia (see Figure 19.1A). On the surface, this makes good sense, given that theories of reading development highlight a multitude of component skills and sources of knowledge to undergird reading (Gough & Tunmer, 1986; Perfetti & Stafura, 2014; Vellutino et al., 2007).

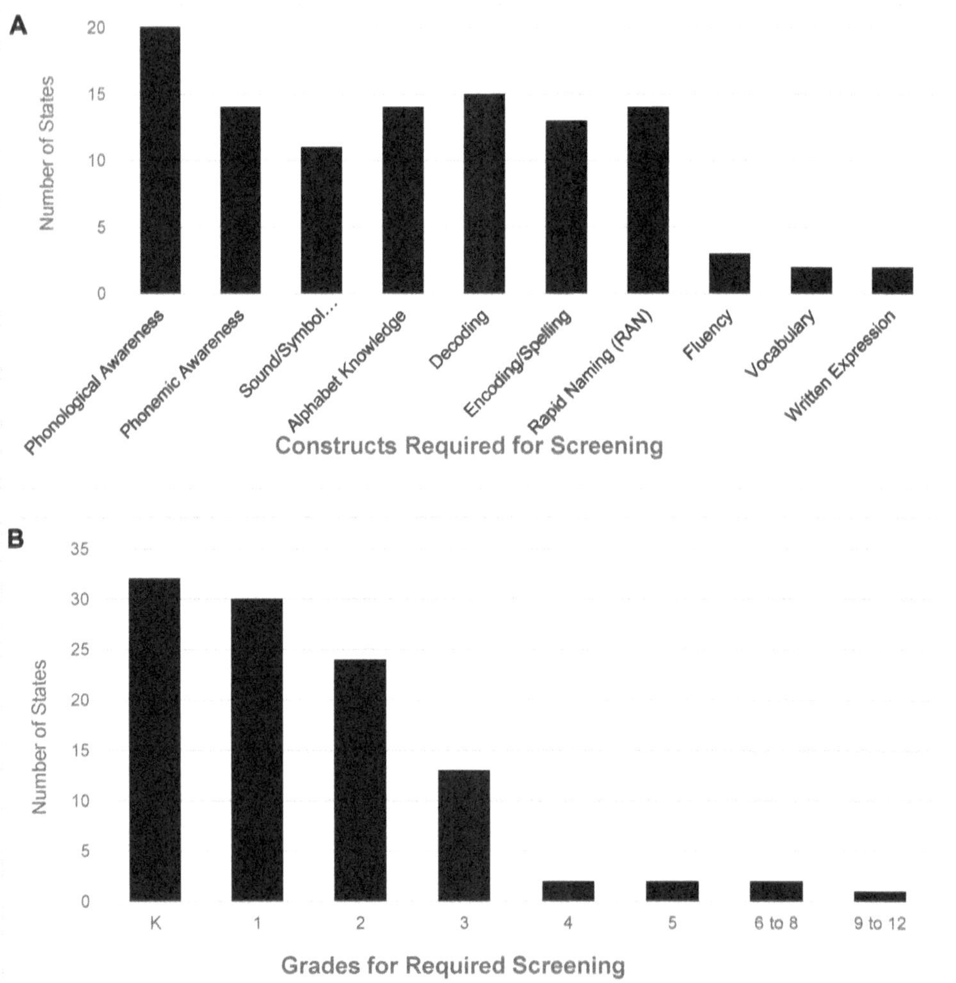

FIGURE 19.1. Constructs included and grades specified in state dyslexia laws screening mandates. Panel A: The number of states requiring each construct to be part of dyslexia screening. Panel B: The number of states that specify the inclusion of each grade in dyslexia screening.

Moreover, the areas specified roughly align with the constructs in the IDA definition of dyslexia. However, when they are to be measured does not necessarily align with what is known about reading and spelling development and what constructs are included in commonly adopted instruments used for screening. In addition, screening mandates focus almost exclusively on kindergarten through third grade (see Figure 19.1B) and rarely state whether the constructs included in dyslexia screening should vary across the specified grades. These characteristics of dyslexia laws create a misalignment, which can hinder efforts to implement them.

Constructs Included in Screening

Based on our review, current state laws that mandate universal screening for dyslexia require schools to measure 2–7 literacy constructs. The areas included in these state-mandated screening procedures correspond to constructs in the IDA definition of dyslexia (see Figure 19.1A). For example, several states require schools to screen students for decoding, encoding, or fluency, all core characteristics of dyslexia in the IDA definition. Moreover, states with screening mandates almost uniformly require schools to screen for phonological processing deficits. In particular, every state that specifies constructs to be measured requires schools to screen phonological awareness, and some states require schools to screen rapid naming.

Other constructs captured in screening mandates include alphabet knowledge and sound-symbol correspondences, emergent and foundational literacy skills critical for developing phonological decoding and word recognition—two reading skills named explicitly in the IDA definition. A few laws require vocabulary and written expression to be measured. Deficits in vocabulary and written expression can be secondary consequences that emerge from reduced access to written language for individuals with dyslexia.

When Screening Happens

In addition to knowing what is to be included in screening, it is essential to consider *when* a construct is included in the screening process. All states with screening mandates require screening to take place in kindergarten (see Figure 19.1B). In many of these states, the process includes first grade. However, far fewer states include second and third grades. After third grade, screening for dyslexia is not required in almost all of these laws. As such, these laws are calibrated for early-grade screening.

Moreover, in every state but Louisiana, all the constructs specified in the law are to be universally screened in all grades named. In Louisiana, alphabet knowledge is only assessed as part of dyslexia screening in kindergarten. In contrast, phonemic awareness and rapid naming are assessed in kindergarten through third grades, whereas decoding, encoding, and fluency are included in dyslexia screening procedures in first through third grades in that state.

When a construct is mandated to be part of universal screening, it is a critically important consideration for at least two reasons. First, the utility of a construct for determining the risk of future reading and spelling deficits or identifying current deficits depends on when a construct is measured (Catts et al., 2015; Schatschneider et al., 2004). Utility is used in this context as commonly understood in the cognitive sciences, where it denotes how useful a piece of information is in supporting a decision. Within the context of screening, measuring a construct has utility when the information adds value to the predictive validity of a constellation of predictors to determine the likelihood of an end state or if an end state has been reached (e.g., word-reading or spelling deficits). For example, in the fall of kindergarten, letter-naming fluency is one of the strongest predictors of word reading and fluency at the end of first grade, but its predictive value decreases considerably past kindergarten (Catts et al., 2015). As a result, letter naming is commonly included in many screening instruments in kindergarten but not in later grade levels. Several universal screening instruments do not include a measure of oral reading fluency or word-reading accuracy after second grade for similar reasons.

Second, valid and reliable screening instruments with accompanying grade-level normative data are not available in kindergarten through third grade for all constructs specified in dyslexia laws. These laws rarely permit changes in the constructs assessed across grades. In contrast, commonly adopted tests used for screening were designed to identify students at risk of future or continued reading struggles without restricting the focus to the word recognition and spelling deficits that are primary characteristics of dyslexia. They are optimized to find a balance between the amount of time it takes to administer them and the value added by measuring each construct. The omission of certain constructs in these assessments is partly due to the convergent nature of reading skills and what the commercially available screening instruments are calibrated to predict. On these instruments, reading struggles are often represented by reading comprehension difficulties after kindergarten and first grade. Moreover, few instruments commonly used for universal screening include an indicator of encoding, despite being a construct commonly named as part of dyslexia screening. As a result, these screeners were not calibrated to identify future word-reading and spelling difficulties, which is partly why parents championed dyslexia laws. The laws are a reaction to screening practices that may not provide a complete picture of a child's reading deficits. As a result, schools may be providing intensified instruction that is not calibrated to students' instructional needs when risk is identified through commonly adopted universal screening practices (Odegard et al., 2020). Regardless, the reality is that normed measures appropriate for universal screening are currently not available in the grades specified in dyslexia laws for all named constructs.

Screening Past Third Grade

There is practically no mention of requirements for dyslexia screening in later elementary, middle, or high school (Figure 19.1B). The lack of inclusion of students in the later grades in the dyslexia screening process may be motivated by an emphasis in the empirical literature on dyslexia risk screening as a means for prevention, early identification, and early intervention (Catts et al., 2015; Fletcher et al., 2020). Additionally, studies illustrate the presence of temporal stability in reading ability relative to same-age peers. These findings include moderate to strong correlations from the end of second to the end of eighth grade for phonological awareness, rapid naming, verbal memory, word reading, spelling, and comprehension (Scarborough, 1998). There is also a consistency in profile membership at the start of kindergarten and end of first grade based on scores in phonological awareness, rapid naming, letter knowledge, and verbal short-term memory (Ozernov-Palchik et al., 2017).

The temporal stability of a student's reading ability compared to same-age peers does not mean that any intervention attempt is futile because many students' reading skills can and do improve in response to intervention (Middleton et al., 2021). Nor does it imply that a student cannot begin to exhibit low achievement in later grades. Students with late-emerging reading difficulties exist and may struggle with reading comprehension and also, or primarily, with word-reading skills (Catts et al., 2012; Leach et al., 2003). It also does not negate the occurrence of persistent difficulties with spelling, word reading, reading fluency, or phonological processing in adults with childhood histories of reading struggles, even when they exhibit some compensation and remediation as evidenced by average range performance on some measures of word reading or comprehension (Nergard-Nilssen & Hulme, 2014; Scarborough, 1984). Regardless of when or if they are ever identified, previous or ongoing struggles with reading may contribute to strains in a child's or an adult's mental health and psychological well-being (Livingston et al., 2018).

Another explanation for the lack of inclusion of students in later grades in the dyslexia screening process is the interconnectedness of dyslexia legislation and other state and federal guidance specifying procedures for reading instruction and assessment within the school system. For example, Tennessee identifies six component areas to be screened, but it does not explicitly specify the grades for which this screening should occur. However, the Tennessee dyslexia law refers to dyslexia screening within the state's required universal screening process for students in kindergarten through 12th grade, as specified by the state's response to instruction and intervention (RTI^2) framework. Thus, it implies that dyslexia screening should include students in all of kindergarten through twelfth grade.

Inclusion of Additional Risk Factors

In addition to component skills and specified grade ranges for screening, Oregon and Washington explicitly acknowledge that a family history of difficulty with reading and language acquisition must be part of the screening process. The inclusion of these additional risk factors is supported by research. Meta-analytic estimates reveal that when a first-degree relative, such as a parent or sibling, has dyslexia, the student is four times more likely to have reading problems than a student without a family history of reading problems (Snowling & Melby-Lervag, 2016). Further, longitudinal studies of children with a risk of dyslexia based on family history highlight the value of considering family history and assessing a child's language abilities in the early school years when identifying reading difficulties

(Muter & Snowling, 2009). Neuroimaging research, including studies with children at risk for dyslexia due to family history, further illustrates that differences in brain structures can be seen very early in life (Zuk et al., 2021).

In contrast, no states that require screening appear to list environmental factors as a screening component. Yet aspects of the home environment, family socioeconomic status, and school quality interact with a genetic predisposition for reading struggles and impact students' reading and early literacy skills (Haughbrook et al., 2017). Moreover, in all of these state dyslexia laws, there is no clear prescription for addressing the exceptionality and unexpected aspects of their adopted definition of dyslexia. This finding indicates a mismatch between the adopted definition of dyslexia and prescribed screening processes. The laws state that dyslexia is not just low achievement, but low achievement that is not due to widespread struggles (i.e., it is exceptional), and that occurs even when empirically validated reading instruction was provided (i.e., it is unexpected). The laws do not describe how to rule out these exclusionary factors.

Thus, although the research base is moving toward a probabilistic view of our understanding of dyslexia that incorporates family history, environmental factors and other language measures, and hybrid models for identification that focus on low achievement and response to intervention, the state dyslexia laws have not followed suit. Instead, the prescriptions for screening in the laws focus only on low achievement in skills that (1) are believed to be the underlying cause of dyslexia, (2) represent the primary characteristics of dyslexia, and (3) support the development of word-reading abilities. Further, the laws focus on kindergarten to third grade, which is the focal area for extensive research on prevention and early intervention of dyslexia (Catts et al., 2015; Fletcher et al., 2020; Muter & Snowling, 2009) and of guiding documents for instructional practices and response to intervention (RTI) (Foorman et al., 2016). In kindergarten, the goal is to find children at risk of future word-reading and spelling issues, and once a child reaches first grade and beyond, they are developmentally expected to be engaging in basic word reading and spelling, allowing for deficiencies in these areas to be identified. However, parents and other stakeholders often conflate screening for and identifying students with dyslexia, which is confounded with established policies and procedures for determining eligibility for educational support and services under IDEA based on an SLD. The prescriptive nature of these laws commonly manifests as mandates for dyslexia-specific intervention for students identified through the dyslexia screening process.

Instruction and Intervention

Legislation in many states outlines how and what should be included as part of a dyslexia-specific intervention. Many of the instructional characteristics specified in state laws align with those traditionally descriptive of the Orton–Gillingham (OG) methodological approach. The OG approach is described as a "direct, explicit, multisensory, structured, sequential, diagnostic, and prescriptive way to teach reading and spelling" (Orton–Gillingham Academy, 2020). These characteristics of reading instruction were codified as characteristics of interventions to be used when teaching students with dyslexia in 29 states.

The inclusion of language consistent with an OG approach to intervention is likely due in part to parent advocates believing that this approach is the most beneficial for individuals identified with dyslexia. However, the relative effectiveness of such practices is unclear and has been a topic of debate for many years. For example, a recent meta-analysis comparing OG interventions to alternative methods of phonics-based instruction reported a small but nonsignificant positive effect for OG methods on foundational reading skills (Stevens et al., 2021)—a finding consistent with previous research suggesting that OG methodologies elicit similar student outcomes compared to alternative systematic phonics instruction (Ritchey & Goeke, 2006). However, it should be noted that much of the instruction classified as alternative methods in these studies also included characteristics of OG interventions. Regardless of the "branding" of the intervention approach, research clearly shows that systematic, code-based instruction is more effective than other methods such as whole-language instruction (see Castles et al., 2018, for review).

More importantly, dyslexia laws that mandate dyslexia-specific intervention prescribe the characteristics of the interventions that must be provided to individuals with dyslexia. The following sections outline intervention characteristics most commonly specified in dyslexia laws. They are grouped into instructional methods and instructional targets (see Figures 19.2A and 19.2B).

Instructional Methods

SYSTEMATIC: STRUCTURED, SEQUENTIAL, CUMULATIVE

Instruction that aligns with descriptors such as *structured* or *sequential* is generally organized such that the presentation of material follows the inherent order of the language in terms of frequency and complexity. The easiest, most fundamental concepts are introduced early in the instructional sequence, progressing systematically to introduce more complex or challenging concepts. Cumulative instruction is designed such that new learning builds on prior learning so that students are prepared to achieve accuracy. The relative effectiveness of these instructional characteristics has not been individually investigated (e.g., to ascertain the optimal number and/or sequence of introduction of phonics concepts). However, a scientific consensus has long supported the efficacy of code-oriented instruction over other instructional approaches (e.g., whole language) (Foorman, 1995).

DIRECT OR EXPLICIT INSTRUCTION

Direct instruction and explicit instruction are commonly used to differentiate intervention pedagogy from typical classroom instruction. At present, 15 states mandate that instruction delivered as part of a dyslexia-specific intervention be direct or explicit. In educational settings, this means that students are given clear and explicit directions in all parts of a learning task, leaving no part of the

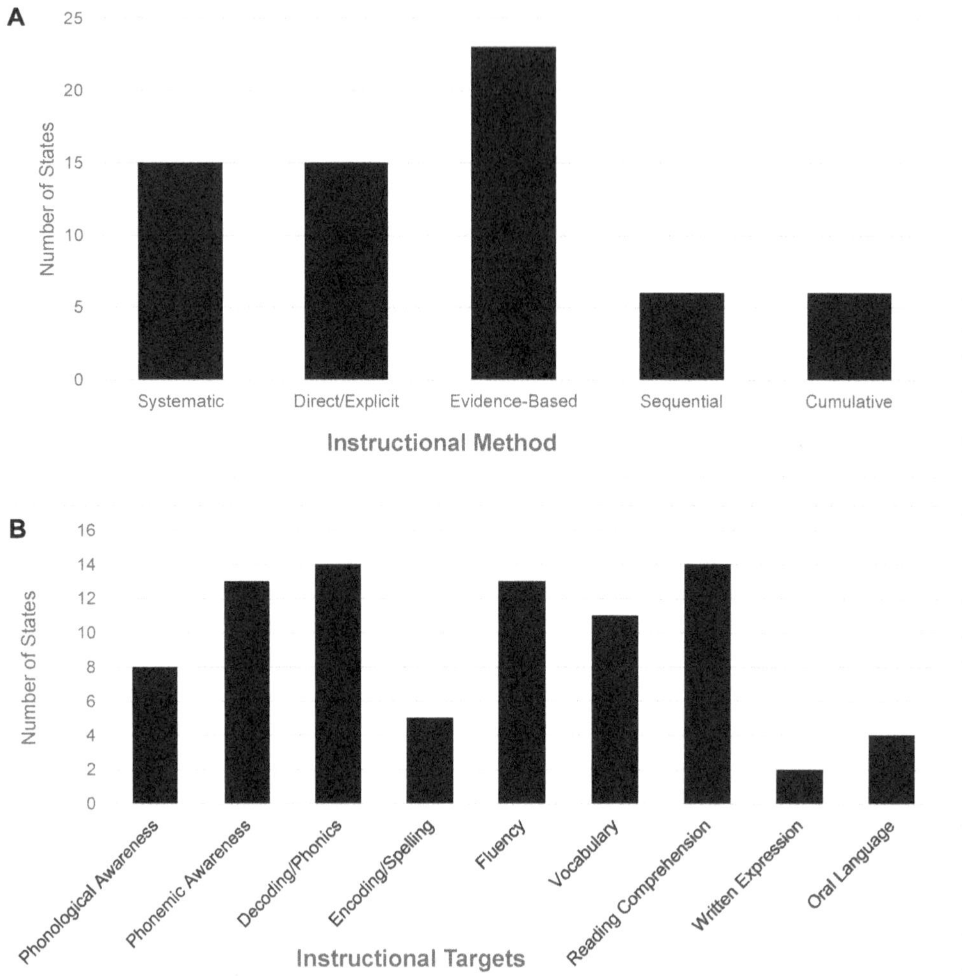

FIGURE 19.2. Instructional methods and targets specified in dyslexia laws. Panel A: The number of states requiring each instructional method to be part of a dyslexia-specific intervention. Panel B: The number of states requiring each instructional method to be part of a dyslexia-specific intervention.

learning process to chance. Direct instruction leverages explicit learning to help students develop an awareness of complex written language structures. This type of instruction is particularly critical for developing early reading skills, as preliterate children do not independently acquire knowledge of the alphabetic principle (Byrne, 2005). Direct instruction also allows for immediate corrective feedback, which may help to thwart the consolidation of incorrect information.

Although explicit instruction is vital for developing accurate and targeted learning, the selective use of this descriptor in characterizing effective pedagogy may downplay the importance of the equally crucial implicit learning mechanism

(Kahneman, 2011; Seidenberg et al., 2020). The explicit learning system is a complementary cognitive system that runs alongside and supports implicit learning. Implicit learning is responsible for much of the subconscious analysis of patterns in the environment (i.e., written language) necessary for building automatic and efficient word-reading skills. Each of these learning systems is valuable—if not requisite—in support of learning. Future research is needed to provide clear and instructive evidence toward the optimal balance between explicit and implicit learning in supporting various types of skill development (e.g., Kearns, 2020; Seidenberg et al., 2020).

EVIDENCE-BASED INSTRUCTION

Requiring instruction to be evidence-based necessarily restricts the type of instructional programming a student may receive. Of the 29 states that specify intervention characteristics, 23 have passed legislation requiring that instruction be evidence-based, but none to our knowledge operationalize the term. In the educational realm, the term *evidence-based* is used to describe programs designed following empirically supported best practices (e.g., NRP's five key components) and programs that have themselves been empirically evaluated. However, the inconsistent use of the term is particularly problematic in that the former interpretation of the term leaves much room for subjectivity in designing instructional courses.

Multisensory Intervention

Every dyslexia law that mandates dyslexia-specific intervention requires that the intervention be multisensory. The nature of any written language intervention is inherently multisensory, requiring the integration of auditory (speech sounds), visual (letter forms), and kinesthetic (motor-writing) language components. However, the term *multisensory* often describes instruction that utilizes other kinesthetic/tactile methods, such as skywriting or tracing letters on textured surfaces, which are intended to emphasize the orthographic features of a letter. There is little evidence to suggest these types of instructional activities have any added benefit when incorporated into explicit, systematic phonics instruction (Al Otaiba et al., 2018). Evidence does suggest that standard handwriting instruction benefits the learning of letters in the early grades (Kersey & Jame, 2013). However, this instruction does not include tracing letters in sand or on a rough surface. Fifteen states specify that instruction be multisensory, though to our knowledge, none of the laws specify an intended interpretation of the term *multisensory* or the types of instructional activities that satisfy this requirement.

Targets of Dyslexia-Specific Intervention

Decades of research investigating the effectiveness of various reading interventions and instructional components support the utility of systematic instruction in phonemic awareness, phonics, decoding, and word recognition (Castles et al.,

2018). Findings of the NRP report have been interpreted as supporting five essential components of reading instruction, despite inherent differences in the types of constructs each represents: some describe knowledge, others describe skills, and yet others describe outcomes (Seidenberg et al., 2020). Many states have codified specific instructional targets required for dyslexia interventions, often structured around these five components and a handful of others.

Phonological Awareness

By our count, 14 state laws require phonological awareness (or, relatedly, phonemic awareness) to be part of a dyslexia-specific intervention. Phonological awareness refers to one's ability to identify the underlying phonological structure of a spoken language and is an essential precursor to understanding the alphabetic principle. Phonological processing has long been specified as a characteristic weakness in dyslexia and is a robust predictor of later reading outcomes (Scarborough, 1998; Schatschneider et al., 2004). Despite the robust relationship between phonological awareness and reading ability, phonological awareness instruction is most effective when integrated with other methods, such as decoding instruction (Hatcher et al., 1994). Furthermore, despite the predictive nature of the relationship between phonological awareness and reading outcomes, it is not predictive of response when provided as part of a comprehensive phonics-based dyslexia-specific intervention (Middleton et al., 2021).

Phonics/Decoding

In alphabetic writing systems, such as English, individual sounds (phonemes) are represented by letters and letter patterns (graphemes). Thus, a critical component of early instruction in alphabetic writing systems is building associations between the language's visual/orthographic (letter) and auditory/phonological (sound) codes. Decades of accumulating evidence support systematic phonics instruction in teaching reading (see Castles et al., 2018, for review). The scientific consensus surrounding the importance of phonics instruction is reflected in the prevalence of this component in 14 states' dyslexia laws. Phonics instruction alone does not equip children to decode irregular words, which stray from conventional spelling patterns. A combination of phonics and sight word instruction may be a more efficient method for developing successful, independent readers (McArthur et al., 2015).

Spelling

Only five states require spelling instruction as part of a dyslexia-specific intervention, and many reading interventions do not include targeted spelling instruction as a component of their intervention structure. While many reading interventions lead to improvements in spelling ability, targeted spelling instruction may provide additional benefits in improving student outcomes (Suggate, 2016). Spelling instruction involves the application of a reciprocal process to reading: translating sounds to letters. This process may support orthographic learning better than reading, leading to greater improvements in accuracy and efficiency (Ouellette, 2010; Ouellette et al., 2017).

Fluency

Fluency deficits are another hallmark of impaired reading that may result from a breakdown in lower-order reading skills. This characteristic weakness of dyslexia is acknowledged in 13 states' dyslexia laws that specify fluency as an instructional target. Although fluency has been conceptualized as both an outcome of skilled reading and a process taught in order to facilitate skilled reading, one thing remains clear: one of the most critical factors in developing reading fluency is exposure. Exposure is a key factor in allowing students to practice applying new knowledge and skills. Reduced reading exposure negatively affects struggling readers (Torgesen & Hudson, 2006). However, evidence suggests that targeted fluency practice can be a beneficial method for increasing fluency and comprehension skills, though effect sizes vary widely (Hudson et al., 2020). The most common instructional method for improving fluency involves scaffolded repeated reading practice. Importantly, these methods provide students with multiple opportunities to read text (i.e., increasing print exposure) in addition to some other instructional supports (e.g., corrective feedback and modeling).

Reading Comprehension

The goal of reading is to comprehend text. Like fluency, comprehension is an outcome of skilled reading. It is a highly complicated, multifactorial ability, which is the end product of various subprocesses supporting understanding (e.g., inference, background knowledge, and vocabulary) (Elleman & Oslund, 2019). Because of this complexity, it can be challenging to teach and measure (Elleman & Oslund, 2019). Strategies to enhance subprocesses are often recommended to improve reading comprehension (NICHD, 2000). There is no scientific consensus on a single method best suited for comprehension instruction. Various strategies tend to have similar outcomes, as most require increased engagement with text and enable metacognitive skills such as comprehension monitoring. At present, 14 states mandate reading comprehension as an instructional target.

Vocabulary and Oral Language

Oral and written language abilities are deeply intertwined and become inextricable as reading skill develops. Oral language skills, such as listening comprehension and vocabulary, are robust predictors of reading comprehension. Generally speaking, greater oral language abilities provide a stronger foundation from which to develop written language abilities. This is reflected in 13 states' laws that specify vocabulary and/or oral language as mandatory instructional targets. Direct and active instruction in vocabulary can be beneficial in supporting reading comprehension and may be particularly important for struggling readers (Elleman & Oslund, 2019; NICHD, 2000). Although word meanings can be explicitly taught, they do not necessarily lead to generalizable improvements in oral language skills. Furthermore, explicit instruction would not be a reasonable method for teaching the meanings of over 40,000 words when children reach high school. Thus, while vocabulary instruction can effectively boost oral language and comprehension skills, instruction for students with dyslexia should be limited to focusing on high-utility word meanings that can be found across academic disciplines and strategically integrated into a comprehensive intervention.

As we look across the instructional targets required for dyslexia-specific intervention, it is striking that just as many states require reading comprehension to be a part of dyslexia-specific intervention as they require phonics instruction. The common perception is that these laws are calibrated to focus exclusively on phonics instruction, but this perception is unjustified. In addition, spelling is a primary characteristic of dyslexia, but only a handful of states mandate that dyslexia-specific intervention directly teach students to spell. As such, the patterns observed across dyslexia laws disconfirm a common misperception that these laws mandate a sole focus on phonics to the exclusion of reading comprehension and point to an area of need—spelling.

Conclusions

This chapter began with a discussion of gains made in a collective understanding of how best to teach foundational literacy skills to students, which transitioned into a discussion of dyslexia—a condition characterized by deficits in foundational literacy skills in the print domain. Starting from this premise allowed us to consider the ramifications of a continued failure to realize the potential of science to improve students' reading outcomes. That failure creates a reality in which far too many kids are born into a context where the potential of public education goes unrealized due to the lack of effective reading instruction in the early grades. This environmental context is a social determinant of an end state—struggling to read and write the English language due to deficits in the basic mechanics that undergird these uniquely human capacities—word reading and spelling. However, many of the kids who wind up at this end state will not have their inability to read and spell words viewed as exceptional.

Within this educational context, dyslexia laws were passed. From our point of view, dyslexia laws are a reaction to the inherent injustice of an educational system struggling to meet its potential to equip children with the skills to thrive in the 21st century. As outlined in dyslexia laws across the United States, the prescription for this problem has been to mandate public schools to universally screen for foundational literacy skills—predominately skills that support reading and spelling. Mandates for screening are coupled with mandates to provide students who, based on that screening, are not meeting developmental expectations with intervention. As such, dyslexia laws are an effort to require schools to screen for emergent print skills and print skills deficits in the early grades and directly teach instructional targets that support word reading, spelling, and reading comprehension to students not meeting expectations based on the screening.

Oddly, schools already must do this as part of RTI and multi-tiered systems of support (MTSS) procedures in states across the country. As such, parents are striving to clarify what schools must do by using a research-informed definition of one form of a reading disability—dyslexia. However, if the issue is implementing existing educational policy, then one might suggest clarifying existing policies and procedures instead of complicating matters with competing mandates because a failure to move existing policies to procedures and provide effective instruction for most students creates a challenge to implementing state dyslexia laws.

Too often, many students within a school struggle to read and spell words. Within the context of these schools, where struggling to read and spell is the norm and not the exception, schools struggle to find students with dyslexia. We observed students to be less likely to be identified through dyslexia screening and provided dyslexia intervention as the percentage of students who struggle to read and spell words increases in a school (Odegard et al., 2020). These were underperforming schools that were majority African American, and over 90% of the students in these schools were eligible for free or reduced lunch. Similar findings have been reported for students qualifying for services and protections under IDEA based on SLD. Minority children are less likely than otherwise similar children to be identified as having an SLD or speech or language impairments (Morgan et al., 2017). Importantly, underrepresentation appears to be a policy issue directly linked to assumptions that undergird identification models. The exclusionary criteria for SLD nationally restrict children from diagnosis whose learning problems are "primarily the result of . . . environmental, cultural, or economic disadvantage" (U.S. Department of Education, 2004). Currently, in the United States, it is challenging to be both poor and be identified with an SLD. If a child is poor and cannot read, it is assumed that it is because the child is poor. Moreover, schools almost entirely populated with economically disadvantaged kids consistently underidentify students with dyslexia (Odegard et al., 2020).

The environment and its impact on neurocognitive development, which we consider to include language, are exclusionary criteria under the current federal policy and the logic inherent to exceptionalism as most commonly implemented in identification models of SLD and dyslexia. This discrepancy led Blanchett (2010) to refer to SLD as "a category of privilege for the privileged." Children most likely to be identified as SLD are White and middle to upper-middle class, and this observation must be understood within the reality that minority and economically disadvantaged students often find themselves within the context of underperforming schools from day 1 of their educational experience. Our findings would suggest this statement extends to a specific form of SLD—dyslexia. As such, we suggest there is a need to reconsider the notion of exceptionality inherent to the model of

SLD and consider the implications of social determinants of SLD and dyslexia. As we highlighted, the modal definition of dyslexia adopted in laws across the United States adheres to an exceptionality model of dyslexia.

An emerging trend suggests that we are not alone in our concerns with an exclusive legislative focus on the needs of the few when the needs of the many appear to be going unmet. In the wake of the dyslexia laws that were the focus of this chapter, a new generation of legislation is emerging. This legislation is focused on mandating foundational literacy skills instruction, universal screening, and teacher training. However, it would seem that continued mandates to change student outcomes through policy alone are not improving reading rates. States already have policies and standards that address foundational literacy skills and require screening to identify students at risk of reading failure. What appears to be missing are practical approaches to guide implementation models that allow current policies, procedures, and standards to be translated into effective support systems that enable educators to provide effective reading instruction to their students. Once effective instruction coupled with ample opportunities to apply and practice what is taught is in place for most students, struggling to read and spell will become the exception, providing an educational context to more effectively identify students with dyslexia. Put simply, we must meet the needs of the many to identify the few who will require more intensive and sustained intervention to thrive and overcome their learning differences.

REFERENCES

Al Otaiba, S., Rouse, A. G., & Baker, K. (2018). Elementary grade intervention approaches to treat specific learning disabilities, including dyslexia. *Language, Speech, and Hearing Services in Schools, 49*(4), 829–842.

American Psychiatric Association. (2013). *Diagnostic and statistical manual of mental disorders* (5th ed.). Author.

Blanchett, W. J. (2010). Telling it like it is: The role of race, class, and culture in the perpetuation of learning disability as a privileged category for White middle class. *Disabilities Studies Quarterly, 30*(2).

Byrne, R. (2005). Theories of learning to read. In M. J. Snowling & C. Hulme (Eds.), *The science of reading: A handbook* (pp. 104–119). Blackwell.

Castles, A., Rastle, K., & Nation, K. (2018). Ending the reading wars: Reading acquisition from novice to expert. *Psychological Science in the Public Interest, 19*(1), 5–51.

Catts, H. W., Compton, D., Tomblin, J. B., & Bridges, M. S. (2012). Prevalence and nature of late-emerging poor readers. *Journal of Educational Psychology, 104*(1), 166–181.

Catts, H. W., Nielsen, D. C., Bridges, M. S., Liu, Y. S., & Bontempo, D. E. (2015). Early identification of reading disabilities within an RTI framework. *Journal of Learning Disabilities, 48*(3), 281–297.

Daane, M. C. (2005). *Fourth-grade students reading aloud: NAEP 2002 special study of oral reading* [Electronic resource]. National Center for Education Statistics, U.S. Department of Education, Institute of Education Sciences, Government Printing Office Catalog. *https://nces.ed.gov/nationsreportcard/pubs/studies/2006469*

Education for All Handicapped Children Act, Pub. L. No. 94–142, 89 Stat. 773 (1975).

Elleman, A. M., & Oslund, E. L. (2019). Reading comprehension research: Implications for practice and policy. *Policy Insights from the Behavioral and Brain Sciences, 6*(1), 3–11.

Elliott, J. G., & Grigorenko, E. L. (2014). *The dyslexia debate.* Cambridge University Press.

Fletcher, J. M. (2009). Dyslexia: The evolution of a scientific concept. *Journal of the International Neuropsychological Society: JINS, 15*(4), 501–508.

Fletcher, J. M., Francis, D. J., Foorman, B. R., & Schatschneider, C. (2020). Early detection of dyslexia risk: Development of brief, teacher-administered screens. *Learning Disability Quarterly, 44*(3), 145–157.

Fletcher, J. M., Lyon, G. R., Fuchs, L. S., & Barnes, M. A. (2018). *Learning disabilities: From identification to intervention* (2nd ed.). Guilford Press.

Fletcher, J. M., & Miciak, J. (2017). Comprehensive cognitive assessments are not necessary for the identification and treatment of learning disabilities. *Archives of Clinical Neuropsychology, 32,* 2–7.

Foorman, B. R. (1995). Research on "the Great Debate": Code-oriented versus whole language approaches to reading instruction. *School Psychology Review, 24*(3), 376–392.

Foorman, B., Beyler, N., Borradaile, K., Coyne, M., Denton, C. A., Dimino, J., et al. (2016). *Foundational skills to support reading for understanding in kindergarten through 3rd grade. Educator's practice guide* (NCEE 2016-4008). National Center for Education Evaluation and Regional Assistance, Institute of Education Sciences, U.S. Department of Education. *https://ies.ed.gov/ncee/wwc/Docs/PracticeGuide/wwc_foundationalreading_040717.pdf*

Garcia, J. R., & Cain, K. (2014). Decoding and reading comprehension: A meta-analysis to identify which reader and assessment characteristics influence the strength of the relationship in English. *Review of Educational Research, 84*(1), 74–111.

Gearin, B., Petscher, Y., Stanley, C., Nelson, N. J., & Fien, H. (2021). Document analysis of state dyslexia legislation suggests likely heterogeneous effects on student and school outcomes. *Learning Disability Quarterly,* 1–13.

Gough, P., & Tunmer, W. (1986). Decoding, reading, and reading disability. *Remedial and Special Education, 7*(1), 6–10.

Hart, B., & Risley, T. R. (1995). *Meaningful differences in the everyday experience of young American children.* Brookes.

Hatcher, P. J., Hulme, C., & Ellis, A. W. (1994). Ameliorating early reading failure by integrating the teaching of reading and phonological skills: The phonological linkage hypothesis. *Child Development, 65*(1), 41–57.

Haughbrook, R., Hart, S. A., Schatschneider, C., & Taylor, J. (2017). Genetic and environmental influences on early literacy skills across school grade contexts. *Developmental Science, 20,* e12434.

Hinshelwood, J. (1917). Congenital word-blindness. *The Lancet, 190*(4922), 980.

Hudson, A., Koh, P., Moore, K. A., & Binks-Cantrell, E. (2020). Fluency interventions for elementary students with reading difficulties: A synthesis of research from 2000–2019. *Education Sciences, 10*(3), 52.

Hussar, B., Zhang, J., Hein, S., Wang, K., Roberts, A., Cui, J., et al. (2020). *The condition of education 2020* (NCES 2020-144). U.S. Department of Education, National Center for Education Statistics. *https://nces.gov/pubsearch/pubsinfo.asp?pubid=2020144*

Kahneman, D. (2011). *Thinking, fast and slow.* Farrar, Strauss, and Giroux.

Kearns, D. M. (2020). Does English have useful syllable division patterns? *Reading Research Quarterly, 55,* S145–S160.

Kersey, A. J., & James, K. H. (2013). Brain activation patterns resulting from learning letter forms through active self-production and passive observation in young children. *Frontiers in Psychology, 4,* 567.

Kim, Y. S. G. (2017). Why the simple view of reading is not simplistic: Unpacking component skills of reading using a direct and indirect effect model of reading (DIER). *Scientific Studies of Reading, 21*(4), 310–333.

Kirk, S. A., & Gallagher, J. J. (1979). *Educating exceptional children* (3rd ed.). Houghton Mifflin.

Leach, J. M., Scarborough, H. S., & Rescorla, L. (2003). Late-emerging reading disabilities. *Journal of Educational Psychology, 95*(2), 211–224.

Livingston, E. M., Siegel, L. S., & Ribary, U. (2018). Developmental dyslexia: Emotional impact and consequences. *Australian Journal of Learning Difficulties, 23*(2), 107–135.

Lyon, G. R., Shaywitz, S. E., & Shaywitz, B. A. (2003). A definition of dyslexia. *Annals of Dyslexia, 53*(1), 1–14.

McArthur, G., Castles, A., Kohnen, S., Larsen, L., Jones, K., Anandakumar, T., & Banales, E. (2015). Sight word and phonics training in children with dyslexia. *Journal of Learning Disabilities, 48*(4), 391–407.

McCandliss, B. D., & Noble, K. G. (2003). The development of reading impairment: A cognitive neuroscience model. *Mental Retardation and Developmental Disabilities Research Reviews, 9*(3), 196–204.

Miciak, J., & Fletcher, J. M. (2020). The critical role of instructional response for identifying dyslexia and other learning disabilities. *Journal of Learning Disabilities, 53*(5), 343–353.

Middleton, A. E., Farris, E. A., Ring, J. J., & Odegard, T. N. (2021). Predicting and evaluating treatment response: Evidence towards protracted response patterns for severely impacted students with dyslexia. *Journal of Learning Disabilities, 55*(4), 272–291.

Morgan, P. L., Farkas, G., Hillemeier, M. M., & Maczuga, S. (2017). Replicated evidence of racial and ethnic disparities in disability identification in U.S. schools. *Educational Researcher, 46*(6), 305–322.

Muter, V., & Snowling, M. J. (2009). Children at familial risk of dyslexia: Practical implications from an at-risk study. *Child and Adolescent Mental Health, 14*(1), 37–41.

National Assessment of Educational Progress. (2019). *The nation's report card.* National Center for Educational Statistics. *www.nationsreportcard.gov*

National Governors Association Center for Best Practices & Council of Chief State School Officers. (2010). *Common Core State Standards for English language arts and literacy in history/social studies, science, and technical subjects.*

National Institute of Child Health and Human Development. (2000). *Report of the National Reading Panel. Teaching children to read: An evidence-based assessment of the scientific research literature on reading and its implications for reading instruction.* U.S. Government Printing Office.

Nergard-Nilssen, T., & Hulme, C. (2014). Developmental dyslexia in adults: Behavioural manifestations and cognitive correlates. *Dyslexia, 20*, 191–207.

Norton, E. S., Beach, S. D., & Gabrieli, J. D. E. (2015). Neurobiology of dyslexia. *Current Opinion in Neurobiology, 30*, 73–78.

Odegard, T. N., Farris, E. A., Middleton, A. E., Oslund, E., & Rimrodt-Frierson, S. (2020). Characteristics of students identified with dyslexia within the context of state legislation. *Journal of Learning Disabilities, 53*(5), 366–379.

Odegard, T. N., Hutchings, T., Farris, E. A., & Oslund, E. L. (2021). External evaluations for dyslexia: Do the data support parent concerns? *Annals of Dyslexia, 71*(1), 50–59.

Office of Special Education and Rehabilitative Services, U.S. Department of Education. (2017). *39th Annual Report to Congress on the Implementation of the Individuals with Disabilities Education Act, 2017.*

Orton, S. T. (1928). Specific reading disability—Strephosymbolia. *Journal of the American Medical Association, 90*, 1095–1099.

Orton–Gillingham Academy. (2020). *What is the Orton-Gillingham approach? www.ortonacademy.org/resources/what-is-the-orton-gillingham-approach*

Ouellette, G. (2010). Orthographic learning in learning to spell: The roles of semantics and type of practice. *Journal of Experimental Child Psychology, 107*(1), 50–58.

Ouellette, G., Martin-Chang, S., & Rossi, M. (2017). Learning from our mistakes: Improvements in spelling lead to gains in reading speed. *Scientific Studies of Reading, 21*(4), 350–357.

Ozernov-Palchik, O., Norton, E. S., Sideridis, G., Beach, S. D., Wolf, M., Gabrieli, J. D. E.,

& Gaab, N. (2017). Longitudinal stability of pre-reading skill profiles of kindergarten children: Implications for early screening and theories of reading. *Developmental Science, 20*(5), e12471.

Pearson, P. D., Palinscar, A. S., Biancarosa, G., & Berman, A. I. (Eds.). (2020). *Reaping the rewards of the reading for understanding initiative.* National Academy of Education.

Perfetti, C., & Stafura, J. (2014). Word knowledge in a theory of reading comprehension. *Scientific Studies of Reading, 18*, 22–37.

Phillips, B. A. B., & Odegard, T. N. (2017). Evaluating the impact of dyslexia laws on the identification of specific learning disability and dyslexia. *Annals of Dyslexia, 67*(3), 356–368.

Ritchey, K. D., & Goeke, J. L. (2006). Orton-Gillingham and Orton-Gillingham-based reading instruction: A review of the literature. *The Journal of Special Education, 40*(3), 171–183.

Sabatini, J., Wang, Z., & O'Reilly, T. (2018). Relating reading comprehension to oral reading performance in the NAEP fourth-grade special study of oral reading. *Reading Research Quarterly, 54*(2), 253–271.

Scammacca, N. K., Roberts, G., Vaughn, S., & Stuebing, K. K. (2015). A meta-analysis of interventions for struggling readers in grades 4–12: 1980–2011. *Journal of Learning Disabilities, 48*(4), 369–390.

Scarborough, H. S. (1984). Continuity between childhood dyslexia and adult reading. *British Journal of Psychology, 75*, 329–348.

Scarborough, H. S. (1998). Predicting the future achievement of second graders with reading disabilities: Contributions of phonemic awareness, verbal memory, rapid naming, and IQ. *Annals of Dyslexia, 48*, 115–136.

Schatschneider, C., Fletcher, J. M., Francis, D. J., Carlson, C. D., & Foorman, B. R. (2004). Kindergarten prediction of reading skills: A longitudinal comparative analysis. *Journal of Educational Psychology, 96*(2), 265–282.

Seidenberg, M. S., Cooper Borkenhagen, M., & Kearns, D. M. (2020). Lost in translation? Challenges in connecting reading science and educational practice. *Reading Research Quarterly, 55*, S119–S130.

Snowling, M. J., & Melby-Lervag, M. (2016). Oral language deficits in familial dyslexia: A meta-analysis and review. *Psychological Bulletin, 142*(5), 498–545.

Stevens, E. A., Austin, C., Moore, C., Scammacca, N., Boucher, A. N., & Vaughn, S. (2021). Current state of the evidence: Examining the effects of Orton–Gillingham reading interventions for students with or at risk for word-level reading disabilities. *Exceptional Children, 87*(4), 397–417.

Suggate, S. P. (2016). A meta-analysis of the long-term effects of phonemic awareness, phonics, fluency, and reading comprehension interventions. *Journal of Learning Disabilities, 49*(1), 77–96.

Torgesen, J. K., & Hudson, R. F. (2006). Reading fluency: Critical issues for struggling readers. In S. J. Samuels & A. E. Farstrup (Eds.), *What research has to say about fluency instruction* (pp. 130–158). International Reading Association.

Turkeltaub, P. E., Gareau, L., Flowers, D. L., Zeffiro, T. A., & Eden, G. F. (2003). Development of neural mechanisms for reading. *Nature Neuroscience, 6*(7), 767–773.

U.S. Department of Education. (2002). *No Child Left Behind (NCLB) Act of 2001* (No. 107–110, § 101, Stat. 1425). *https://files.eric.ed.gov/fulltext/ED556108.pdf*

U.S. Department of Education. (2004). *Individuals with Disabilities Education Improvement Act* (20 U.S.C. § 1400). *https://sites.ed.gov/idea/statute-chapter-33/subchapter-i/1400*

U.S. Department of Education. (2006). 34 CFR Parts 300 and 301: Assistance to states for the education of children with disabilities and preschool grants for children with disabilities. Final Rules. *Federal Register, 71*, 46540–46845.

Vellutino, F. R. (1979). *Dyslexia: Theory and research.* MIT Press.

Vellutino, F. R., Tunmer, W. E., Jaccard, J. J., & Chen, R. (2007). Components of reading ability: Multivariate evidence for a convergent skills model of reading development. *Scientific Studies of Reading, 11*(1), 3–32.

Wagner, R. K., Zirps, F. A., Edwards, A. A., Wood, S. G., Joyner, R. E., Becker, B. J., et al. (2020). The prevalence of dyslexia: A new approach to its estimation. *Journal of Learning Disabilities, 53*(5), 354–365.

Wender, P. H. (1975). The minimal brain dysfunction syndrome. *Annual Review of Medicine, 26*, 45–62.

White, T. G., Sabatini, J. P., & White, S. (2021). What does "below basic" mean on NAEP reading? *Educational Researcher, 50*(8), 570–573.

Zuk, J., Yu, X., Sanfilippo, J., Figuccio, M. J., Dunstan, J., Carruthers, C., et al. (2021). White matter in infancy is prospectively associated with language outcomes in kindergarten. *Developmental Cognitive Neuroscience, 50*, 100973.

CHAPTER 20

Advances in Assessment to Monitor Progress and Performance

Matthew K. Burns, Monica E. Romero, McKinzie D. Duesenberg-Marshall, Hoi Ting Wan, and Heba Z. Abdelnaby

Advances in Assessment to Monitor Progress and Performance

School practitioners have engaged in monitoring of student progress for at least 50 years, and those efforts have intensified over the past 15 years as part of collaborative problem solving and multi-tiered systems of support (MTSS). School-based progress monitoring was rooted in precision teaching and was outlined as the foundation for data-based program modification (DBPM) (Deno & Mirkin, 1977). Progress monitoring is defined as frequent and repeated data collection used to indicate if students will meet curriculum and state objects based on their current level of performance (Stecker et al., 2005), and doing so increases student academic outcomes if time series data are collected with psychometrically sound approaches and evaluated with predefined rules of decision making (Christ et al., 2012). However, when teachers were trained to implement progress monitoring and began to do so, they reportedly did not use assessments other than oral reading fluency (Greenfield et al., 2010), and a lack of understanding of how to use progress-monitoring data was frequently listed as a barrier to implementing tiered interventions and supports (Castro-Villarreal et al., 2014). Given the documented efficacy of progress monitoring, as well as challenges with its implementation, there has been considerable research on progress monitoring in the past 15 years. The purpose of this chapter will be to discuss various approaches to progress monitoring, describe research supporting each, and present a comprehensive approach that is based on research and can address the needs of students with learning disabilities.

Approaches to Progress Monitoring

When special education was formally institutionalized in this country by Public Law 94-142 in 1975, there were no established methods to determine how much progress students were making toward individual goals. Deno and Mirkin (1977) proposed a method to objectively monitor student progress with data collected at regular intervals over time (e.g., once each week) because these time series data were "uniquely appropriate" (p. 11) for evaluating the effects of instruction and intervention. In other words, in order to evaluate how well a student is doing, data must be systematically collected over time. Deno went on to develop curriculum-based measurement (CBM) (Deno, 1985) as a method to conduct weekly progress-monitoring assessments based on an objective per-minute rate measure and normative goals. The terms *CBM* and *progress monitoring* have since become almost synonymous, but there are other ways to monitor progress beyond CBM. Next, we will discuss CBM, computer-adapted testing, and subskill mastery measures as tools to monitor progress. Readers are encouraged to examine the Academic Progress Monitoring Tools chart from the National Center on Intensive Intervention (2021) for more information about specific progress-monitoring tools.

Curriculum-Based Measurement

CBM was developed to monitor progress in the basic skill areas of reading, mathematics, written expression, and spelling (Deno, 2003; Deno & Mirkin, 1977). In the initial stages of research and development, the priorities were to develop progress-monitoring measures that were (1) reliable and valid, (2) simple and efficient for use to frequently assess and evaluate instructional effects, (3) easily understood by educators to guide instructional decisions, and (4) inexpensive to use (Deno, 1985). In each academic area, CBM usually consists of short measures conducted weekly to assess students' performance development over time. CBM also relies on a traditional psychometric framework by incorporating conventional notions of reliability and validity so that standardized assessments yield accurate and significant data (Fuchs, 2004).

CBM in Reading

Research has shown that CBM in reading (CBM-R) is a valid indicator of general reading proficiency as measured by standardized tests (Wayman et al., 2007). Two types of CBM-R have received the most attention in research literature and school settings. The first, reading aloud, often called oral reading fluency (ORF), requires students to read aloud a passage of meaningful text for 1 minute. Student performance is measured by counting the number of words read correctly. The second, a maze, requires students to read passages and select word choices. A maze passage is developed by deleting every seventh word of a reading passage and replacing it with three response choices (Vannest et al., 2011). Both approaches to CBM-R can be considered a proxy of general reading proficiency as measured by standardized achievement tests, with correlations reported to range from r = .60 to .75 (Nese et al., 2011) or over .80 (Wayman et al., 2007) for ORF and between .58 (LeRoux et al., 2020) and .65 (Conoyer et al., 2022) for maze.

CBM in Mathematics

There are two types of math CBM measures that are well researched and recognized as tools for progress-monitoring students for academic difficulty: math computation probes (M-CBM) and math concepts and application probes (M-CAP). M-CBM includes 1- to 2-minute timed assessments of students' math fact fluency, with scores reported as digits correct per minute (DCM). Probes can be easily and quickly administered to get an idea of overall math fact fluency. There are free online resources available that can automatically create math CBM probes (e.g., AplusMath, EasyCBM, and Intervention Central). Foegen et al. (2007) reviewed progress-monitoring measures in mathematics and found 32 studies published between 1983 and 2005 that addressed CBM in mathematics. They found that most CBM mathematics studies explored Stage 1 research (reliability and validity of data and decisions made from an assessment at one time point), but those that examined progress-monitoring decisions resulted in reliable data and valid decisions. Many studies since the Foegen et al. (2007) review have analyzed M-CBM data and have consistently shown moderate to high predictive validity (Codding et al., 2016; Keller-Margulis et al., 2008; Methe et al., 2015).

CBM in Writing and Spelling

Writing CBM is a simple yet efficient tool that is consistently proven to be effective in measuring and progress-monitoring students' writing and spelling ability (Datchuk et al., 2022). There are two types of writing CBM: CBM in written expression (CBM-WE) and CBM in spelling (CBM-S). CBM in writing expression is used to monitor students' writing fluency. Students receive either picture-word prompts or story prompts, and they are given either 3, 5, or 7 minutes to write, depending on their grade level. All writing prompts are scored through total words written (TWW), words spelled correctly (WSC), correct word sequences (CWS), or correct minus incorrect word sequences (CIWS). CBM in spelling is used to monitor students' spelling progress. Students are required to spell about 20 words in 2 minutes. The spellings are scored through correct letter sequences (CLS) or incorrect letter sequences (ILS).

Data from 21 studies regarding writing CBM showed convincing evidence for the validity of writing CBM scored with CIWS, with moderate validity coefficients for CWS, WSC, and TWW (Romig et al., 2017). CBM writing has also been shown to be highly reliable, with mean coefficients of approximately .90 (Amato & Watkins, 2011; Gansle et al., 2002). There is considerably less research on CBM spelling, but there are high reliabilities and initial validity evidence reported for spelling metrics such as WSC (Amato & Watkins, 2011; Gansle et al., 2002; Romig et al., 2017).

CBM: Psychometrics

Three states of CBM development are commonly cited (Fuchs, 2004), with the first stage establishing the technical adequacy of data collected at one point in time. This research emphasizes the reliability and criterion validity of the measures and the extent to which scores can be used to predict future performance (Foegen et al., 2007). The second stage consists of assessing the technical features of slope or growth rates over time. The third stage includes consideration of how the tool can be used for instructional purposes. When assessing the psychometric properties of CBM, a preliminary step involves examining empirical studies investigating both reliability and validity (Stage 1) of use for CBMs. According to the National Center on Intensive Intervention (NCII), measures having "convincing evidence" must include multiple studies and have a lower bound of confidence interval (CI) of .70 in the area of reliability and at least .60 in validity (American Institutes for Research, 2018).

CBMs have been systematically reviewed recently in reading (Shin & McMaster, 2019; Yeo, 2011), math (Gersten et al., 2012), writing (Romig et al., 2017), and science and social studies (Conoyer et al., 2020). Yeo (2011) reviewed 28 studies examining the reliability of read-aloud measures and reported a mean correlation of .89. Shin and McMaster (2019) conducted a meta-analysis to examine the validity of CBMs in the area of ORF and maze compared with state achievement assessments. A total of 61 studies met criteria, and results indicated an overall mean validity coefficient of .63 for ORF and .60 for maze measures. Romig et al. (2017) examined writing CBMs, and results showed a mean of .55. Science and social studies CBMs were found to demonstrate a mean correlation of .59 for criterion validity. There are multiple standards with which validity coefficients for progress-monitoring measures can be evaluated, but the NCII (2021) uses a criterion of r = .60 or higher as convincing evidence for validity for progress-monitoring measures. Many CBM tools have been developed to provide psychometrically rigorous data (Graney et al., 2010; VanDerHeyden & Broussard, 2021), such as Acadience Learning (2018), AIMSweb (Pearson, 2010), the Dynamic Indicators of Basic Early Literacy (DIBELS) (Good et al., 2002), and FastBridge (Illuminate Education, 2022).

Computer-Adapted Tests

Computer-adapted tests (CATs) provide an alternative approach to measuring student progress by employing algorithms and item response theory (IRT) to estimate student ability (Weiss & Kingsbury, 1984). Unlike CBM, most CATs rely on multiple-choice items that are highly objective and efficient, and the items that a student completes are individualized based on performance on earlier items within the test (Papanastasiou, 2003). The Measures of Academic Progress (MAP) (Northwest Evaluation Association [NWEA], 2019) is a CAT and considers item difficulty and test-taker ability to estimate the probability that a student will be successful on a given item. Additionally, STAR-Reading and STAR-Math are

CATs that are commonly used for screening and progress monitoring (Renaissance, 2015). CATs are easy to administer and often with a reduced number of questions (e.g., STAR-Reading typically requires 10 minutes to complete [Renaissance, 2015]), with automatic computer scoring while measuring a wider range of skills than is possible with CBM.

CAT: Implementation

CATs are typically used periodically to monitor student progress, with assessments at seasonal benchmarks (e.g., January and May), three times during the benchmark duration, or monthly (five times), with more frequent assessments leading to better estimates of growth (Nelson et al., 2017). Weekly administration of STAR-Math led to adequate reliable estimates of growth after 16 weeks and adequate predictions of actual growth after 8 to 10 weeks (Van Norman et al., 2017). Research with STAR-Reading found that data collected five times over 20 weeks (every 4 weeks) led to psychometrically sound decisions (Bulut & Cormier, 2018). Thus, data collected with CATs at least monthly can lead to valid decisions (Van Norman & Ysseldyke, 2020).

CAT: Psychometrics

In addition to time-efficient assessments, CAT data can lead to psychometrically sound decisions. For example, progress monitoring with STAR-Early Literacy led psychometrically sound data at the beginning of kindergarten, with higher reliability than scores from early literacy CBMs (Clemens et al., 2019). Moreover, slope data from STAR-Math predicted math outcomes in third and fourth grades better than math CBMs (Shapiro et al., 2015). However, there are substantially fewer studies regarding the technical adequacy of progress-monitoring decisions with STAR-Reading data and other CAT approaches than there are for CBM. Thus, additional research is probably needed to better understand how to progress monitor with CATs.

Subskill Mastery Measurement

CBMs and CATs are considered general outcome measures (GOM), which are designed to provide a global index of a student's current level and degree of improvement. GOMs may not be sensitive to improvement in more narrow skills that contribute to the general outcome (Burns, 2010; Shapiro, 2010). For example, a student receiving an intervention that focuses on phonics may be doing well in learning to decode the words but may not show large growth in a GOM such as CBM-R, which could lead to an interventionist incorrectly interpreting that the intervention is not working. Thus, school-based personnel may use subskill mastery measures (SMMs) to monitor student improvement in more targeted skills, which may be helpful in better interpreting student growth and making instructional decisions.

SMM: Implementation

SMMs sample academic behavior in more narrow slices as they align to current instruction or intervention and change the measures when the student masters the skill being measured (Solomon et al., 2022). Reading SMMs usually involves 1-minute samples of student behavior, such as reading words that contain target graphemes being taught, providing sounds that correspond to letters, or phonemic awareness skills (e.g., isolating sounds for beginning, ending, and middle sounds; blending and segmenting words). The data usually consist of the number or percentage of correct responses in the 1-minute assessment. Math SMMs are usually 1- to 4-minute assessments of specific curricular objectives, which again are scored according to correct responses per minute. SMM can be used to identify if students are making sufficient progress (Ysseldyke & Bolt, 2007), and using the data to identify areas needing instruction has led to increased student achievement (Burns, Scholin, et al., 2010), even among students who struggled with math (Burns et al., 2012).

SMM: Psychometrics

Mastery measures have been used in intervention research for decades and can result in reliable decision making for math (Solomon et al., 2022; VanDerHeyden et al., 2017) and reading (Burns et al., 2000; Van Norman et al., 2018). Multiple studies have demonstrated SMM to be a psychometrically sound approach to progress monitoring. For example, word lists that contain target phonemes taught during phonics interventions (Olinghouse et al., 2006; Van Norman et al., 2018), measures of phonemic awareness and decoding (Oslund et al., 2012), letter-sound fluency (Ritchey, 2008), letter naming, rhyming, and sound blending (McConnell & Wackerle-Hollman, 2015) all led to psychometrically sound data that were at least equal to or preferable to GOM data in reading. Moreover, 1- to 4-minute measures of specific objectives in math led to sufficiently reliable data that more frequently exceeded thresholds for adequacy than GOM measures (Solomon et al., 2022). SMMs examine a sequence of narrower skills than GOMs, which requires multiple forms to reduce familiarity with the assessments that are equal in content focus and task difficulty for each skill (VanDerHeyden & Broussard, 2021) while building using a validated hierarchy of skills across domains (VanDerHeyden et al., 2021).

Decision-Making Rules

Student progress should be judged by evaluating performance at one point in time as compared to a standard and by evaluating the slope of improvement, also compared to a meaningful standard (Fuchs, 2004; Fuchs et al., 2021). Next, we will discuss how to interpret data by evaluating performance at a point in time for CBM, CATs, and SMMs and how to interpret rates of improvement.

Point-in-Time CBM and CAT

The first strand in interpreting progress-monitoring data is to examine the data at one point in time, which is crucial to understanding where student performance is compared to expected performance, hypothesis generation, and intervention selection. It makes most sense to compare student CBM scores in reading, writing, and math to seasonal benchmark criteria such as those published by DIBELS (*https://dibels.uoregon.edu/sites/dibels1.uoregon.edu/files/2021-06/DIBELS8thEdition-Goals.pdf*) or EasyCBM (*https://help.easycbm.com/wp-content/uploads/2021/01/easycbm_percentile_lookup_table.pdf*). Scores that fall below the 25th percentile certainly indicate difficulty, but scores below the 40th percentile may also suggest a potential problem and a need for further assessment or intervention.

CAT data are often interpreted with a detailed report provided by the test publisher that provides standard scores, percentile ranks, and rates of improvement (ROI). An example of a report can be found at *www.renaissance.com/star-scores*. Much like CBM, a score at or below the 40th percentile might suggest a low score, but a score at or below the 25th percentile should almost certainly be interpreted as an indication of student difficulty.

Because CATs provide GOM data, practitioners should be careful about interpreting domain scores that indicate percent mastery of specific domains (e.g., key ideas details, vocabulary, integration of knowledge and ideas, number and operations, measurement and data, and geometry) for individual students. CAT assessments are designed to select questions based on performance on items presented early in the test based on probability that the student will continue to perform well or not on similar items. Thus, it is possible for domain scores to contain few items, which could result in a reliable overall score that correlates well with important outcomes (Shapiro et al., 2015; Shapiro & Gebhardt, 2012). However, the utility of the domain scores remains less clear. Moreover, practitioners are discouraged from interpreting grade-equivalent scores because of psychometric difficulties and promotion of typological thinking that is not actually reflected in the score (Salvia et al., 2016).

Point-in-Time SMM

SMMs are based almost completely on assessing an instructional level, or optimal level of challenge, in which task demands and student performance are balanced so that the task is not too difficult or too easy for learning to occur (Burns & Parker, 2014). Assessments with reading of connected text are usually interpreted by computing the percentage of words read correctly ([Number of Words Read Correctly / Total Number of Words] × 100) and comparing it to a criterion for an instructional level of 93% to 97%. Most other tasks, such as spelling, word lists, letter sounds, math facts, and so forth, can be interpreted by computing the percentage of items answered correctly and comparing it to a criterion of 90% correct (Burns, 2004; Burns et al., 2022). Tasks that represent an instructional level are appropriate intervention targets.

There is a unique approach for computing an instructional level for math computation tasks within SMM. As described early and outlined in Table 20.1, a SMM of math computation involves creating a brief sample of the specific problem being assessed (e.g., addition of two double-digit numbers, subtraction of a single-digit number from a double-digit number without regrouping, multiplication of two single-digit numbers, etc.) and having the student complete the task for 1 to 4 minutes depending on the complexity of the skill. The data are then converted to a DCM metric by counting the number of correct digits in the answer (e.g., 4 × 4 = 16 would be 2 digits correct, 12 × 12 = 144 would be 3 digits correct, and 13 × 13 = 168 (correct answer 169) would be 2 digits correct out of 3). The number of digits correct per minute is then compared to the instructional level criteria outlined in Table 20.1 of 14 to 31 DCM for second and third grades and 24 to 49 DCM for fourth and fifth grades (Burns et al., 2006).

There is considerable research to demonstrate that being able to read 93% to 97% of words correctly (Parker & Burns, 2014; Treptow et al., 2007), correctly responding to 90% of items (Burns, 2004; Burns et al., 2022), and completing math tasks at a DCM that falls within the instructional-level range (Burns, Codding, et al., 2006; Burns et al., 2010) increases student learning. When students are capable of completing tasks that represent an instructional level, they consistently demonstrate increased rates of learning, task comprehension, task completion, and

TABLE 20.1. Subskill Mastery Measures and Interpretive Criteria in Words Read Correctly/Minute or Digits Correct/Minute

Skill domain	Measures	Data	Instructional-level criteria	Mastery criteria
Phonemic awareness	1-minute measures of isolating sounds (e.g., initial sound fluency), blending sounds, or segmenting sounds (e.g., phoneme segmentation fluency)	Number or percentage of correct responses in 1 minute	90% correct	Proficiency scores on CBM norms for correct responses/minute
Phonics	1-minute measures of word lists that contain target graphemes or letter-sound fluency	Number or percentage of WCM or LSM	90% correct	Proficiency scores on CBM norms
Fluency	1-minute fluency score from an instructional-level reading probe	Number or percentage of WCM	93–97% correct	Proficiency scores on CBM norms for the student's grade
Math	1- to 4-minute assessments of specific math objectives		2nd and 3rd grades = 14–31 DCM 4th and 5th grades = 24–49 DCM	Proficiency scores on CBM norms

Note. WCM = words read correctly per minute; DCM = digits correct per minute.

time on task (Burns, Codding, et al., 2010; Burns & Parker, 2014; Treptow et al., 2007). Moreover, multiple studies have shown that the criteria outlined here led to reliable estimates of an instructional level (Burns et al., 2000, 2006, 2022).

Rate of Improvement

The second approach to interpreting progress-monitoring data involves evaluating the slope or ROI. Interventionists employ different approaches in interpreting ROI. Hintze et al. (2018) described two approaches, *data point decision rules* and *trendline decision rules.*

Data Point Decision Rules

Data point decision rules interpret student growth by examining where individual data points fall in relation to desired growth (Hintze et al., 2018). According to this approach, as shown in Figure 20.1, interventionists first need to set an aimline for the student based on peer performance or standard scores. For example, if CBM norms indicate that students should be reading 69 words per minute by the second

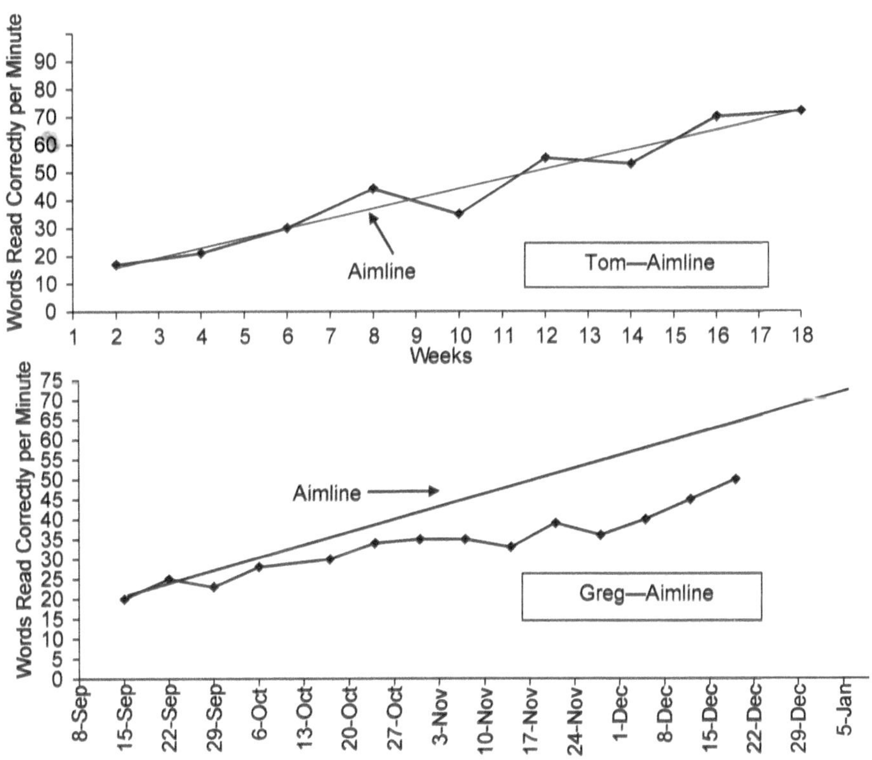

FIGURE 20.1. Sample progress-monitoring data interpreted with data point rule.

benchmark assessment, typically conducted the second week of January, but the student is reading 17 words per minute during the second week of September, then the interventionist would draw an aimline from 17 words per minute in week 2 to 69 words per minute 16 weeks later. Then intervention data points are collected and compared to the aimline. The desired outcome is for the progress-monitoring data points to approximate the aimline. If 4 consecutive data points fall below the aimline, then the goal was not set high enough and should be reconsidered, but 4 consecutive data points below the aimline suggest that the intervention is not effective and the intervention should be reconsidered (Fuchs et al., 1990). The data in the top panel of Figure 20.1 (Tom) suggest an effective intervention because the data fall around the aimline, but the data in the bottom half (Greg) suggest an ineffective intervention.

Burns, Codding, et al. (2010) found that data point decision rules led to inaccurate decisions, with reliability estimates ($\kappa = .29$) that fell far below what is considered acceptable for instructional decisions, which has been a consistent finding for data point decision rules based on 3 data points (Van Norman & Christ, 2016) or 4 data points (Hintze et al., 2018). That does not mean that data point decision making has no place in progress monitoring; it simply means that the types of decisions that can be made are limited. In other words, an interventionist who was informally monitoring progress to assess the effects of their efforts, or a special educator who was monitoring progress toward a goal in a student's individualized educational program, could certainly use a data point decision rule to evaluate their instruction. However, resource allocation decisions (e.g., identifying a child with a disability and providing special education or moving a child from a Tier 2 intervention to a Tier 3 intervention with an MTSS) require a higher standard for psychometric rigor (Salvia et al., 2016), which is rarely met by data point decision making. For those types of higher-stakes decisions, a trendline rule is probably more appropriate.

Trendline Rules

According to the trendline decision rules, the estimated growth of a student is determined by regressing the student's CBM score onto time. Then the estimated growth is compared to the goal line slope (Hintze et al., 2018). The data presented in Figure 20.2 show this approach in which the data were graphed with graphing software or with MS Excel. When creating a graph with MS Excel, trendlines are easily inserted into a line graph by (1) selecting the intervention data, (2) selecting Add Chart Element, (3) selecting Trendline, and (4) selecting Linear. The data for the goal line represent the criteria for proficiency at each benchmark assessment for CBM-R for a student in second grade of 49 words per minute in the fall and 94 words per minute in the spring (*https://dibels.uoregon.edu/sites/dibels1.uoregon.edu/files/2021-06/DIBELS8thEditionGoals.pdf*). Plotting a trendline and goal line allows for visual analysis of the data, which results in accurate decisions as long as there were at least 6 weeks' worth of data (Van Norman & Christ, 2016).

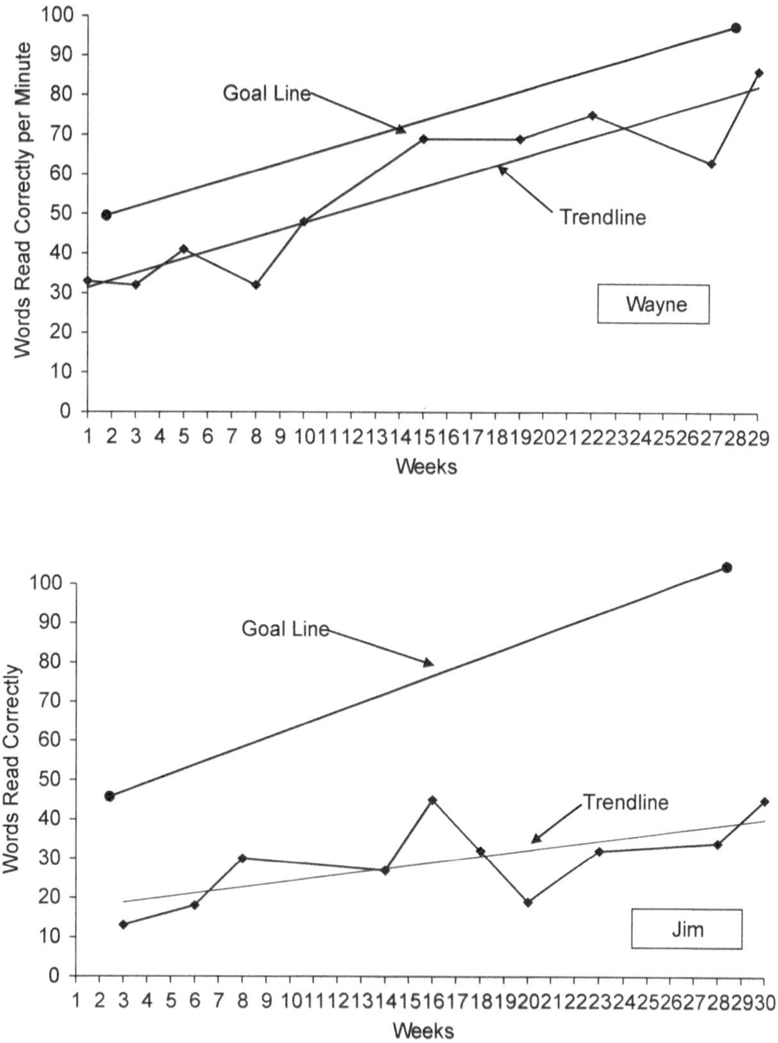

FIGURE 20.2. Sample progress monitoring data interpreted with trendline.

The data shown in the top panel of Figure 20.2 (Wayne) represent an effective intervention because the data in the trendline run at least parallel to the goal line that is made up of the benchmark proficiency scores for Wayne's grade. The data in the bottom half (Jim) indicate an ineffective intervention because the student is not progressing at a rate that matches his grade-level peers. The data in Figure 20.2 can be interpreted by visually examining the slope of the trendline compared to the slope of the goal line. Alternatively, the trendline can be computed with the slope function in MS Excel by (1) selecting the SLOPE function, (2) selecting the array that represents the data as the dependent variable, (3) selecting the array that represents the week number as the independent variable, and (4) clicking OK.

Many progress-monitoring systems report the ROI, which can be interpreted by computing the slope/ROI of the data with the criteria for proficiency for the fall, winter, and spring benchmarks using the weeks that represent the week of the year in which the data were collected. For example, benchmark assessments collected at the second week of the school year, and 16 weeks later in the winter benchmark and 16 weeks after that would be weeks 2, 18, and 34. The benchmark criteria represented in Figure 20.2 with Wayne were 49 words correct per minute in the fall (week 2), 78 words correct per minute in the winter (week 18), and 94 words correct per minute in the spring (week 34), which equals a slope of 1.41. As demonstrated in Table 20.2, ROIs or slopes should be 1.41 to demonstrate sufficient progress. Basing criteria for ROIs based on growth of typically developing peers may seem somewhat problematic, but Deno et al. (2001) found that students with learning disabilities progress at median ROI of 1.53 when provided effective treatments, and Burns et al. (2020) found that second- and third-grade students with severe reading difficulties grew at a rate (ROI = 1.24) that exceeded their peers with average reading skills (ROI = 1.08). Trendline decision making is preferable over data point rules for important decisions because they take into account all of the data and are compared to criteria for proficiency.

TABLE 20.2. Sample Slope Data for a Second-Grade Classroom

Student	Number of weeks	Last score	Score criterion	Slope	Slope criterion	Decision
MA	8	75	94	1.01	1.41	Intervention not working—intensify the intervention
SB	24	101	94	1.55	1.41	Intervention worked—discontinue the intervention
TB	16	84	94	1.75	1.41	Intervention working—continue as-is
JH	27	45	94	0.78	1.41	Intervention did not work—intensify the tier
TK	16	71	94	3.37	1.41	Intervention working—continue as-is
IM	25	65	94	1.54	1.41	Intervention working—continue as-is
RS	12	45	94	0.95	1.41	Intervention did not work—intensify the tier
MT	18	98	94	1.65	1.41	Intervention worked—discontinue the intervention
WS	29	86	94	1.81	1.41	Intervention working—continue as-is
GW	15	50	94	0.26	1.41	Intervention did not work—intensify the tier

Decision Outcomes

The primary goal of progress monitoring is to evaluate the effects of an intervention based on student growth. As described earlier, data can start to be evaluated after approximately 6 data points (Van Norman & Christ, 2016). However, resource allocation decisions require more psychometric rigor than what is typically seen after 6 data points. Seminal research by Christ (2006) found that slopes of data, as interpreted with data point and trendline decision rules, had standard errors of estimate that were so large as to be uninterpretable until approximately 12 data points. Thus, a school team can examine data after 6 weeks of weekly progress monitoring to decide if they need to make any modifications to the intervention, but changes in tiers that add resources (e.g., Tier 2 to Tier 3) or remove them (e.g., Tier 2 to Tier 1) probably require at least 12 data points.

Intervention Working or Worked

Decision outcomes from progress-monitoring data are outlined in Table 20.3 and are used to interpret the data presented in Table 20.2. The first decision outcome is that the intervention worked, which would result in the student having resources removed and would require at least 12 GOM data points to reach that decision. The intervention is judged to have worked if the slope of growth exceeds the criterion and at least two consecutive individual data points exceed the criterion for proficiency (i.e., benchmark standard), as is the case for Student SB in Table 20.2.

TABLE 20.3. Progress Monitoring Outcomes and Types of Data Needed

Outcome	Action	Data
Intervention worked	Discontinue the intervention and transition back to previous tier (i.e., from Tier 3 to Tier 2, or Tier 2 to Tier 1)	At least 12 GOM data points with a slope that is above criterion AND At least two individual data points above criterion for proficiency
Intervention working	Continue the intervention as-is	Slope of GOM data is above criterion BUT Individual data points are not above criterion for proficiency
Intervention not working	Intensify the intervention within the tier (e.g., add more modeling, dosage, or training for transfer)	Slope of GOM data is below criterion, and Individual data points are not above criterion for proficiency, BUT Have not collected enough data yet (e.g., less than 12 data points)
Intervention did not work	Intensify the tier (i.e., move from Tier 2 to Tier 3 or from Tier 3 to special education evaluation)	Slope of GOM data is below criterion, and Individual data points are not above criterion for proficiency, and Have collected enough data (i.e., at least 12 data points)

If the slope of growth meets or exceeds the criterion but individual data points are not yet reaching the criterion for proficiency, then the intervention is judged to be working (e.g., Student TB in Table 20.2). In this decision outcome, the intervention would simply continue as-is until reaching the criterion for proficiency.

It is also possible for a school team to judge the intervention as working when the slope of the GOM data does not meet or exceed the criterion for growth. For example, a student may be receiving an intervention that focuses on a foundational skill like phonemic awareness or phonics and the student is doing quite well, but the growth is yet to be adequately transferred to be detectable in a GOM like CBM-R that focuses on reading fluency. The team may see evidence in the SMMs, such as mastering the lesson (e.g., at least 90% correct on immediate assessments of phonics skills that were taught, Table 20.1) or making growth on a more precise measure like Nonsense Word Fluency (phonics) or Phoneme Segmentation Fluency (phonemic awareness). In this case, the team may decide to wait a few more weeks to see if transfer occurs to the GOM before changing the intervention or reducing resources.

Intervention Not Working or Did Not Work

Slope data that fall below the criterion for growth indicate that the intervention is not working and a change is needed. If there are fewer than 12 progress-monitoring data points and the slope of growth does not meet or exceed the criterion, then the team cannot be certain that the low score is not measurement error and should not change resources allocated to support the student. The team can determine that the data suggest that the intervention is not yet working (e.g., Student MA, Table 20.3) but would elect to modify the intervention without changing resources. For example, they could provide more modeling, dosage, or training for transfer in the intervention sessions (Fuchs et al., 2017). SMM data may help determine which approach is best in that students who continue to demonstrate low accuracy after being taught the skill may need more modeling, those who have high accuracy but do not retain the skill or perform it fluently may need more dosage, and those with high accuracy, retention, and rate but who struggle to apply the skill would likely need additional training for transfer (Burns, 2021; Burns et al., 2025).

The final decision outcome requires at least 12 GOM data points because it entails adding resources. If the slope of growth and individual data points both fall below criteria and there are sufficient data, then the team can identify the intervention as not working and begin moving the student to a more intensive intervention, such as transferring from Tier 2 to Tier 3 or from Tier 3 to a special education evaluation.

Progress Monitoring in Action

Next, we will provide some examples of progress monitoring and the resulting decisions. The first example will be a student who is being progress-monitored for reading. This example illustrates a situation where GOM data are not suggesting sufficient growth, but SMM data indicate that learning is occurring. The second example shows how SMM data are used to monitor progress in math.

Reading

Ryan was a third-grade student receiving an intervention that focused on phonics. His benchmark assessment reading screener assessed CBM-R with DIBELS, which resulted in a score of 55 words read correctly per minute (DIBELS fall benchmark criterion = 73), with 83% of the words read accurately. He received phonics intervention four times per week, and his progress was monitored with weekly third-grade DIBELS (8th ed.) CBM-R. The CBM-R data served as the GOM. His progress was also monitored at the end of each intervention session (total of 40 each week) with SMM. He read word lists that contained 10 words with the sounds that were being taught. Finally, progress was monitored each week with DIBELS-8 Nonsense Word Fluency. As can be seen in Figure 20.3, his progress on the CBM-R GOM was adequate over the 16-week intervention period. However, the team met after 6 weeks of intervention (at week 7) because the slope for Ryan's GOM data was 0.54 words per minute per week and the goal based on standards for benchmark proficiency was 1.28 words per minute per week. Fortunately, the team had two sources of SMM data. Ryan's Nonsense Word Fluency score increased from 55 correct letter sounds per minute to 79 correct letter sounds per minute, which was an average increase of 4.2 correct letter sounds per minute per week. He also correctly read at least 36 (out of 40, 90%) words correctly during the post-intervention session wordlist assessments.

The school team examined the data and concluded that the intervention was not working according to the GOM data, but the two sets of SMM data suggested that the intervention was having a positive effect. They then decided to increase dosage and train for transfer to try to ensure better application of the phonics skills that he was learning. After making the intervention change, Ryan's GOM slope increased to 2.66 words correct per minute per week, which was well above the criterion of 1.28. He had not quite reached the winter benchmark by the 18th week, so the team decided that the intervention was working and to continue the intervention.

Math

Dave was a second-grade student receiving a math intervention. He scored at the 22nd percentile on the STAR-Math, which immediately triggered the school team to conduct a series of 2-minute assessments sampling from the following sequence of math skills based on VanDerHeyden and Broussard (2021), (1) addition sums to 12, (2) add/subtract 0–20, (3) add three-digit numbers with and without regrouping, (4) subtracting three-digit numbers with and without regrouping, and (5) multiplication 0 to 9. Each 2-minute assessment was scored as DCM and compared to the instructional level criterion of 14 to 31 DCM. Dave scored within the

Ryan's Curriculum-Based Measurement of Reading General Outcome Measure

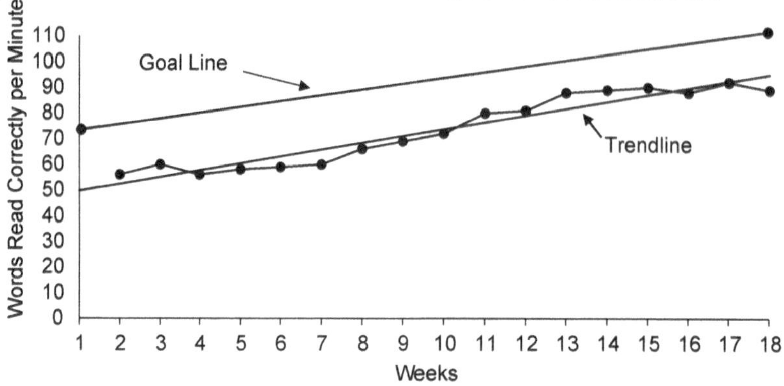

Ryan's Nonsense Word Fluency Skill Measures as Subskill Mastery Measure of Phonics

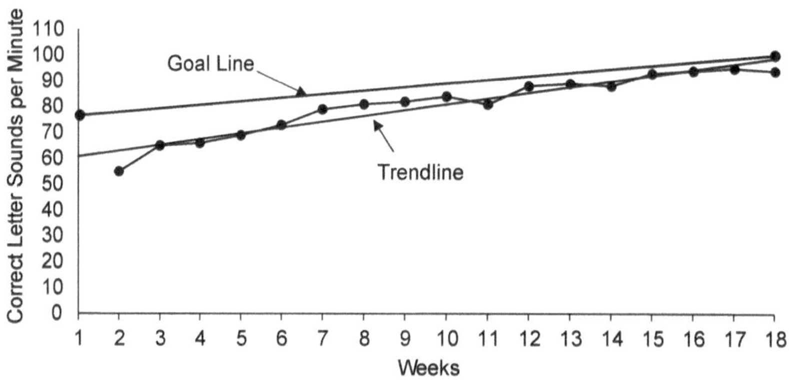

Weekly Totals (out of 40) of Words Read Correctly from Subskill Mastery Measure of Phonics

Week	1	2	3	4	5	6	7	8	9	10	11	12	13	14	15	16	17	18
Number Correct	38	36	39	40	38	40	39	40	37	40	38	36	39	38	40	39	38	39

FIGURE 20.3. General outcome measure and subskill mastery measurement progress-monitoring data for Ryan.

instructional level on addition sums to 12, but at a frustration level (i.e., less than 14 DCM) on add/subtract 0–20 and adding three-digit numbers with and without regrouping. The intervention focused on increasing conceptual understanding of numbers and procedural fluency for basic fact addition, and progress was monitored with a weekly SMM of addition to sums of 12.

As can be seen in Figure 20.4, he quickly increased his responding on addition of sums to 12, and his score fell within the independent range (i.e., more than 31 DCM) in just 3 weeks. The intervention continued until Dave scored in the independent range for two consecutive weeks, when the intervention and SMM

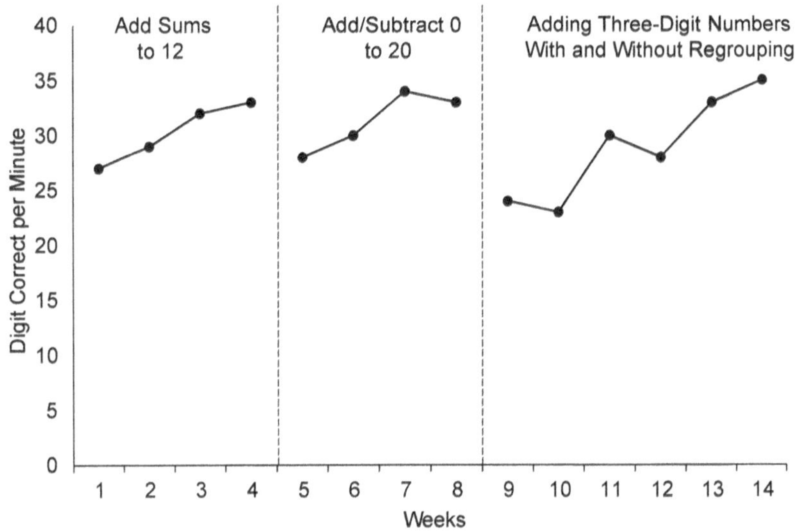

FIGURE 20.4. Subskill mastery measurement progress-monitoring data for Dave.

switched to add/subtract 0 to 20. Dave once again demonstrated independent level scores on two consecutive weekly progress-monitoring assessments after just 4 weeks. The final phase of intervention included in Figure 20.4 intervened for and assessed adding three-digit numbers with and without regrouping. Dave scored in the independent range on two consecutive weekly SMM progress-monitoring probes after 6 weeks. After the intervention period of 14 weeks, Dave completed the winter benchmark assessment on the STAR-Math and scored at the 48th percentile, and the intervention ended.

Conclusion

There has been considerable research in progress monitoring since 2004 when federal law allowed the use of student response to intervention to evaluate students for a specific learning disability. Some of the most important findings include the number of data points necessary to make a low-stake (6) (Van Norman & Christ, 2016) or high-stake (12) (Christ, 2006) decision, the low reliability of data point decision rules based on aimlines (Burns, Scholin, et al., 2010; Hintze et al., 2018), the utility of CAT for progress monitoring (Clemens et al., 2019; Shapiro et al., 2015), and the important role of SMMs in progress monitoring (Burns, 2010; Solomon et al., 2022; Van Norman et al., 2018). Using well-constructed measures with established decision rules can lead to sound decision making, but different types of data may be needed for different decisions. The guidance provided in this chapter may be a solid place for school-based teams to make more sound data-based decisions in designing progress-monitoring tools and interpreting the resulting data.

REFERENCES

Acadience Learning (2018). *The DIBELS Next assessment is now Acadience Reading. https://acadiencelearning.org/the-dibels-next-assessment-is-now-acadience-reading*

Amato, J. M., & Watkins, M. W. (2011). The predictive validity of CBM writing indices for eighth-grade students. *The Journal of Special Education, 44*(4), 195–204.

American Institutes for Research. (2018). *National Center for Intensive Intervention: Academic progress monitoring tools chart. https://charts.intensiveintervention.org*

Bulut, O., & Cormier, D. C. (2018). Validity evidence for progress monitoring with STAR-Reading: Slope estimates, administration frequency, and number of data points. *Frontiers in Education, 3*, 68.

Burns, M. K. (2004). Empirical analysis of drill ratio research: Refining the instructional level for drill tasks. *Remedial and Special Education, 25*(3), 167–173.

Burns, M. K. (2010). Formative evaluation in school psychology: Fully informing the instructional process. *School Psychology Forum, 4*(1), 22–33.

Burns, M. K. (2021). Intensifying reading interventions through a skill-by-treatment interaction: What to do when nothing else worked. *Communiqué, 50*(4), 30–32.

Burns, M. K., Codding, R. S., Boice, C. H., & Lukito, G. (2010). Meta-analysis of acquisition and fluency math interventions with instructional and frustration level skills: Evidence for a skill-by-treatment interaction. *School Psychology Review, 39*(1), 69–83.

Burns, M. K., Kanive, R., & DeGrande, M. (2012). Effect of a computer-delivered math fact intervention as a supplemental intervention for math in third and fourth grades. *Remedial and Special Education, 33*(3), 184–191.

Burns, M. K., Maki, K. E., Brann, K. L., McComas, J. J., & Helman, L. A. (2020). Comparison of reading growth among students with severe reading deficits who received intervention to typically achieving students and students receiving special education. *Journal of Learning Disabilities, 53*(6), 444–453.

Burns, M. K., & Parker, D. C. (2014). *Curriculum-based assessment for instructional design: Using data to individualize instruction.* Guilford Press.

Burns, M. K., Scholin, S. E., Kosciolek, S., & Livingston, J. (2010). Reliability of decision-making frameworks for response to intervention for reading. *Journal of Psychoeducational Assessment, 28*(2), 102–114.

Burns, M. K., Tucker, J. A., Frame, J., Foley, S., & Hauser, A. (2000). Interscorer, alternate-form, internal consistency, and test-retest reliability of Gickling's model of curriculum-based assessment for reading. *Journal of Psychoeducational Assessment, 18*(4), 353–360.

Burns, M. K., VanDerHeyden, A. M., & Jiban, C. L. (2006). Assessing the instructional level for mathematics: A comparison of methods. *School Psychology Review, 35*(3), 401–418.

Burns, M. K., Welland, J. B., Singell, E. L., & Graves, K. A. (2025). Effects of intensifying reading interventions with a skill-by-treatment interaction framework: A contraindication single-case design. *Learning Disabilities: A Multidisciplinary Journal, 30*(1), 1–12.

Burns, M. K., Young, H., McCollom, E. M., Stevens, M. A., & Izumi, J. T. (2022). Predicting intervention effects with preintervention measures of decoding: Evidence for a skill-by-treatment interaction with kindergarten and first-grade students. *Learning Disability Quarterly, 45*(4), 320–330.

Castro-Villarreal, F., Rodriguez, B. J., & Moore, S. (2014). Teachers' perceptions and attitudes about response to intervention (RTI) in their schools: A qualitative analysis. *Teaching and Teacher Education, 40*, 104–112.

Christ, T. J. (2006). Short-term estimates of growth using curriculum-based measurement of oral reading fluency: Estimating standard error of the slope to construct confidence intervals. *School Psychology Review, 35*(1), 128–133.

Christ, T. J., Zopluoglu, C., Long, J. D., & Monaghen, B. D. (2012). Curriculum-based measurement of oral reading: Quality of progress monitoring outcomes. *Exceptional Children, 78*(3), 356–373.

Clemens, N. H., Hsiao, Y. Y., Simmons, L. E., Kwok, O. M., Greene, E. A., Soohoo, M. M., et al. (2019). Predictive validity of kindergarten progress monitoring measures across the school year: Application of dominance analysis. *Assessment for Effective Intervention, 44*(4), 241–255.

Codding, R. S., Mercer, S., Connell, J., Fiorello, C., & Kleinert, W. (2016). Mapping the relationships among basic facts, concepts and application, and common core curriculum-based mathematics measures. *School Psychology Review, 45*(1), 19–38.

Conoyer, S. J., Therrien, W. J., & White, K. K. (2020). Meta-analysis of validity and review of alternate form reliability and slope for curriculum-based measurement in science and social studies. *Assessment for Effective Intervention, 47*(2), 101–111.

Datchuk, S. M., Rodgers, D. B., Wagner, K., Hier, B. O., & Moore, C. T. (2022). Effects of writing interventions on the level and trend of total words written: A meta-analysis. *Exceptional Children, 88*(2), 145–162.

Deno, S. L. (1985). Curriculum-based measurement: The emerging alternative. *Exceptional Children, 52*(3), 219–232.

Deno, S. L. (2003). Developments in curriculum-based measurement. *The Journal of Special Education, 37*(3), 184–192.

Deno, S. L., Fuchs, L. S., Marston, D., & Shin, J. (2001). Using curriculum-based measurement to establish growth standards for students with learning disabilities. *School Psychology Review, 30*(4), 507–524.

Deno, S. L., & Mirkin, P. (1977). *Data-based program modification: A manual.* Council for Exceptional Children.

Foegen, A., Jiban, C., & Deno, S. (2007). Progress monitoring measures in mathematics: A review of the literature. *The Journal of Special Education, 41*(2), 121–139.

Fuchs, L. S. (2004). The past, present, and future of curriculum-based measurement research. *School Psychology Review, 33*(2), 188–192.

Fuchs, L. S., Fuchs, D., Hamlett, C. L., & Stecker, P. M. (1990). The role of skills analysis in curriculum-based measurement in math. *School Psychology Review, 19*(1), 6–22.

Fuchs, L. S., Fuchs, D., Hamlett, C. L., & Stecker, P. M. (2021). Bringing data-based individualization to scale: A call for the next-generation technology of teacher supports. *Journal of Learning Disabilities, 54*(5), 319–333.

Fuchs, L. S., Fuchs, D., & Malone, A. S. (2017). The taxonomy of intervention intensity. *Teaching Exceptional Children, 50*(1), 35–43.

Gansle, K. A., Noell, G. H., VanDerHeyden, A. M., Naquin, G. M., & Slider, N. J. (2002). Moving beyond total words written: The reliability, criterion validity, and time cost of alternate measures for curriculum-based measurement in writing. *School Psychology Review*, 31(4), 477–497.

Gersten, R., Clarke, B., Jordan, N. C., Newman-Gonchar, R., Haymond, K., & Wilkins, C. (2012). Universal screening in mathematics for the primary grades: Beginnings of a research base. *Exceptional Children, 78*(4), 423–445.

Good, R. H., Gruba, J., & Kaminski, R. A. (2002). Best practices in using Dynamic Indicators of Basic Early Literacy Skills (DIBELS) in an outcomes-driven model. In A. Thomas & J. Grimes (Eds.), *Best practices in school psychology IV* (pp. 699–720). National Association of School Psychologists.

Graney, S. B., Martinez, R. S., Missall, K. N., & Aricak, O. T. (2010). Universal screening of reading in late elementary school: R-CBM versus CBM maze. *Remedial and Special Education, 31*(5), 368–377.

Greenfield, R., Rinaldi, C., Proctor, C. P., & Cardarelli, A. (2010). Teachers' perceptions of a response to intervention (RTI) reform effort in an urban elementary school: A consensual qualitative analysis. *Journal of Disability Policy Studies, 21*(1), 47–63.

Hintze, J. M., Wells, C. S., Marcotte, A. M., & Solomon, B. G. (2018). Decision-making accuracy of CBM progress-monitoring data. *Journal of Psychoeducational Assessment, 36*(1), 74–81.

Illuminate Education. (2022). *FastBridge. www.illuminateed.com/products/fastbridge*

Keller-Margulis, M. A., Shapiro, E. S., & Hintze, J. M. (2008). Long-term diagnostic accuracy of curriculum-based measures in reading and mathematics. *School Psychology Review, 37*(3), 374–390.

LeRoux, M., Zvoch, K., & Biancarosa, G. (2020). Using curriculum-based measurement to predict student performance on an eighth-grade state reading assessment. *Assessment for Effective Intervention, 45*(4), 277–287.

McConnell, S., & Wackerle-Hollman, A. (2015). Can we measure the transition to reading? General outcome measures and early literacy development from preschool to early elementary grades. *AERA Open, 2*(3), 2332858416653756.

Methe, S. A., Briesch, A. M., & Hulac, D. (2015). Evaluating procedures for reducing measurement error in math curriculum-based measurement probes. *Assessment for Effective Intervention, 40*(2), 99–113.

National Center on Intensive Intervention. (2013). *Data-based individualization: A framework for intensive intervention. www.intensiveintervention.org/sites/default/files/DBI_Framework.pdf*

National Center on Intensive Intervention. (2021). *Academic progress monitoring tools chart. https://charts.intensiveintervention.org/aprogressmonitoring?_ga=2.229162268.1613499225.1663004498-802156250.1663004498*

Nelson, P. M., Van Norman, E. R., Klingbeil, D. A., & Parker, D. C. (2017). Progress monitoring with computer adaptive assessments: The impact of data collection schedule on growth estimates. *Psychology in the Schools, 54*(5), 463–471.

Nese, J. F., Park, B. J., Alonzo, J., & Tindal, G. (2011). Applied curriculum-based measurement as a predictor of high-stakes assessment: Implications for researchers and teachers. *The Elementary School Journal, 111*(4), 608–624.

Northwest Evaluation Association. (2019). *MAP Growth technical manual. www.nwea.org/uploads/2021/11/MAP-Growth-Technical-Report-2019_NWEA.pdf*

Olinghouse, N. G., Lambert, W., & Compton, D. L. (2006). Monitoring children with reading disabilities' response to phonics intervention: are there differences between intervention aligned and general skill progress monitoring assessments? *Exceptional Children, 73*(1), 90–106.

Oslund, E. L., Elleman, A. M., & Wallance, K. (2012). Factors related to data-based decision-making: examining experience, professional development, and the mediating effect of confidence on teacher graph literacy. *Journal of Learning Disabilities, 54*(4), 243–255.

Papanastasiou, E. (2003, July). Computer-adaptive testing in science education. In C. P. Constantinou & Z. C. Zacharia (Eds.), *Proceedings of the 6th International Conference on Computer Based Learning in Science, Nicosia, Cyprus* (pp. 965–971). Odegetes Publications.

Pearson. (2010). *AIMSweb: Assessment and data management for RTI.*

Renaissance Learning (2015). *STAR Reading technical manual.*

Ritchey, K. D. (2008). Assessing letter sound knowledge: A comparison of letter sound fluency and nonsense word fluency. *Exceptional Children, 74*(4), 487–506.

Romig, J. E., Therrien, W. J., & Lloyd, J. W. (2017). Meta-analysis of criterion validity for curriculum-based measurement in written language. *The Journal of Special Education, 51*(2), 72–82.

Salvia, J., Ysseldyke, J., & Witmer, S. (2016). *Assessment in special and inclusive education.* Cengage Learning.

Shapiro, E. S. (2010). *Academic skills problems* (4th ed.) Guilford Press.

Shapiro, E. S., Dennis, M. S., & Fu, Q. (2015). Comparing computer adaptive and curriculum-based measures of math in progress monitoring. *School Psychology Quarterly, 30*(4), 470–487.

Shapiro, E. S., & Gebhardt, S. N. (2012). Comparing computer-adaptive and curriculum-based measurement methods of assessment. *School Psychology Review, 41*(3), 295–305.

Shin, J., & McMaster, K. (2019). Relations between CBM (oral reading and maze) and reading comprehension on state achievement tests: A meta-analysis. *Journal of School Psychology, 73*, 131–149.

Solomon, B. G., VanDerHeyden, A. M., Solomon, E. C., Korzeniewski, E. R., Payne, L. L., Campaña, K. V., & Dillon, C. R. (2022). Mastery measurement in mathematics and the Goldilocks effect. *School Psychology, 37*(3), 213–224.

Stecker, P. M., Fuchs, L. S., & Fuchs, D. (2005). Using curriculum-based measurement to improve student achievement: Review of research. *Psychology in the Schools, 42*(8), 795–819.

Treptow, M. A., Burns, M. K., & McComas, J. J. (2007). Reading at the frustration, instructional, and independent levels: The effects on students' reading comprehension and time on task. *School Psychology Review, 36*(1), 159–166.

Van Norman, E. R., & Christ, T. J. (2016). How accurate are interpretations of curriculum-based measurement progress monitoring data? Visual analysis versus decision rules. *Journal of School Psychology, 58*, 41–55.

Van Norman, E. R., Maki, K. E., Burns, M. K., McComas, J. J., & Helman, L. (2018). Comparison of progress monitoring data from general outcome measures and specific subskill mastery measures for reading. *Journal of School Psychology, 67*(1), 179–189.

Van Norman, E. R., Nelson, P. M., & Parker, D. C. (2017). Technical adequacy of growth estimates from a computer adaptive test: Implications for progress monitoring. *School Psychology Quarterly, 32*(3), 379.

Van Norman, E. R., & Ysseldyke, J. E. (2020). The impact of data collection frequency and trend estimation method on the consistency of growth estimates from two computer-adaptive tests. *School Psychology Review, 49*(1), 20–30.

VanDerHeyden, A. M., & Broussard, C. (2021). Construction and examination of math subskill mastery measures. *Assessment for Effective Intervention, 46*(3), 188–196.

VanDerHeyden, A. M., Broussard, C., & Burns, M. K. (2021). Classification agreement for gated screening in mathematics: Subskill mastery measurement and classwide intervention. *Assessment for Effective Intervention, 46*(4), 270–280.

VanDerHeyden, A. M., Codding, R. S., & Martin, R. (2017). Relative value of common screening measures in mathematics. *School Psychology Review, 46*(1), 65–87.

Vannest, K. J., Parker, R., & Dyer, N. (2011). Progress monitoring in grade 5 science for low achievers. *The Journal of Special Education, 44*(4), 221–233.

Wayman, M., Wallace, T., Wiley, H. I., Tichá, R., & Espin, C. A. (2007). Literature synthesis on curriculum-based measurement in reading. *The Journal of Special Education, 41*(2), 85–120.

Weiss, D. J., & Kingsbury, G. G. (1984). Application of computerized adaptive testing to educational problems. *Journal of Educational Measurement, 21*(4), 361–375.

Yeo, S. (2011). Reliability generalization of curriculum-based measurement reading aloud: A meta-analytic review. *Exceptionality, 19*(2), 75–93.

Ysseldyke, J., & Bolt, D. M. (2007). Effect of technology-enhanced continuous progress monitoring on math achievement. *School Psychology Review, 36*(3), 453–467.

CHAPTER 21

Child × Instruction Interactions

Using Technology to Support Differentiated Instruction

Ashley M. Adams Sanabria and Sarah W. Siegal

Individualization of instruction is a foundational element of special education as well as a core component of the services supporting children with language and learning disabilities. The mechanism by which free and appropriate public education is provided to children with diagnosed learning disabilities is through the creation of the Individualized Education Program or Plan (IEP). Part B of the Individuals with Disabilities Education Act (IDEA, 2004) indicates that "to the maximum extent appropriate, children with disabilities, including children in public or private institutions or other care facilities, are educated with children who are nondisabled." As administrators and general and special educators have grappled with how to best provide instruction to learners of all different skill levels in the least restrictive environment (i.e., the same classroom), the need for understanding how to implement differentiated instruction has become indispensable.

Accumulating research supports that one crucial reason that students of varying levels of ability may not achieve proficient reading skills is because they may require differing amounts and types of reading instruction depending on the individual skills they bring to the classroom (Connor, Morrison, & Katch, 2004). When children enter the classroom, they bring varying constellations of cognitive, linguistic, and social–emotional skills. Multiple sources of influence, including home, formal schooling, parent education levels, preschool experience, baseline ability levels, and community resources, impact children's literacy development (Bronfenbrenner & Morris, 2006; Connor et al., 2016). Differentiated instruction allows for teachers to respond to differences in students' reading skills and their learning profiles so that all students in the classroom may be more successful (Tomlinson & Jarvis, 2009). Importantly, as the field of special education has moved toward the use of an inclusion model for educating children with learning disabilities and as classrooms have become more ethnically diverse and poverty has increased over the past two decades (Kena et al., 2016), educators have been pushed to thoughtfully consider how to provide instruction that meets the individual needs of all children.

Despite the growing evidence that individualized instruction may be more beneficial for students, delivering individualized instruction has still proven to be quite difficult (Tomlinson, 2014). Providing students with differentiated instruction requires flexibility in grouping, instruction, and assessment in order to foster the optimal learning environment for each student. However, delivering individualized instruction can be overwhelming for many teachers who already feel pressure from increased teaching demands and larger class sizes. Effective and high-quality differentiated instruction also often requires professional development training, administrative support, and additional materials—all of which contribute to the challenges for schools and teachers to provide individualized instruction.

A response-to-intervention (RTI) model has been a widely used approach to differentiated instruction since the reauthorization of IDEA in 2004 (Watts-Taffe et al., 2012). While research on RTI programs has mostly focused on improving the more intensive Tiers 2 and 3, much less work has prioritized core Tier 1 instruction. Nevertheless, providing more effective and differentiated core instruction at Tier 1 can prevent students from having to move to Tier 2 or Tier 3 intervention levels (Jones et al., 2012); thus, tailoring instruction to meet the individual needs of students at Tier 1 is also an important consideration. While individualizing instruction for an entire classroom of children with varying abilities may seem a daunting task, easy-to-administer, economical, and data-driven assessment and intervention tools for teachers can be used to help target and individualize instruction at Tier 1 more accurately and efficiently (Yeh, 2010).

Theoretical Considerations in Individualizing Literacy Instruction

A thoughtful discussion of how best to individualize instruction for children learning to read requires a clear conceptualization of what is meant by reading. Some have advocated for a narrow view of reading, confining the discussion of reading to a discussion of word or character recognition (e.g., Kamhi, 2009), arguing that comprehension is difficult to quantify in any kind of domain-general way. This is because a substantial amount of the variance in how well a student understands a given text is explained by how much they already know (i.e., their background knowledge) about the content of that text (Kendeou et al., 2003; Hirsch, 2006; Willingham, 2006), the text itself (what they are reading), and the activity (why they are reading) (Collins et al., 2020). Comprehension outcomes may also vary widely depending on the measure of comprehension used (Cutting & Scarborough, 2006; Keenan et al., 2008). Indeed, comprehension is a much broader and more difficult-to-measure construct than word reading, being likened by Perfetti (1986) to *thinking guided by print*. In contrast, Snow and Mathews (2016) refer to word reading and the skills that underlie it as constrained skills, in that they are finite and there is a clear scope and sequence for teaching them. We find the narrow view of reading attractive for its clarity, simplicity, and acknowledgment of the complexities of measuring reading comprehension. However, when thinking about the implications of this theoretical model for teaching reading, there is concern that this narrow conception would lead to neglect of the decades of research establishing the foundational nature of oral language skills for successful reading (Hogan et al., 2014; Snow, 1991; Snowling & Hulme, 2012; Storch & Whitehurst, 2002).

Related to both the conceptualization of what reading is and the relative ease of measurement of decoding skills compared to comprehension skills, the idea of screening for reading disabilities has historically focused on screening for word-reading difficulties (Coyne & Harne, 2006; Good et al., 2004). However, there is good evidence to support that screening for oral language difficulties can lead to identification of children who will struggle with reading due to weaknesses in their oral language (Adlof & Hogan, 2012; Catts et al., 2001). In early grades, children with underlying language difficulties may appear to be typical readers because the texts children are asked to read tend to consist of very simple language, and decoding skills capture the majority of variance in reading comprehension (Catts et al., 2005; García & Cain, 2014; Language and Reading Research Consortium [LARRC], 2015).

When children transition to reading more decontextualized and complex texts in third grade and beyond, the demands on oral language increase dramatically, and expectedly, oral language begins to explain more variance in reading comprehension (Catts et al., 2006; Foorman et al., 2018; LARRC, 2015). This is also a time when children who had previously seemed to be typically developing readers may suddenly begin to struggle with reading comprehension. Many times, this struggle is related to undetected weaknesses in language that may have been identified with an early screening of oral language abilities (Adlof & Hogan, 2019; Catts et al., 2012) and attended to via appropriately individualized instruction.

We then turn to perhaps the most well-known theory of reading comprehension—the Simple View of Reading (SVR) (Hoover & Gough, 1990). Substantial support exists for the SVR that holds that reading comprehension is the product of readers' skills within *two* major domains, decoding skills and linguistic comprehension (e.g., Catts et al., 2003; Gough & Tunmer, 1986; Hoover & Gough, 1990). Simply put, if one could validly and reliably measure a student's ability to read words and their ability to understand oral language of a complexity akin with that found in written text, one could explain almost all of the variance in student's reading comprehension (LARRC, 2015; Lervåg et al., 2018; Petersen et al., 2020). Snow and Mathews (2016) refer to the types of language abilities that underlie reading comprehension, such as vocabulary and background knowledge, as a set of unconstrained skills that will be learned across the lifespan but that are essential to students' long-term reading outcomes.

With a good grasp on the predictors of reading comprehension, there is a strong theoretical foundation for recommending what reading instruction should look like. In accordance with the SVR, Connor and colleagues (Connor, Morrison,

& Katch, 2004) conceptualized reading instruction as either pertaining to code-focused (CF) or meaning-focused (MF) skills. CF teaching encompasses phonological awareness, alphabet knowledge, phonics, word reading, and reading fluency—essentially everything that is needed to "crack the code" of how written language maps to its spoken form. There is extensive evidence that explicitly teaching CF skills leads to improved reading comprehension via improved word reading in English (Castles et al., 2018; National Reading Panel, 2000; Rayner et al., 2001; Rose, 2006). MF teaching encompasses the array of skills children need to extract and construct meaning from text (Snow, 2002). Vocabulary, grammar, building background knowledge, asking comprehension questions, discussion of texts read in class, silent independent reading, and any activity that requires interacting with the meaning of written language would fall under the umbrella of MF instruction. MF instruction is certainly broader and has less clear starting and stopping points, but there is good evidence that it is also an important lever for improving reading comprehension (Beck et al., 1982; Cabell & Hwang, 2020; Clarke et al., 2010; Elleman et al., 2009; Goldman et al., 2016; LARRC et al., 2019; LARRC & Logan, 2017; National Reading Panel, 2000; Williams et al., 2009). Perhaps the conclusion seems simplistic—if we know that reading comprehension is a product of word-reading and language comprehension skills, then teach children how to read words and understand language. Although indeed this is an oversimplified statement, it serves as a foundational guiding principle of teaching reading. However, as any teacher will tell you, children come to the classroom with varying language abilities and emergent literacy skills, meaning that the exact same instruction will impact children differently. That is, there are child × instruction interactions that need to be considered in the context of teaching reading.

Child-by-Instruction Interactions in Reading

Originally conceived as aptitude-by-treatment interactions (ATI) (Cronbach & Snow, 1969), research on child characteristics-by-instruction (CXI) interactions has grown over the past decade. Research has strongly supported the importance of understanding the impact that individual child differences and CXI interactions have on the effect of reading instruction (Connor, Morrison, & Petrella, 2004; Tobin & McInnes, 2008; Connor, Jakobsons, et al., 2009; Al Otaiba et al., 2011; Connor & Morrison, 2016; Förster et al., 2018; Bondie et al., 2019; Lyon et al., 2020).

While the idea of students having individual or unique needs does not sound groundbreaking, finding empirical evidence for these individual differences amongst students is not a simple task. While the concept and potential importance of aptitude X treatment interactions were introduced in the late 1960s, it was not until much later that study results began to reveal how this interaction may play out for students during literacy instruction. In one of the earliest studies to report these types of interactions, Foorman and colleagues (1998) reported that students entering the school year with weak phonemic awareness skills showed more growth in CF (decoding) skills over a school year when compared to their peers beginning the year with higher phonological awareness. Similarly, Juel and Minden-Cupp (2000) found that the first-grade children with weaker reading skills made more progress when instruction was focused on word recognition, and children with stronger reading skills demonstrated better literacy outcomes when the teacher focused on more text-based instruction, with less emphasis on foundational (CF) skills.

The next iteration of this work involved the creation of classroom observation systems capable of recording the instructional experiences of individual students in a classroom. Maintaining a focus on the experience of the child was critical. While many observation systems capture instruction at the classroom or teacher level, this observational coding system (what would evolve into the Individualizing Student Instruction [ISI] classroom observation system) was unique in that it focused on the instruction received by individual students (Connor, Morrison, et al., 2009). Through this observational system, it was revealed that different students, even if they are in the same classroom, can have different instructional experiences. In turn, these differences in the amounts and type of instruction received led to predictable differences in student outcomes, that is, child × instruction interactions (read as "child-by-instruction" interactions).

In addition to solving the challenge of observing multiple students at the same time in a classroom, multiple iterations of the ISI classroom observation system were required to determine precisely what to capture in order to accurately identify and record meaningful units of literacy instruction. The macro-categories established by the ISI system allowed a framework to be established that could be used to describe which child-level and instruction-based characteristics were driving the interactions. This framework, also guided in part by the SVR proposed by Gough and Tunmer (1986), provides a useful way to summarize the impact of students' entry-level skills on their reading progress.

Connor and colleagues ultimately settled on a set of four variables that formed a two-by-two matrix of important types of instruction. As mentioned, the final consensus was consistent with the SVR and divided the "content of instruction" into two types, MF and CF. Two instructional groupings were also used, distinguished by who managed children's attention in learning—the child or the teacher. By identifying both the content of instruction and who was managing the students' learning, reading instruction could be placed into one of four quadrants. Figure 21.1 provides examples of each of the four types of instruction. While this final result is a relatively simple taxonomy, important amounts of variance in children's reading growth can be predicted simply by knowing how much of each type of instruction children had received across a school year. The final iteration of the coding system for classroom observations tracked the amount of time students spent in each of these four areas (Connor, Morrison, et al., 2009).

Using Algorithms to Guide Instruction and Predict Child-by-Instruction Interactions

Once the four dimensions of literacy instruction were identified as the potential drivers for identifying child × instruction interactions, the next step was to

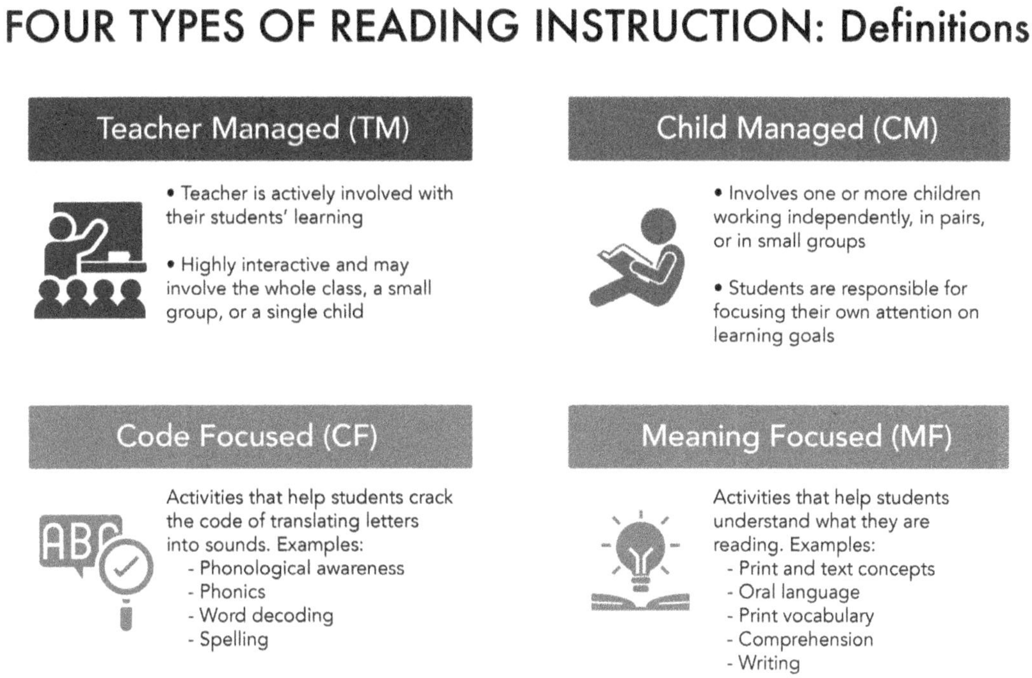

FIGURE 21.1. The four types of reading instruction.

determine what combination of code- and meaning-focused instruction, delivered during child- or teacher-managed time (CM or TM), was most beneficial for students of varying skill profiles. To do this, a series of algorithms were created and tested to determine how best to differentiate instruction for students, and these algorithms were embedded into a new software called Assessment to Instruction (A2i) (Connor et al., 2007). The algorithms were based on student ability in decoding, comprehension, and vocabulary, and multiple assessments were successfully used to quantify these skills and serve as inputs for the algorithms (e.g., the Woodcock-Johnson III sub-tests, the Gates-MacGinitie Reading Test, DIBELS, GRADE, and the A2i Online Assessments).

The algorithms that utilize the assessment information were generated using classroom observation data. The observational codes for the four dimensions of reading instruction, along with student assessment data across the school year, were used to reverse-engineer the ideal amounts and types of instruction students received in the classroom, resulting in the best literacy outcomes by the end of the school year. This work revealed that instructional needs changed across the school year and, in many cases, were not linear between content areas or time, as shown in Figure 21.2.

Once the algorithms had been created and student assessment data was available (for decoding, comprehension, and vocabulary skills), it was possible to test how child × instruction interactions could actually impact student achievement. These studies utilized a novel metric, called "distance from recommendation," that

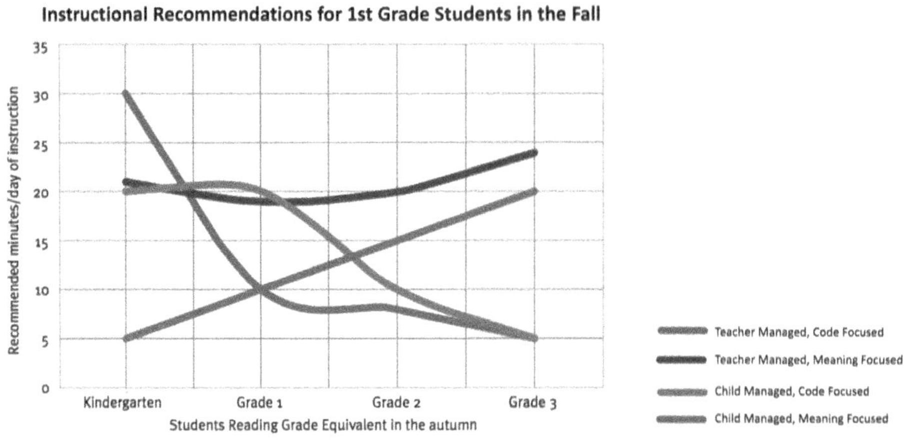

FIGURE 21.2. Instructional recommendations for first-grade students in the fall. *Note:* This figure demonstrates how student instructional needs can vary within a single classroom or grade. The *x*-axis indicates possible reading-levels for students entering first grade in the fall (beginning) of the school year. The *y*-axis indicates the daily instruction recommendations in minutes. Grade 1 students entering first grade on-level need approximately 10 minutes of TM-CF instruction per day. In contrast, first-grade students beginning the school year reading at a kindergarten level need 30 minutes per day of TM-CF time.

was calculated by determining the difference between the instructional time a student actually spent in each of the four dimensions of instruction and the amount of instructional time the algorithms predicted would be most effective. For example, a student in a classroom observation may be recorded as receiving 15 minutes of TM-CF instruction, while the algorithms reported the ideal instructional time for that same student was actually 25 minutes of TM-CF instruction. In this example, the distance from recommendation value would be 10 minutes.

In addition to the child × instruction interactions focused on the time in either meaning- or CF instruction, research has also shown that, in kindergarten through third grade classrooms, teachers who provided individualized instruction by utilizing small groups (rather than just whole-class instruction) and varying the amount of code- and meaning-focused instruction based on students' needs had students who made greater gains in reading. In classrooms where the A2i software platform was used with associated professional development (called the ISI intervention in most studies), students made greater gains when compared to students who received instruction without guidance from A2i, especially when it was delivered in a small-group setting (Connor, Morrison, et al., 2009; Al Otaiba et al., 2011; Connor, Morrison, Fishman, et al., 2011). This demonstrates that, while both meaning- and code-focused instruction are important for learning to read, the effect of instruction may also vary depending on the individual skills and needs of students in the classroom as well as the context or delivery of said instruction.

As described earlier, proficient reading ability is driven by both language comprehension and decoding ability. These constructs not only represent the possible profiles of students learning to read but are also the key components used to predict what amounts and types of instruction would benefit a student most during literacy instruction. To illuminate this in more detail, the following sections outline the evidence for child × instruction interactions in detail for both code- and meaning-focused instruction.

Evidence for Code-Focused Child × Instruction Effects

Multiple studies focused on providing students with tailored amounts of CF instruction have consistently demonstrated the impact this individualization of instruction has on student outcomes in word reading. In 2007, Connor and colleagues found that first graders who participated in classrooms where A2i was used demonstrated more growth in decoding skills across the school year when compared to children in control classrooms where A2i was not used; this was particularly true for children who started the school year with lower language skills. With another group of first graders, Connor, Piasta, and colleagues (2009) found that students who got TM-CF instruction that aligned well with the recommended amounts from the A2i algorithms demonstrated more growth in decoding skills across the school year than children who received instruction misaligned to their instructional needs. Children with weaker fall word recognition skills (i.e., below grade expectations) demonstrated more growth in decoding skills when they were in classrooms where teachers provided greater amounts of TM-CF instruction than did children with similar skills in classrooms where smaller amounts of this type of instruction were observed. In contrast, children with stronger fall word recognition skills showed less progress in classrooms where greater amounts of TM-CF instruction were observed.

In the largest study of the effects of the use of A2i on reading outcomes, Connor and colleagues (2013) found that children in first, second, and third grade all benefited from the ISI intervention as measured by their accelerated growth in word-reading skills across the school year as compared to a control group (d = 0.32, d = 0.44, and d = 0.25, respectively). Additionally, this study followed students who had been provided A2i in 0, 1, 2, or 3 years while they progressed from first to third grade. Results showed that reading gains continued to accumulate for children when the child × instruction interactions (via the A2i algorithms) were provided to teachers and used to guide instruction across multiple grades. Students who had been in A2i classrooms for 3 years in a row showed average reading achievement results well above grade level in third grade (grade equivalent of 5.0 on a nationally standardized reading test). Within intervention classrooms, the relative importance of distance from recommendation was greatest for students beginning the year well above or well below grade level, that is, the students least likely to receive instruction precisely aligned to the algorithm recommendations (Connor, Morrison, Fishman, et al., 2011). The most recent work exploring the impact of A2i use on children's outcomes demonstrates promise that A2i is also effective at improving the CF skills of children who are English learners (Connor et al., 2022).

These studies led to evidence-based recommendations for provision of CF instruction in early elementary grades; that is, students whose decoding skills are above grade level need relatively small amounts of daily, TM-CF instruction. In contrast, students whose skills fall below grade level require exponentially more time in CF instruction, especially as they fall further behind grade-level expectations. In addition, while instruction can be provided in small groups or to the whole class, teacher-managed/code-focused (TM-CF) instruction is 4 to 10 times more effective when provided in small groups (Connor, 2014; Connor et al., 2006). Finally, for code-focused instruction, it does appear possible to have "too much of a good thing," as students who received CF instruction in amounts well above the recommended time actually showed reduced rates of growth on reading skills (Connor, Morrison, Fishman, et al., 2011).

Evidence for Meaning-Focused Child × Instruction Effects

Instruction on the meaning and understanding of both spoken and written language is critical as students learn to read and, not surprisingly, is also impacted by child × instruction interactions. For *teacher-managed* instruction on MF lessons, the total (raw) amount of instruction received predicted better student outcomes on passage comprehension. However, time spent on *child-managed*/meaning-focused (CM-MF) activities impacted students' passage comprehension growth differently, depending on their vocabulary skills at the beginning of the school year (Connor et al., 2007).

More specifically, when first-grade teachers provided students with CM-MF lessons close to the A2i algorithm-recommended amounts, more growth was observed in their students' decoding and comprehension scores across the school year (Connor, Piasta, et al., 2009). Students who started first grade with lower vocabulary skills demonstrated greater growth in word recognition skills when they received smaller amounts of CM-MF instruction in the fall, with steady increases for the rest of the school year. Conversely, students with low vocabulary skills at the beginning of the school year who received greater amounts of CM-MF instruction consistently all year long showed weaker gains. These results reveal that the management of MF instruction appears to be particularly important consideration for maximizing student growth.

Receiving opportunities for CM-MF time was also impacted by child × instruction interactions in older (third-grade) students (Connor, Morrison, Fishman, et al., 2011). The magnitude of students' gains increased with increased teacher-managed/meaning-focused instruction precision as it relates to the instructional algorithm minute recommendations; the more aligned the actual instructional MF time was to the A2i recommendations, the greater their growth on the reading comprehension measure. In general, it appears that MF instruction has a positive effect on reading skills for most students (regardless of differences they may have in reading skills), especially when the instruction is teacher-managed. Some studies have revealed preliminary evidence of child × instruction interactions for TM-MF instruction (Connor, Morrison, & Katch, 2004; Connor, Jakobsons, et al., 2009), although differences in whole-class versus small-group instruction make it difficult to fully understand the interactions. Regardless, the MF results clearly demonstrate the importance of this type of instruction for all students.

CHILD × INSTRUCTION INTERACTION: EXAMPLE 1

This first example, depicted in Figure 21.3, illustrates how the same amount of child-managed instruction can be associated with very different outcomes for first graders who enter the grade with different levels of vocabulary knowledge. The *x*-axis is the average amount of child-managed instruction observed per day in different classrooms (e.g., silent reading, journaling, students working in pairs, and workbooks). As is evident in the figure, classrooms varied widely in how much time children spent working on their own (16–37 minutes, see numbers on the *x*-axis). The *y*-axis is children's decoding score in the spring—their word-identification skills as measured on a nationally standardized test. For students who entered first grade with a high level of vocabulary knowledge (scoring better than 75% of their peers), more time spent in child-managed instruction was associated with better reading outcomes (Connor, Morrison, & Katch, 2004). This finding is indicated by the steep incline in the solid line depicting how reading outcomes varied at different amounts of minutes spent in child-managed instruction.

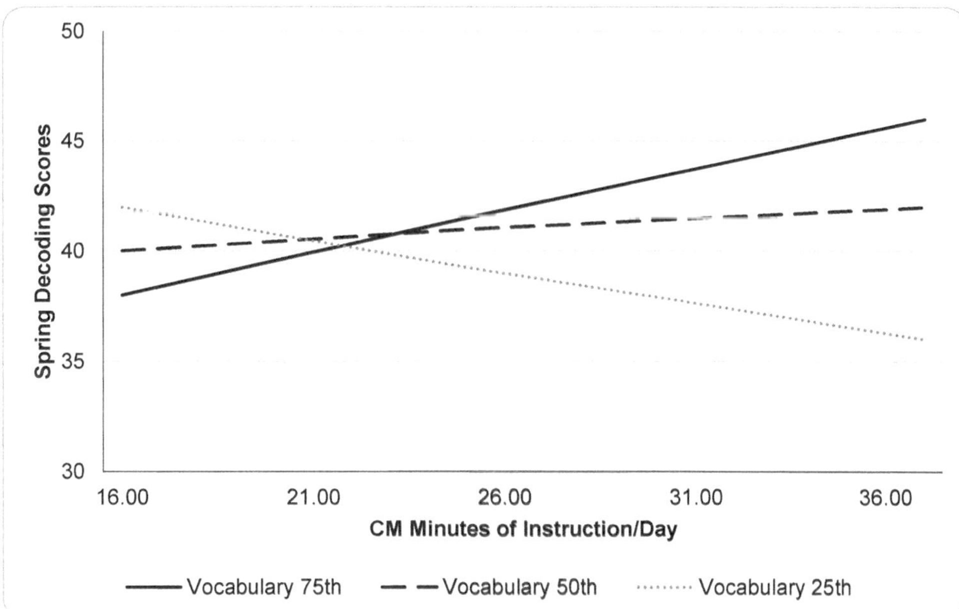

FIGURE 21.3. Child × instruction type interaction effect for spring decoding raw scores.

Conversely, for students who entered with low vocabulary skills (scoring better than only 25% of their peers), more time spent in child-managed instruction was associated with lower word-reading skills, as indicated by the steep decline in the dotted line linking reading outcomes and minutes of child-managed instruction for this group. Children who were in the average range (50th percentile) in vocabulary skills had similar word-reading skills regardless of the minutes of child-managed instruction. Note that only at about 22 minutes of child-managed instruction per day did the three lines showing the relationship between minutes in child-managed instruction and decoding scores for the three groups of students with different entry-decoding skills intersect, indicating similar word-reading outcomes for all groups of students.

CHILD × INSTRUCTION INTERACTION: EXAMPLE 2

This second example, shown in Figure 21.4, illustrates the extent to which the "fit" of an instructional pattern with a child's needs can be associated with better or poorer reading outcomes. In this example, gains in decoding skills are contrasted but only for the subgroup of first graders who had low fall vocabulary scores and low decoding skills (25th percentile for each skill). Although the entire group started at the same place at the beginning of the year (scoring about half a year below grade level), where children ended the year varied systematically with the pattern of instruction they received during the year, children who got smaller amounts of teacher-managed explicit instruction (e.g., instruction in word segmentation and letter sounds) and greater amounts of child-managed

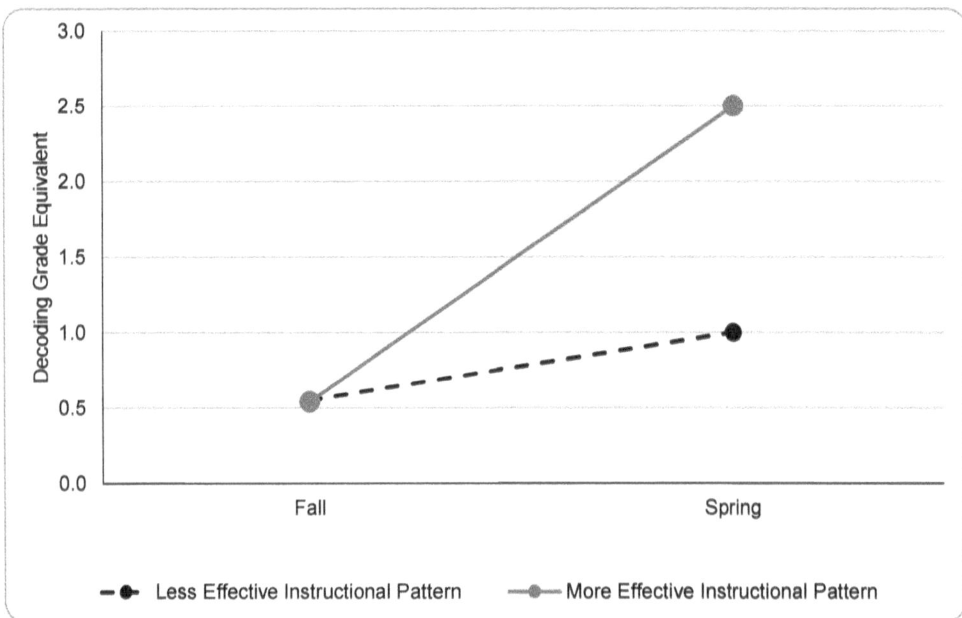

FIGURE 21.4. Growth in decoding skill over a school year by effectiveness of instruction.

implicit instruction (e.g., reading or writing on their own or in groups) made very modest gains and ended the year further behind their peers (Connor, Morrison, & Katch, 2004). The decoding skill gain for children who got this ineffective pattern is depicted in Figure 21.4 with the dashed line. Children who received substantial amounts of teacher-managed explicit instruction, paired with smaller amounts of child-managed implicit instruction that increased across the year made large gains in decoding skills. By the end of the year, the students who had this pattern now scored an average grade equivalent of 2.5 in decoding. The decoding skill gain for students who got this more effective pattern is depicted in Figure 21.4 by the solid line.

It is important to note that these particular patterns of instruction and student outcomes only hold for a specific group of students. Said another way, the specific group of students who entered first grade with higher levels of decoding and language skills made more growth in decoding skills if they had greater amounts of child-managed implicit instruction. This means that the patterns of amounts and types of reading instruction across the year were only more or less effective when considered with the children's initial decoding and language skills.

Using Child × Instruction Interactions to Improve Practice

Including the first experimental field test of A2i published in 2007, seven articles summarizing the results of randomized controlled trials of A2i have now been published. These rigorous studies demonstrate the efficacy of the strategy for using assessment and child × instruction interaction information to guide instruction and the importance of moving beyond a one-size-fits-all model of reading instruction. Three of the studies have been reviewed by the *What Works Clearinghouse*, and all met the standards, two without reservations (Connor, Morrison, Fishman, et al., 2011; Connor, Morrison, Schatschneider, et al., 2011; Connor et al., 2013).

The level of research accumulated on this topic serves as a critical point of reference for elementary school teachers looking for effective instructional practices to follow during their literacy block. The potential impact goes beyond the individual study results, as the longitudinal results also reveal; there is a cumulative impact of using child × instruction to guide instruction over multiple years. However, these findings have additional implications as well. One critical implication to consider is the fact that instructional methods that do not incorporate a dynamic approach that can be customized to meet the individual needs of students will be less effective at meeting the needs of all students (i.e., a traditional curriculum that does not include opportunities for differentiation). In the same way, instructional methods that adhere to a one-size-fits-all model or claims that more instructional time is always better have been disproven by the body of work Dr. Connor and colleagues have compiled (Connor, 2017).

Beginning in 2017, the A2i Professional Support System became a central component of one of the largest early literacy scale-up projects in the United States, focused on how to effectively bring proven evidence-based solutions into the classroom (Grant U411A170011). Funded by the U.S. Department of Education, this work is focused on bringing rigorously tested interventions to practice at scale. The A2i recommendations have been used in classrooms across the United States that are extremely diverse and multifaceted. A2i has supported teachers to respond to this range of student needs through better individualization and planning for small-group instruction based on the recommendations informed by the child × instruction interactions. A preliminary analysis conducted in 2022, based on data from 3,741 students across 29 schools, revealed that teachers with consistent A2i usage (at least logging on every 10 days) had 22% higher average growth rates for their students (on the A2i Online Assessment called Letters2Meaning) when compared to teachers logging on less consistently. Additional reports and results of this work will be available when the final United2Read report is published.

Implications for Child × Instruction Interactions and Students with Disabilities

Implementing our knowledge of child × instruction interactions and using the framework of recommending minutes of instruction tailored to each child's learning needs may be supportive of children with disabilities. We can think about this impact in several ways. First, if a child's teacher is meeting the recommended minutes but the child is not advancing at the expected pace, this information could inform the decision to provide additional small-group and individualized opportunities for learning in a multi-tiered system of support (MTSS) framework (Tier 2). Alternatively, if the results of the child assessments lead to a recommendation for more minutes of instruction in a given area (e.g., TM-CF activities) than what is feasible in the general education classroom, this may provide evidence to support Tier 3 intervention. Ongoing work to evaluate the Dynamic Forecasting Intervention (DFI) algorithms with children with severe literacy disabilities is using extant assessment and observation data to run simulations of the impact of various algorithms on students' gains during the school year. As part of these simulations, investigators are evaluating whether the predictability of DFI algorithms can be improved by changing the coefficients for language and literacy ability, adding other child characteristics (e.g., family history, writing skills, social skills, executive function, self-regulation, more complex aspects of oral language [lexical knowledge is already used in the DFI models], and family history) or other types of intervention, including assistive technologies (e.g., text-to-speech, speech-to-text, and keyboarding). The goal of this body of work continues to be supporting each child in reaching their full potential for successful reading.

Final Thoughts: The Importance of Individualizing Instruction

Educational research often validates reading practices for particular types of learners, such as children reading at grade level, children at risk for learning disabilities, or children who are English language learners (ELLs) (Scammacca et al., 2015; Al Otaiba et al., 2008; Swanson et al., 2017). But what if all these children are in the same class? Knowing to whom research findings apply and then figuring out how to integrate research-based practices into a busy classroom where children have very different needs can be difficult. The dilemma of which research-based practices to implement, and for whom, is one facet of the implementation gap that often prevents research-based practices from improving outcomes for children when they are implemented in real-world classrooms (Fixsen et al., 2005).

To support teachers in meeting this challenge, rigorous studies (as described earlier) have investigated and established both the existence of child × instruction interactions (Connor et al., 2007, 2013; Connor, Jakobsons, et al., 2009; Connor, Morrison, et al., 2009; Connor, Piasta, et al., 2009; Foorman et al., 1998) and highlighted the beneficial role technology can play in supporting teachers' response to these interactions (Connor, 2017). Ultimately, the accumulation of this work can be summarized by stating that, when teachers are given instructional recommendations based on child × instruction interactions, they are able to effectively use this information to guide their instructional moves and improve student reading outcomes.

REFERENCES

Adlof, S. M., & Hogan, T. P. (2019). If we don't look, we won't see: Measuring language development to inform literacy instruction. *Policy Insights from the Behavioral and Brain Sciences, 6*(2), 210–217.

Al Otaiba, S., Connor, C. M., Folsom, J. S., Greulich, L., Meadows, J., & Li, Z. (2011). Assessment data-informed guidance to individualized kindergarten reading instruction: Findings from a cluster-randomized control field trial. *The Elementary School Journal, 111*(4), 535–560.

Al Otaiba, S., Connor, C., Lane, H., Kosanovich, M. L., Schatschneider, C., Dyrlund, A. K., et al. (2008). Reading First kindergarten classroom instruction and students' growth in phonological awareness and letter naming-decoding fluency. *Journal of School Psychology, 46*(3), 281–314.

Beck, I. L., Perfetti, C. A., & McKeown, M. G. (1982). Effects of long-term vocabulary instruction on lexical access and reading comprehension. *Journal of Educational Psychology, 74*(4), 506.

Bondie, R. S., Dahnke, C., & Zusho, A. (2019). How does changing "one-size-fits-all" to differentiated instruction affect teaching? *Review of Research in Education, 43*(1), 336–362.

Bronfenbrenner, U., & Morris, P. A. (2006). The bioecological model of human development. In W. Damon & R. M. Lerner (Eds.), *Handbook of child psychology, Vol. 1: Theoretical models of human development* (6th ed., pp. 793–828). Wiley.

Cabell, S. Q., & Hwang, H. (2020). Building content knowledge to boost comprehension in the primary grades. *Reading Research Quarterly*, 55(S1), S99–S107.

Castles, A., Rastle, K., & Nation, K. (2018). Ending the reading wars: Reading acquisition from novice to expert. *Psychological Science in the Public Interest, 19*(1), 5–51.

Catts, H. W., Adlof, S. M., Hogan, T., & Weismer, S. E. (2005). Are specific language impairment and dyslexia distinct disorders? *Journal of Speech, Language, and Hearing Research, 48*(6), 1378–1396.

Catts, H. W., Adlof, S. M., & Weismer, S. E. (2006). Language deficits in poor comprehenders: A case for the Simple View of Reading. *Journal of Speech, Language, and Hearing Research, 49*(2), 278–293.

Catts, H. W., Compton, D., Tomblin, J. B., & Bridges, M. S. (2012). Prevalence and nature of late-emerging poor readers. *Journal of Educational Psychology, 104*(1), 166.

Catts, H. W., Fey, M. E., Zhang, X., & Tomblin, J. B. (2001). Estimating the risk of future reading difficulties in kindergarten children: A research-based model and its clinical implementation. *Language Speech and Hearing Services in Schools, 32*, 38–50.

Catts, H. W., Hogan, T. P., & Fey, M. E. (2003). Subgrouping poor readers on the basis of individual differences in reading-related abilities. *Journal of Learning Disabilities, 36*(2), 151–164.

Clarke, P. J., Snowling, M. J., Truelove, E., & Hulme, C. (2010). Ameliorating children's reading-comprehension difficulties: A randomized controlled trial. *Psychological Science, 21*(8), 1106–1116.

Collins, A. A., Compton, D. L., Lindström, E. R., & Gilbert, J. K. (2020). Performance variations across reading comprehension assessments: Examining the unique contributions of text, activity, and reader. *Reading and Writing, 33*(3), 605–634.

Connor, C. M. (2014). Individualizing teaching in beginning reading. In *Better: Evidence-based education* (pp. 3–7). Institute for Effective Education, University of York.

Connor, C. M. (2017). Using technology and assessment to personalize instruction: Preventing reading problems. *Prevention Science, 20*, 89–99.

Connor, C. M., Day, S. L., Phillips, B., Sparapani, N., Ingebrand, S. W., McLean, L., et al. (2016). Reciprocal effects of self-regulation, semantic knowledge, and reading comprehension in early elementary school. *Child Development, 87*(6), 1813–1824. Connor, C. M., Jakobsons, L. J., Crowe, E. C., & Meadows, J. G. (2009). Instruction, student engagement, and reading skill growth in reading first classrooms. *Elementary School Journal, 109*(3), 221–250.

Connor, C. M., May, H., Sparapani, N., Hwang, J. K., Adams, A., Wood, T. S., et al. (2022). Bringing Assessment-to-Instruction (A2i) technology to scale: Exploring the process from development to implementation. *Journal of Educational Psychology, 114*(7), 1495.

Connor, C. M., & Morrison, F. J. (2016). Individualizing student instruction in reading implications for policy and practice. *Policy Insights from the Behavioral and Brain Sciences, 3*(1), 54–61.

Connor, C. M., Morrison, F. J., Fishman, B., Crowe, E. C., Al Otaiba, S., & Schatschneider, C. (2013). A longitudinal cluster-randomized controlled study on the accumulating effects of individualized literacy instruction on students' reading from first through third grade. *Psychological Science, 24*(8), 1408–1419.

Connor, C. M., Morrison, F. J., Fishman, B., Giuliani, S., Luck, M., Underwood, P. S., et al. (2011). Testing the impact of child characteristics × instruction interactions on third graders' reading literacy instruction. *Reading Research Quarterly, 46*(3), 189–221.

Connor, C. M., Morrison, F. J., Fishman, B. J., Ponitz, C. C., Glasney, S., Underwood, P. S., et al. (2009). The ISI classroom observation system: Examining the literacy instruction provided to individual students. *Educational Researcher, 38*(2), 85–99.

Connor, C. M., Morrison, F. J., Fishman, B. J., Schatschneider, C., & Underwood, P. (2007). Algorithm-guided individualized reading instruction. *Science*, 315(2007), 464–465.

Connor, C. M., Morrison, F. J., & Katch, L. E. (2004). Beyond the reading wars: Exploring the effect of child-instruction interactions on growth in early reading. *Scientific Studies of Reading, 8*(4), 305–336.

Connor, C. M., Morrison, F. J., & Petrella, J. (2004). Effective reading comprehension instruction: Examining child × instruction interactions. *Journal of Educational Psychology, 96*, 682–698.

Connor, C. M., Morrison, F. J., Schatschneider, C., Toste, J. R., Lundblom, E., Crowe, E. C., & Fishman, B. (2011). Effective classroom instruction: Implications of child characteristics by reading instruction interactions on first graders' word reading achievement. *Journal of Research on Educational Effectiveness, 4*(3), 173–207.

Connor, C. M., Morrison, F. J., & Slominski, L. (2006). Preschool instruction and children's emergent literacy growth. *Journal of Educational Psychology, 98*(4), 665–689.

Connor, C. M., Piasta, S. B., Fishman, B., Glasney, S., Schatschneider, C., Crowe, E., et al.

(2009). Individualizing student instruction precisely: Effects of child × instruction interactions on first graders' literacy development. *Child Development, 80*(1), 77–100.

Coyne, M. D., & Harne, B. (2006). Promoting beginning reading success through meaningful assessment of early literacy skills. *Psychology in the Schools, 43*, 33–43.

Cronbach, L. J., & Snow, R. E. (1969). *Individual differences in learning ability as a function of instructional variables. Final report. https://eric.ed.gov/?id=ED029001*

Cutting, L., & Scarborough, H. S. (2006) Prediction of reading comprehension: Relative contributions of word recognition, language proficiency, and other cognitive skills can depend on how comprehension is measured. *Scientific Studies of Reading, 10*(3), 277–299.

Elleman, A. M., Lindo, E. J., Morphy, P., & Compton, D. L. (2009). The impact of vocabulary instruction on passage-level comprehension of school-age children: A meta-analysis. *Journal of Research on Educational Effectiveness, 2*(1), 1–44.

Fixsen, D. L., Naoom, S. F., Blasé, K. A., Friedman. R. M., & Wallace, F. (2005). *Implementation matters: A synthesis of the literature* (FMHI Publication #231). University of South Florida, Louis de la Oarte Florida Mental Health Institute, National Implementation Research Network.

Foorman, B. R., Francis, D. J., Fletcher, J. M., Schatschneider, C., & Mehta, P. (1998). The role of instruction in learning to read: Preventing reading failure in at risk children. *Journal of Educational Psychology, 90*, 37–55.

Foorman, B. R., Petscher, Y., & Herrera, S. (2018). Unique and common effects of decoding and language factors in predicting reading comprehension in grades 1–10. *Learning and Individual Differences, 63*, 12–23.

Förster, N., Kawohl, E., & Souvignier, E. (2018). Short- and long-term effects of assessment-based differentiated reading instruction in general education on reading fluency and reading comprehension. *Learning and Instruction, 56*, 98–109.

García, J. R., & Cain, K. (2014). Decoding and reading comprehension: A meta-analysis to identify which reader and assessment characteristics influence the strength of the relationship in English. *Review of Educational Research, 84*(1), 74–111.

Goldman, S. R., Snow, C., & Vaughn, S. (2016). Common themes in teaching reading for understanding: Lessons from three projects. *Journal of Adolescent & Adult Literacy, 60*, 255–264.

Good, R. H., Kaminski, R. A., Shinn, M., Bratten, J., Shinn, M., Laimon, D., et al. (2004). *Technical adequacy of DIBELS: Results of the Early Childhood Research Institute on measuring growth and development* (Technical Report, No. 7). University of Oregon.

Gough, P. B., & Tumner, W. E. (1986). Decoding, reading, and reading disability. *Remedial and Special Education, 7*, 6–10.

Hirsch, E. D. (2006). *The knowledge deficit: Closing the shocking education gap for American children*. Houghton Mifflin.

Hogan, T. P., Adlof, S. M., & Alonzo, C. N. (2014). On the importance of listening comprehension. *International Journal of Speech-Language Pathology, 16*(3), 199–207.

Hoover, W. A., & Gough, P. B. (1990). The Simple View of Reading. *Reading and Writing: An Interdisciplinary Journal, 2*(2), 127–160.

Individuals with Disabilities Education Act, 20 U.S.C. § 1400 (2004).

Jones, R. E., Yssel, N., & Grant, C. (2012). Reading instruction in Tier 1: Bridging the gaps by nesting evidence-based interventions within differentiated instruction. *Psychology in the Schools, 49*(3), 210–218.

Juel, C., & Minden-Cupp, C. (2000). Learning to read words: Linguistic units and instructional strategies. *Reading Research Quarterly, 35*, 458–492.

Kamhi, A. (2009). The case for the narrow view of reading. *Language, Speech, and Hearing Services in Schools, 40*, 174–177.

Keenan, J. M., Betjemann, R. S., & Olson, R. K. (2008). Reading comprehension tests vary in the skills they assess: Differential dependence on decoding and oral comprehension. *Scientific Studies of Reading, 12*(3), 281–300.

Kena, G., Hussar, W., de Bray, C., Musu-Gillette, L., Wang, X., Zhang, J., & Dunlop Velez, E. (2016). *The condition of education 2016* (No. NCES 2016-144). U.S. Department of Education, National Center for Education Statistics. *http://nces.ed.gov/pubsearch*

Kendeou, P., Rapp, D. N., & van den Broek, P. (2003). The influence of reader's prior knowledge on text comprehension and learning from text. In R. Nata (Ed.), *Progress in education* (Vol. 13, pp. 189–209). Nova Science Publishers.

Language and Reading Research Consortium. (2015). Learning to read: Should we keep things simple? *Reading Research Quarterly, 50*(2), 151–169.

Language and Reading Research Consortium, Jiang, H., & Logan, J. (2019). Improving reading comprehension in the primary grades: Mediated effects of a language-focused classroom intervention. *Journal of Speech, Language, and Hearing Research, 62*(8), 2812–2828.

Language and Reading Research Consortium, & Logan, J. (2017). Pressure points in reading comprehension: A quantile multiple regression analysis. *Journal of Educational Psychology, 109*(4), 451–464.

Lervåg, A., Hulme, C., & Melby-Lervåg, M. (2018). Unpicking the developmental relationship between oral language skills and reading comprehension: It's simple, but complex. *Child Development, 89*(5), 1821–1838.

Lyon, C., Hogan, E. K., & Kearns, D. M. (2020). Individualizing literacy instruction in co-taught classrooms through a station teaching model. *Intervention in School and Clinic, 56*(4), 224–232.

National Reading Panel (U.S.), & National Institute of Child Health and Human Development (U.S.). (2000). *Report of the National Reading Panel: Teaching children to read: An evidence-based assessment of the scientific research literature on reading and its implications for reading instruction.* U.S. Department of Health and Human Services, Public Health Service, National Institutes of Health, National Institute of Child Health and Human Development.

Perfetti, C. A. (1986). Continuities in reading acquisition, reading skill, and reading disability. *RASE: Remedial & Special Education, 7*(1), 11–21.

Petersen, D. B., Spencer, T. D., Konishi, A., Sellars, T. P., Foster, M. E., & Robertson, D. (2020). Using parallel, narrative-based measures to examine the relationship between listening and reading comprehension: A pilot study. *Language, Speech, and Hearing Services in Schools, 51*(4), 1097–1111.

Rayner, K., Foorman, B. R., Perfetti, C. A., Pesetsky, D., & Seidenberg, M. S. (2001). How psychological science informs the teaching of reading. *Psychological Science in the Public Interest, 2*(2), 31–74.

Rose, J. (2006). *Independent review of the teaching of early reading.* DfES Publications.

Scammacca, N. K., Roberts, G., Vaughn, S., & Stuebing, K. K. (2015). A meta-analysis of interventions for struggling readers in grades 4–12: 1980–2011. *Journal of Learning Disabilities, 48*(4), 369–390.

Snow, C. E. (1991). The theoretical basis for relationships between language and literacy in development. *Journal of Research in Childhood Education, 6*(1), 5–10.

Snow, C. (2002). *Reading for understanding: Toward an R&D program in reading comprehension.* Rand Corporation.

Snow, C. E., & Matthews, T. J. (2016). Reading and language in the early grades. *The Future of Children, 26*(2), 57–74.

Snowling, M. J., & Hulme, C. (2012). Interventions for children's language and literacy difficulties. *International Journal of Language & Communication Disorders, 47*(1), 27–34.

Storch, S. A., & Whitehurst, G. J. (2002). Oral language and code-related precursors to reading: evidence from a longitudinal structural model. *Developmental Psychology, 38*(6), 934–937.

Swanson, H., Orosco, M., & Kudo, M. (2017). Do specific classroom reading activities predict English language learners' later reading achievement? *Reading and Writing Quarterly, 33*, 199–210.

Tobin, R., & McInnes, A. (2008), Accommodating differences: Variations in differentiated literacy instruction in grade 2/3 classrooms. *Literacy, 42*, 3–9.

Tomlinson, C. A. (2014). *The differentiated classroom: Responding to the needs of all learners* (2nd ed.). Association for Supervision and Curriculum Development.

Tomlinson, C. A., & Jarvis, J. (2009). Differentiation: Making curriculum work for all students through responsive planning and instruction. In J. S. Renzulli, E. J. Gubbins, K. S. McMillen, R. D. Eckert, & C. A. Little (Eds.), *Systems and models for developing programs for the gifted and talented* (pp. 599–628). Creative Learning Press.

Watts-Taffe, S., Laster, B. P., Broach, L., Marinak, B., McDonald Connor, C., & Walker-Dalhouse, D. (2012). Differentiated instruction: Making informed teacher decisions. *The Reading Teacher, 66*(4), 303–314.

Williams, J. P., Stafford, K. B., Lauer, K. D., Hall, K. M., & Pollini, S. (2009). Embedding reading comprehension training in content-area instruction. *Journal of Educational Psychology, 101*(1), 1.

Willingham, D. T. (2006). How knowledge helps. *American Educator, 30*(1), 30–37.

Yeh, S. S. (2010). Understanding and addressing the achievement gap through individualized instruction and formative assessment. *Assessment in Education: Principles, Policy & Practice, 17*, 169–182.

CHAPTER 22

Trends in Research Methods in the Learning Disabilities Field

Bryan G. Cook, Jesse I. Fleming, William J. Therrien, and Vivian C. Wong

Trends in Research Methods in the Learning Disabilities Field

Using research findings to inform policy and practice has long been a hallmark of special education (e.g., Carnine, 1997) and the field of learning disabilities (LD) in particular (Crockett, 2004). Indeed, legislative and policy reforms emphasizing evidence-based practices are premised on the notion that research can validly identify generally effective instructional methods that should be prioritized in policy and practice (Cook et al., 2012, 2020). The importance of using research—rather than tradition, personal experience, or anecdotes—as a basis for instruction seems particularly important for students with LD, given that these learners have unique needs and characteristics requiring instruction that is different and more intensive than for typical learners. Accordingly, research in the LD field is replete with applied studies and syntheses aiming to identify effective approaches for instructing learners with and at risk for LD (e.g., Ciullo et al., 2020; Swanson, 1999). Given the important role research plays in the LD field, it is critical to maximize the validity of research evidence and the application of the research base in practice. In this chapter, we (1) discuss recent progress toward increasing the validity of the LD research base and then (2) identify ongoing threats to validity of research in the field (i.e., infrequent and nonsystematic replication studies, insufficient power and representativeness of participant samples, questionable research practices, and limited impact and reach of research) and recommend emerging approaches for addressing these threats.

Progress Toward a More Valid Research Base

Special education has made great strides in advancing the rigor of research used to inform practice and policy in recent decades by, for example, increasing use of true experimental designs and systematic reviews and meta-analyses, as well as developing and applying criteria for conducting and reporting rigorous research. These trends have been applied in the LD field, with the effect of reducing error and bias in study results and, in turn, increasing the trustworthiness of research evidence that guides policy and practice.

Although studies that do not address causal questions contribute to the knowledge base in the LD field in important ways, one critical area of applied research involves examining whether instructional practices and intervention cause improved learner outcomes. True group experiments (i.e., randomized controlled trials, or RCTs) and single-case designs are designed to answer causal questions with a high level of internal validity. Thus, publication of studies using these designs provides the field with important evidence regarding what practices cause improved outcomes for students with LD. As a coarse indicator of change in the frequency with which these designs are applied in the LD field, we searched titles and abstracts of three LD journals (*Journal of Learning Disabilities*, *Learning Disabilities: Research and Practice*, and *Learning Disability Quarterly*) in the Web of Science database for (1)*"random* control* trial*," *RCT*, or *experiment** and (2) *single-case* or *single-subject*. Although these searches likely missed many studies that did not use these specific terms in their titles or abstracts, clear trends emerged. Our search for terms related to RCTs identified 1 article published prior to the 1990s, 6 in the 1990s, 11 in the 2000s, and 25 since 2010. Similarly, we identified 2 articles with single-case or single-subject in the title or abstract published prior to 1990, 6 in the 1990s, 5 in the 2000s, and 16 since 2010. We interpret the increasing number of publications targeting these experimental designs as positive trends that support the validity and impact of the LD research base.

Because all studies contain error, no matter their design, research consumers should consider findings from multiple studies across entire research bases rather than make up their minds after reading one study (Santangelo et al., 2015). Accordingly, systematic reviews and meta-analyses have become popular approaches to objectively synthesize findings across studies. If error in studies reviewed is primarily random, meta-analyses of many studies should, in theory, provide relatively unbiased estimates of effects because random error in one direction in some studies will be canceled out by random error in the other direction in other studies. Our Web of Science search of the same three LD journals indicated increasing publication of meta-analyses in the field. We found that 6 articles were published in the 1980s with *meta-analy** in the title or abstract, 7 in the 1990s, 10 in the 2000s, and 42 since 2010. Thus, similar to trends related to publication of experimental research across time, we interpret these results as a positive trend indicating greater availability of reliable syntheses of research in the LD literature.

Finally, the development and application of standards for conducting and reporting research in education (What Works Clearinghouse, 2020) and special education (Council for Exceptional Children, 2014; Odom et al., 2005) constitute another positive development contributing to the validity of the LD research base. Researchers in the LD field use these standards to guide the design, conduct, and reporting of their studies to enhance the rigor, validity, and transparency of their research. The standards are also commonly applied to describe and evaluate the quality of studies included in systematic reviews and meta-analyses to (1) assess overall rigor and validity and (2) identify areas of strengths and limitations of studies included in the review.

These and other developments in the field reflect ongoing efforts of researchers to improve the validity of the LD research base. Nonetheless, as in other fields, the research base continues to contain threats to validity. Indeed, difficulty in replicating study findings in multiple fields, presumably due to study error and bias, has precipitated a replication crisis in scientific research broadly (Baker, 2016). Following the lead of fields such as psychology (e.g., Nosek et al., 2021), LD researchers have begun to consider additional threats to validity and new approaches for minimizing them.

Threats to Validity and Approaches for Addressing Them

Despite continuing efforts to strengthen the LD research base, threats to validity still exist. In this section, we briefly identify and discuss the implications of four threats to validity of the LD research base (i.e., insufficient and nonsystematic replication research, unrepresentative samples in insufficiently powered studies, questionable research and reporting practices, and limited reach and impact of research) and make recommendations for approaches to help address each threat.

Insufficient and Nonsystematic Replications

Although rigorously designing and conducting research reduces bias, threats to validity and error are present in every study. As such, replication is an important part of the scientific process (Schmidt, 2009). *Direct replications* seek to reproduce an original study effect as faithfully as possible to test the validity of previous findings, whereas *conceptual replications* seek to evaluate the replicability of findings across systematic sources of variation in populations, settings, outcomes, and treatments. The importance of replication is reflected in standards for evidence-based practices that require intervention effects to be replicated across multiple high-quality studies (Cook et al., 2020).

Despite the central role of replication in establishing scientific knowledge, explicit replications are conducted infrequently in special education. Makel et al. (2016) and Lemons et al. (2016) independently reviewed the special education literature base and respectively found that explicit replication studies comprised only 0.5% and 0.4% of the published literature. Lemons and colleagues also reported that (1) the vast majority of explicit replication studies in special education were conceptual replications, (2) most replications were conducted by the same authors as the studies being replicated, and (3) only 17 explicit replication studies had been conducted in the LD field. A search of the same three LD journals noted previously in Web of Science showed that, though still relatively scarce, the frequency of replication studies may be increasing. We found that 1.7% of publications (10 of

592 total publications) in these three journals were explicitly identified as replications in the title or abstract since 2016, when Makel et al. and Lemons et al. were published.

Though studies explicitly identified as replications are rare in the special education literature, Cook et al. (2016) and Therrien et al. (2016) found that special education researchers often examine the effects of interventions investigated in previous research. However, these studies seldom (1) clearly indicate which elements of a previous study were and were not reproduced or (2) systematically examine whether results were consistent with previous research (Coyne et al., 2016). As such, systematic lines of conceptual replications that establish the boundaries of intervention effectiveness across populations, outcomes, and variations in the intervention are rare in special education.

Recommendations

The scarcity of replication studies (1) limits the confidence that stakeholders have in the findings of unreplicated studies and (2) hampers the ability of researchers to identify the boundaries of effectiveness for interventions and the critical elements of effective interventions. Challenges with planning, conducting, and reporting systematic replication studies include lack of consensus on what replication means, how high-quality replication studies should be implemented in field settings, and what inferences can be made from a replication study.

To remedy this situation, we recommend that researchers in the field of LD plan and conduct replication studies within systematic replication frameworks. Steiner et al. (2019; see also Wong & Steiner, 2018) introduced the Causal Replication Framework, which defines replication as a research design that tests whether two or more studies reproduce estimates of the same well-defined causal estimand—or the causal effect of a well-defined treatment-control contrast for a clearly determined target population—within the limits of sampling error. Steiner et al. described sets of replication–design and individual–study–design assumptions under which replication success can be expected. Replication–design assumptions ensure that the same causal effect for treatment–control contrast, target population, and setting is targeted across studies. Individual–study assumptions are standard in most individual causal studies and ensure valid research designs are used for identifying study-specific effects, unbiased estimators are used for estimating effects, and effects are correctly reported. Failing to meet one or more of the replication–design or individual–study assumptions results in replication failure.

Steiner et al. (2019) showed that replication failure is not inherently "bad" so long as the source of the replication failure can be identified. This is because replication failure resulting from violations in replication assumptions (e.g., the target population in the replication is different from the original study) is evidence of effect variation, which is essential for understanding whether and how intervention effects generalize to broader target populations of interest (Stuart et al., 2011; Tipton, 2012). Prospective research designs can be used to assess the replicability of effects and to evaluate potential sources of effect heterogeneity when study results do not replicate (Wong et al., 2022). Here, researchers introduce planned variations in replication assumptions, including systematic differences in treatment conditions, population characteristics, settings, or outcome measures. For example, conceptual replication designs include multisite designs with variations in participant or setting characteristics across sites, switching replication designs with variations in settings across alternating intervention intervals, multiple cohorts, and stepped-wedge designs with variations in when treatments are introduced across time and multi-arm treatment designs with variations in treatment dosage levels (Wong et al., 2022). In each of these designs, if replication failure is observed, it is because of systematic differences in units, treatments, outcomes, settings, or time.

As described by Coyne et al. (2016), we recommend that researchers prioritize conducting carefully planned lines of replication studies on interventions with initial evidence of effectiveness. These lines of replication studies would begin with closely aligned replication studies that replicate the intervention study as directly as possible to verify efficacy of intervention effects for a specific target population in a specific outcome area. Researchers would then conduct more distal conceptual replications using the Causal Replication Framework to explore whether the intervention is effective for other populations of learners and for other outcome areas and which elements of the intervention are critical for improving outcomes. We are encouraged by a growing recognition of the importance of replication research in education and special education research (see Chhin et al., 2018) and multiple recent examples of replication studies conceptualized within systematic frameworks of replication research in the LD field (e.g., Doabler et al., 2019; Toste et al., 2019).

To facilitate the ability of researchers to independently replicate one another's work, we encourage LD researchers to (1) fully and explicitly report study methods, (2) share their materials and data, and (3) use crowdsourcing to conduct concurrent replications. To meaningfully replicate a study, other researchers need to know detailed specifics of how the original study was conducted, which will be facilitated by clear and detailed reporting of study methods and sharing of study materials, such as instruments, survey questions, stimuli, and intervention protocols (see Cook, Fleming, et al., 2021). If page limits prohibit providing extensive details in the published article, most journals now allow authors to post supplementary materials on the journal website. Additionally, supplementary material can be posted to online repositories such as the Open Science Framework (OSF) and Figshare. Sharing one's data on a repository like LDBase or OSF (van Dijk et al., 2021) also facilitates other researchers' abilities to (1) statistically analyze the degree to which findings of subsequent replication studies are consistent with those of the original studies and (2) meta-analyze findings across studies. Finally, one form of crowdsourcing research involves multiple teams or labs of researchers concurrently conducting replication studies across different sites and samples (Makel et al., 2019; see following section for a more detailed discussion of crowdsourcing in research). By involving many research teams in the conduct of systematic lines of replication studies, large-scale crowdsourcing can establish the effects of interventions across planned variations in populations, outcomes, settings, and treatment variations over perhaps a few years instead of decades that it might take one or a few researchers working in isolation.

Unrepresentative Samples and Insufficiently Powered Studies

Another core issue related to the validity of the LD research base is adequacy of sampling. This section focuses on two issues related to sampling that pose threats to study validity: unrepresentative samples and small samples that result in inadequate statistical power.

External validity refers to the degree to which study findings apply or generalize to other settings and individuals within a population. When researchers conduct studies with the intent of generalizing findings to a broader population, they can employ probability sampling methods, such as randomly sampling from the target population, to enhance the likelihood that the study sample represents the target population and study findings will generalize to others in that population (see Cook & Cook, 2017). However, probability sampling approaches are seldom used in education research, especially in studies that examine the effectiveness of instructional interventions. For example, Tipton and Matlen (2019) observed, "in most education RCTs, the sample of schools included is recruited based on convenience, potentially compromising a study's ability to generalize to an intended population" (p. 414). As a consequence of researchers using convenience samples, small school districts in rural areas as well as students from culturally diverse groups tend to be underrepresented in the experimental studies that identify effective instructional practices (Carrero et al., 2017; Tipton et al., 2021; West et al., 2016). Therefore, it is not always clear the degree to which practices identified as evidence-based are effective for these underrepresented groups of learners.

Statistical power is "the probability that a research study avoids a Type II error by correctly rejecting a null hypothesis of zero treatment effect" (Hedges & Rhoads, 2010, p. 1). Intervention studies that are adequately powered have large enough samples to detect statistically significant findings if the expected effect is observed. Underpowered studies run the risk of Type II error, in which meaningful effects do not yield statistically significant results. Power is a function of effect size, sample size, and alpha level. Given that alpha is typically set at .05, the two remaining variables for determining power are effect size and sample size, which are related reciprocally—small effects require large samples to be detected, whereas large effects can be detected in smaller samples. In education, effect sizes tend to be small. For example, Kraft (2020) reported an average effect size of 0.10 for 747 RCTs that evaluated educational interventions with standardized test outcomes for PreK through 12th-grade students. Due to small effects and insufficiently large samples, Lortie-Forgues and Inglis (2019) reported that most of the 141 large-scale RCTs in K–12 education they reviewed were underpowered (23% power on average). Research examining the effects of instructional practices for students with LD may be at even greater risk for inadequate power because of the relative scarcity of students with LD in most schools and classrooms, resulting in significant challenges for recruiting large study samples.

Although we did not identify a review of statistical power specific to research on students with LD, evidence of low power exists in special education historically (Sindelar et al., 1988) and in recent reviews in related fields. Gaeta and Brydges (2020) reviewed >1,000 studies in the field of audiology and speech–language pathology. They found that median sample size in experimental and control conditions in the group-difference studies reviewed was 18 and 14, respectively, which is insufficient to detect even large effects. Indeed, only ~10% of group-difference studies reviewed were adequately powered to detect medium effects. Thus, small samples and inadequate power may result in some truly effective interventions going undetected in the LD research base.

Recommendations

Crowdsourcing, or combining resources across researchers to conduct studies that could not be accomplished individually (Uhlmann et al., 2019), is a potential solution to the unrepresentative samples and low power often found in LD research. Crowdsourcing can take many forms, such as many researchers (1) collecting data for one large-*N* study (e.g., Jones et al., 2021), (2) replicating one or multiple studies (e.g., Klein et al., 2018), and (3) analyzing the same data set (e.g., Silberzahn et al., 2018). As Uhlmann and colleagues (2019) argued, crowdsourcing is powerful because it "flips research planning from, what is the best we can do with the resources we have to investigate our question, to what is the best way to investigate our question, so that we can decide what resources to recruit" (p. 713).

Conducting well-powered, representative studies is expensive and requires resources that most LD researchers do not have on their own. However, by combining resources (e.g., human capital, expertise, and monetary funds) via crowdsourcing across many researchers, what seemed impossible alone can become possible as a group. Although a new approach in the LD field, crowdsourcing has been used to great effect in fields such as physics and psychology. For example, in the Many Labs 2 project, crowdsourcing was used to conduct high-powered replications of 28 influential psychology studies across 186 researchers with over 15,000 participants (Klein et al., 2018). By utilizing crowdsourcing, well-powered, large-*N* studies in the field of LD are possible as well. For example, an individual researcher may only be able to recruit and work with a moderate number of students with LD, say 30. However, in a crowdsourced study involving 15 researchers recruiting the same number of students, the total *N* is 450. Involving multiple researchers in different locations in data collection likely increases the diversity and representativeness of research participants as well.

To further address external validity, we recommend LD researchers use the Generalizer (*www.thegeneralizer.org*), a web-based platform that examines and can be used to improve generalizability of applied research studies. The Generalizer can be used two ways: (1) to determine if and where the results of an already conducted study are likely generalizable and (2) to help design a recruitment plan to increase the likelihood that study results will generalize (Tipton, 2021). For completed studies, the Generalizer compares the characteristics of schools included in a study against schools throughout the United States. The Generalizer then summarizes how similar the schools included in the study are to the population at large (Tipton, 2021). When designing a new study via the Generalizer, researchers first define their inference population using a variety of variables (e.g., geographic, school characteristics, and student demographics). The Generalizer then creates a stratified recruitment plan and provides the researcher with the names and contact information of schools that match their stated criteria in each of the relevant stratum (Tipton, 2014). Thus, LD researchers can use the Generalizer to select schools to participate in studies that maximize generalization to a targeted population. For example, we used the Generalizer to develop a school recruitment plan for an observational study to ascertain the quantity and quality of science instruction fourth- and fifth-grade students with LD receive across the United States. Previous research shows that science achievement varies based on school socioeconomic status, urbanicity, percentage of non-White students, and percentage of English learners (Curran & Kitchin, 2019). In creating our sampling plan, we therefore selected these factors as core considerations in the Generalizer. The Generalizer then provided us with four strata of schools (including school names and contact information for potential schools) that varied on these dimensions with target numbers of schools to recruit in each stratum.

Questionable Research and Reporting Practices

Fabricating data, falsifying results, and making errors in data analysis are broadly recognized as research misconduct. Conversely, quality indicators (e.g., Council for Exceptional Children, 2014; Odom et al., 2005) provide guidelines for best practices in conducting and reporting research in special education. However, many research behaviors are neither clearly forbidden nor endorsed. Researchers have suggested that many of these practices, which we refer to as questionable research and reporting practices (QRPs), may introduce significant error into research results and bias entire research bases if used commonly (Cook et al., 2018; Makel et al., 2021; Simmons et al., 2011).

Because studies reporting large, positive effects and statistically significant results are more likely to be published (Therrien & Cook, 2018), researchers may—consciously or unconsciously—engage in behaviors to increase the likelihood of such findings. QRPs that advantage large and statistically significant findings include but are not limited to p-hacking, selective-outcome reporting, and hypothesizing after results are known (HARKing) (Makel et al., 2021). Typically, data can be analyzed to address a research question in multiple ways. For example, covariates can be included or excluded, and different approaches for dealing with outlying and missing data can be taken. P-hacking occurs when researchers analyze data in many ways and decide which analyses to report based on whether they yield statistically significant findings. Although single-case and qualitative studies do not typically involve the use of p-values, researchers can explore different data analytic approaches in these fields to optimize the likelihood of obtaining desired results (Cook, Johnson, et al., 2021). With selective-outcome reporting, researchers who collect and analyze data for multiple different outcome measures in a study selectively exclude some outcomes when statistically significant (or otherwise desirable) findings are not achieved. Finally, HARKing occurs when researchers conduct exploratory analyses by analyzing relations between many variables in a data set without making *a priori* hypotheses and, when an interesting result is found, pose and report a retroactive hypothesis in the final research report as if it was made beforehand.

We are not suggesting that researchers engage in QRPs to purposefully distort research finding. We suspect that researchers are frequently unaware that they engage in QRPs and there is a lack of consensus on whether and when QRPs should be used. Indeed, we have engaged in some QRPs ourselves. Additionally, page limits in journals may make it impossible to fully report all decisions and behaviors made during the course of a study. Nonetheless, QRPs can introduce bias into research results. For example, Simmons et al. (2011) estimated that engaging in four QRPs (i.e., determining whether to include or combine outcome measures, add more study participants, control for gender and interaction of gender with the treatment, and drop one of three conditions based on how decisions impacted statistical significance) resulted in an astounding 61% false positive rate. Thus, Makel and colleagues' (2021) findings that 46% of approximately 1,500 educational researchers surveyed reported engaging in HARKing, 50% in p-hacking, and 62% in selective-outcome reporting at least once raise important questions about the validity of education research studies and, potentially, entire research bases.

Recommendations

Simmons et al. (2011) framed QRPs in the context of researcher degrees of freedom. In other words, researchers have considerable flexibility regarding how they conduct and report their studies such that they might engage in QRPs and not report doing so, resulting in threats to the validity of the study of which research consumers are unaware. Two related approaches for introducing greater transparency into the research process to limit researcher degrees of freedom and discourage QRPs are preregistration and registered reports.

Preregistration involves researchers publicly posting study plans before the study is conducted, typically on a registry such as the Registry of Efficacy and Effectiveness Studies (*https://sreereg.icpsr.umich.edu/sreereg*) or the Open Science Framework (*https://osf.io/prereg*) (see Gehlbach & Robinson [2018] and Nosek et al. [2018] for additional information on preregistration). Preregistration enables research consumers to compare plans for key study elements with research reports (e.g., published articles) and determine if unexplained discrepancies exist that may indicate a QRP. For example, if the hypothesis in a published study differs meaningfully from the preregistered hypothesis, it is possible that HARKing occurred. Similarly, suppose researchers stated they planned to collect and analyze three outcome variables in a preregistration but reported only two in the published article. In that case, it is possible that selective-outcome reporting occurred. Finally, a mismatch between data analysis plans in the preregistration and the analysis reported in the article suggests the possibility of p-hacking. Of course, research plans change in the course of a study for myriad reasons that often are unrelated to QRPs (e.g., a principal asked to reduce the time commitment of teachers and students, so the researcher eliminated one of the planned outcome measures). In such cases, researchers can post updates to their preregistrations to explain and justify deviations from preregistered plans. Importantly, preregistration does not prevent QRPs, but it makes QRPs potentially discoverable by journal editors, reviewers, and other researcher consumers—which may discourage researchers from engaging in them. Preregistered studies have been found to have smaller effect sizes than non-preregistered studies in medicine and psychology (Kaplan & Irvin, 2015; Schäfer & Schwarz, 2019), which may be due to researchers engaging in fewer QRPs after preregistering.

One potential limitation of preregistration is that it requires research consumers (e.g., journal editors and peer reviewers) to find and compare preregistrations with final research reports to identify discrepancies, which is not common practice (Claesen et al., 2021). Registered reports address this issue by embedding examination of preregistration in the peer review process (see Chambers, 2019; Cook, Maggin, et al., 2021). In registered reports, researchers submit complete but prospective introduction and method sections to a journal for peer review before conducting the study. The proposed study is reviewed based on its importance and the rigor of the proposed methods (Stage 1 review). If and when reviewers and the editor feel that the proposed study merits publication, the study is accepted in principle, and the accepted version of the proposal is preregistered. Researchers then conduct the study, updating the preregistration when deviations from the accepted protocol are necessitated. After completing the study and writing up the results and discussion, the completed paper is then submitted for final acceptance (Stage 2 review). At this point, the reviewers and editor compare the accepted preregistration with the final research report to make sure any meaningful discrepancies are identified and justified. Importantly, the paper cannot be rejected because of small, uninteresting, or null effects at this point, thereby removing the primary incentive for researchers to engage in QRPs (i.e., generating results that are likely to result in publication). Similar to preregistration, registered reports are associated with a greater likelihood of null effects (Allen & Mehler, 2019; Scheel et al., 2020; Wiseman et al., 2019), potentially due to reduced use of QRPs.

Limited Social Validity and Implementation of Research

In this section, we focus on threats to social validity, or the degree to which research procedures and findings are practical. Social validity is a broad concept that includes acceptability of treatment procedures by stakeholders (e.g., teachers and students), feasibility of treatment procedures, treatments meeting a defined need, and the implementation of treatments with fidelity by typical intervention agents (e.g., teachers) in typical settings (e.g., classrooms) (Horner et al., 2005). As in other fields, special education has grappled with bridging the divide between research findings and practice (Cook & Odom, 2013; Onken et al., 2014). The research-to-practice gap is influenced by multiple factors related to social validity, including the accessibility, relevance, and feasibility of research.

Access is inclusive of both openness and usability of research reports. Research findings or materials that are open access (OA) have no financial, technical, or legal barriers preventing practitioners and other stakeholders from accessing them. Most articles published in professional journals are behind a paywall that requires those not affiliated with an institution that has paid for a subscription with the publisher to pay to access each individual article of interest. Teachers and other stakeholders cannot apply research findings and materials to which they do not have access. Usability refers to materials that have been translated into a format that is easily understood and easy to apply for practitioners (Higgins & Boone, 2016). Generally, original reports of research (1) are not easily understood by practitioners and other stakeholders who do not have advanced training in research design and statistical analysis and (2) do not include materials that are ready to be used in classrooms. Although some professional journals focus on disseminating strategies and practices from intervention research to practitioner audiences in the fields of LD and special education (e.g., *Intervention in School and Clinic*, the practice section of *Learning Disabilities Research & Practice*, and *Teaching Exceptional Children*), most of these articles also lie behind a paywall.

Relevant research meets a specific need or answers a question of interest for practitioners (Carnine, 1997). Finding effective interventions for specific students with LD can be especially challenging because of the variability in individual characteristics and unique learning needs. To further complicate this issue, the values, priorities, and vocabularies of academics and practitioners are often misaligned (Smith et al., 2013) such that researchers sometimes (1) conduct studies on questions and issues that are not a priority to practitioners and (2) develop and examine interventions that are not feasible to implement in typical classrooms (Greenwood & Abbott, 2001).

Feasibility is the degree to which typical teachers and other intervention agents can implement an intervention with fidelity. When planning a study, researchers should assess and report whether research is conducted in a typical setting, the cost (in both resources and time) to implement the intervention, the type and level of support required to implement the intervention with fidelity, and whether practitioners can implement the intervention after supports are removed (Ledford et al., 2016). Even if they have been shown by bodies of research to be effective at increasing outcomes for students with LD, if interventions are not feasible, they are unlikely to be implemented with fidelity in the absence of external supports and may be abandoned entirely after supports are removed (Jones, 2009).

Recommendations

To improve the accessibility, relevance, and feasibility of research, we recommend adopting lessons from the implementation-science literature and making research findings and materials openly accessible. Implementation science is the study of how and why research findings are understood, adopted, and maintained by practitioners in classrooms and schools (Cook & Odom, 2013; Fixsen et al., 2005). Researchers can draw on implementation-science frameworks and include opportunities for practice to inform research and consider implementation challenges across multiple stages of research. Practice-based evidence is derived from real-world settings under typical conditions, which results in greater feasibility, relevance, and external validity of findings (Cook & Cook, 2016). Practice-based evidence is drawn from a breadth of research designs, including true experiments, quasi-experiments, single-case design, mixed-method, and qualitative research. Generally, these studies involve (1) practitioners who implement practices under real-world conditions as interventionists and (2) collecting and reporting data to document practitioners' implementation, adaptation, and/or perceptions of the practice (Cook & Cook, 2016; Doabler et al., 2021). Thus, the essential element of practice-based research is valuing and including practitioners as partners in the research process.

Rather than relying on a top-down approach where researchers inform practitioners of best practices, we recommend the field foster bidirectional partnerships between researchers and practitioners. Examples of these researcher–practitioner collaborations include research–practice partnerships and communities of practice (Cook & Cook, 2016; Smolkowski et al., 2019). The goals of these partnerships are to remove the traditional barriers between researchers and practitioners, improve implementation and sustainability of evidence-based practice, and enhance long-term collaboration to improve practice-based evidence and evidence-based practice. Researcher–practitioner partnerships can facilitate the development of interventions that are feasible to implement, the conduct of studies that (1) address questions and issues that are important to practitioners and (2) examine the effects of intervention when implemented by real teachers in typical settings, and the creation of accessible materials and practice-based evidence.

Another way that implementation science can inform the reach and impact of research is by considering challenges associated with implementation at each stage of research. Although implementation efforts often become a focus after conducting research, Smolkowski and colleagues (2019) described how findings from implementation-science literature can be applied throughout the research process. Implementation challenges can be addressed within the (1) development, (2) efficacy in controlled settings, (3) efficacy in real-world settings, (4) effectiveness, and (5) implementation, dissemination, and scale-up stages of research. For example, during the development stage, researchers can consider the feasibility and acceptability of a planned intervention and solicit stakeholder input before conducting pilot studies. In the efficacy in real-world settings and effectiveness stages, practitioners can implement the intervention and provide feedback on the feasibility and acceptance of the intervention to inform potential adaptations to optimize the likelihood of the intervention being adopted, maintained over time, and scaled up in classrooms and schools. Researchers' efforts to implement, disseminate, and scale up research-based interventions should also involve practitioners (e.g., creating practice-based evidence).

Open access (OA) publishing and open materials can also help address the problem of limited implementation of research. OA publishing involves researchers publishing manuscripts that are freely and openly available (Piwowar et al., 2018). Gold OA is a peer-reviewed journal that is completely open and accessible. These journals are rare in education, but *AERA Open* is one example. To publish in a gold OA journal, researchers pay an article processing fee (APC) to cover publishing costs. Diamond OA journals make all publications freely available without charging an AOC to authors. *Research in Special Education* and *Journal of Special Education Preparation* are two examples of diamond OA journals in special education. Hybrid OA provides researchers the option to pay an APC to publish an article as OA in an otherwise closed journal. In special education, hybrid OA is more common than gold OA, and the APCs generally cost around $3,000 (Fleming & Cook, 2022). Green OA is when researchers post completed, author-formatted manuscripts to an online repository such as EdArXiv (*https://edarxiv.org*). Green OA is inclusive of preprints (manuscripts posted prior to peer review) and postprints (manuscripts poster after peer review). In some cases, researchers must wait a period of one to 3 years before posting their postprint to an online repository (i.e., embargo period).

For practitioners, administrators, and policymakers without institutional or organizational subscriptions to professional journals, accessing research can be expensive. In some instances, accessing a single research article can cost upwards of $40, and readers must pay before knowing the usefulness or relevance of the findings (Rosenau, 2016). Simply put, teachers and other practitioners cannot implement research findings that they cannot access. Open access democratizes access to research findings by providing free access to those who are tasked with applying research findings in practice (Fleming et al., 2021). Additionally, preprints allow researchers to immediately disseminate their findings without waiting for the often-lengthy process of peer review, which can be especially important for time-sensitive research. However, given that green OA papers may not have been peer-reviewed, research consumers should be cautious about interpreting and applying findings.

As discussed previously, researchers can openly share study materials by posting them on a journal website or open repository for other researchers to use when conducting replication or other research. Shared materials can also be used to support practitioners' understanding and implementation of research-based practices featured in articles. For example, researchers can share worksheets, intervention protocols and procedures, lesson plans, training manuals, implementation fidelity checklists, student assessments, and other materials that practitioners can use. Availability of these materials facilitates the feasibility of practitioners implementing evidence-based practices with fidelity without external support. To further enhance the positive effects of open materials, researchers should provide (1) clear and detailed instructions for using materials and (2) materials in easily accessible formats (e.g., .txt or .html) that allow others to access and edit the materials (Cook, Fleming, et al., 2021).

Implementation science, OA, and open materials can improve the social validity and implementation of research findings in the field of special education. With an increased emphasis on addressing the issues of accessibility, usability, relevance, and feasibility, researchers can improve the social validity of the research base and help bridge the research-to-practice gap.

Conclusion

To meet the unique learning needs of students with LD, educators have sought to inform practice and policy with valid research evidence. In an ongoing effort to address threats to validity in research evidence, in recent decades, researchers in the field of LD specifically and special education more broadly have embraced trends related to increased use of rigorous experimental designs, development and application of rigorous quality indicators for reporting and conducting research of various designs, and synthesizing findings across bodies of research. Although these trends have increased the validity of research in the LD field, threats to validity remain, such as those identified in this chapter:

- Insufficient and nonsystematic replications, which result in lack of clarity regarding the accuracy of study findings, the critical elements of interventions, and the boundaries of intervention effectiveness,
- Small and non-representative study samples that result in inadequately powered studies with findings that may not generalize broadly,
- Use of QRPs that may inflate findings of specific studies and potentially entire research bases, and
- Limited research and impact of research findings, resulting in a gap between research and practice that restricts the application of research findings in applied settings.

For each of these threats to validity, we suggested multiple practices and approaches researchers in the LD field can consider to further improve the validity of research in the field.

It is important to recognize that neither the threats to validity nor the recommendations for addressing them described in this chapter are exhaustive. Regardless of the specific strategies the field seeks to adopt to further improve the validity of its research base, broad and lasting change will require the development of additional infrastructure and supports, incentives for change, and new norms and policies for research behavior (Mellor, 2021). We hope that such change will occur from the bottom up (e.g., researchers in the field updating quality indicators that include open practices to address QRPs) and from the top down (e.g., journal editors and funding agencies requiring open practices as a condition for publication and funding) to effect positive changes in research, practice, and the outcome of individuals with LD.

REFERENCES

Allen, C., & Mehler, D. M. (2019). Open science challenges, benefits and tips in early career and beyond. *PLOS Biology, 17*(5), e3000246.

Baker, M. (2016). Reproducibility crisis? *Nature, 533*(26), 353–366.

Carnine, D. (1997). Bridging the research-to-practice gap. *Exceptional Children, 63*(4), 513–521.

Carrero, K. M., Collins, L. W., & Lusk, M. E. (2017). Equity in the evidence base: Demographic sampling in intervention research for students with emotional and behavior disorders. *Behavioral Disorders, 43*, 253–261.

Chambers, C. (2019). What's next for registered reports? *Nature, 573*, 187–189.

Chhin, C. S., Taylor, K. A., & Wei, W. S. (2018). Supporting a culture of replication: An examination of education and special education research grants funded by the Institute of Education Sciences. *Educational Researcher, 47*(9), 594–605.

Ciullo, S., Collins, A., Wissinger, D. R., McKenna, J. W., Lo, Y. L., & Osman, D. (2020). Students with learning disabilities in the social studies: A meta-analysis of intervention research. *Exceptional Children, 86*(4), 393–412.

Claesen, A., Gomes, S., Tuerlinckx, F., & Vanpaemel, W. (2021). Comparing dream to reality: An assessment of adherence of the first generation of preregistered studies. *Royal Society Open Science, 8*(10).

Cook, B. G., Collins, L. W., Cook, S. C., & Cook, L. H. (2016). A replication by any other name: A systematic review of replicative intervention studies. *Remedial and Special Education, 37*(4), 223–234.

Cook, B. G., Collins, L. W., Cook, S. C., & Cook, L. (2020). Evidence-based reviews: How evidence-based practices are systematically identified. *Learning Disabilities Research & Practice, 35*(1), 6–13.

Cook, B. G., & Cook, L. (2016). Leveraging evidence-based practice through partnerships based on practice-based evidence. *Learning Disabilities: A Contemporary Journal, 14*(2), 143–157.

Cook, B. G., & Cook, L. (2017). Sampling and special education research: Examining whether and how study results apply to you. *Learning Disabilities Research & Practice, 32*(2), 78–84.

Cook, B. G., Fleming, J. I., Hart, S. A., Lane, K. L., Therrien, W. J., van Dijk, W., & Wilson, S. E. (2021). A how-to guide for open-science practices in special education research. *Remedial and Special Education, 43*(4), 270–280.

Cook, B. G., Johnson, A. H., Maggin, D. M., Therrien, W. J., Barton, E. E., Lloyd, J. W., Reichow, B., et al. (2021). Open science and single-case design research. *Remedial and Special Education, 43*(5), 359–369.

Cook, B. G., Lloyd, J. W., Mellor, D., Nosek, B. A., & Therrien, W. J. (2018). Promoting open science to increase the trustworthiness of evidence in special education. *Exceptional Children, 85*(1), 104–118.

Cook, B. G., Maggin, D. M., & Robertson, R. E. (2021). Registered reports in special education: Introduction to the special series. *Remedial and Special Education, 42*(3), 131–139.

Cook, B. G., & Odom, S. L. (2013). Evidence-based practices and implementation science in special education. *Exceptional Children, 79*(3), 135–144.

Cook, B. G., Smith, G. J., & Tankersley, M. (2012). Evidence-based practices in education. In K. R. Harris, S. Graham, & T. Urdan (Eds.), *APA educational psychology handbook, volume* 1 (pp. 495–528). American Psychological Association.

Council for Exceptional Children. (2014). Standards for evidence-based practices in special education. *Exceptional Children, 80*(4), 504–511.

Coyne, M. D., Cook, B. G., & Therrien, W. J. (2016). Recommendations for replication research in special education: A framework of systematic, conceptual replications. *Remedial and Special Education, 37*(4), 244–253.

Crockett, J. B. (2004). Taking stock of science in the schoolhouse: Four ideas to foster effective instruction. *Journal of Learning Disabilities, 37*(3), 189–199.

Curran, F. C., & Kitchin, J. (2019). Early elementary science instruction: Does more time on science or science topics/skills predict science achievement in the early grades? *AERA Open, 5*(3), 2332858419861081.

Doabler, C. T., Clarke, B., Kosty, D., Kurtz-Nelson, E., Fien, H., Smolkowski, K., & Baker, S. K. (2019). Examining the impact of group size on the treatment intensity of a tier 2 mathematics intervention within a systematic framework of replication. *Journal of Learning Disabilities, 52*(2), 168–180.

Doabler, C. T., Clarke, B., Kosty, D., Turtura, J. E., Sutherland, M., Maddox, S. A., & Smolkowski, K. (2021). Using direct observation to document "practice-based evidence" of evidence-based mathematics instruction. *Journal of Learning Disabilities, 54*(1), 20–35.

Fixsen, D. L., Naoom, S. F., Blase, K. A., Friedman, R. M., & Wallace, F. (2005). *Implementation research: A synthesis of the literature* (FMHI Publication #231). University of South Florida, Louis de la Parte Florida Mental Health Institute, National Implementation Research Network. *https://nirn.fpg.unc.edu/sites/nirn.fpg.unc.edu/files/resources/NIRN-MonographFull-01-2005.pdf*

Fleming, J. I., & Cook, B. G. (2022). Open access in special education: A review of journal and publisher policies. *Remedial and Special Education, 43*(1), 3–14.

Fleming, J. I., Wilson, S. E., Hart, S. A., Therrien, W. J., & Cook, B. G. (2021). Open accessibility in education research: Enhancing the credibility, equity, impact, and efficiency of research. *Educational Psychologist, 56*(2), 110–121.

Gaeta, L., & Brydges, C. R. (2020). An examination of effect sizes and statistical power in speech, language, and hearing research. *Journal of Speech, Language, and Hearing Research, 63*(5), 1572–1580.

Gehlbach, H., & Robinson, C. D. (2018). Mitigating illusory results through preregistration in education. *Journal of Research on Educational Effectiveness, 11*(2), 296–315.

Greenwood, C. R., & Abbott, M. (2001). The research to practice gap in special education. *Teacher Education and Special Education, 24*(4), 276–289.

Hedges, L. V., & Rhoads, C. (2010). *Statistical power analysis in education research* (NCSER 2010-3006). National Center for Special Education Research, Institute of Education Sciences, U.S. Department of Education. *https://files.eric.ed.gov/fulltext/ED509387.pdf*

Higgins, K., & Boone, R. (2016). Research to practice: Accepting the challenge of innovation. *Intervention in School and Clinic, 51*(3), 135–136.

Horner, R. H., Carr, E. G., Halle, J., McGee, G., Odom, S., & Wolery, M. (2005). The use of single-subject research to identify evidence-based practice in special education. *Exceptional Children, 71*, 165–179.

Jones, B. C., DeBruine, L. M., Flake, J. K., Liuzza, M. T., Antfolk, J., Arinze, N. C., et al. (2021). To which world regions does the valence–dominance model of social perception apply? *Nature Human Behaviour, 5*(1), 159–169.

Jones, M. L. (2009). A study of novice special educators' views of evidence-based practices. *Teacher Education and Special Education, 32*(2), 101–120.

Kaplan, R. M., & Irvin, V. L. (2015). Likelihood of null effects of large NHLBI clinical trials has increased over time. *PLOS One, 10*(8), Article e132382.

Klein, R. A., Vianello, M., Hasselman, F., Adams, B. G., Adams Jr, R. B., Alper, S., et al. (2018). Many Labs 2: Investigating variation in replicability across samples and settings. *Advances in Methods and Practices in Psychological Science, 1*(4), 443–490.

Kraft, M. A. (2020). Interpreting effect sizes of education interventions. *Educational Researcher, 49*(4), 241–253.

Ledford, J. R., Hall, E., Conder, E., & Lane, J. D. (2016). Research for young children with autism spectrum disorders: Evidence of social and ecological validity. *Topics in Early Childhood Special Education, 35*(4), 223–233.

Lemons, C. J., King, S. A., Davidson, K. A., Berryesa, T. L., Gajjar, S. A., & Sacks, L. H. (2016). An inadvertent concurrent replication: Same roadmap, different journey. *Remedial and Special Education, 37*(4), 213–222.

Lortie-Forgues, H., & Inglis, M. (2019). Rigorous large-scale educational RCTs are often uninformative: Should we be concerned? *Educational Researcher, 48*(3), 158–166.

Makel, M. C., Hodges, J., Cook, B. G., & Plucker, J. A. (2021). Both questionable and open research practices are prevalent in education research. *Educational Researcher, 50*(8), 493–504.

Makel, M. C., Plucker, J. A., Freeman, J., Lombardi, A., Simonsen, B., & Coyne, M. (2016). Replication of special education research: Necessary but far too rare. *Remedial and Special Education, 37*(4), 205–212.

Makel, M. C., Smith, K. N., McBee, M. T., Peters, S. J., & Miller, E. M. (2019). A path to greater credibility: Large-scale collaborative education research. *AERA Open, 5*(4).

Mellor, D. (2021). Improving norms in research culture to incentivize transparency and rigor. *Educational Psychologist, 56*(2), 122–131.

Nosek, B. A., Ebersole, C. R., DeHaven, A. C., & Mellor, D. T. (2018). The preregistration revolution. *Proceedings of the National Academy of Sciences, 115*(11), 2600–2606.

Nosek, B. A., Hardwicke, T. E., Moshontz, H., Allard, A., Corker, K. S., Almenberg, A. D., et al. (2021, February 9). Replicability, robustness, and reproducibility in psychological science. *Annual Review of Psychology, 73*, 719–748.

Odom, S. L., Brantlinger, E., Gersten, R., Horner, R. H., Thompson, B., & Harris, K. R. (2005). Research in special education: Scientific methods and evidence-based practices. *Exceptional Children, 71*(2), 137–148.

Onken, L. S., Carroll, K. M., Shoham, V., Cuthbert, B. N., & Riddle, M. (2014). Reenvisioning clinical science: Unifying the discipline to improve the public health. *Clinical Psychological Science, 2*(1), 22–34.

Piwowar, H., Priem, J., Larivière, V., Alperin, J. P., Matthias, L., Norlander, B., Farley, A., West, J., & Haustein, S. (2018). The state of OA: A large-scale analysis of the prevalence and impact of open access articles. *PeerJ, 6*, Article e4375.

Rosenau, J. (2016, March 17). *For teachers, access to the scientific literature is priceless. https://ncse.ngo/teachers-access-scientific-literature-priceless*

Santangelo, T., Novosel, L., Cook, B. G., & Gapsis, M. (2015). Using the 6S Pyramid to identify research-based instructional practices for students with learning disabilities. *Learning Disabilities Research and Practice, 30*(2), 91–101.

Schaeffer, T., & Schwarz, M. (2019). The meaningfulness of effect sizes in psychological research: Differences between sub-disciplines and the impact of potential biases. *Frontiers in Psychology, 10*, Article 813.

Scheel, A. M., Schijen, M., & Lakens, D. (2020, February 5). An excess of positive results: Comparing the standard psychology literature with registered reports. *Advances in Methods and Practices in Psychological Science, 4*(2), Article 251524592110074.

Schmidt, S. (2009). Shall we really do it again? The powerful concept of replication is neglected in the social sciences. *Review of General Psychology, 13*(2), 90–100.

Silberzahn, R., Uhlmann, E. L., Martin, D. P., Anselmi, P., Aust, F., Awtrey, E., et al. (2018). Many analysts, one data set: Making transparent how variations in analytic choices affect results. *Advances in Methods and Practices in Psychological Science, 1*(3), 337–356.

Simmons, J. P., Nelson, L. D., & Simonsohn, U. (2011). False-positive psychology: Undisclosed flexibility in data collection and analysis allows presenting anything as significant. *Psychological Science, 22*(11), 1359–1366.

Sindelar, P. T., Allman, C., Monda, L., Vail, C. O., Wilson, C. L., & Schloss, P. J. (1988). The power of hypothesis testing in special education efficacy research. *Journal of Special Education, 22*(3), 284–296.

Smith, G. J., Schmidt, M. M., Edelen-Smith, P., & Cook, B. G. (2013). Pasteur's quadrant as the bridge linking rigor and relevance. *Exceptional Children, 79*(3), 147–161.

Smolkowski, K., Crawford, L., Seeley, J. R., & Rochelle, J. (2019). Introduction to implementation science for research on learning disabilities. *Learning Disability Quarterly, 42*(4), 192–203.

Steiner, P. M., Wong, V. C., & Anglin, K. L. (2019). A causal replication framework for designing and assessing replication efforts. *Zeitschrift Für Psychologie/Journal of Psychology, 227*(4), 280–292.

Stuart, E. A., Cole, S. R., Bradshaw, C. P., & Leaf, P. J. (2011). The use of propensity scores to assess the generalizability of results from randomized trials. *Journal of the Royal Statistical Society: Series A (Statistics in Society), 174*(2), 369–386.

Swanson, H. L. (1999). Reading research for students with LD: A meta-analysis of intervention outcomes. *Journal of Learning Disabilities, 32*(6), 504–532.

Therrien, W. J., & Cook, B. G. (2018). Null effects and publication bias in learning disabilities research. *Learning Disabilities Research & Practice, 33*(1), 5–10.

Therrien, W. J., Matthews, H. M., Hirsch, S. E., & Solis, M. (2016). Progeny review: An alternative approach for examining the replication of intervention studies in special education. *Remedial and Special Education, 37*(4), 235–243.

Tipton, E. (2012). Improving generalizations from experiments using propensity score subclassification. *Journal of Educational and Behavioral Statistics, 38*(3), 239–266.

Tipton, E. (2014). How generalizable is your experiment? An index for comparing experimental samples and populations. *Journal of Educational and Behavioral Statistics, 39*(6), 478–501.

Tipton, E. (2021, October 5). *The generalizer. www.bethtipton.com/generalizations*

Tipton, E., & Matlen, B. J. (2019). Improved generalizability through improved recruitment: Lessons learned from a large-scale randomized trial. *American Journal of Evaluation, 40*(3), 414–430.

Tipton, E., Spybrook, J., Fitzgerald, K. G., Wang, Q., & Davidson, C. (2021). Toward a system of evidence for all: Current practices and future opportunities in 37 randomized trials. *Educational Researcher, 50*(3), 145–156.

Toste, J. R., Capin, P., Williams, K. J., Cho, E., & Vaughn, S. (2019). Replication of an experimental study investigating the efficacy of a multisyllabic word reading intervention with and without motivational beliefs training for struggling readers. *Journal of Learning Disabilities, 52*(1), 45–58.

Uhlmann, E. L., Ebersole, C. R., Chartier, C. R., Errington, T. M., Kidwell, M. C., Lai, C. K., et al. (2019). Scientific utopia III: Crowdsourcing science. *Perspectives on Psychological Science, 14*(5), 711–733.

van Dijk, W., Schatschneider, C., & Hart, S. A. (2021). Open science in education science. *Journal of Learning Disabilities, 54*(2), 139–152.

West, E. A., Travers, J. C., Kemper, T. D., Liberty, L. M., Cote, D. L., McCollow, M. M., & Stansberry Brusnahan, L. L. (2016). Racial and ethnic diversity of participants in research supporting evidence-based practices for learners with autism spectrum disorder. *Journal of Special Education, 50*, 151–163.

What Works Clearinghouse. (2020). *Standards handbook, version 4.1.* U.S. Department of Education, Institute of Education Sciences, National Center for Education Evaluation and Regional Assistance. *https://ies.ed.gov/ncee/wwc/Docs/referenceresources/WWC-Standards-Handbook-v4-1-508.pdf*

Wiseman, R., Watt, C., & Kornbrot, D. (2019). Registered reports: An early example and analysis. *PeerJ*, 7, e6232.

Wong, V. C., Anglin, K., & Steiner, P. M. (2022). Design-based approaches to causal replication studies. *Prevention Science, 23*(5), 723–738.

Wong, V. C., & Steiner, P. M. (2018). *Replication designs for causal inference.* EdPolicyWorks Working Paper Series. *https://education.virginia.edu/sites/default/files/uploads/epw/62_Replication_Designs.pdf*

CHAPTER 23

Beyond Demography

Integrating Mind, Culture, and Equity in LD Research

Amy L. Ferrell and Alfredo J. Artiles

Students with specific learning disabilities (SLD) constitute the largest population of learners served under the Individuals with Disabilities Education Act (IDEA), representing about one-third of the special education system in the United States (National Center for Education Statistics, 2020). The idea of SLD clusters a heterogeneous group of learning difficulties purportedly comprising cognitive and linguistic dimensions. The U.S. Department of Education (2018) defines SLD as

> a disorder in one or more of the basic psychological processes involved in understanding or in using language, spoken or written, that may manifest itself in the imperfect ability to listen, think, speak, read, write, spell, or to do mathematical calculations, including conditions such as perceptual disabilities, brain injury, minimal brain dysfunction, dyslexia, and developmental aphasia.
>
> [SLD] does not include learning problems that are primarily the result of visual, hearing, or motor disabilities, of intellectual disability, of emotional disturbance, or of environmental, cultural, or economic disadvantage. (para. i–ii)

Throughout its history, the SLD definition has been debated and revised (Hallahan et al., 2013; Tefera & Artiles, 2023). Enduring points of contention include the interfacing of biological and cultural facets of SLDs. Related controversies cover equity questions affecting learners from racialized backgrounds and students whose first language is not English, most prominently questions germane to identification disparities (Connor et al., 2016; Skiba et al., 2008).

This category has been described as "subjective" or a "soft" form of disability (Dickman, 2017; Gersten et al., 2001; Macmann et al., 1989) due to the significant role that professional judgments play in identification decisions. To illustrate, researchers have conducted assessments of school-identified SLD students and found that their profiles did not clearly align with SLD diagnostic criteria; in fact, many of these students had profiles associated with intellectual disabilities (ID) (Donovan & Cross, 2002).

To mitigate these trends, the LD field has sought precision in diagnosis and classification (Danforth, 2011; Klingner & Boardman, 2011). However, continued efforts toward parsimony have resulted in problems with understanding the complexities of learning. At the same time, LD scholars have raised concerns about limited reliability within actuarial methods for identification due to correlational inconsistencies across measures and especially because measures do not adequately account for variations in instruction (Fletcher et al., 2013; Macmann et al., 1989). Further, scholars highlighted the arbitrary nature of cutoff scores because individuals on either side of the point were similar (Fletcher et al., 2013). These criticisms led to increasing skepticism about the discrepancy formula to identify SLD.

We argue that limitations in the view of learning underlying the SLD definition have had a significant influence on these conceptual polemics. For this reason, we present in this chapter considerations germane to a *cultural conception of learning* that systematically accounts for individual, interpersonal, institutional, and historical forces. The unprecedented demographic changes in schools and beyond and the deepening of inequalities in society at large (Bobo, 2011) require more complex understandings of learning. Moreover, this conceptual shift enables researchers to engage considerations of equity that are urgently needed in the 21st century. We sketch in the next section a historical overview of the conceptual fractures in views of SLD with an emphasis on the role of culture. Next, we outline a sociocultural view of learning and discuss research on learning strategies that is grounded in these principles. We conclude with a brief discussion of the implications of a cultural view of learning for future research in this field.

What Is SLD? Enduring Tensions with Culture, Race, and Other Difference Markers

An earlier version of the SLD definition quoted previously was included in the federal definition passed in 1975 when IDEA was initially approved. The SLD literature has consistently acknowledged the role of biological underpinnings that impair psychological functioning. The definition also includes an exclusionary clause that suggests "environmental, cultural, or economic disadvantage" is orthogonal to SLD. Given the meanings attributed to these keywords in the 1960s and 1970s, this clause specifies that SLDs cannot be the result of context [environmental], racial [cultural], or poverty [economic disadvantage] factors.[1] This exclusionary

[1]The concepts of context, environment, and culture have been treated in problematic ways in social sciences. This has been the case in this literature as well. For instance, culture is often used as a proxy for race, as in "culturally and linguistically diverse learners." "Context" is also used interchangeably with "environment" even though context is more complex and dynamic (see Erickson, 2004). We address some of these conceptual issues, particularly about culture, on page 491.

statement implies that culture and psychological processing are independent of one another, that the individual is separate from the environment, and that economic disadvantage and advantage may impact access to educational opportunities.

The policy message encoded in the exclusionary clause is intriguing, considering the persistent presence of racialized and low-income students in this disability category. At the same time, these ambiguities have complicated the work of practitioners and raise the question about a possible link between SLD's conceptual vagueness and racial disparities in this category. For instance, in the 2019–2020 school year, American Indian/Alaska Native students were 1.16 times as likely to become eligible for special education with an SLD, compared to all other disabilities, while White students were only 0.88 times as likely to be identified for an SLD (U.S. Department of Education, 2021). Similarly, dual-language learners (DLLs) are more likely to be placed in restrictive learning environments than their White monolingual peers and less likely to receive instruction that supports their full linguistic repertoires than their non-disabled peers (González & Artiles, 2015; Sullivan, 2011). Of note, these disparities transcend social class considerations—for example, Black and Latinx students are more likely to be identified for special education compared to White students when income levels are held constant (Grindal et al., 2019).

Biology–culture tensions have a long history in the LD field; in fact, these issues date back to the 19th century. The early work of European researchers stressed the biological (i.e., neurological) origins of verbal language disorders, including studies with military personnel with brain injuries. Early research also covered reading disorders that were assumed to have congenital or hereditary causes (Hallahan et al., 2013). Attention to the brain and other biological causes has persisted to this day. This early line of research eventually spread to the United States by the beginning of the 20th century. Investigators were increasingly interested in children with reading difficulties who were assumed to have "brain dysfunctions," even in the absence of brain injuries. By the 1940s, such cases were classified as having two main kinds of causes, namely brain injuries or poor learning backgrounds (Werner & Strauss, 1941). In short, notwithstanding the preeminence of the medical model in this field, this distinction made visible longstanding tensions we have seen in the LD field between biology and environment to explain difficulties associated with learning and language (Danforth, 2009).

LD research gradually moved from observation studies to explain these conditions to the development of assessments and interventions. Kirk first used the term *learning disabilities* in the early 1960s during a conference talk to parents of children with reading disorders. His conceptualization was instrumental in the development of the federal definition approved in 1975. Of significance, Kirk included in his definition an exclusionary clause: "It is not the result of mental retardation, sensory deprivation, or cultural and instructional factors" (Kirk as cited in Hallahan et al., 2013, p. 22). Again, although the biological underpinnings of this condition remained central, a concern with "cultural" or environmental ("sensory deprivation") influences was mentioned as alternative explanations of learning difficulties. As we stated earlier, this exclusionary reasoning was kept in the federal definition of SLD. Some commentators argue that this differentiation was made in part to secure resources for this emerging category and minimize competition for federal policy support with other groups that were vying for recognition and resources at this point in history through various social movements—for example, racialized communities, low-income groups (E. Martin, personal communication, November 29, 2020; Fletcher et al., 2013; Whittaker & Ortiz, 2019).

Beyond this resource competition thesis, we find other historical undercurrents surrounding biology–culture tensions to explain learning difficulties. For instance, as part of the project of nation building, certain groups have been used as the referent over time, that is, White, male, able-bodied, and middle class. "Backwardness" is an illustration of categories of difference that emerged in the early 20th century to privilege some groups and marginalize others. Backwardness was applied to children and youth who were deemed to have average intelligence but struggled academically in schools (Franklin, 1980). Poverty and cultural explanations (deficits and deprivation) were central factors contributing to backwardness; racialized others, low-income White groups, and immigrants have been typically identified as struggling to meet expectations of what is considered competent performance (Deschenes et al., 2001).

Aligned with these historical trends, the idea of "culture" has been used in problematic ways in contemporary LD research. Specifically, culture has been deployed to index demographic groups as well as signal negative influences on child development (Artiles et al., 2011). To illustrate, Artiles and colleagues (2010) described the problems with the ways culture is addressed in disproportionality research. Though culture is not explicitly named in much of the disproportionality literature, unacknowledged assumptions about the presumed cultures of minoritized groups pervade many studies, including, for example, the negative role of culture in the development of students of color (e.g., language, cognition, and self-regulation skills), deficit views of families' cultural practices at home (e.g., "culture of poverty or disadvantage"), stereotypical presumptions about student cultures and their links to school failure when making special education referrals, and assumptions about the role of language in instruction for multilingual learners. Interestingly, the exclusionary clause of the LD definition does call attention to culture (though still in a deficit mode) by stipulating that students' learning problems should *not* be "the result of . . . environmental, cultural, or economic disadvantage" (U.S. Department of Education, 2018, para. ii). Despite the good intentions behind the clause, the lack of a robust understanding of the cultural nature of learning in LD research has introduced ambiguities and uncertainties in educators' practices (e.g., in referrals, assessments, and diagnostic decisions) (Artiles et al., 2020).

From their analysis on the ways the notion of culture is used in explanations of disproportionality, Artiles and colleagues (2010) found that culture tends to be framed as an *essentializing* concept—that is, all members of a cultural group behave and think the same way—and/or a *deterministic* idea—that is, members of cultural groups are socialized into "ways of life" (e.g., beliefs, values, cognitive skills, emotions, and behaviors); thus, culture governs how people do things in the world (Artiles et al., 2020). Culture is often equated with demographic markers as reflected in terms like "culturally and linguistically diverse" learners to describe *racially* minoritized students and DLLs. Although demographic markers provide insights into broad patterns according to various social categories, demographics are static and incomplete representations of the human experience when treated as categorical variables. Implicit in this perspective is the assumption that cultural groups are homogeneous, thus discounting in-group diversity. Associated with this presumption of cultural groups' cohesion is the idea that culture does not change; that is, the "ways of life" of cultural groups and institutional cultures are invariable (Artiles et al., 2020). This vision of culture implies that racialized groups do possess culture, while the referent category (i.e., Whites) does not. Moreover, if the norms for child development and learning are *a*-cultural, the developmental and learning pathways of students of color (including DLLs) constitute exceptions to the norm. A consequence of these assumptions is that the role of culture in learning theory is underspecified in traditional LD scholarship, despite evidence of cross-cultural variations in LDs, sometimes associated with the structures of languages or with cultural–historical influences (Kalyanpur, 2022; Tannok, 2012).

The limits of this traditional view of culture have important consequences for the ways questions about equity are framed and answered in LD policy and research. Equity research questions and policy concerns cannot be addressed by isolating disparities according to singular, unitary categories (e.g., ability differences), nor can learning be understood by focusing exclusively on cognition (Nasir et al., 2021). Contrary to what is emerging in other disciplines, most researchers in the LD field are not asking questions about the interdependence of the cultural and biological threads of human development (Artiles et al., 2020).

"Culture" has also been used in the LD field to describe socialization processes in child development, typically with a negative spin. Terms like "cultural deprivation" and "culture of poverty" have been generally applied to groups living in poverty and racialized communities since the 1960s, though their lineage can be traced to comparative research among racial groups most prominently visible in the 1800s and early 1900s (Valencia, 2011). These terms belong in the tradition of deficit thinking that has permeated characterizations of communities of color. It is troubling that scholars are noting a resurgence in the use of these notions (Darity, 2011; McDermott & Vossoughi, 2020). A core assumption of this pernicious vision of culture is that families and communities of color and low-income groups have beliefs and values and rely on routines and practices that deprive their offspring of the appropriate linguistic, cognitive, and socioemotional experiences and tools to function effectively in institutions and society at large (Tefera & Artiles, 2023). In this reductive paradigm, the poor and communities of color are envisioned as socializing their upcoming generations to detrimental learning and developmental repertoires; of note, these groups are characterized as devoid of cultural assets and resilience. These meanings of culture have predominated in the identification of ID and emotional/behavioral disorders (E/BD), which is considerably apparent in the context of racial disparities in these categories (Artiles et al., 2010). In turn, the SLD exclusionary clause seems to be grounded in these cultural perspectives as well.

A related cultural–historical consideration in the evolution of the LD field is the changing status of this category. For instance, SLD had a high status in the emerging landscape of special education as it was largely populated by White students in the early years of the field. But due to equity-related litigation in the ID category, among other factors, we witnessed the migration of White students to other categories (e.g., OHI) and of African Americans and other groups of color to an SLD diagnosis. In short, the historical evolution of constructs like "culture"—and their stratifying consequences—must be considered in the analysis of SLD, its changing status, and the meanings and implications of the exclusionary clause. When culture implies deficiencies in social practices or people outside the White, monolingual, English-speaking norm, demographic markers connote false distinguishers between groups, thus confounding any analysis of the nebulous shifts within SLD membership. Greater heterogeneity exists within racialized and otherwise minoritized groups than across them (Gutiérrez et al., 1999; Gutiérrez & Rogoff, 2003).

Intersectional Considerations and Implications for SLD Knowledge Production

The definition of SLD favors a "universalistic perspective in which one 'variable' or marker of difference . . . is assumed to be both more important than the others and stable" (Artiles, 2013, p. 337). That is, disturbances in psychological or linguistic factors define the nature of this category. But the persistent presence of racialized and linguistic minoritized groups in this classification raises questions about students who embody *double-bind* identities as racialized *and* disabled (Artiles, 2011; Harry & Klingner, 2006; Skiba et al., 2008). School leaders and practitioners have grappled with this issue for generations, but the SLD definition—particularly the exclusionary clause—has generated ambiguities and confusion in identification processes.

Instead of relying on a unitary perspective (Hancock, 2007) that focuses on single factors at a time, we contend that an intersectional lens affords new opportunities to understand the interlocking of SLD with other identity markers such as race, social class, gender, and language. This perspective compels us to realize, for example, that minoritized male learners with SLD have distinctively unique experiences from White female students with SLD or racialized gay learners without SLD (Artiles, 2013). In other words, an intersectional prism enables researchers to document how institutional infrastructures, such as policies, practices, and social conventions, are not experienced in the same way by everyone, nor are they neutral (Hankivsky & Cormier, 2011). This perspective also helps us uncover that minoritized learners can be placed in more segregated programs than their White peers *with the same diagnosis* (Fierros & Conroy, 2002). Because social systems interlock (e.g., the effects of housing discrimination on educational funding), challenges compound for people with multiple oppressed social identities.

The deployment of an intersectional standpoint also calls attention to the historical sedimentations of categories. Historians of disability have documented over the years the entanglements of disability with race, poverty, and national origin, among others (Baynton, 2001; Schweik, 2009; Stiker, 2009). Categories have status and are used to build hierarchies of access and opportunities for participation that mediate educational experiences and outcomes. The legacies of comparative racial research in intelligence, health status, and anatomical traits that defined status as human or subhuman are examples of problematic intersections with disabilities that SLD researchers and practitioners need to remain vigilant (Artiles, 2019; Krieger, 2011; Valencia, 2011).

It is necessary, therefore, that researchers produce study reports with careful intersectional descriptions of samples. This is a foundational practice in the conduct of research. In fact, major LD organizations (e.g., NJCLD and CLD) have called for thorough documentation of study samples to describe research participants (e.g., in terms of gender, race, ethnicity, language background, social class, etc.). Yet comprehensive reviews of research covering considerable periods of time have documented the consistent neglect of these basic research requirements in the special education and psychology fields (Artiles & Trent, 1997; Donovan & Cross, 2002; Graham, 1992; Lindo, 2006; Reed et al., 2012; Santos de Barona, 1993; Trent et al., 2014). This systematic inattention to equity-related phenomena in SLD research, like racism in education and the cultural nature of learning, could be a result of "boundary work" within the field, or processes of maintaining demarcations around what constitutes LD scholarship and practice, particularly that which is neutral, objective, *a*-cultural, non-ideological, and so forth (Artiles et al., 2011). In short, the SLD (and special education) knowledge base is colorblind.

The same logic applies to intervention research; that is, this scholarship should be designed and implemented with explicit attention to students' intersectional identities. In contrast, a unitary logic pervades in this knowledge base. Let us consider, for instance, response to intervention (RTI). Early formulations of RTI, though not grounded in an intersectional perspective, promised to reduce the overidentification of racialized students in special education. Nevertheless, research evidence suggests RTI has not delivered on this promise (Bouman, 2010; Hartlep & Ellis, 2012).

A combination of experimental/generalizing and descriptive/particularizing approaches (Cole, 2002) suits great possibilities in LD research because of the dual mission in special education toward both generalized efficacy and individuality in educational programming. Individualized education, a hallmark of special education, aligns to epistemologies that envision learning according to the particulars of the human experience, beyond static characterizations of demography. Methodologies such as naturalistic histories, longitudinal case studies, and clinical science can, in fact, support the evidence base of instructional methods, even a numeric scale that is generalizable to predictive outcomes across a large population of students (Leko et al., 2021). Qualitative methodologies should be used to help generalize quantitative methods and to help explain the complexities of quantitative patterns beyond causal inferences of grand scales (Klingner & Boardman, 2011), with demographic categories less as statistical variables and more as potential indices of historical and intersectional marginalization (Artiles et al., 2020).

We echo the calls of scholars who are beginning to argue for heterogeneity, not replicability, when studying interventions (Bryan et al., 2021; Walton & Yeager, 2020). Walton and Yeager (2020) propose that more adaptive belief systems are analogous to good seeds, and a context created by appropriate learning affordances can be symbolized by fertile soil. Intervention wisdom, to them, involves examinations of variations of context because heterogeneity allows for a better understanding of boundary conditions, especially when considering populations most affected by social problems. We agree. After all, two hallmarks of special education are adaptive, individualized programming and multidisciplinary, collective contexts of discernment, a good seed within fertile soil.

To summarize, SLD research knowledge production can be enriched with the use of an intersectional mindset. First, it is a good research practice. Second, an intersectional frame allows for contextualization of the qualitatively different experiences of students with SLD who have disparate identity intersections. Third, it empowers researchers to contextualize the historical baggage of particular identities that have historically intersected with SLD. Finally, it challenges the SLD research community to ask crucial questions about the standard epistemological practices in this field—for example, how do we maintain the invisibility of SLD's intersections with race in research studies while SLD–race intersections remain present in many schools and school districts? What are the ideological assumptions about the competence of students of color that permeate research and identification practices (Artiles, 2022)?

A corollary to the preceding discussion is that an intersectional standpoint can be complemented with a cultural conceptualization of learning. We outline core ideas about this vision in the next section.

Expanding Conceptualizations of SLD: The Critical Role of a Cultural View of Learning

We argue that a cultural view of learning makes significant contributions that address some of the issues and challenges we identified in the preceding sections. We start with the premise that culture is the very mechanism through which humans learn (Cole, 2003; Vygotsky, 1978). Rather than either a demographic proxy (e.g., race) or an *externally imposed* set of values or practices, culture manifests as dynamic everyday practices that humans build, transform, and enact together when learning how to engage with their social worlds (Gutiérrez & Rogoff, 2003). Culture can be identified by members' changing participation within systems of activity, which also evolve and intersect across social formations (Rogoff, 2003).

However, the activity of learning is never neutral. A framework of culture affords an understanding of how structures of power affect learning, whether institutionalized political systems or dynamics within a classroom. In recent years, learning scientists have noted "the pressing need for engaging the political dimensions of learning" (Politics of Learning Writing Collective, 2017, p. 92), especially given the rise of nationalism built on bigotry against minoritized groups in the United States and in other countries across the globe. Vygotsky's theories were informed by the shifting political climate, one in which access to education had opened for the proletariat, while educational research was heavily influenced by state ideologies, with restrictions against publications that used epistemologies and ideological frameworks deemed unfavorable to the state (Smagorinksy, 2009). Positioning children as agents who develop in socially mediated contexts, rather than as recipients of correct forms of knowledge, was considered a political threat.

Distinguishing assumptions of a cultural conception of learning include its social origins and cultural mediation. In his early work, Vygotsky studied learning in individuals with cognitive and sensory disabilities (Englert & Mariage, 2013). He observed growth when interventionists focused on how students employed compensatory processes and used tools that emerged from collaborative interactions. He did not consider the learning context as distinct from the learner nor culture from biology, as he states: "Insofar as physical development takes place in a cultural medium, it becomes a historically conditioned biological process" (Vygotsky, 1929/1987, p. 42). The Latin *contextere,* from which the word *context* derives, means "weaving together" (Cole, 1996). Context's origins connote the reciprocal nature of the mind, cultural tools, the activity through which the learning occurs, and the institutional milieu in which the activity takes place. This is described as the "activity system," which is used as the unit of analysis. Contradictions within the system serve as the integral focus of analysis because such tensions are considered the source of potential development (Engeström, 1991). Context represents the process of weaving together a person's mind and the cultural tools made relevant to their activity. As context, cultural tools mediate, or weave together, humans with their social worlds, much in the same way that intersectionality highlights patterned experiences woven together with threads of various social identities.

Cultural tools can be material artifacts that facilitate specific cultural functions when engaging in meaningful activities with the social world, whether a walking cane, alarm clock, or assistive technology. What good is an alarm clock in a society that measures time according to the sun and seasons? Or an office landline phone when an employee works remotely and communicates virtually? Or the exclusive use of learning materials that contain isolated letters, words, or even sentences when a fourth grader with a learning disability wants to understand the wonders of telescopes because his grandfather tells him stories about the stars?

Vygotsky explored the qualitative changes in how cognitive processes are modifiable when implementing interventions or with mediational supports (Englert & Mariage, 2013, p. 548). Stated differently, the tools used in a mental circuit are cultural artifacts; cognition cannot be separated from culture. In addition to examining the performance of children with disabilities according to various tasks, Vygotsky examined how children themselves modified the stimulus in challenging learning situations by resolving them through artifacts or with the help of more competent others. In this way, Vygotsky positioned children as agents who leveraged difficulties to compensate for their impairments, creating alternate ways to understand child development (Smagorinksy, 2012).

In sociocultural research with students with disabilities, the focus of analysis targets the social organization of the learning context: the learning materials, the children, and the languages used. Vygotsky and his contemporaries, Luria and Leontiev, considered language as the tool of tools (Cole & Engeström, 1993). Discourse is precisely what constitutes the learning environment because it weaves people together in shared activity, which indexes underlying belief systems (Cole & Wertsch, 1996; McDermott et al., 1978). For example, in homes where adults only pose questions to children that solicit information unknown to the adult (e.g., Who were you with? Where is your brother?), children become socialized into positions of knowers and information givers in everyday learning activities. This social practice stands in contrast to the known-answer display questions predominantly posed by adults in schools (e.g., What sound does *t* make? Who is the main character?), creating an assumption that children are passive recipients of knowledge (Cazden, 2001). These presumptions inform the ways people constitute their environments together using communication in concerted activity, situated within broader presumptions of activities that constitute school success and failure (McDermott et al., 1978). Collaborative participation structures are important for students with learning disabilities when students can use some sort of procedural tool, like mnemonics, a cue sheet, role descriptions, or image prompts during reading and writing processes (Biancarosa & Snow, 2004; Fuchs & Fuchs, 2011; Klingner et al., 2012; Palincsar & Brown, 1984). Collective work is enhanced by independent work in which students consider how the content is relevant to their own contributions and performance.

In addition to their material dimension, tools are also ideational. Thus, it is important to examine the goals, values, emotions, and beliefs that operate within any activity system. Tools such as values, belief systems, and emotions relevant to a given group of people can inform the extent to which learning occurs. We highlight the role of emotions because they have been under-examined in learning theories. In a sociocultural perspective, emotions afford connections with others and with ideas and are associated with neurological development, suggesting that youth must have opportunities for exploration, interest, and emotionally supported endeavors to develop their brain functioning (Lee et al., 2020; Nasir et al., 2021). Within a paradigm that integrates cognition with emotion, scientific endeavors become commensurate with literary ones in which larger quests toward learning affirm each individual's whole, intersectional being.

Nasir (2004) described the notion of *halal* (permissible) as relevant to an African American Muslim child in an urban Muslim school when considering his otherwise deemed "resistance" and "opposition" at school. The family's and school's orientation to Muslim spiritual practices allowed Nasir to explain the teachers' attention to the child's emotions, spirituality, and culture in the co-construction of resistance rather than isolating resistance as an intrinsic cognitive property of the child. Similarly, a sociocultural view of students as experts and teachers affords expansive notions of learning when considering students' intersectional experiences and histories, for example, as young, immigrant, multilingual girls of color with disabilities (Ferrell, 2021). Leveraging students' values and cultural practices through authentic or relevant texts similarly reflects a process that employs ideational tools to facilitate growth (Englert et al., 2009).

The SLD definition constitutes an ideational tool used to mediate educational programming decisions. Despite historical shifts in definitions of SLD, the field has tightly held two premises within its belief system: (1) a learning disability reflects unexpected underachievement in reading, writing, and/or mathematics due to psycholinguistic processing (Fletcher et al., 2013), and (2) "culture" connotes a factor that is extraneous to the nature of learning. As we explained earlier, these premises were already reflected in Kirk's foundational description of this category, in which he framed cultural or instructional factors as orthogonal to SLD (Hallahan et al., 2013).

More recently, Dickman (2017) proposed, "Learning disabilities reflect natural variations in brain function that predict unexpected difficulty learning skills and concepts valued by the culture in which the individual is expected to perform (e.g., academic achievement, social competence)" (para. 1 under "Proposed Construct"). Here, culture is not presumed as orthogonal to biology, but the definition does construe culture as a monolithic set of values and practices prevalent in U.S. schools. In contrast, we advance a cultural–historical perspective of learning in which the very nature of learning is conceptualized as cultural. In our view of culture, power plays a central role. Thus, missing in Dickman's framing is the fact that distinct cultural repertoires are historically endowed with more (or less) prestige, status, and, thus, power. Neglecting the role of power only maintains greater advantage for unmarked and presumably *a*-cultural groups, such as those whose cultural repertoires align to the institution of schooling's dominant Eurocentric values and practices. In other words, the idea of unexpected achievement must be situated in the context of crucial interrogations such as whose normative expectations. Which cultural communities are advantaged in official psychological and linguistic indicators of competence? In what ways do expectations reinforce benefits for already-advantaged groups? Ultimately, a cultural conception of learning requires that researchers and practitioners be guided by contextualized understandings of educational performance: "What works with whom, in what contexts, what for what purposes?" (Ferri et al., 2011; Klingner & Boardman, 2011).

The Cultural Nature of Learning: Illustrations from Reading Comprehension Strategy Instruction

To make visible the application of a cultural conception of learning that is already being used in LD research, we highlight multi-strategic, collaborative models of reading comprehension strategy instruction. Intervention research has increasingly leveraged sociocultural theory in its application of metacognitive strategy instruction (Englert & Mariage, 2013; McVee et al., 2005; Watkins, 2012), which has facilitated positive learning outcomes for learners with and without disabilities (Biancarosa & Snow, 2004; Edmonds et al., 2009; Kamil et al., 2008). Strategy instruction is built upon both cognitive psychology (Flavell, 1979) and the sociocultural nature of learning (Vygotsky, 1978), specifically with respect to mediation and collaborative participation structures, as readers learn to use before-, during-, and after-strategies to support active comprehension monitoring (Deshler et al., 2007; Kamil et al., 2008; National Reading Panel, 2000).

Reading comprehension is a complex activity that necessarily involves both cognitive functions, like working memory and knowledge development (Cutting & Scarborough, 2006; McMaster et al., 2014), as well as sociocultural ones, like collective sensemaking, experience with the content, multiple linguistic tools, heterogeneity of resources, intergenerational practices and rituals with text, and the extent to which text is epistemically used as authoritative (Gutiérrez et al., 1999; Moje, 2007). Explaining reading "failure" as an individual processing problem or lack of linguistic facility based solely on individual measures neglects the important role of social and cultural practice. Rather than determining readers' achievement relative to a normed, fixed level (e.g., on grade level or at benchmark), we agree with others who place more importance on examining how readers perform in varied reading activities or practices (Catts & Kamhi, 2017). For example, in addition to examining outcomes on achievement measures, teachers may ask, "What happens when a student reads with loved ones? With a familiar text? When using multiple languages? When using the text with others to solve an authentic problem? When asked to critique or argue with the author?" Toward attention to intersectionality, teachers might consider using texts that reflect the differing histories, practices, and experiences among various groups of students socially organized in some way (e.g., SLD, race, ethnicity, linguistic background, gender, etc.).

Uses of text, such as for argumentation and knowledge development, vary according to disciplines, like the natural sciences, math, or literature (Shanahan & Shanahan, 2008). This variability reflects the cultural nature of learning because comprehending text requires more than acquiring knowledge through cognitive processing; it also requires an orientation to the social *practices* established across generations within a given field (Moje, 2007; Shanahan & Shanahan, 2008). Studies that examine models that focus on the cognitive or metacognitive aspects of reading comprehension, like summarizing, clarifying, and questioning, have yet to consider how content and discipline-specific practices can be incorporated into the frameworks of strategy instruction, as well as how strategies can be used in approaches to literacy as a tool for enacting social justice (Boardman et al., 2018; Moje, 2007). Strategy instruction has also been critiqued because of its implementation as procedural, rote, or behavioral surveillance (Handsfield & Jiménez, 2009). However, scholars have shown the potential for flexibility within strategy models when applied as mediational tools and appropriated for readers' purposes (Boardman et al., 2018; Palincsar & Schutz, 2011).

Strategy instruction affords heterogeneity, multiplicity, and flexibility in collaborative learning structures. Rather than rigid methods with a set scope and sequence, collaborative strategy instruction models can allow for attention to disciplinary and epistemic variability when treating the model as flexible framework rather than a script to follow (Boardman et al., 2018). This flexibility allows teachers to consider student interest and familiarity with the content while also using explicit instruction and modeling (Biancarosa & Snow, 2006; Linan-Thompson et al., 2003). Studies report that incorporating multiple strategies over time and with a gradual release of teacher-led applications supports comprehension better than teaching one strategy in isolation (Kamil et al., 2008). Additionally, multiplicity and flexibility of tools, like mnemonics of acronyms and imagery, afford students with disabilities contexts through which to critique mainstream academic knowledge, merging practices from theoretical traditions of critical literacy and sociocultural theory (Ferrell, 2021).

Collaborative models of strategy instruction create contexts in which cognition can be distributed among group members (Rogoff, 2003) during dialogic meaning construction using rich, diverse language practices (Boardman et al., 2018; Brevik, 2019; Englert & Mariage, 1996; Ferrell, 2021; Klingner et al., 2012). Boardman and colleagues (2018) found that Collaborative Strategic Reading (CSR), a multicomponent strategy reading comprehension model, allowed for increased discussion of text with demonstrations of reasoning and debate among students, when compared to business-as-usual modes of instruction. CSR models additionally incorporate the application of cognate knowledge for multilingual learners as a strategy related to morphological awareness (Klingner et al., 2012). Similarly, Handsfield and Jiménez (2009) note that despite one novice teacher's procedural implementation of cognitive strategy instruction and orientation to reading as an individual activity, she incorporated the languages and experiences of her immigrant students to capitalize on their linguistic repertoires, utilizing Spanish in an English-dominant context. Certainly, teachers' role in soliciting and facilitating varied linguistic practices depends upon their knowledge of culturally responsive pedagogy when supporting students' bilingual development and engagement (Orosco & O'Connor, 2014). Because certain discourse practices enacted by marginalized groups are treated as unacceptable in school, like signifying, code-switching, or using African American Vernacular English (Lee, 1995), it is crucial that teachers critique mainstream presumptions about what counts as knowledge, thereby reversing such dismissals of discursive practices that facilitate student success (Ladson-Billings, 1995). Still, students themselves will help each other understand word meanings through code-switching and other intentionally accessed linguistic repertoires when placed in heterogeneous collaborative groupings during comprehension strategy instruction (Klingner & Vaughn, 2000).

Discourse practices make evident the various cultural practices aligned with disciplinary knowledge (Moje, 2007). How knowledge is represented, the kinds of acceptable interactions, or how ideas may be defended depend upon the particular conventions and communication practices to which students are socialized, whether at school, home, or elsewhere (Englert & Mariage, 1996). For disciplines that place importance on reasoning, like scientific inquiry, the application of comprehension strategies to text incorporates textual evidence for claims (Jadallah et al., 2011). Additionally, authentic teacher questions allow for deeper comprehension processes because they mitigate expectations to display correct responses and create a context for modes of inquiry (Soter et al., 2008).

In sum, we highlight the scholarship of reading comprehension strategy instruction because it exemplifies possibilities for reframing equity in LD, given its flexible application to employ a variety of mediational resources, especially language. Within multicomponent collaborative strategy models, learning can be reframed as involving both cognition and culture, woven together by the various tools employed in the activity, allowing for the integration of not only disciplines but also epistemic and ideological orientations to knowledge generation (e.g., critical literacy with comprehension strategies). Flexibility within collaborative strategy instruction models allows teachers to attend to matters of power, whether according to the content of texts, distributed expertise among students, or by leveraging students' languages and discursive practices.

Conclusions

We have advanced a vision for LD scholarship that weaves together culture and biology, considers the intersectional nature of learning disabilities, and realizes culture's role in learning and development. To better understand equity in the field of learning disabilities, we suggest that scholars move beyond static, separative conceptions of demography that falsely homogenize minoritized groups. Instead, complexities of learning disabilities can be better understood with investigations that attend to the ways that systemic injustices are built into the structures of pervasive material and ideational tools used in education, whether basing expected achievement on assessment instruments normed to monolingual White U.S. English speakers or discursive patterns in schools that mirror the dominant group, for example. Cultural theories of learning frame students as active agents with expertise who generate their own practices toward building knowledge.

In sum, we provide the following recommendations for the field:

1. In the continued conceptual refinement of learning disabilities, draw from theories of learning that integrate the mind, emotions, culture, and power. Individual, cognitively-based presumptions of learning, and, thus, learning difficulties are misrepresentations of learning as an activity. Consider not only the interaction within the learner and more competent others inside of a school setting, but also interactions that are present as a result of her intergenerational and naturalistic histories, as well as her social, cultural, and political environment. Interrogate the meaning of unexpected achievement in the criteria for LD. From where has the expectation come, and whose values are imposed in those expectations? Presumptions of competence are socially, culturally, and politically situated, often benefiting the groups in power: White, monolingual English-speaking, middle-class, cisheteronormative groups.

2. Forgo notions of culture that imply a reference to groups outside of U.S. dominant norms, especially when the implication is one of deficiency. Examine the heterogeneity within groups organized by social identity, and position children as active creators of knowledge in systems of activity. Consider how their cognition and emotions are woven together with their histories and positions of power

toward holistically comprising the learning environment. Integrate culture as critical to understanding learning rather than a factor to be excluded from it.

3. Employ research that highlights the intersectional nature of demography within interlocking social systems. Design studies using frameworks that account for legacies of racism that shape the field's presumptions about what counts as learning and what counts as disability, especially when attempting to explain inequities in special education. Refrain from using participant demographics in LD studies as only variables for output. Treating social identity as quantifiable labels removes the broader sociopolitical narratives of entire groups of people (Artiles, 2015). Work toward understanding the rich histories and expansive ways that demographics index larger social structures of power imbalances.

4. Examine responsiveness to instruction as beyond the causal efficacy of a given method. Rather, investigate learning with the activity system as the unit of analysis. When examining what works, consider Messick's (1987) validity as a matter of an instrument's use and consequences of the score. For example, more restrictive settings and decreased access to language support for students identified as both ELL and LD render problems with the validity of the measures used in determining eligibility because the consequences lead to practices that hinder learning (Shepard, 2021). Move toward heterogeneity when understanding the efficacy of interventions rather than an exactitude of measures or replicability (Bryan et al., 2021; Walton & Yeager, 2020). Examine the multidimensionality within common instructional methods for students with LD. For example, in a single-case design study that examines explicit instruction of phonological processing, highlight the social and cultural nature of the instructional activities, where the discourse is the environment, and provide the natural histories of each of the students. Consider how power operates in everyday school activity, such as presumptions that students' culture implies a kind of deficiency to rectify.

If the construct of learning is understood beyond narrow notions of achievement, then perhaps the construct of learning disability can be as well. What could a learning disability be if learning means leveraging both the mechanics of the code and also the soul of the logos? We impose our modes of representing learning to the extent to which a gardener plants a seed (Cole, 1996; Walton & Yeager, 2020), certainly a disruption to the soil's former way of being, though the engagement between the two is rich with potential. The gardener's faith has no certainty in the events to follow, no control over how the elements will receive the seed. However, the simple act indicates the gardener's self-expression of trust in complexities across relationships: her hand, the seed, the elements, and the mystery.

ACKNOWLEDGMENTS

The second author acknowledges the support of the Stanford Center for Opportunity Policy in Education (SCOPE), the Stanford Center for Comparative Studies in Race and Ethnicity, and the Equity Alliance.

REFERENCES

Artiles, A. J. (2011). Toward an interdisciplinary understanding of educational equity and difference: The case of the racialization of ability. *Educational Researcher, 40*, 431–445.

Artiles, A. J. (2013). Untangling the racialization of disabilities: An intersectionality critique across disability models. *DuBois Review, 10*, 329–347.

Artiles, A. J. (2015). Beyond responsiveness to identity badges: Future research on culture in disability and implications for response to intervention. *Educational Review, 67*(1), 1–22.

Artiles, A. J. (2019). Re-envisioning equity research: Disability identification disparities as a case in point. *Educational Researcher, 48*, 325–335.

Artiles, A. J. (2022). Interdisciplinary notes on the dual nature of disability: Disrupting ideology–ontology circuits in racial disparities research. *Literacy Research: Theory, Mind, and Practice*, 1–20.

Artiles, A. J., King Thorius, K., Bal, A., Neal, R., Waitoller, F., & Hernandez Saca, D. (2011). Beyond culture as group traits: Future learning disabilities ontology, epistemology, and inquiry on research knowledge use. *Learning Disability Quarterly, 34*, 167–179.

Artiles, A. J., Kozleski, E., Trent, S., Osher, D., & Ortiz, A. (2010). Justifying and explaining disproportionality, 1968–2008. *Exceptional Children, 76*, 279–299.

Artiles, A. J., Rose, D., Gonzalez, T., & Bal, A. (2020). Biology and culture in learning disabilities research: Legacies and possible futures. In N. S. Nasir, C. Lee, R. Pea, & M. M. de Royson (Eds.), *Handbook of the cultural foundations of learning* (pp. 160–177). Routledge.

Artiles, A. J., & Trent, S. C. (Eds.). (1997). Building a knowledge base on culturally diverse students with learning disabilities: The need to enrich research with a sociocultural perspective. *Learning Disabilities Research & Practice, 12*, 80–144.

Baynton, D. (2001). Disability and the justification of inequality in American history. In P. K. Longmore & L. Umansky (Eds.), *The new disability history* (pp. 33–57). New York University Press.

Biancarosa, C., & Snow, C. E. (2004). *Reading next—A vision for action and research in middle and high school literacy: A report to Carnegie Corporation of New York* (2nd ed.). Alliance for Excellent Education.

Boardman, A. G., Boelé, A. L., & Klingner, J. K. (2018). Strategy instruction shifts teacher and student interactions during text-based discussions. *Reading Research Quarterly, 53*, 2, 175–195.

Bobo, L. D. (2011). Somewhere between Jim Crow and post-racialism: Reflections on the racial divide in America today. *Daedalus, 140*(2), 11–36.

Bouman, S. H. (2010). *Response-to-intervention in California public schools: Has it helped address disproportionality placement rates for students with learning disabilities?* [Unpublished dissertation]. Claremont Graduate University.

Brevik, L. M. (2019). Explicit reading strategy instruction or daily use of strategies? Studying the teaching of reading comprehension through naturalistic classroom observation in English L2. *Reading and Writing, 32*, 2281–2310.

Bryan, C. J., Tipton, E., & Yeager, D. S. (2021). Behavioural science is unlikely to change the world without a heterogeneity revolution. *Nature Human Behaviour, 5*(8), 980–989.

Catts, H. W., & Kamhi, A. G. (2017). Prologue: Reading comprehension is not a single ability. *Language, Speech, and Hearing Services in Schools, 48*(2), 73–76.

Cazden, C. (2001). *Classroom discourse: The language of teaching and learning* (2nd ed.). Teachers College Press.

Cole, M. (1996). *Cultural psychology: A once and future discipline.* Harvard University Press.

Cole, M. (2002). Alexander Luria, cultural psychology, and the resolution of the crisis in psychology. *Journal of Russian & East European Psychology, 40*(1), 4–16.

Cole, M. (2003). Cultural and cognitive science. *Critical Practice Studies, 5*(1), 3–15.

Cole, M., & Engeström, Y. (1993). A cultural-historical approach to distributed cognition. In

G. Salomon (Ed.), *Distributed cognitions: Psychological and educational considerations* (pp. 1–46). Cambridge University Press.

Cole, M., & Wertsch, J. V. (1996). Beyond the individual-social antimony in discussions of Piaget and Vygotsky. *Human Development, 39*, 250–256.

Connor, D., Ferri, B., & Annamma, S. (2016). *DisCrit: Disability studies and critical race theory in education*. Teachers College Press.

Cutting, L. E., & Scarborough, H. S. (2006). Prediction of reading comprehension: Relative contributions of word recognition, language proficiency, and other cognitive skills can depend on how comprehension is measured. *Scientific Studies of Reading, 10*(3), 277–299.

Danforth, S. (2011). The actuarial turn in the science of learning disabilities. *Learning Disability Quarterly, 34*(2), 123–136.

Darity, W., Jr. (2011). The new (incorrect) Harvard/Washington consensus on racial inequality. *DuBois Review, 8*, 467–495.

Deschenes, S., Cuban, L., & Tyack, D. (2001). Mismatch: Historical perspectives on schools and students who don't fit them. *Teachers College Record, 103*, 527–547.

Deshler, D. D., Palincsar, A. S., Biancarosa, G., & Nair, M. (2007). *Informed choices for struggling adolescent readers: A research-based guide to instructional programs and practices.* International Reading Association.

Dickman, E. (2017, May). *Learning disability: What the heck is it?* International Dyslexia Association. *https://dyslexiaida.org/learning-disability-what-the-heck-is-it*

Donovan, M. S., & Cross, C. T. (2002). *Minority students in special education and gifted education*. National Academy Press.

Edmonds, M. S., Vaughn, S., Wexler, J., Reutebuch, C., Cable, A., Tackett, K. K., & Schnakenberg, J. W. (2009). A synthesis of reading interventions and effects on reading outcomes for older struggling readers. *Review of Educational Research, 79*(1), 262–300.

Engeström, Y. (1991). *Non scolae sed vitae discimus*: Toward overcoming the encapsulation of school learning. *Learning and Instruction, 1*, 243–259.

Englert, C. S., & Mariage, T. (2013). The sociocultural model as a framework in instructional intervention research. In H. L. Swanson, K. R. Harris, & S. Graham (Eds.), *Handbook of learning disabilities* (2nd ed., pp. 545–564). Guilford Press.

Englert, C. S., Mariage, T. V., & Okolo, C. M. (2009). The learning-to-learn strategies of adolescent students with disabilities: Highlighting, note taking, planning, and writing expository texts. *Assessment for Effective Intervention, 34*, 147–161.

Erickson, F. (2004). *Talk and social theory: Ecologies of speaking and listening in everyday life*. Polity.

Ferrell, A. L. (2021). Exploring critical literacy for elementary students with disabilities. *Equity, Excellence, & Education, 54*(4), 393–408.

Ferri, B. A., Gallagher, D., & Connor, D. J. (2011). Pluralizing methodologies in the field of LD: From "what works" to what matters. *Learning Disability Quarterly, 34*(3), 222–231.

Fierros, E. G., & Conroy, J. W. (2002). Double jeopardy: An exploration of restrictiveness and race in special education. In D. J. Losen & G. Orfield (Eds.), *Racial inequity in special education* (pp. 39–70). Harvard Education Press.

Flavell, J. H. (1979). Metacognition and cognitive monitoring: A new area of cognitive developmental inquiry. *American Psychologist, 34*(10), 906–911.

Fletcher, J. M., Stuebing, K. K., Morris, R. D., & Lyon, G. R. (2013). Classification and definition of learning disabilities: A hybrid model. In H. L. Swanson, K. R. Harris, & S. Graham (Eds.), *Handbook of learning disabilities* (2nd ed., pp. 33–50). Guilford Press.

Franklin, B. M. (1980). From backwardness to LD: Behaviorism, systems theory, and the learning disabilities field historically reconsidered. *Journal of Education, 162*(4), 5–22.

Fuchs, L. S., & Fuchs, D. (2011). *Using CBM for progress monitoring in reading*. National Center on Student Progress Monitoring. *https://files.eric.ed.gov/fulltext/ED519252.pdf*

Gersten, R., Fuchs, L. S., Williams, J. P., & Baker, S. (2001). Teaching reading comprehension strategies to students with learning disabilities: A review of research. *Review of Educational Research, 71*(2), 279–320.

González, T., & Artiles, A. J. (2015). Reframing venerable standpoints about language and learning differences: The need for research on the literate lives of Latina/o language minority students. *Journal of Multicultural Education Research, 6*(3), 9–34.

Graham, S. (1992). Most of the subjects were White and middle class: Trends in published research on African Americans in selected APA journals. *American Psychologist, 47,* 629–639.

Grindal, T., Schifter, L. A., Schwartz, G., & Hehir, T. (2019). Racial difference in special education identification and placement: Evidence across three states. *Harvard Educational Review, 89*(4), 525–553.

Gutiérrez, K., Baquedano-López, P., & Tejeda, C. (1999). Rethinking diversity: Hybridity and hybrid language practices in the third space. *Mind, Culture, and Activity, 6*(4), 286–303.

Gutiérrez, K., & Rogoff, B. (2003). Cultural ways of learning: Individual traits of repertoires of practice. *Educational Researcher, 32*(5), 19–25.

Hallahan, D. P., Pullen, P. C., & Ward, D. (2013). A brief history of the field of learning disabilities. In H. L. Swanson, K. R. Harris, & S. Graham (Eds.), *Handbook of learning disabilities* (2nd ed., pp. 15–32). Guilford Press.

Hancock, A-M. (2007). When multiplication doesn't equal quick addition: Examining intersectionality as a research paradigm. *American Political Science Association, 5*(1), 63–79.

Handsfield, L. J., & Jiménez, R. T. (2009). Cognition and misrecognition: A Bourdieuian analysis of cognitive strategy instruction in a linguistically and culturally diverse classroom. *Journal of Literacy Research, 41,* 151–195.

Hankivsky, O., & Cormier, R. (2011). Intersectionality and public policy: Some lessons from existing models. *Political Research Quarterly, 64*(1), 217–229.

Harry, B., & Klingner, J. K. (2006). *Why are so many minority students in special education? Understanding race and disability in schools.* Teachers College Press.

Hartlep, N. D., & Ellis, A. L. (2012). Just what is response to intervention and what's it doing in a nice field like education? A critical race theory examination of RTI. In J. Gorlewski, B. Porfilio, & D. Gorlewski (Eds.), *Using standards and high-stakes testing for students: Exploiting power with critical pedagogy* (pp. 87–108). Peter Lang.

Jadallah, M., Anderson, R. C., Nguyen-Jahiel, K., Miller, B. W., Kim, I. H., Kuo, L. J., & Wu, X. (2011). Influence of a teacher's scaffolding moves during child-led small-group discussions. *American Educational Research Journal, 48*(1), 194–230.

Kalyanpur, M. (2022). *Development, education and learning disability in India.* Palgrave Macmillan.

Kamil, M. L., Borman, G. D., Dole, J., Kral, C. C., Salinger, T., & Torgesen, J. (2008). *Improving adolescent literacy: Effective classroom and intervention practices: A practice guide* (NCEE 2008-4027). Center for Education Evaluation and Regional Assistance, Institute of Education Sciences, U.S. Department of Education.

Klingner, J. K., & Boardman, A. G. (2011). Addressing the "research gap" in special education through mixed methods. *Learning Disability Quarterly, 34*(3), 208–218.

Klingner, J. K., & Vaughn, S. (2000). The helping behaviors of fifth graders while using collaborative strategic reading during ESL content classes. *TESOL Quarterly, 34*(1), 69–98.

Klingner, J. K., Vaughn, S., Boardman, A., & Swanson, E. (2012). *Now we get it! Boosting comprehension with collaborative strategic reading.* John Wiley & Sons.

Krieger, N. (2011). *Epidemiology and the people's health: Theory and context.* Oxford University.

Ladson-Billings, G. (1995). But that's just good teaching! The case for culturally relevant pedagogy. *Theory into Practice, 34*(3), 159–165.

Lee, C. D. (1995). Signifying as a scaffold for literary interpretation. *Journal of Black Psychology, 21*(4), 357–381.

Lee, C. D., Meltzoff, A. N., & Kuhl, P. K. (2020). The braid of human learning and development: Neuro-physiological processes and participation in cultural practices. In N. S. Nasir, C. D. Lee, R. Pea, & M. McKinney de Royston (Eds.), *Handbook of the cultural foundations of learning* (pp. 24–43). Routledge.

Leko, M. M., Cook, B. G., & Cook, L. (2021). Qualitative methods in special education research. *Learning Disabilities Research & Practice, 36*(4), 278–286.

Linan-Thompson, S., Vaughn, S., Hickman-Davis, P., & Kouzekanani, K. (2003). Effectiveness of supplemental reading instruction for second-grade English language learners with reading difficulties. *The Elementary School Journal, 103*(3), 221–238.

Lindo, E. J. (2006). The African American presence in reading intervention experiments. *Remedial and Special Education, 27*, 148–153.

Macmann, G. M., Barnett, D. W., Lombard, T. J., Belton-Kocher, E., & Sharpe, M. N. (1989). On the actuarial classification of children: Fundamental studies of classification agreement. *Journal of Special Education, 23*, 127–149.

McDermott, R. P., Gospodinoff, K., & Aron, J. (1978). Criteria for an ethnographically adequate description of concerted activities and their contexts. *Semiotica, 24*, 245–276.

McDermott, R. P., & Vossoughi, S. (2020). The culture of poverty, again. *Diaspora, Indigenous, and Minority Education, 14*(2), 60–69.

McMaster, K. L., Espin, C. A., & Van Den Broek, P. (2014). Making connections: Linking cognitive psychology and intervention research to improve comprehension of struggling readers. *Learning Disabilities Research & Practice, 29*(1), 17–24.

McVee, M. B., Dunsmore, K., & Gavelek, J. R. (2005). Schema theory revisited. *Review of Educational Research, 75*(4), 531–566.

Messick, S. (1987). Validity. *ETS Research Report Series*, p. i-208.

Moje, E. B. (2007). Chapter 1. Developing socially just subject-matter instruction: A review of the literature on disciplinary literacy teaching. *Review of Research in Education, 31*(1), 1–44.

Nasir, N. S., Lee, C. D., Pea, R., & McKinney de Royston, M. (2021). Rethinking learning: What the interdisciplinary science tells us. *Educational Researcher, 50*, 557–565.

Nasir, N. S. (2004). "Halal-ing" the child: Reframing identities of resistance in an urban Muslim school. *Harvard Educational Review, 74*, 153–174.

National Center for Education Statistics. (2020). *The condition of education. Students with disabilities.* Author. *https://nces.ed.gov/programs/coe/indicator_cgg.asp*

National Reading Panel. (2000). *Teaching children to read: An evidence-based assessment of the scientific research literature on reading and its implications for reading instruction: Reports of the subgroups.* National Institute of Child Health and Human Development.

Orosco, M. J., & O'Connor, R. (2014). Culturally responsive instruction for English language learners with learning disabilities. *Journal of Learning Disabilities, 47*(6), 515–531.

Palincsar, A. S., & Brown, A. L. (1984). The reciprocal teaching of comprehension-fostering and comprehension-monitoring activities. *Cognition and Instruction, 1*(2), 117–175.

Palincsar, A. S., & Schutz, K. M. (2011). Reconnecting strategy instruction with its theoretical roots. *Theory into Practice, 50*(2), 85–92.

Politics of Learning Writing Collective. (2017). The learning sciences in a new era of US nationalism. *Cognition and Instruction, 35*(2), 91–102.

Reed, D. K., McCray, Sorrelis, A. M., Cole, H. A., & Takakawa, N. N. (2012). The ecological and population validity of reading interventions for adolescents: Can effectiveness be generalized? *Learning Disability Quarterly, 36*(3), 131–144.

Rogoff, B. (2003). *The cultural nature of human development.* Oxford University Press.

Santos de Barona, M. (1993). The availability of ethnic materials in psychology journals: A review of 20 years of journal publication. *Contemporary Educational Psychology 18*, 391–400.

Schweik, S. M. (2009). *The ugly laws: Disability in public.* New York University Press.

Shanahan, T., & Shanahan, C. (2008). Teaching disciplinary literacy to adolescents: Rethinking content-area literacy. *Harvard Educational Review, 78*(1), 40–59.

Shepard, L. (2021). Ambitious teaching and equitable assessment: A vision for prioritizing learning, not testing. *American Educator, 45*(3), 28–37.

Skiba, R. J., Simmons, A. B., Ritter, S., Gibb, A. C., Rausch, M. K., Caudrado, J., & Chung, C. (2008). Achieving equity in special education: History, status, and current challenges. *Exceptional Children, 74*, 264–288.

Smagorinsky, P. H. (2009). The culture of Vygotsky. *Reading Research Quarterly, 44*(1), 85–95.

Soter, A. O., Wilkinson, I. A., Murphy, P. K., Rudge, L., Reninger, K., & Edwards, M. (2008). What the discourse tells us: Talk and indicators of high-level comprehension. *International Journal of Educational Research, 47*(6), 372–391.

Stiker, H. J. (2009). *A history of disability*. University of Michigan Press.

Sullivan, A. L. (2011). Disproportionality in special education identification and placement of English language learners. *Exceptional Children, 77*, 317–334.

Tannok, R. (2012). *DSM-5 changes in diagnostic criteria for specific learning disabilities (SLD)1: What are the implications?* International Dyslexia Association. *https://dyslexiaida.org/dsm-5-changes-in-diagnostic-criteria-for-specific-learning-disabilities-sld1-what-are-the-implications*

Tefera, A. A., & Artiles, A. J. (2023). Learning disabilities' unsettling intersections: Disrupting learning, cultural, socioeconomic, and environmental deficits. In R. Tierney, F. Rizvi, K. Ercikan, & G. Smith (Eds.), *International encyclopedia of education* (4th ed). Elsevier.

Trent, S. C., Driver, M. K., Rodriguez, D., Oh, K., Stewart, S., Kea, C., & Artiles, A. J. (2014). Beyond Brown: Empirical research on diverse learners with or at-risk for specific learning disabilities from 1994–2012. *Multiple Voices, 14*(2), 12–29.

U.S. Department of Education. (2018). *IDEA. Sec. 300.8 (c) (10). https://sites.ed.gov/idea/regs/b/a/300.8/c/10*

U.S. Department of Education. (2021). *OSEP fast facts: race and ethnicity of children with disabilities served under IDEA Part B*. Office of Special Education Programs. *https://sites.ed.gov/idea/osep-fast-facts-race-and-ethnicity-of-children-with-disabilities-served-under-idea-part-b*

Valencia, R. R. (Ed.). (2011). *Chicano school failure and success: Past, present, and future* (3rd ed.). Routledge/Falmer.

Vygotsky, L. S. (1978). *Mind in society: The development of higher psychological processes*. Harvard University Press.

Vygotsky, L. S. (1987). *Fundamentals of defectology. The collected works of L. S. Vygotsky* (Vol. 2). Plenum Press. (Original work published 1929)

Walton, G. M., & Yeager, D. S. (2020). Seed and soil: Psychological affordances in contexts help to explain where wise interventions succeed or fail. *Current Directions in Psychological Science, 29*(3), 219–226.

Watkins, C. (2015). Meta-learning in classrooms. In D. Scott & E. Hargreaves (Eds.), *The SAGE handbook of learning* (pp. 321–330). SAGE.

Werner, H., & Strauss, A. A. (1941). Pathology of figure-background relation in the child. *Journal of Abnormal and Social Psychology, 36*, 236–248.

Whittaker, M., & Ortiz, S. O. (2019). *What a specific learning disability is not: Examining exclusionary factors* [White paper]. National Council for Learning Disabilities. *www.ncld.org/wp-content/uploads/2019/11/What-a-Specific-Learning-Disability-Is-Not-Examining-Exclusionary-Factors.12192019.pdf*

CHAPTER 24

Integrated Multi-Tiered Systems of Support (I-MTSS)

New Directions for Supporting Students with or at Risk for Learning Disabilities

Allison Gruner Gandhi, Nathan H. Clemens, Michael D. Coyne, Steve Goodman, Kathleen Lynne Lane, Erica S. Lembke, and Brandi Simonsen

In this chapter, we discuss integrated multi-tiered systems of support (I-MTSS), including its historical roots, policy context, benefits, and considerations for the relationship between I-MTSS and students with disabilities. We pay particular attention to implementation challenges and lessons learned from recent research, specifically as it relates to the expanded notion of *integrating* what has traditionally been operationalized as separate academic and behavioral-tiered systems of support. We conclude with a call to action to ensure researcher and practitioner communities are collaboratively engaged in productive cycles of inquiry that lead to improved outcomes for all students, including especially those at risk for or with disabilities.

The authors of this chapter represent four projects funded by the Institute of Education Sciences (IES) as a *network* to investigate I-MTSS. These projects collectively are investigating the implementation and impact of MTSS frameworks that coordinate evidence-based practices to meet the academic, social, emotional, and behavioral needs of all students. Although these projects are separate, research teams meet regularly to share emerging findings and lessons learned and collaborate on dissemination and activities to build the capacity of the next generation of I-MTSS scholars. The four projects are described next.

Cohesive Integration of Behavior Support within a Process of Data-Based Intervention Intensification (BASIC)[1]

This project involves a related set of investigations that focus on the cohesive integration of support for academic engagement as a keystone behavior within a system of intervention intensification for students struggling in reading or math in second and third grades. A Sequential Multiple Assignment Randomized Trial (SMART) design is used to evaluate whether self-regulation strategies, embedded within reading and math interventions, have positive effects on academic and behavioral skills.

Enhancing Ci3T: Building a Professional Capacity for High-Fidelity Implementation to Support Students' Educational Outcomes (Project Enhance)[2]

In Project ENHANCE, we partner with districts to engage in a rapid iterative design approach to identify critical opportunities and develop professional learning structures for bringing to scale a single, coherent integrated MTSS framework—Comprehensive, Integrated, Three-Tiered (Ci3T)—to meet students' academic, behavioral, and social and emotional well-being needs. We identified three focus areas for this design inquiry: (1) Developing Leadership Skills and Structures Needed to Support Ci3T; (2) Building the Capacity of Ci3T Leadership Teams to Support Implementation; and (3) Facilitating the Installation of Systematic Screening for Behavior.

Integrated MTSS Fidelity Rubric (IMFR)[3]

This project aims to develop a fully validated rubric, including accompanying scoring instructions and materials for schools to use as a self-assessment and for researchers to use in studies about integrated MTSS. The project will identify the essential components of an integrated MTSS framework as well as understand the analytic evidence to support the validity and reliability of the IMFR. Finally, the project aims to identify the cost of the IMFR relative to its perceived benefit.

---

[1]Clemens, Vaughn, Roberts, and Doabler; University of Texas at Austin.

[2]Lane, Oakes, Chafouleas, Briesch, Royer, and Common; University of Kansas, Arizona State University, University of Connecticut, Northeastern University, University of Louisville—Kentucky, University of Michigan—Flint.

[3]Gandhi, Lembke, and Riley-Tillman; American Institutes for Research, University of Missouri.

Evaluating the Impact of Integrated Behavior and Reading Multi-Tiered Systems of Support in Elementary School (I-MTSS)[4]

The goal of this project is to rigorously evaluate the impact of integrated behavior and reading practices in kindergarten through grade 2 within a comprehensive, MTSS framework. The project examines the impacts of integrating reading and behavior support at Tiers 1, 2, and 3 of an MTSS framework on students' reading and behavior outcomes as well as teachers' practice. This project involves a randomized controlled trial to evaluate the impact of integrated Tier 1 classroom instruction, a regression discontinuity study to evaluate the impact of integrated Tier 2 supplemental intervention, and a series of single-case design studies to evaluate the impact of individualized integrated Tier 3 behavior and reading intervention on students' behavior and reading outcomes. The project also examines whether there are school, teacher/classroom, or student factors that moderate outcomes. Finally, the project supports schools and districts to build their capacity to implement integrated schoolwide MTSS leadership team training, professional development, and coaching.

The goal of this chapter is to discuss I-MTSS as an important contextual component that guides the education of students with learning disabilities. Understanding its origins, benefits, and current challenges is critical for researchers and practitioners who study and serve this population of students. In particular, the emphasis that I-MTSS frameworks place on supporting the overall social, emotional, behavioral, and academic health of all students has implications for how schools can most effectively serve students who are identified with learning disabilities. The following sections provide general background information on the topic of I-MTSS, as well as specific information and lessons learned from the four IES-funded I-MTSS research network projects.

The History of Tiered Systems

Prior to 1996, most—if not all—educators and school psychologists engaged in what is now referred to as the refer–test–place model (Walker et al., 2004). Specifically, when the discrepancy between current and desired levels of students' academic performance became too great or when students' social and behavioral patterns impeded their academic performance, teachers referred students for assessment to determine special education eligibility (Lane et al., 2020). In many instances, these multidisciplinary teams identified students for special education services, which, in theory, afforded students a customized learning experience based on their individualized needs (Kauffman, 2020).

Practitioners and researchers began to realize this model appeared to result in over—or unnecessary—identification of students with disabilities (Lloyd et al., 1991). These concerns led researchers in the field of school psychology to introduce a new approach to meeting students' needs: refer–consult–intervene (Bergan

[4]Coyne, Simonsen, and McCoach; University of Connecticut.

& Kratochwill, 1990). In this problem-solving approach, teachers could access a general education-led prereferral intervention process to design, implement, and evaluate interventions generated by this team, which included educators and family members. In theory, these prereferral intervention teams (e.g., student study teams and child study teams) functioned to support teachers in meeting students' academic, behavioral, and social skills by adjusting instruction and/or classroom environments (Lane et al., 2003; Lloyd et al., 1991). Yet teachers—through no fault of their own—tended to implement interventions developed by these teams without attention to treatment intensity (Codding & Lane, 2015), treatment integrity (the degree to which it was implemented as planned), or social validity (stakeholders views regarding goals, procedures, and intended outcomes) (Wolf, 1978). These important elements of intervention design were in their infancy. As such, interventions tended to fall short of meeting identified goals.

Bergan and Kratchowill (1990) refined this problem-solving model with the introduction of a four-step problem-solving module: problem identification, problem analysis, implementation, and plan evaluation. This was an important advancement in refining intervention efforts. However, the overall approach focused primarily on within-child characteristics rather than a larger system view (Lane et al., 2020).

Thankfully, in 1996, an important shift occurred: moving away from reactive, within-child approaches to responding to learning and behavior challenges and toward a systems-level approach for meeting students' academic, behavioral, and social learning needs using proactive and reactive components (Lane et al., 2011; Lane et al., 2014; McIntosh & Goodman, 2016; Yudin, 2014). In a seminal 1996 article, Walker and colleagues borrowed important structures from the mental health community and introduced the educational community to tiered systems. In this article, they introduced an integrated model of universal (Tier 1), selected (Tier 2), and indicated (Tier 3) organized to facilitate primary, secondary, and tertiary prevention in schools. This important article paved the path for Positive Behavior Interventions and Support (PBIS) (Horner & Sugai, 2015)—the cornerstone of most tiered systems and featured prominently in the *Individuals with Disabilities Education Improvement Act* (IDEA, 2004).

Over the last 25 years, educational leaders across the country have embraced system-level approaches to prevention and responding to challenging behaviors. During this time, researchers and practitioners have designed, implemented, and tested a variety of tiered systems addressing various learning domains such as PBIS (Sugai & Horner, 2002), response to intervention (RTI) (Fuchs et al., 2012), Interconnected Systems Framework (ISF) (Barrett et al., 2013), multi-tiered system of support (MTSS) (McIntosh & Goodman, 2016), and Ci3T (Lane et al., 2009) models of prevention. These models have been studied widely, with a range of descriptive and experimental inquiry suggesting these models can be implemented with integrity and yield shifts in important academic outcomes for students (e.g., improved reading skills, decreases in internalizing and externalizing behaviors, and improvements in school climate) (Bradshaw et al., 2008, 2010; Common et al., 2019; Lane et al., 2019; McIntosh et al., 2014), as well as improvements for teacher well-being (e.g., lower levels of teacher burnout and higher sense of self-efficacy) (Oakes et al., 2013, 2021).

As these models have been introduced, refined, and sustained, there has been an increased emphasis on *integrated tiered systems* in practice and policy (McIntosh & Goodman, 2016; IES, 2018; Lane et al., 2020; Sugai & Horner, 2009). For example, MTSS initially featured integrating reading, math, and behavioral domains, ISF featured behavioral and mental health domains, and Ci3T featured academic, behavioral, as well as social and emotional well-being domains. It is important to note that PBIS remains a core feature of all integrated domains, with a substantial body of evidence supporting its efficacy and effectiveness. While each integrated system has unique features, there are also several common features, such as the use of treatment integrity and systematic screening to inform decision-making efforts (e.g., Buckman et al., 2021; Lane et al., 2021). In the next section, we explore core characteristics and discuss the benefits of integrated MTSS, highlighting how these complex systems facilitate equity and educational access—important priorities as we navigate the pandemic era (Lane et al., 2021).

Rationale, Definition, and Benefits of I-MTSS

The shift to an *integrated* MTSS framework is particularly critical in an increasingly complex educational landscape. For example, during and after crisis experiences (e.g., natural disasters, school or community violence, social unrest, and COVID-19 global pandemic), state and local education agencies are challenged to implement measures to promote public health and prioritize safety while simultaneously meeting students' elevated social, emotional, behavioral (SEB) (i.e., mental health), and academic needs. An I-MTSS framework allows states, districts, and schools to efficiently and effectively organize, implement, monitor, and enhance supports, with a goal of maximizing benefit for students, families, and educators.

I-MTSS Definition

As members of the national I-MTSS Research Network, we define I-MTSS as "a comprehensive prevention framework for improving the outcomes of all students, including students with or at risk for disabilities, through integrated academic and behavioral support" (I-MTSS Research Network, n.d., para. 1). Within that definition, we further describe the I-MTSS framework in terms of the following five core features.

Integrated Continuum of Research-Informed Practices

Schools implementing an MTSS framework organize practices within a continuum of support that includes universal (Tier 1) support for all (100%), targeted (Tier 2) support for some (~15%) students, and intensive and individualized (Tier 3) support for a few (≤5%) students (e.g., Walker et al., 1996). Within an I-MTSS framework, schools intentionally integrate practices and systems to improve the efficiency and effectiveness of implementation.

Comprehensive Data-Driven Decision Making

Within an MTSS framework, educators collect and use data (i.e., existing school/community data, screening, fidelity monitoring, progress monitoring, and outcome data) to guide all decisions. Within an integrated framework, educators review and make decisions based on multiple streams of academic and behavioral data.

Integrated Teaming and Coaching Structures

Within a traditional MTSS framework, schools and districts invest in systems to support educators' implementation fidelity and sustainability. Within an integrated framework, among the critical systems are representative leadership teaming and effective coaching structures.

Integrated Professional Development

Another critical systems-level support within an I-MTSS framework is job-embedded training in evidence-based practices and ongoing coaching to prompt and provide data-based performance feedback to enhance implementation. Although many states, districts, and schools have established routines for professional development, many approaches are siloed—requiring educators to learn unique practices and programs in isolation (e.g., training in new reading or math curriculum and training in mental health support) and then work to integrate practices at the department, grade, or individual classroom levels. Instead, the I-MTSS Research Network recommends integrated professional development to maximize efficiency while promoting effective implementation.

Additional Systems

In addition to integrated leadership teaming, training, and coaching systems, states, districts, and schools invest in other key systems to enable sustained and scaled implementation. As described in a recent guide, additional considerations include (1) active and authentic engagement of all interested parties (e.g., educators, students, families, and community partners); (2) intentional alignment of funding to support long-term capacity building; (3) consideration of policy to support implementation and outcomes; and (4) developing capacity within the workforce (e.g., preservice through in-service support) (Center on PBIS et al., 2020).

Benefits of I-MTSS

By implementing support within an I-MTSS framework with fidelity, states, districts, and schools may promote equitable access and benefit. Though additional research is needed to document benefits of integrated support within an I-MTSS framework, the following points summarize (1) extensive empirical support for implementing SEB support within an MTSS framework, like PBIS; (2) promise of integrating SEB and school mental health support within a tiered framework; (3) research demonstrating the promise of RTI or MTSS frameworks for implementing academic support; and (4) emerging evidence demonstrating the potential benefit of an I-MTSS approach to integrated academic and behavior support. Consider the following areas of empirical support.

- Organizing SEB support within a MTSS framework, like PBIS, is associated with improved student SEB skills, decreased exclusionary discipline, improved academic outcomes, reduced perceptions of bullying and substance abuse, increased attendance, and improved school climate (Bastable et al., 2015; Bradshaw et al., 2008; Bradshaw et al., 2009; Bradshaw et al., 2010; Bradshaw et al., 2012; Freeman et al., 2016; Gage et al., 2019; Horner et al., 2009; Lee & Gage, 2020; Ross & Horner, 2009; Simonsen et al., 2012; Waasdorp et al., 2012). In addition, educators experience improved self-efficacy and decreased stress and burnout when schools implement PBIS (Kelm & McIntosh, 2012; Ross et al., 2012).

- Integrating school-based SEB support (PBIS) and school mental health support SMH), through an ISF, is associated with enhanced student access to and potential benefit from school mental health support (Splett et al., 2018; Weist et al., 2018).

- Organizing academic support within an RTI or MTSS framework is associated with improved academic outcomes (e.g., improved reading outcomes) (Grapin et al., 2019; Leonard et al., 2019; Swanson et al., 2017).

- Integrating reading and SEB support within an I-MTSS framework is associated with improved reading and SEB outcomes (Algozzine et al., 2012; Chaparro et al., 2012; Chaparro et al., 2012; Chaparro et al., 2020).

- Integrating academic, behavior, and social and emotional well-being in Ci3T models is associated with decreased levels of risk in internalizing and externalizing behaviors (e.g., Lane et al., 2008; Lane et al., 2012), which were, in turn, predictive of academic (e.g., reading measures, grade point averages, and course failures) as well as behavioral and social skills outcomes (e.g., ODRs, suspension, and self-control skills) (e.g., Ennis et al., 2012; Lane et al., 2008; Lane et al., 2019; Oakes et al., 2010).

Integrated MTSS and Students in Special Education

Although MTSS is traditionally thought of as a schoolwide model of tiered intervention, it is important to keep in mind that its impetus was RTI, an effort to improve how students with learning disabilities (LD) are identified. RTI is a decision-making process for identifying disability/determining need for special education. But the core features of MTSS (strong, evidence-based core instruction; system of screening/early identification of risk; some level of intensifying support in addition to core instruction; and methods for monitoring progress) provide the structure that makes RTI decisions possible.

MTSS helps educators determine (1) whether difficulties are the result of inadequate core support, (2) the extent to which core supports are sufficient or if more ongoing, intensive intervention is needed, and (3) what intervention/supports should look like for that student. Perhaps most key, MTSS also provides data that can be utilized in subsequent eligibility evaluation decisions, thus supporting a more informed decision that can be clearly tied to Individualized Education Plan (IEP) goals. MTSS also offers a way to more immediately provide intervention for students in need, whereby supplemental intervention can be provided as soon as risk is identified. If students are later referred for a formal evaluation, an MTSS model allows them to receive intervention while the process unfolds.

For example, if a student with LD is provided Tier 2 supplemental intervention in reading using a standard, validated intervention, ongoing progress monitoring should be implemented to determine whether the intervention is effective. If the data indicate the intervention is effective, it can be continued. However, if not effective, more intensive intervention should be considered. This more intensive intervention, oftentimes provided as part of Tier 3, should be specifically tailored to the student's needs. Whereas typical intervention might involve a standard, validated intervention (i.e., "off-the-shelf") provided to several students in a small group who all have similar needs, intensive intervention is more likely to involve strategies and programs that are (1) tailored specifically to the needs of individual students, and (2) further tailored and adjusted based on frequent analysis of progress-monitoring data.

I-MTSS, through the integration of academic and behavior supports and data sources, may further improve the ways in which LDs are identified compared to an MTSS model focused only on academic skills. I-MTSS involves establishing core behavior instruction and supports, which allows for ruling out the possibility that a student's behavior difficulties are the result of inadequate core behavior support. Behavior data, collected through universal screening and additional assessments for students experiencing behavior difficulties, can be used in an LD evaluation to inform the extent to which challenging behaviors are playing a role in the students' academic difficulties. For students referred for behavioral difficulties, the academic skills data provided by the I-MTSS system informs the extent to which behavior problems may be motivated or maintained by academic difficulties. For students in need of additional supports, I-MTSS system provides a way to structure intensive interventions that target multiple domains of need for a student (academic, behavior, and motivation), thus offering greater chances for success than only targeting one domain.

An I-MTSS system also provides a better context for supporting comprehensive, intensive interventions across settings and times of day. Stronger core behavior support in general education can improve student engagement and reduce disruptions to instruction, thereby providing students with LD as well as other disabilities (e.g., emotional disturbances) better opportunities for learning and success in core instruction (Lane et al., 2020). For students with more intensive needs, greater communication among general and special education teachers and shared awareness of a student's needs and support plan allows supplemental behavior supports to be embedded across settings (e.g., resource room, core instruction, and nonclassroom settings) rather than remaining limited to just one location.

Role of I-MTSS in LD Identification

Currently, special education law allows for the use of academic RTI data in decision making to determine whether a student has an LD. The following is an example of how the structures and data sources in an I-MTSS model support an RTI decision-making process for the identification of LD. Hector was a second-grade student who was new to his school at the beginning of the year. The school's gradewide fall screening assessments identified him as performing low in reading. Gradewide behavior screening also indicated difficulties in behavior, such as disruptive and off-task behavior during core instruction. The grade-level team identified him for Tier 2 intervention in reading. As part of the school's I-MTSS model, behavior intervention was integrated within academic intervention, which included teaching behavior expectations and a token economy to reinforce behaviors consistent with those expectations. These expectations and the token economy are consistent with those used in Hector's core instruction, thereby providing a cohesive link in the behavior support across settings. The Tier 2 intervention also included progress-monitoring data in reading and behavior.

Following implementation of the Tier 2 intervention for six weeks, the grade-level decision-making team determined that Hector was in need of Tier 3 intervention in reading, based on very little progress in reading. However, Hector's behavior had improved considerably during the intervention; progress-monitoring data indicated significant improvement in his on-task behavior, and his classroom teacher reported similar engagement to that of his peers and very few instances of disruptive behavior. This information was critical in demonstrating that (1) Hector's reading difficulties were due to more than difficulties staying on-task during instruction and (2), because he was highly responsive to Tier 1 and Tier 2 behavior support strategies, he is likely not in need of specially designed intervention for behavior.

As part of the Tier 3 intervention routine, Hector received an evidence-based intervention, delivered with fidelity, as part of a small group that included two other students with similar reading skill needs. Fidelity data were collected on intervention implementation via a checklist that is completed by a coach or school psychologist in the building. Progress monitoring continued during the Tier 3 intervention, but at greater frequency than during the Tier 2 support. Based on a predetermined length of intervention implementation (typically 6 weeks), the grade-level team met to evaluate Hector's progress. Although Hector's behavior remained consistent with expectations (and was not a cause of continued reading difficulties), his reading had improved only slightly and was still considerably below the goal the team had targeted for him. At this point, the intervention was intensified (see following section and Table 24.1), and data collection continued. A few weeks into the intensified intervention saw Hector making some progress, but still below his target. The team decided to refer Hector for an evaluation to determine whether he qualified for special education as a student with an LD. At this stage, the school psychologist conducted a brief evaluation using standardized tests of relevant academic skills and considered the universal screening and progress-monitoring data collected throughout the process in making a determination.

There are several important components of this process that are worth pointing out. First, an I-MTSS system provides screening and progress-monitoring data on academic skills and behavior, thus allowing schools to (1) identify students at risk in either area (or both) and (2) monitor responsiveness to intervention aimed at improving either domain. Interventions that *integrate* behavior support within academic skills intervention and align supports across settings offer a greater likelihood of success and a stronger basis for evaluating student responsiveness to intervention in academic skills and behavior. Overall, integration of academic and behavior data sources and interventions provides educators with a better basis for ruling out behavior as a cause of a student's learning difficulties and a stronger basis for determining whether a behavior disorder co-occurs with an LD. In a school without an I-MTSS model, a student like Hector might be referred for an evaluation as a student with a behavior disorder (in addition to LD), whereas the I-MTSS structure and data sources revealed specially designed instruction in behavior for Hector was not necessary. Additionally, as mentioned earlier, a clear benefit to this process is that if students are later referred for a formal evaluation, they are already receiving intervention throughout the process (which usually takes over several weeks).

Role of I-MTSS in Intervention and Specially Designed Instruction for LD

I-MTSS offers a way to structure interventions to meet students' needs in a more comprehensive way. Attention difficulties and challenging behaviors are among the primary variables associated with students' inadequate responsiveness to academic interventions (Al Otaiba & Fuchs, 2002; Nelson et al., 2003). Better integrating behavior support within academic skills interventions for students with LD may improve behaviors and skills, such as academic engagement and self-regulation, which are critical for learning and may enhance academic skill growth. Additionally, I-MTSS allows behavior support to be better integrated across multiple school settings, thus providing greater consistency in expectations and support approaches for students with LD who traverse multiple academic and non-academic contexts during the day.

One consideration when utilizing MTSS with students with LD is to make certain that students who are identified for special education services are receiving intensive, specialized intervention within the tiered system. In some cases, students with IEPs are provided intervention as part of Tier 3 services with other students who are not on IEPs. While these students may have similar needs, it is critical that students with LD, for example, are receiving specialized services targeting their areas of need according to their IEP. Utilizing an intensification framework (see Fuchs et al., 2018), the current intervention program can be refined in one of the dimensions listed in column 1 of Table 24.1.

This intensification process utilizes I-MTSS to provide a specialized intervention model that is tailored to individual student need, which is exactly what is needed for students with LD and particularly for those students for whom typical intervention has failed in the past.

TABLE 24.1. Intensification Guidelines and Examples

Dimension	Guidelines and examples
Strength: Is the intervention designed or validated for this population?	Include more error correction Include additional practice options
Dosage: Is the intervention amenable to dosage increase or change?	Deliver more one-to-one activities Increase duration or frequency by continuing activities until the student can quickly and consistently produce the correct target skill
Alignment: Is the intervention targeted towards the student's specific skill strengths and needs?	Align instruction to each student's specific skill deficit Build on a student's strengths by interleaving known skills with new skills (two known to one new)
Transfer: Does the intervention have high transfer potential?	Help students transfer the skills they learn from this instruction to other related or broader skills
Complexity: Is the intervention sufficiently complex?	Provide more direct, explicit instructional principles, such as modeling the steps or providing enough practice opportunities until they generate more correct responses Incorporate systematic cumulative review
Behavioral support: Is it easy or feasible to integrate appropriate behavioral supports with this intervention?	Incorporate attention, motivation, or self-regulated learning components (e.g., goal setting with the student) Use strategies to minimize nonproductive (i.e., distracting or disruptive) behavior
Individualization: Does this intervention lend itself to being adapted to individual student needs?	Systematically tailor the activities over time based on the student's progress monitoring data (i.e., CBM) to address the student's specific needs Modify instruction (e.g., providing more opportunities for practice, more modeling, more instructional time, more one-to-one opportunities), keep as is, or increase the goal depending on the progress monitoring data

Note. Based on Fuchs et al. (2018).

Implementation of Integrated MTSS: Current Challenges and Research

Integrated MTSS is a relatively new concept. Understandably, schools struggle with operationalizing what it means and setting up the infrastructure to support its effective implementation. We know that setting up effective academic-tiered systems, such as RTI, or behavioral-tiered systems, such as PBIS, takes many years, and sustaining them requires ongoing financial and strategic support (McIntosh et al., 2018; Scaletta & Tejero Hughes, 2020; Ward et al., 2021). It is reasonable to assume, therefore, that setting up and sustaining effective tiered systems that *integrate* academic and behavioral supports is even more complicated. Indeed, setting up integrated systems sometimes requires dismantling or adjusting practices that schools have grown accustomed to when implementing tiered systems that only focus on academics *or* behavior.

Each of the I-MTSS Research Network projects has observed challenges among their participating schools in the implementation of I-MTSS. For example, among schools participating in the IMFR project, few demonstrate strong, sustained implementation of integrated MTSS. Instead, most schools in the IMFR sample could be described as "aligning" their tiered systems, but not yet fully integrating. Making the shift from alignment to integration requires a change in mindset and infrastructure that is particularly difficult, and among the IMFR schools, this was reflected most notably in school-teaming structures and school or district-level supports. With respect to teams, the IMFR project observed significant variation across the schools in the participating sample with respect to the number of teams and their functions. For example, some schools had teams organized by tier. Some had teams organized by content (academic and behavior). Some had teams organized by tier and content area together. Some had teams at each grade level or grouped grade levels together. Some had overall building-level teams in addition to many of these other teams. In many cases, it was clear that combining teams could lead to efficiencies and a more seamless way to conduct data-based decision making using both academic and behavioral data. Furthermore, the IMFR project found siloed infrastructure in that school-level or district-level supports, such as professional development, staffing, resources, and leadership, were rarely set up to promote integration. On the contrary, these kinds of supports focused either on academic-tiered systems or behavioral-tiered systems, and it was up to the schools to piece these supports together in a way that best supports their implementation of an integrated MTSS model. For example, the district might offer comprehensive professional development on tiered intervention in reading but not have a parallel offering for behavior, or if they do offer both, staff might be required to choose one or the other. Similarly, the data systems that schools use in their tiered systems are a combination of separate academic, behavior, and social–emotional screening, progress monitoring, and diagnostic tools. School staff must work to bring data from these sources together to conduct effective integrated decision making. Implementation of integrated MTSS will benefit from systems that intentionally support the examination of these multiple data sources together.

Project BASIC investigated a process of intensifying supplemental intervention that integrates academic and behavior support. Although intervention was implemented entirely by well-resourced and highly trained project staff, there were challenges similar to what schools commonly experience in implementing tiered interventions. These challenges included (1) the need to rapidly process screening data to identify students for intervention, (2) scheduling intervention at times in which staff are available but do not conflict with academic instruction or other necessary classroom/school activities, (3) finding physical space in school buildings to conduct small-group intervention, (4) balancing student data and logistical constraints in creating heterogenous student groups, (5) allocating resources for progress monitoring and conducting with minimal disruptions to interventions, (6) rapidly processing student data to determine for which students intervention intensity should increase or decrease, and (7) regular observations of intervention groups by project leadership to observe implementation and, when needed, provide coaching and booster training. Learning from Project BASIC suggests that navigating these challenges requires strong leadership and coordination at the project (i.e., district) and building levels, good communication, as well as staff flexibility and the ability to adjust on the fly. Efficient integration of academic and behavior intervention may reduce burdens associated with attempting to implement parallel supports. However, the challenges that schools face in implementing and sustaining MTSS suggest that its common conceptualization requires reconsideration, with an effort toward simpler systems.

Project ENHANCE worked with partner district- and school-site leaders in their capacity to use their Ci3T structures to pivot to remote and hybrid learning environments as they navigate the pandemic. The Project ENHANCE researchers collaborated with district leaders and Ci3T Leadership Team members to facilitate positive, productive environments for students, families, educators, and administrators during the pandemic (Lane et al., 2021). The iterative design inquiry taking place as part of Project ENHANCE has provided schools with immediate, on-demand professional learning resources (e.g., ebooks, videos, practice guides, infographics, and interactive resources) using input from descriptive studies taking place in the first year (e.g., professional learning priorities) (Common et al., 2021). Educators use these resources to support students' continued learning and welcome students in returning to schools. Amidst these successes, there are also challenges: negotiating changes in district and school-site leaders, balancing the need for timely data collection with the multiple demands educators face daily, and being cautious not to overwhelm or alienate the very people we seek to serve.

When working with schools and districts to implement integrated reading and behavioral practices at Tiers 1, 2, and 3, the I-MTSS Research Team at UConn encountered many of the same challenges identified by the other Network projects, particularly related to schools wanting to integrate academic and behavior practices and systems, but facing structural barriers to accomplishing true integration. We also found that the instructional materials that schools use to teach reading and behavior often pose a challenge to integration. Even when teachers and schools have committed to combining practices, instructional materials do not always lend themselves to integration. For example, a school may have an evidence-based small-group reading intervention as well as explicit routines for teaching and supporting behavioral engagement. However, because these instructional materials are highly scripted and specified, it is very difficult for interventionists to integrate these in a cohesive way. Therefore, one goal of the I-MTSS project is to develop strategies to embed explicit instruction in behavior engagement strategies directly into scripted reading lessons.

Next Steps: Call to Action

We believe that I-MTSS offers a promising approach for meeting the needs of students with LD in schools. First, through universal screening, early intervention for students experiencing academic difficulties, and ongoing progress monitoring, teachers and schools have access to important information about students that can support timely and valid identification of students with LD. This information includes not only assessment data but also students' response to evidence-based interventions, a central feature of current models of LD identification. Access to information about students' behavioral and social and emotional needs within I-MTSS frameworks also provides planning and placement teams with additional information that can help with decisions about identification and IEP development.

Second, and more importantly, schools that implement comprehensive I-MTSS are able to provide students with LD with more effective and efficient academic and behavioral support. Because I-MTSS is a preventative schoolwide approach that encompasses both general and special education, there is less possibility that support for students with LD will be siloed, generic, or delayed. Instead, I-MTSS frameworks ensure all students identified as at risk through universal screening measures, including students with as-yet-undiagnosed LD, receive timely evidence-based academic and behavioral interventions. Tiers of support within I-MTSS frameworks also provide students with access to increasingly more intensive intervention options based on progress-monitoring data. Often, information about lack of response to I-MTSS interventions triggers a comprehensive special education evaluation. When a student is determined eligible for special education services with a learning disability in a school that is implementing I-MTSS, that student will already be receiving academic and behavioral support aligned with their needs. Instead of special education eligibility initiating supplemental support for students in a separate special education system, developing an IEP for a student who is already accessing I-MTSS provides an opportunity to better align, individualize, intensify, and protect supports that are already partially in place.

Although we believe that I-MTSS offers teachers and schools a powerful framework for better meeting the needs of students with LD, we also recognize that, as a field, we are still learning about both the evidence that supports I-MTSS as well as how schools can best implement I-MTSS. Next, we propose some next steps for practitioners and researchers.

Implications for Practitioners

I-MTSS is complex, yet we believe that it is essential for schools to implement the practices and systems associated with I-MTSS with high levels of fidelity and consistency, especially to meet the needs of students with LD. There is evidence that partial and inconsistent implementation of I-MTSS practices may not lead to effects on important student outcomes (e.g., Balu, 2015). In addition, in our experience, schools underestimate the systems and infrastructure needed to implement and sustain I-MTSS practices (Coyne et al., 2016). Therefore, schools need to work to ensure that there is a comprehensive schoolwide plan for implementing I-MTSS with fidelity. This includes both identifying and adopting evidence-based practices in assessment, instruction, and intervention, as well as working to establish the systems and structures (e.g., school leadership teams, data-meeting processes, and coaching capacity) that are necessary to coordinate and align these academic and behavioral practices across grades and tiers, facilitate ongoing data-based decision making, support teachers and staff, and monitor the fidelity and quality of implementation).

Despite the challenges of implementing comprehensive I-MTSS, many of which were identified earlier in this chapter, our experience working with schools and districts across the country has shown us that schools can implement the practices and systems associated with I-MTSS frameworks with high levels of quality and fidelity. In our different programs of research, we have seen high-quality implementation of I-MTSS in schools of different sizes in different types of districts (small, large, urban, suburban, and rural) and across tiers of instruction, grade levels, academic areas (e.g., mathematics and reading), and behavior support models (e.g., PBIS and social and emotional learning approaches). However, to implement an integrated MTSS model correctly and consistently, educators need necessary conditions in place. They need guidance on what to do and why it is important to do it. Educators need to know what to do, how to do it, and why they should be doing it. In our observations and research, one of the most important factors associated with high-quality implementation is skilled and consistent leadership.

A leadership team at the school and district level helps support implementation by developing and maintaining an infrastructure to support staff in their use of effective practices. The team reviews data and engages in data-informed action. The teams also provide communication with different groups/teams within the school and across the district to promote visibility and priority for this work. A leadership team can help promote the purpose and importance for the work of integrating MTSS. The leadership helps to guard against staff feeling that this work is a temporary project and will go away when a new initiative appears (Adelman & Taylor, 2007). This may focus on facilitating action that promotes proper implementation, such as providing priority, policy, and guidance. Facilitating also means providing clear, positive, and specific feedback to implementers for their work. Promoting the integration work also means removing barriers to implementation. Such barriers may include lack of direction, competing initiatives, or limited resources for implementation of the I-MTSS practices. Competing initiatives are aligned, integrated, or removed. A leadership team at the school and the district level should help to drive forward the effective implementation of integrated MTSS while also removing resistance to implementation efforts. The following is a quick checklist for supporting educators in the implementation of effective practices:

- Urgency and priority for the practices are communicated by leadership.
- Competing initiatives are aligned, integrated, or removed.
- Adequate training and coaching are provided.
- Necessary resources and materials are provided to implement the practices.
- Information is provided for implementing staff and leadership on student outcomes, fidelity of implementation, and performance feedback.
- Staff are provided with time to plan, review information, and act on the data.

Although I-MTSS is complex and requires a dedicated and strong leadership, schoolwide commitments, and ongoing supports for teachers and staff, we believe that I-MTSS is both a feasible and promising framework that can help schools better meet the needs of all students, particularly students with LD.

Implications for Research

As part of the research network, we have been working across teams and sites to develop a framework for both understanding existing research related to I-MTSS as well as guiding current and future research on I-MTSS. Because I-MTSS is complex, dynamic, and flexible and includes multiple components, we believe that different types of research designs and methodologies are needed to accumulate rigorous and trustworthy evidence on the effects of I-MTSS. First, I-MTSS is built on a foundation of existing evidence-based academic and behavioral practices in assessment, instruction, intervention, and data-based decision making. For example, the field has converging evidence on the positive impacts of the use of specific screening and progress-monitoring measures, classroom instructional approaches, and intervention programs on student academic and behavioral outcomes. However, we have fewer studies on the effects of these evidence-based academic and behavioral practices when they are integrated.

The research network is currently conducting experimental and quasi-experimental studies examining the effects of just such integrated practices. Key research questions for studies evaluating integrated academic and behavioral practices include whether the effects of integrated practices are similar to, or larger than, the effects of those practices implemented separately. Findings of similar effects would suggest that integrated practices may be equally effective but more efficient. For example, if an intervention that included both reading and behavioral engagement instruction produced effects on reading and behavioral outcomes comparable to the effects of these interventions implemented separately (and were of comparable time and duration), it would suggest efficiencies for integrated interventions. Findings of larger effects would suggest a facilitative and interactive relationship between the academic and behavioral components of integrated intervention. For example, the behavioral engagement component of the intervention described previously might facilitate students' response to the reading instruction, while the fast pace and successful learning opportunities associated with the reading instruction might facilitate increased behavioral engagement. Similar research could be conducted on the utility, feasibility, and predictive power of screening models that include both academic and behavior data.

Although conducting experimental research on the impacts of specific integrated practices in assessment, instruction, and intervention is essential for accumulating evidence on the effects of I-MTSS, it is not sufficient. Systems, structures, and routines for aligning, coordinating, and supporting implementation are also central to I-MTSS frameworks. Therefore, research investigating how these systems-level components contribute to the effectiveness, feasibility, and sustainability of I-MTSS is also essential. Some of the systems that are integral to I-MTSS frameworks, and all MTSS frameworks, include the role and function of school teams (e.g., leadership, data, grade level, and intervention), the process for making data-based instructional decisions, the availability of professional development and coaching activities, and the alignment and coordination of supports across tiers (and across general and special education). Experimental research designs may be appropriate for examining the contributions of some of these systems components, but other methodologies could also provide more targeted and nuanced information, for example, research questions and designs informed by implementation science as well as descriptive and mixed-methods approaches. Finally, evaluations of comprehensive schoolwide, or districtwide, implementations of I-MTSS are important to provide evidence on the effects of I-MTSS implemented at scale in real-world applied settings.

In summary, there is strong, compelling evidence that supports the specific academic and behavioral practices that provide the foundation for I-MTSS frameworks, and current research being conducted by the network is evaluating the effects of integrating some of these practices across different tiers and across different academic and behavioral domains. To continue to build a strong and convergent evidence base on the effects, implementation, and sustainability of I-MTSS frameworks, however, researchers should continue to carry out rigorous experimental studies on integrated practices as well as conceptualize and conduct research using more diverse designs and methodologies to investigate the contribution of the systems and structures that are central to I-MTSS.

REFERENCES

Adelman, H. S., & Taylor, L. (2007). Systemic change for school improvement. *Journal of Educational and Psychological Consultation, 17,* 55–77.

Al Otaiba, S., & Fuchs, D. (2002). Characteristics of children who are unresponsive to early literacy intervention: A review of the literature. *Remedial and Special Education, 23*(5), 300–316.

Algozzine, B., Wang, C., White, R., Cooke, N., Marr, M. B., Algozzine, K., et al. (2012).

Effects of multi-tier academic and behavior instruction on difficult-to-teach students. *Exceptional Children, 79*, 45–64.

Balu, R., Zhu, P., Doolittle, F., Schiller, E., Jenkins, J., & Gersten, R. (2015). *Evaluation of response to intervention practices for elementary school reading* (NCEE 2016-4000). National Center for Education Evaluation and Regional Assistance, Institute of Education Sciences, U.S. Department of Education.

Bastable, E., Kittelman, A., & McIntosh, K. (March 2015). *Do high schools implementing SWPBIS have lower rates of illegal drug and alcohol use?* Center on PBIS, University of Oregon. *www.pbis.org*

Bergan, J., & Kratochwill, T. (1990). *Behavioral consultation and therapy.* Plenum Press.

Bradshaw, C. P., Koth, C. W., Bevans, K. B., Ialongo, N., & Leaf, P. J. (2008). The impact of school-wide Positive Behavioral Interventions and Supports (PBIS) on the organizational health of elementary schools. *School Psychology Quarterly, 23*, 462–473.

Bradshaw, C. P., Koth, C. W., Thorton, L. A., & Leaf, P. J. (2009). Altering school climate through school-wide Positive Behavioral Interventions and Supports: Findings from a group-randomized effectiveness trial. *Prevention Science, 10*, 100–115.

Bradshaw, C. P., Mitchell, M. M., & Leaf, P. J. (2010). Examining the effects of schoolwide Positive Behavioral Interventions and Supports on student outcomes. *Journal of Positive Behavior Interventions, 12*, 133–148.

Bradshaw, C., Waasdorp, T., & Leaf, P. (2012). Effects of school-wide Positive Behavioral Interventions and Supports on child behavior problems. *Pediatrics, 130*, 1136–1145.

Buckman, M. M., Lane, K. L., Common, E. A., Royer, D. J., Oakes, W. P., Allen, G. E., et al. (2021). Treatment integrity of primary (Tier 1) prevention efforts in tiered systems: Mapping the literature. *Education and Treatment of Children, 44*(3), 145–168.

Center on Positive Behavioral Interventions and Supports, State Implementation and Scaling Up of Evidence-Based Practices Center, National Integrated Multi-Tiered Systems of Support Research Network, National Center on Improving Literacy, & Lead for Literacy Center. (2020, June). *Returning to school during and after crisis: A guide to supporting states, districts, schools, educators, and students through a multi-tiered systems of support framework during the 2020–2021 school year.* University of Oregon. *www.pbis.org*

Chaparro, E. A., Jackson, K. R., Baker, S. K., & Smolkowski, K. (2012). Effective behavioural and instructional support systems: An integrated approach to behaviour and academic support at the district level. *Advances in School Mental Health Promotion, 5*(3), 161–176.

Chaparro, E. A., Smolkowski, K., Baker, S. K., Hanson, N., & Ryan-Jackson, K. (2012). A model for system-wide collaboration to support integrated social behavior and literacy evidence-based practices. *Psychology in the Schools, 49*(5), 465–482.

Chaparro, E. A., Smolkowski, K., & Jackson, K. R. (2020). Scaling up and integrating Effective Behavioral and Instructional Support Systems (EBISS): A study of one state's professional development efforts. *Learning Disability Quarterly, 43*(1), 4–17.

Codding, R. S., & Lane, K. L. (2015). Spotlight on treatment intensity: An important and often overlooked component of intervention inquiry. *Journal of Behavioral Education, 24*, 1–10.

Common, E. A., Buckman, M. M., Lane, K. L., Leko, M., Royer, D. J., Oakes, W. P., & Allen, G. E. (2019). Exploring solutions to address students' social competencies to facilitate school success: A usability and feasibility study. *Education and Treatment of Children, 42*(4), 489–514.

Common, E. A., Buckman, M. M., Lane, K. L., Oakes, W. P., Royer, D. J., Chafouleas, S., et al. (2021). Project ENHANCE: Assessing professional learning needs for implementing Comprehensive, Integrated, Three-Tiered (Ci3T) Models of Prevention. *Education and Treatment of Children, 44*, 125–144.

Coyne, M. D., Oldham, A., Leonard, K., Burns, D., & Gage, N. (2016). Delving into the details: Implementing multitiered K–3 reading supports in high-priority schools. *New Directions for Child and Adolescent Development, 154*, 67–85.

Ennis, R. P., Lane, K. L., & Oakes, W. P. (2012). Score reliability and validity of the Student Risk Screening Scale: A psychometrically sound, feasible tool for use in urban elementary schools. *Journal of Emotional and Behavioral Disorders, 20*, 241–259.

Freeman, J., Simonsen, B., McCoach, D. B., Sugai, G., Lombardi, A., & Horner, R. (2016). Relationship between school-wide positive behavior interventions and supports and academic, attendance, and behavior outcomes in high schools. *Journal of Positive Behavior Interventions, 18*, 41–51.

Fuchs, L. S., Fuchs, D., & Compton, D. L. (2012). Smart RTI: A next-generation approach to multilevel protection. *Exceptional Children, 78*(3), 236–279.

Fuchs, L. S., Fuchs, D., & Malone, A. S. (2018). The taxonomy of intervention intensity. *Teaching Exceptional Children, 50*(4), 194–202.

Gage, N. A., Grasley-Boy, N., George, H. P., Childs, K., & Kincaid, D. (2019). A quasi-experimental design analysis of the effects of school-wide positive behavior interventions and supports on discipline in Florida. *Journal of Positive Behavior Interventions, 21*, 50–61.

Grapin, S. L., Waldron, N., & Joyce, B. D. (2019). Longitudinal effects of RTI implementation on reading achievement outcomes. *Psychology in the Schools, 56*(2), 242–254.

Horner, R. H., & Sugai, G. (2015). School-wide PBIS: An example of applied behavior analysis implemented at a scale of social importance. *Behavior Analysis in Practice, 8*, 80–85.

Horner, R. H., Sugai, G., Smolkowski, K., Eber, L., Nakasato, J., Todd, A. W., & Esperanza, J. (2009). A randomized, wait-list controlled effectiveness trial assessing school-wide positive behavior support in elementary schools. *Journal of Positive Behavior Interventions, 11*, 133–144.

Institute of Education Sciences. (2018). *Request for applications: Research networks focus on critical problems of policy and practice in special education* (CFDA 84.324N). U.S. Department of Education.

Kauffman, J. M. (Ed.). (2020). *On educational inclusion: Meanings, history, issues, and international perspectives*. Routledge.

Kelm, J. L., & McIntosh, K. (2012). Effects of school-wide positive behavior support on teacher self-efficacy. *Psychology in the Schools, 49*(2), 137–147.

Lane, K. L., Buckman, M. M., Oakes, W. P., & Menzies, H. M. (2020). Tiered systems and inclusion: Potential benefits, clarifications, and considerations. In J. M. Kauffman (Ed.). *On educational inclusion: Meanings, history, issues, and international perspectives* (pp. 85–106). Routledge.

Lane, K. L., Harris, K., Graham, S., Driscoll, S. A., Sandmel, K., Morphy, P., et al. (2011). Self-regulated strategy development at tier-2 for second grade students with writing and behavioral difficulties: A randomized control trial. *Journal of Research on Educational Effectiveness, 4*, 322–353.

Lane, K. L., Kalberg, J. R., Bruhn, A. L., Mahoney, M. E., & Driscoll, S. A. (2008). Primary prevention programs at the elementary level: Issues of treatment integrity, systematic screening, and reinforcement. *Education and Treatment of Children, 31*, 465–494.

Lane, K. L., Kalberg, J. R., & Menzies, H. M. (2009). *Developing schoolwide programs to prevent and manage problem behaviors: A step-by-step approach.* Guilford Press.

Lane, K. L., Mahdavi, J. N., & Borthwick-Duffy, S. A. (2003). Teacher perceptions of the prereferral intervention process: A call for assistance with school-based interventions. *Preventing School Failure, 47*, 148–155.

Lane, K. L., Menzies, H. M, Oakes, W. P., & Kalberg, J. R. (2012). *Systematic screenings of behavior to support instruction: From preschool to high school.* Guilford Press.

Lane, K. L., Oakes, W. P., Cantwell, E. D., Royer, D. J., Leko, M., Schatschneider, C., & Menzies, H. M. (2019). Predictive validity of Student Risk Screening Scale for Internalizing and Externalizing scores in secondary schools. *Journal of Emotional and Behavioral Disorders, 27*, 86–100.

Lane, K. L., Oakes, W. P., & Menzies, H. M. (2014). Comprehensive, Integrated, Three-Tiered

(CI3T) Models of Prevention: Why does my school—and district—need an integrated approach to meet students' academic, behavioral, and social needs? *Preventing School Failure, 58*, 121–128.

Lane, K. L., Oakes, W. P., & Menzies, H. M. (2021). Considerations for systematic screening PK-12: Universal screening for internalizing and externalizing behaviors in the COVID-19 era. *Preventing School Failure: Alternative Education for Children and Youth, 65(3)*, 275–281.

Lee, A., & Gage, N. A. (2020). Updating and expanding systematic reviews and meta-analyses on the effects of schoolwide positive behavior interventions and supports. *Psychology in the Schools, 57*(5), 783–804.

Leonard, K. M., Coyne, M. D., Oldham, A. C., Burns, D., & Gillis, M. B. (2019). Implementing MTSS in beginning reading: Tools and systems to support schools and teachers. *Learning Disabilities Research & Practice, 34*(2), 110–117.

Lloyd, J., Kauffman, J., Landrum, T., & Roe, D. (1991). Why do teachers refer pupils for special education: An analysis of referral records. *Exceptionality, 2*, 115–126.

McIntosh, K., & Goodman, S. (2016). *Integrating multi-tiered systems of support: Blending RTI and PBIS.* Guilford Press.

McIntosh, K., Mercer, S. H., Nese, R. N. T., Strickland-Cohen, M. K., Kittelman, A., Hoselton, R., & Horner, R. H. (2018). Factors predicting sustained implementation of a universal behavior support framework. *Educational Researcher, 47*(5), 307–316.

McIntosh, K., Ty, S. V., & Miller, L. D. (2014). Effects of school-wide positive behavioral interventions and supports on internalizing problems: Current evidence and future directions. *Journal of Positive Behavior Interventions, 16*(4), 209–218.

Nelson, R. J., Benner, G. J., & Gonzalez, J. (2003). Learner characteristics that influence the treatment effectiveness of early literacy interventions: A meta-analytic review. *Learning Disabilities Research & Practice, 18*, 255–267.

Oakes, W. P., Lane, K. L., Jenkins, A., & Booker, B. B. (2013). Three-tiered models of prevention: Teacher efficacy and burnout. *Education and Treatment of Children, 36*, 95–126.

Oakes, W. P., Lane, K. L., Royer, D. J., Menzies, H. M., Buckman, M. M., Brunsting, N. C., et al. (2021). Elementary teachers' self-efficacy during initial implementation of comprehensive, integrated, three-tiered models of prevention. *Journal of Positive Behavior Interventions, 23*, 93–105.

Oakes, W. P., Wilder, K., Lane, K. L., Powers, L., Yokoyama, L., O'Hare, M. E., & Jenkins, A. B. (2010). Psychometric properties of the Student Risk Screening Scale: An effective tool for use in diverse urban elementary schools. *Assessment for Effective Intervention, 35*, 231–239.

Ross, S., & Horner, R. (2009). Bully prevention in positive behavior support. *Journal of Applied Behavior Analysis, 42*, 747–759.

Ross, S. W., Romer, N., & Horner, R. H. (2012). Teacher well-being and the implementation of school-wide positive behavior interventions and supports. *Journal of Positive Behavior Interventions, 14*, 118–128.

Scaletta, M., & Tejero Hughes, M. (2020). Sustained Positive Behavioral Interventions and Supports implementation: School leaders discuss their processes and practices. *Journal of Positive Behavior Interventions, 23*(1), 30–41.

Simonsen, B., Eber, L., Black, A., Sugai, G., Lewandowski, H., Sims, B., & Myers, D. (2012). Illinois state-wide positive behavior interventions and supports: Evolution and impact on student outcomes across years. *Journal of Positive Behavior Interventions, 14*, 5–16.

Splett, J. W., Trainor, K. M., Raborn, A., Halliday-Boykins, C. A., Garzona, M. E., Dongo, M. D., & Weist, M. D. (2018). Comparison of universal mental health screening to students already receiving intervention in a multitiered system of support. *Behavioral Disorders, 43*, 344–356.

Sugai, G., & Horner, R. (2002). The evolution of discipline practices: School-wide positive behavior supports. *Child & Family Behavior Therapy, 24*(1–2), 23–50.

Sugai, G., & Horner, R. H. (2009). Responsiveness-to-intervention and school-wide positive behavior supports: Integration of multi-tiered system approaches. *Exceptionality, 17*(4), 223–237.

Swanson, E., Stevens, E. A., Scammacca, N. K., Capin, P., Stewart, A. A., & Austin, C. R. (2017). The impact of tier 1 reading instruction on reading outcomes for students in Grades 4–12: A meta-analysis. *Reading and Writing: An Interdisciplinary Journal, 30*(8), 1639–1665.

Waasdorp, T. E., Bradshaw, C. P., & Leaf, P. J. (2012). The impact of schoolwide positive behavioral interventions and supports on bullying and peer rejection: A randomized controlled effectiveness trial. *Archives of Pediatrics and Adolescent Medicine, 166*(2), 149–156.

Walker, H. M., Horner, R. H., Sugai, G., Bullis, M., Sprague, J. R., Bricker, D., & Kaufman, M. J. (1996). Integrated approaches to preventing antisocial behavior patterns among school-age children and youth. *Journal of Emotional and Behavioral Disorders, 4*, 194–209.

Walker, H., Ramsey, E., & Gresham, G. (2004). *Antisocial behavior in schools: Evidence-based practices.* Cengage.

Ward, C. S., Kittelman, A., & Rowe, D. A. (2021). Supporting evidence-based practices: What implementation activities are needed when for success? *Teaching Exceptional Children, 53*(5), 332–335.

Weist, M. D., Eber, L., Horner, R., Splett, J., Putnam, R., Barrett, S., et al. (2018). Improving multitiered systems of support for students with "internalizing" emotional/behavioral problems. *Journal of Positive Behavior Interventions, 20*, 172–184.

Wolf, M. M. (1978). Social validity: The case for subjective measurement or how applied behavior analysis is finding its heart. *Journal of Applied Behavior Analysis, 11*, 203–214.

Yudin, M. (2014). *PBIS: Providing opportunity. A keynote address presented at the National PBIS Leadership Forum.* Keynote address presented at the PBIS Building Capacity & Partnerships to Enhance Educational Reform, Rosemont, IL.

CHAPTER 25

Understanding and Developing Expert Teachers for Students with Learning Disabilities

Mary T. Brownell, Melinda M. Leko, and Amber E. Benedict

Successful education of students with specific learning disabilities (SLD) depends on knowledgeable and skilled teachers who can craft high-quality instruction designed to support these students' learning and social–emotional needs (Brownell et al., 2012; Brownell & Leko, 2018). Since most, if not all, students with SLD are educated for a portion of time in general education environments, special and general education teachers must have the knowledge and skill to implement such instruction and be able to collaboratively leverage that knowledge and skill. Doing so supports their ability to craft instruction that enables students with disabilities to access the general education curriculum while also designing and implementing intensive interventions that complement and support learning in the general education curriculum (Benedict et al., 2020). To effectively educate students with SLD, general and special education teachers must have adequate opportunities to learn how to use and interpret validated classroom assessments (e.g., oral reading fluency probes) and implement evidence-based practices (EBPs) that can support learning needs identified in assessments (Leko, Kiely, et al., 2015; Lemons et al., 2018). Special education teachers must have additional knowledge and skills that allow them to implement data-based individualized interventions (Brownell et al., 2010; Fuchs et al., 2014).

Special education literature is replete with discussions of what general and special education teachers need to know and be able to do (e.g., Lemons et al., 2018; Vaughn & Linan-Thompson, 2003). These discussions focus mostly on how teachers need to be able to implement EBPs (i.e., strategies whose efficacy has been established according to guidelines set forth by the Council for Exceptional Children [CEC], 2014). Yet results of observational studies demonstrate that general and special education teachers do not implement EBPs with regularity or fidelity, though teachers have shown some improvements in doing so since the early 2000s (Ciullo et al., 2016; Gage et al., 2018; Klingner et al., 2010).

Implications from studies of teachers' EBP implementation (or lack thereof) point to the need to better address the research-to-practice gap by delving deeper into issues of implementation (Brownell et al., 2014; Leko, Roberts, et al., 2015). As a result, scholars within the field began conducting studies using an implementation-science framework to understand the factors that facilitated or hindered teachers' use of EBPs with fidelity. Findings shed light on many factors affecting implementation, including the critical role of preservice teacher education and ongoing professional development (PD) in advancing implementation fidelity (e.g., Odom et al., 2013; Scheeler et al., 2016). Researchers employing an implementation-science framework promulgate professional coaching as a mechanism for training teachers to use practices with fidelity (Fixsen et al., 2005); yet they simultaneously recognize that training teachers to use strategies will be insufficient. Schools and districts interested in improving the research-to-practice gap need to also consider contextual factors shown to support teachers' EBP implementation, such as school culture, leadership, support for general and special education collaboration, schoolwide analysis of student data, and fiscal resources that support training and collaboration (Cook & Odom, 2013).

Need for More Complex Views of Teaching Quality and Learning

Research on implementation science presents a complex picture of contextual supports that teachers need to enact practices with fidelity, but the perspective of teacher learning implied in this literature base is underdeveloped. Researchers interested in improving teachers' use of EBPs argue for a type of coaching that is skill-focused (e.g., Odom et al., 2013) and oriented to EBP use. They are relatively silent, however, about how personal and contextual factors, such as teacher knowledge and curriculum structure and content, contribute to teachers' use of EBPs and how coaching promotes teachers' capacity for future learning (Brownell et al., 2020). Although we are gaining new research insights into teachers' knowledge, we still have insufficient understanding about what general and special education teachers need to know (individually and collectively) about the content (e.g., place value in mathematics and the orthography and phonology of the English language) underlying an EBP, how the EBP fits within the broader content domain, and how students learn the content (e.g., misconceptions students might have about how place value works in multi-digit multiplication). Perhaps this is why we observe teachers who focus entirely on decoding strategies they have been taught and do not recognize a need to simultaneously emphasize students' semantic knowledge of words to fully develop students' word-level abilities. We also know little about how general and special education teachers' beliefs about content, instruction, and students with disabilities influence the EBPs they choose to implement; how they adapt them to meet students' needs; or how curriculum enables teachers to learn and use EBPs in ways that are responsive to students' learning needs. Finally, we do not understand the role teacher collaboration plays in learning about EBPs and how to coordinate their use across core and intervention instruction.

It is fascinating that special education researchers have adopted a seemingly atheoretical approach to teacher learning when special education has relied on theory to design and validate student interventions (Brownell et al., 2020), particularly within academic content domains. Brownell et al. (2020) argue that the field of special education teacher education needs stronger theoretical grounding. They assert, "Theory is essential for linking the concepts and ideas about preparing teachers with concrete actions that operationalize these concepts and ideas" (p. 36). Further, theories of teaching and teacher learning should be informed by theories of and research on student learning. Without theory, it is difficult to forge studies that build on each other and help the field understand the knowledge, beliefs, skill fluency, and contextual conditions teachers need to learn and transfer their learning to instructional scenarios that present novel demands.

Purpose of the Chapter

In our chapter, we describe the role that teacher knowledge, beliefs, instructional skill, curriculum, and other contextual factors play in efforts we, and other scholars, have undertaken over the past several decades to understand teaching quality and develop it in general and special education teachers. Specifically, we delineate and explain our efforts to understand teaching quality, to prepare and develop teachers instructing students with SLD, and to understand the role curriculum and other contextual factors play in teaching quality and how teachers learn. Underlying our research efforts are multiple perspectives that account for the complex nature of teaching quality and how it develops. We assert that being clear about these theoretical perspectives is important for moving science forward in the field. We conclude by discussing how current efforts to improve teaching quality for students with SLD are likely to be insufficient if we do not dramatically revise our systems for preparing and developing teachers.

Perspectives Undergirding Our Research

Researchers in general education and, to a lesser extent, special education have shown that teaching is a complex act informed by knowledge, dispositions, beliefs, and individual teachers' command of instructional pedagogy and the context in which teachers work, including their opportunities to learn from each other in formal and informal learning situations (Cohen et al., 2003; Brownell et al., 2007, 2014). Findings from this research suggest the need for a multi-theoretical approach to understanding teaching quality and how to promote it. The research we summarize in this paper, including our own, is based on theories of expertise and its development, as well as sociocultural, situated, and ecological learning theories.

Effective teachers are those with domain expertise (Brownell et al., 2007, 2009). They have specialized, highly integrated knowledge for teaching that includes an understanding of the content they are teaching; how students learn that content, including the misconceptions they develop and challenges they encounter; and how they might best enact that content. Beyond this, general and special education teachers must have the knowledge and skills needed to coordinate their instruction, which likely involves a shared understanding of curriculum and instruction, and how to collaboratively plan and intensify instruction. If research on professional expertise applies to teaching, this highly integrated knowledge of content, pedagogy, students, and collaboration likely takes seven or more years to acquire (Ericsson, 2014) but allows teachers to be responsive to student learning, something necessary to support students with SLD.

The integrated knowledge that characterizes domain expertise is situated; that is, it is acquired through opportunities to enact knowledge in simulated and authentic classroom settings where teachers interact with the different learning needs of students (Dall'Alba & Sandberg, 2006), the curriculum and materials of teaching, and, in many cases, their peers. Thus, what teachers learn is influenced by the structure of their learning opportunities, attempts to apply what they are learning to particular students and students' responses to those attempts, and attempts to apply new learning within the curriculum they are employing. Additionally, when professional collaboration is a component of those opportunities, the demonstrations and dialogue that ensue collectively shape what teachers learn and their expertise (Benedict et al., 2021; Lefstein et al., 2020). Finally, people teach within an ecological system that furthers or hinders their ability to teach and improve. For teachers and teacher candidates, factors that influence teachers' opportunities to enact, discuss, and reflect on what they are learning might include the expectations of teacher evaluation systems; the content of state assessments and expectations surrounding them; how school leaders support collaborative learning opportunities and their expectations for accountability, knowledge, and skill of their colleagues; time constraints due to teaching assignments and responsibilities; and how the job of educating teachers is perceived by the institutions in which they learn and work (e.g., Bishop et al., 2010; Desimone & Hill, 2017).

What Underlies Teaching Quality for Students with Disabilities?

Domain Knowledge

Effective teachers have a high degree of domain knowledge or knowledge that is specialized and inclusive of content, pedagogy, and individual learner needs (Ball et al., 2008; Hudson, 2002). Couched in constructivist views of learning, teachers acquire domain knowledge through a situated learning process wherein they construct new knowledge from social interactions within authentic settings. The components of domain knowledge are complex, highly integrated, and not best learned in isolated or siloed ways, a point to which we return later in our discussion on practice-based preparation.

Over the past several decades, special education teacher education researchers have conducted a small number of studies of domain knowledge for literacy instruction. Brownell et al. (2007, 2009) studied 92 third-, fourth-, and fifth-grade special education teachers, 34 of whom were in their first 3 years of teaching, and their knowledge of teaching word analysis and comprehension to elementary students with SLD. The knowledge assessments, developed by Phelps and Schilling (2004), measured the specialized knowledge teachers use to inform instruction—knowledge that involved an understanding of content, pedagogy, and student needs. Across both studies, teachers' knowledge of how to teach word analysis, but not comprehension, accounted for small to moderate levels of variance in teachers' instructional practice. The strongest relationship was between teachers' word-level knowledge and quality of decoding instruction. Knowledge scores, however, did not predict students' achievement in decoding or comprehension. Spear-Swerling and Zibulsky (2014) also found that elementary and special education teachers' knowledge of teaching reading, particularly of phonemic awareness and phonics, affected the time they allowed during planning for instruction in vocabulary, assessment, phonemic awareness, and spelling.

These findings were also supported in one study examining the relationship between teachers' knowledge of fluency, their instructional practices, and student outcomes on reading fluency measures (Park et al., 2019). In the Park et al. study, researchers assessed 42 third-, fourth-, and fifth-grade special education teachers' fluency practices and knowledge of fluency, why it is important, and how to teach it. Results indicated that teachers' knowledge of fluency and skill in teaching it predicted student outcomes.

In a qualitative study of three expert secondary teachers' pedagogical schemas for teaching literacy to students with SLD, Lauterbach et al. (2020) illustrated the integrated knowledge expert teachers possess. They found experts had deep knowledge of content coupled with well-integrated knowledge of literacy instructional skills, particularly those that meet the learning needs of students with SLD. Further, these teachers understood how to apply what they knew to help students achieve knowledge and skills that would be required in post-secondary environments. Collectively, findings from these studies, though small in number, demonstrate that domain knowledge likely plays a role in teaching quality.

Finally, in a quantitative study of 42 general and special education fourth-grade teachers, Sohn and colleagues (2025) found that a measure of teachers' content knowledge for multi-tiered systems of support (MTSS) instruction, multisyllabic decoding, morphological awareness, vocabulary, comprehension, and systematic explicit instruction was related to content-agnostic measures of effective teaching. Specifically, scores on knowledge assessment were moderately correlated with effective implementation of explicit systematic instruction ($r' = .24$) and responsiveness to student learning ($r' = .39$).

Instructional Skill

Instructional skill is considered one of the most important dimensions of effective teaching, yet few researchers have attempted to identify teaching practices that best predict academic achievement for students with SLD. A small number of studies show that explicit instruction, operationalized and measured differently across the studies, is an instructional practice that captures differences between teachers and provides some evidence for predicting achievement gains of students with SLD (Brownell et al., 2009; Johnson et al., 2021; Pua et al., 2021). Johnson and colleagues found that teachers' performance on the most challenging items comprising explicit instruction, as determined through Rasch measurement analysis, predicted 4.4% of the variance in student achievement.

Brownell and colleagues (2007, 2009), in their study of 92 third-, fourth-, and fifth-grade special education teachers providing reading instruction, discovered complex relationships among knowledge for teaching content, instructional practice, and student achievement. They found that overall classroom practice, effective classroom management, and general instructional environment (i.e., instruction that promotes active student engagement, fosters student interest, and is continuous and intensive) were the strongest predictors of oral reading fluency, and in the 2007 study, explicit instruction in decoding accounted for the greatest variance in word identification skills. As mentioned previously, content knowledge for teaching reading accounted for a small to moderate amount of variance in decoding skills, and that relationship was significant in the 2007 study. Interestingly, post hoc analyses showed that the most experienced colleagues demonstrated significantly more content knowledge for teaching reading and stronger instructional practice, suggesting that experienced teachers had more domain expertise, a finding that is supported by research on professional expertise (e.g., Ericcson, 2014).

Beliefs and Dispositions

Teaching quality for students with SLD is also influenced by teachers' beliefs and dispositions. We refer to dispositions as attitudes and values that are demonstrated through behavior. Beliefs, on the other hand, are convictions or opinions that can be present irrespective of a person's behavior. Teacher beliefs have been studied more extensively than other dimensions of teacher quality. Yet drawing conclusions from this research remains elusive (Risko et al., 2008), partly due to the complexity of teacher beliefs. Leko, Kulkarni, et al. (2015) studied special education preservice teachers and found that the construct of teacher beliefs is multidimensional. Different types of beliefs were more or less stable and developed from varying sources, including personal experiences, practical teaching experiences, or access to pedagogical content knowledge (e.g., coursework or PD). Beliefs that were accessed within specific content areas and instructional tasks seem most amenable to change but only if preservice teachers had practice-based learning opportunities (Risko et al., 2008). Leko and Brownell (2011), in their qualitative study of six preservice special education teachers participating in practicum, found that opportunities to apply knowledge about teaching reading to students with SLD played a role in how these teachers' beliefs changed over time.

Urbach et al. (2015) qualitatively analyzed interviews from 41 special education teachers whose scores on the *Reading Instruction in Special Education (RISE)* observation instrument were in the upper (more accomplished) or lower (less accomplished) third of the total sample of 59 teachers. The research team was interested in learning how the two groups of teachers differed in terms of their beliefs about their roles and responsibilities. Findings indicated that the more and less accomplished teachers' beliefs about what constituted effective reading instruction for students with SLD did not differ in meaningful ways; most believed reading instruction should target individualized student needs and be explicit and systematic. More accomplished teachers, however, believed instruction should be intense, while less accomplished teachers believed instruction should not be intense but rather flexible and open to fun and creativity. Perhaps the most compelling difference was that the more accomplished teachers had a high degree of self-efficacy, believing they were competent educators whose actions, irrespective of how much outside support they received, led to positive student outcomes. These findings are supported in two studies of general education teachers. General education teachers who held more interventionist beliefs than their peers believed students with disabilities could learn despite the nature of their disability and, in turn, provided more explicit instruction (Jordan et al., 2010; Stanovich and Jordan, 1998).

Other researchers have found that more effective teachers for students with disabilities, compared to their less effective peers, seem to have dispositions that enable them to persist despite challenging teaching situations. Bishop et al. (2010) conducted a mixed-methods study of beginning special education teachers who taught reading to students with SLD in grades 3–5. Data sources included participant interviews, classroom observations, and survey responses. The study found that the most accomplished teachers, as measured by a classroom practice instrument, possessed a series of positive dispositions, including being relentless, resourceful, and reflective.

Collaborative Skill

High-quality instruction for students with LD is contingent primarily upon coordinated efforts of skilled general and special educators who can collaboratively execute a cohesive instructional plan and monitor students' progress in relation to their instructional, behavioral, and social goals (Brownell et al., 2018). A foundation for effective collaboration is shared knowledge of evidence-based practice and content; however, the field has little research on how to promote such shared knowledge (Benedict et al., 2020). Current preparation systems are often bifurcated. General educators are prepared as content area experts and special educators as experts in the needs of students with disabilities, providing accommodations and intensifying instruction (Brownell et al., 2005). Understanding how to engage in collaboration so that it advances their peers' knowledge and skill is not intuitive to most teachers. Benedict et al. (2020) found it took some time for general and special education teachers, participating in a collaborative PD effort, to understand the different roles they played in supporting multi-tiered approaches to instruction and to plan for evidence-based instruction that was coordinated across the tiers. Leko, Kiely, et al. (2015) qualitatively studied the discourse patterns of nine elementary special educators teaching reading to students with SLD who participated in a multifaceted PD innovation that included coaching and a learning cohort. Even though all participants worked as elementary special educators who taught reading to students with SLD, their varying levels of domain knowledge and instructional skill made it difficult for the group to engage in discussions that moved beyond basic sharing of resources. Discussions that provided the richest learning opportunities were instigated by teachers who displayed advanced domain knowledge and a strong tendency for inquiry, but these instances were limited and often required facilitation by experts providing the PD. These findings point to why it would be difficult, without intentional support, for general educators and special educators to develop shared knowledge and skill for working in concert to design and enact instruction to meet the needs of all learners, including students with disabilities, across multi-tiered settings.

Contextual Factors

Ecological theories of learning posit that teachers' instruction and implementation of interventions cannot be considered apart from the broader ecosystems in which they work (Wideen et al., 1998). In essence, teachers' ability to enact their knowledge and instructional skill depends on their environment, or context, and the multiple players within it. Contextual factors include school-level factors such as availability of resources and curriculum, administrative support, time to plan, and service delivery model, as these factors have bearing on how effective implementation efforts will be (Fixsen et al., 2005).

The role of contextual factors on teacher quality was evident in a study of 25 beginning elementary special educators. Bishop et al. (2010) found these teachers often struggled to find appropriate reading curricula and materials to meet their students' needs. The most accomplished teachers, as measured by high scores on the RISE observation instrument (Brownell et al., 2007), however, exhibited resourcefulness and relentlessness in overcoming contextual challenges. These teachers sought appropriate curricular materials even when they were not readily available and took full responsibility for students' learning rather than blaming families or unsupportive school contexts.

In a study of five secondary teachers' implementation of a reading intervention program, some teachers were unable to carry out the program with a high degree of fidelity due to several contextual constraints (i.e., large class sizes, limited instructional time, and inadequate technology support) (Leko, Roberts, et al., 2015). Although these teachers had a vision for how they should implement the program, their efforts were often stymied due to environmental conditions beyond their control. The most skilled teachers, as measured by a program implementation fidelity score, however, were able to address the contextual constraints and deliver the program in ways that met their students' needs. Bishop et al. (2010) and Leko, Roberts et al. (2015) studies suggest that contextual variables may impede teaching quality in nuanced ways. More accomplished and skilled teachers may feel stymied by contextual challenges, but they also have strategies that enable them to more easily overcome them.

If findings from literature on professional expertise apply to teachers (Ericcson, 2014), then teachers who possess the knowledge, skills, beliefs, and dispositions discussed earlier have a high degree of expertise that develops neither by chance nor overnight. High-quality teachers for students, particularly those with SLD, are experienced and well-prepared, and they work in conditions that support the execution of evidence-based instruction. In the following section, we review and discuss research that we and others have conducted on teacher education and the theories of teacher learning that have influenced our work.

Approaches to Developing Special and General Education Teachers

Given the complex influences on teaching quality, how should teacher educators and school districts, engaged in educating teachers, develop special and general educators to better educate students with SLD? What practices and strategies can be employed, and how should these practices and strategies be crafted to address the complex set of influences on teaching quality? In the following sections, we summarize research that provides some response to these questions, as well as persistent issues related to educating teachers for students with SLD. In referring to the term *teacher education*, we include initial preparation and ongoing PD, as we view teacher education as a broader enterprise that spans a teacher's career continuum.

Practice-Based Approaches

The concept of a practice-based approach to teacher education emerged originally in the general education literature to describe a core curriculum for teaching that could be used to bring focus to efforts to educate teachers over time (McDonald et al., 2013). The premise for practice-based approaches comes from the literature on expertise and its development. According to Ericsson and other scholars, expertise is the result of repeated exposure to deliberate practice, where professionals and those seeking to become professionals have opportunities to employ their knowledge in simulated and authentic settings and receive feedback on performance (Chernikova et al., 2020; Ericsson, 2014). These deliberate practice opportunities must focus on the key features of expert performance if novice professionals are to develop into experts. The assumption is that repeated, deliberate practice, coupled with feedback, enables teachers and candidates opportunities to acquire situated knowledge and develop fluent performance, allowing them to be more responsive to novel situations encountered during teaching (Brownell et al., 2019).

Focusing Practice-Based Opportunities

To design repeated, coherent practice opportunities, teacher educators and PD providers (hereafter referred to as *teacher educators*) need a focus for their practice-based curriculum. In special education, researchers have amassed an impressive literature base about how to teach content-specific strategies to students with LD, such as summarizing text, writing a persuasive essay, and solving mathematical word problems (see Klingner et al., 2016). These practices form an evidence base for teaching students with SLD that could be used as the basis for practice opportunities. Hundreds of EBPs, however, exist, and teacher candidates and novice teachers cannot, in the limited time they have to learn, deploy them fluently or in ways that are responsive to the needs of students with SLD in specific content areas. Thus, those who are preparing candidates and novice teachers to educate students with SLD face a practical conundrum. How can they design sufficient practice opportunities to allow candidates and novice teachers to learn to implement EBPs in ways that recognize students' needs within a content area?

Scholars argue that practice-based approaches should center on the critical aspects of effective instruction or high-leverage practices (HLPs) to create a coherent focus for teacher learning (Grossman & McDonald, 2008; McLeskey et al., 2017). HLPs are high-frequency practices that can be enacted across different instructional content, instructional approaches, and settings and are foundational to effective teaching. HLPs form the foundation for effective instruction while preserving the complexity of teaching and include such strategies as scaffolding student learning, providing feedback, and providing explicit instruction. Scholars have some evidence to demonstrate that HLPs can be decomposed into smaller components to consider how they can be modeled, rehearsed, and analyzed with teachers, particularly teacher candidates and beginning teachers. Further, some combination of simulated and authentic teaching situations can be crafted to support candidates and novice teachers in recomposing HLPs to reflect the complexity of effective teaching (Brownell et al., 2019). Through this decomposition and recomposition process, scholars believe that effective teaching is developed.

Effective teaching, however, is not a content-neutral exercise. Practice opportunities need to address content in ways that support the needs of students with SLD, particularly as teacher candidates learn to use HLPs in methods courses such as those traditionally offered in reading and mathematics. EBPs, at least in the academic realm, often represent the intersection of content and HLPs. For example, schema-based strategy instruction, an EBP in mathematics, requires teachers to integrate knowledge of mathematics content (e.g., recognizing when a word problem requires you to combine numbers), the procedures involved in implementing schema-based strategy instruction for solving word problems, and HLPs (e.g., explicit instruction, feedback, and scaffolding) to support effective implementation of the selected EBP.

How might teacher educators create a continuum of focused, repeated, practice-based opportunities, particularly for those learning to teach, that integrate use of EBPs, HLPs, and content knowledge, especially when so many EBPs exist? As teacher educators curate practice opportunities, they can choose the most efficacious EBPs that address critical content in a curricular area (e.g., decoding and summarization in reading and schema-based instruction in mathematics) and select HLPs (e.g., explicit instruction, active engagement, and feedback) to be the focus of practice opportunities (Brownell et al., 2018). The selected HLPs can be addressed repeatedly as candidates practice using EBPs across content areas in simulated and authentic settings. The research on the role of deliberate practice (i.e., repeated practice that involves thoughtful analysis of performance) in developing expertise suggests that as candidates repeatedly practice HLPs using different EBPs, they should develop fluent and nuanced use of HLPs, thus enabling them to develop the integrated knowledge characteristic of domain expertise. Yet exactly how should such effective practice opportunities be constructed?

Research on Effective Practice Opportunities

Research on the role of deliberate practice in developing professional expertise shows that effective practice opportunities are defined by modeling, performance feedback, and analysis of performance. Brock and Carter (2017) conducted a meta-analysis of group design research, and Brock et al. (2017) conducted a comprehensive review of single-subject research examining the efficacy of PD interventions for teachers and paraprofessionals educating students with disabilities. Across the two analyses, they found that modeling and performance feedback were important features of effective PD interventions. Scheeler et al. (2016) and Rock et al. (2009), through individual studies and reviews of research on special education teacher preparation (see Brownell et al., 2020, for a summary of this research), supported Brock and Carter's findings about performance feedback. These researchers showed that bug-in-the-ear coaching, an intervention that relies on observation of classroom practice and immediate performance feedback, consistently improved teachers' instructional practice in single-subject design and quasi-experimental studies. Additionally, a meta-synthesis of coaching research in general education, mostly in reading and literacy (Kraft et al., 2018), and a recent summary of effective PD research in general education (Hill & Papay, 2022) and a review of research in special education research (Cornelius & Nagro, 2014) further supported the role of performance feedback in teacher learning. Although coaching interventions varied in studies reviewed and often included PD workshops and institutes to develop teacher knowledge, they always incorporated direct observation of instruction and performance feedback. Results from the meta-analysis and Hill and Papay's research summary showed that coaching was effective in improving instructional practice and, in some cases, student achievement. However, Kraft and colleagues noted that effective interventions were always those implemented by researchers. It seems that when coaching is implemented at scale in districts, it loses potency for improving teacher and student outcomes. Challenges associated with securing large numbers of well-qualified coaches, teachers' openness to feedback, and a school climate that promotes trusting relationships and risk taking might be some of the factors influencing district-level implementation (Kraft et al., 2018).

Analysis is the third feature of effective practice opportunities. In video analysis, teachers and teacher candidates develop instruction that is responsive to student needs by analyzing video of instruction, either their own or that of another teacher. In their synthesis of quasi-experimental and experimental studies of structured video analysis, Nagro and Cornelius (2013) found that this PD strategy could be effective in improving teachers' and teacher candidates' instructional practice, particularly when they were taught to use a structured observation protocol or provided coaching feedback on specific aspects of instruction. Findings from this review are supported by more recent studies of structured video analysis in general and special education (Hiebert et al., 2017; van Es et al., 2014). Hiebert and colleagues found that structured video analysis focused on teaching mathematics content in ways that addressed students' emerging conceptions and misconceptions of mathematical concepts resulted in improved instructional practice for the first 3 years of a teacher's career. This study is important because it documents how repeated, practice-based opportunities, focused on a core mathematical practice, have a lasting impact on teacher candidates' ability to teach, guiding how learning opportunities should be constructed in initial teacher education.

The three features of effective practice, used either alone or in some combination, form the basis of teacher education interventions that are supported by empirical research, such as coaching, video analysis, teacher study groups, and lesson study. Each of these interventions includes two or more of the three features of effective practice, suggesting that these features are important to include in the design of any teacher education intervention. Exactly how these features promote teacher learning in different interventions, however, is difficult to ascertain. Teacher education interventions differ considerably in how they approach the cognitive and social aspects of learning (Kennedy, 2016). For instance, even one of the most well-researched PD innovations, coaching, varies in how content knowledge for teaching is addressed and how coaches work with teachers to learn new strategies. Kraft et al. (2018) described how working definitions of coaching often varied widely from one study to the next. Some researchers viewed coaching as a vehicle for helping teachers implement the steps of EBPs, often with little to no attention to content and its role in teachers' use of EBPs. Other researchers used coaching to help teachers understand why and how certain strategies might be appropriate for students. Coaches also played different roles in studies, sometimes providing direct feedback on how to implement an instructional practice and other times helping teachers reflect on their instruction.

Kennedy (2016) argued that these variations in how PD innovations foster teacher learning make it difficult to compare their relative effectiveness or discern effective features of innovations; in other words, they make it difficult to build a science of teacher learning (Brownell & Leko, 2018). Hence, Brownell and Leko (2018) and Brownell et al. (2020) called for researchers to clearly articulate a theory of change that emphasizes the learning mechanism or mechanisms needed to promote changes in teacher and student outcomes. Brownell and colleagues argued that these theories of change should parallel learning theories that have been supported through research. For Brownell and her colleagues, their PD efforts have helped teachers acquire strategic knowledge of why, when, and how to use EBPs and HLPs along with some of the content knowledge needed for teaching those strategies—a view that recognizes the role of domain expertise and deliberate practice in teaching. They also assert that teachers construct their new knowledge through collaborative opportunities with colleagues and, thus, simultaneously embrace a sociocultural approach to learning. In the following detailed examples, we outline how these various perspectives undergird their PD approaches aimed at improving special and general education teachers' reading instruction and how information acquired in one study led to the construction of a second PD approach.

Literacy Learning Cohorts

Brownell et al. (2017) developed a content-focused professional learning innovation founded in theories of domain expertise and sociocultural learning to teach third-, fourth-, and fifth-grade special education teachers knowledge and skills for providing word-level and fluency instruction to students with SLD. The PD incorporated four main components: (1) a PD institute that helped teachers, through a combination of lecture, live demonstration, video models, role-plays, and discussion, to understand how students acquire word knowledge, become aware of the challenges students with disabilities confront in learning to decode and read text fluently, and strategies for improving decoding and fluency; (2) literacy learning cohort (LLC) meetings that helped teachers collaboratively analyze data and plan for implementing strategies acquired in the PD institute; (3) video self-analysis combined with coaching that helped teachers analyze and receive feedback on their use of PD strategies and student learning that ensued; and (4) a teacher's manual that supported teachers in integrating content knowledge with pedagogical or strategy knowledge. The PD institute occurred early in the school year and was followed by five monthly cohort meetings. Video analysis and coaching sessions were conducted between cohort meetings to help teachers effectively implement selected EBPs using HLPs, such as explicit instruction.

Special education teachers (n = 42) were randomly assigned at the school level to treatment or a comparison group. Both groups received the PD institute, but comparison-group teachers did not participate in follow-up activities. Pre- and posttest teacher measures were administered and included surveys of content knowledge for teaching word study and fluency and an observation protocol designed to assess the quality of word study, word fluency, and text fluency instruction and time spent in EBPs. Students with SLD were assessed on the Oral Reading Fluency and Nonsense Word Fluency subsections of the *Dynamic Indicators of Basic Early Literacy Skills* and the Word Attack and Word Identification subtests of the *Woodcock Reading Mastery Test—Revised.* Results showed complex relationships between treatment and teacher outcomes. Both treatment and comparison groups significantly increased their use of EBPs in word study and fluency (ES = .36). More complicated differences, however, emerged for quality of instruction; treatment teachers who began the study 1 standard deviation below the mean on quality of word-level instruction had significantly higher posttest scores than comparison teachers. There were no significant differences for teachers who began the study 1 standard deviation above the mean. Treatment teachers outperformed control teachers on quality of fluency instruction and posttest measures of fluency knowledge, but not word-level knowledge. Finally, multilevel analyses showed the LLC treatment had a significant and moderate effect on word-level skills for students with SLD, but there were no significant effects for fluency. These results provide some support for a content-focused approach to improving teachers' instructional skills that employs three features of effective practice (modeling, feedback, and analysis) and professional collaboration.

The Role of the Individual, Context, and Collaboration in Fostering Teacher Change

Implementing the LLC, however, was not without challenge. Qualitative studies furthered our understanding of how teachers' individual and contextual factors supported or hindered their learning and were used to strengthen the LLC intervention. In three separate studies, Brownell and colleagues (Brownell et al., 2014; Dingle et al., 2011; Leko, Kiely, et al., 2015) found that individual factors, such as knowledge for teaching reading, ability to demonstrate explicit instruction, ability to reflect on one's practice, and motivation to change, seemed to buffer some teachers against constraints in their environment that could affect integration of EBPs into reading instruction. Contextual factors, such as special education teachers' time for providing intensive instruction, use of curriculum that supported EBPs and HLPs learned in PD, and general education colleagues' expectations for intervention instruction played a role in how well teachers integrated EBPs into their instruction.

Individual factors seemed to influence how teachers responded to contextual factors. For instance, if teachers had more knowledge for teaching reading or stronger initial instruction than their peers, they did not let time constraints, available curriculum, or general education colleagues' expectations for their role interfere. Instead, they created new curriculum materials, took advantage of whatever time they had to implement strategies, or advocated with their colleagues about the need for word study and fluency instruction. Teachers, however, who did not have that knowledge or strong instruction saw themselves as more bound to their existing curriculum and the instructional role their general education colleagues expected of them (e.g., simply repeating general education instruction to "catch students with SLD up").

In addition, we found that collaborative learning opportunities within the group seemed to vary depending on the knowledge teachers communicated and how their colleagues responded. Analysis of special education teachers' discourse revealed that teachers who demonstrated integrated knowledge and a proclivity for inquiry (i.e., teacher talk that suggested a desire to learn more about content and/or how to apply it) provided better and more opportunities for colleagues to learn. What we found from the study of teachers' collaborative discourse, along with findings from previously mentioned studies of contextual and individual factors, led to changes in our LLC innovation and future research. To strengthen teachers' knowledge for teaching reading, we incorporated a teacher's manual that helped teachers use content accurately, such as decoding rules, and provided them with word lists and passages that they could use to develop lessons. We also incorporated video analysis with coaching and supported teachers in using their student data and curriculum during planning portions of LLC cohort meetings. Further, we incorporated the knowledge we were acquiring about the constraints of the general education curriculum into our next study, designed to improve the collaborative instruction of general and special education teachers.

Lesson Study: A Practice-Based Approach for Improving Collaborative, Evidence-Based Instruction

Our research on the LLC intervention helped us realize that PD focused solely on special education teachers was problematic. Without intentional collaborative planning, students with disabilities received intervention instruction that was disconnected from general education instruction. Yet ensuring students with SLD attain positive outcomes within response-to-intervention (RTI) frameworks necessitates coordination within and across tiers (Benedict et al., 2020; Harn et al., 2011; Stevens et al., 2020). In an RTI framework, general educators are responsible for delivering strong core Tier 1 and supplemental Tier 2 instruction to students whose reading achievement data suggest they need additional support. Special educators provide more intensive, data-driven, evidence-based interventions in Tier 3 intended to help SLD achieve in Tier 1 general education curricula.

Such coordinated instruction depends on opportunities general and special educators have to design instruction and analyze student data collaboratively and the knowledge and skill they have for doing so (Brownell et al., 2018). Creating conditions that support coordination is not an easy feat. In addition to lacking the preparation and shared knowledge of EBPs and HLPs, the curriculum teachers use at each tier is often different, making the coordination of a student's overall instructional plan challenging. Further, the time needed to plan, collaborate, and coordinate instruction is in short supply within schools, and special education teachers often are asked to do multiple tasks during the school day that interfere with planning and teaching.

Our next approach to PD attempted to address some of these realities. Project InSync included fourth- and fifth-grade special *and* general educators in a collaborative approach to PD called lesson study (LS) (Benedict et al., 2021). LS has long been promulgated as an intervention for improving teaching (Stigler & Heibert, 1999) that has been validated for elementary general education teachers in mathematics (e.g., Lewis & Perry, 2017). The premise behind LS is that teachers analyze student data to set instructional goals. From there, they collaboratively plan a lesson that they then implement and videotape. After implementing the lesson, they observe the lesson, debrief, and jointly evaluate its effectiveness and how future instruction might be improved. In Project InSync, we coupled LS with content-focused PD on word study over a school year, drawing on sociocultural learning theory to promote teachers' domain knowledge in reading. Findings from qualitative analysis of teachers' talk during LS planning and debriefing sessions showed that teachers' learning and understanding progressed across three phases. In Phase 1, teachers' discussions centered on understanding the new content and how it might be implemented within their instruction and less on how content could address students' needs or how they would develop coordinated, tiered lessons using the new content. After completing their first cycle of LS, teachers moved into Phase 2. Here, they began to deliberate about how instructional strategies could be adapted to meet students' individual needs. The act of planning, executing, and then debriefing about a lesson seemed to allow teachers to connect their knowledge of content, pedagogy, and student needs. At this point, however, they did not make comments about how they could coordinate their instruction. In Phase 3, teachers began to describe how the content could be coordinated across the tiers. As they planned lessons, using a framework focused on coordinating tiered instruction, they demonstrated more integrated knowledge of word study content, pedagogy, and student. In planning and debriefing conversations, they analyzed the impact strategies had on student learning and brainstormed ways they could better support their learning of content.

Over time, teachers' talk demonstrated that they made stronger connections between the strategies they were learning, challenges students might encounter, how curriculum materials could be constructed, and how lessons could be designed to support students' acquisition of foundational skills and strategies across the instructional tiers. Teachers also needed ongoing support from the PD facilitator; even when given the time to collaborate, teachers did not instinctively know how best to support one another's learning.

In a subsequent study, Benedict and colleagues (2024) assessed the impact of Project Coordinate, a PD innovation informed by Project InSync. Project Coordinate, a project funded by the Institute of Education Sciences, was designed for fourth-grade general and special educators to support teams of educators in acquiring shared knowledge and skills for effective MTSS literacy instruction. Project Coordinate coupled LS with online content modules to improve teachers' knowledge for teaching reading, collaborative tiered practice, and use of evidence-based strategies (e.g., cognitive strategies for analyzing morphologically complex, multisyllabic words and summarization).

Forty-three fourth-grade general and special education teachers, working in teams of two to four, were randomly assigned to treatment and control. Although the study was paused because of the COVID-19 pandemic, researchers were able to collect some posttest data and pre-post comparison data for treatment teachers. Using multilevel modeling, researchers found no significant differences in treatment teachers' knowledge compared to control; however, the treatment effect was small to moderate (.29). Results of multiple analyses of covariance (ANCOVA) showed that treatment teachers improved in their collaborative practices for MTSS reading instruction compared with control, and although all results were not significant, the effect sizes were moderate to large (partial η^2 ranged from .07 to .18). Further, subgroup post hoc analyses revealed that gains were larger for special (partial η^2 ranged from 0.06 to .54) compared with general education teachers (partial η^2 ranged from 0.01 to .10), with one exception. General education teachers made larger gains (partial η^2 = 0.10) on perceptions of collaborative planning practices for reading instruction compared with special education teachers (partial η^2 = 0.06). Although posttest instructional data were not available for control-group teachers, data gleaned from implementation videos showed that teachers increased their use of EBPs from an average of 1% to 74% of the time. Additionally, a multivariate analysis of variance showed that Project Coordinate teachers made significant, large gains from pretest to implementation on two practices that supported effective implementation of EBPs: explicit, systematic instruction (Hedges' g = 1.03) and responsiveness to individual student learning (e.g., specific feedback, monitoring for student learning) (Hedges' g = .77).

Our studies of Project Coordinate and InSync show that well-structured, content-focused collaborative PD efforts can improve general and special education teachers in ways that support the learning of students with SLD. However, our earlier research (Brownell et al., 2014; Leko, Kulkarni, et al., 2015) revealed many thorny contextual issues that will challenge efforts to implement such collaborative PD successfully. Teachers are often pulled in too many directions to be fully present for collaborative PD meetings, and this is particularly true of special education teachers. Further, teachers do not always have available curricula that support them in implementing EBPs, particularly word-learning strategies. The lack of available curricula compounds the challenge that many general and special education teachers already experience when they have insufficient knowledge for teaching reading, particularly word study. Despite these challenges, it is neither effective nor efficient to prepare general and special educators separately if these teachers are to have access to the intensive, collaborative, content-focused PD they need to plan and implement effective, coordinated, evidence-based instruction for students with SLD.

Future Directions for Research, Practice, and Policy

Findings from research demonstrate a clear need to provide teachers with practice opportunities that are defined by modeling effective instruction, providing feedback, and fostering analysis of instruction. When these features are present, teachers often grow in instructional skill and ability to promote student achievement. These results help craft teacher education efforts for teacher candidates and practicing teachers. Although less established, we do have evidence in general education and, to a lesser degree, in special education research that teachers' knowledge of teaching content can influence their instruction and student achievement and that teacher education interventions can be designed to increase this knowledge. Two decades ago, we did not have this empirical knowledge of teacher improvement, but we do now; thus, progress has been made. Yet work remains to establish a science of teacher learning, including the collaborative learning of teachers from different disciplines and the creation of cohesive systems of teacher education. At this point, we offer some insights about how to improve efforts in research and consider some directions practice and policy might take to develop general and special education teachers' expertise for educating students with SLD.

Future Research

Insights from our work, and that of other scholars, point to areas in need of further attention if we are to improve the science of teacher learning (e.g., Brownell & Leko, 2018; Brownell et al., 2020). Our field needs to address several major issues related to theory, measurement, and PD implementation. Brownell and Leko (2018), Kraft et al. (2018), and Kennedy (2016) indicate challenges researchers confront when trying to compare PD interventions that may share similar features but differ dramatically in their approach to promoting teacher learning and assessment of teacher outcomes (e.g., instructional practice and knowledge). For example, it is difficult to determine how a coaching intervention designed to increase teachers' implementation of a discrete EBP (e.g., behavior-specific praise) provides a learning opportunity that is similar in nature and outcomes to a coaching intervention that helps teachers elicit students' mathematical thinking and respond to clarify misconceptions.

To address these challenges, researchers in general and special education need to articulate theories of teacher change that underlie their PD innovations, as well as measures of teacher learning that align with those theories (Brownell et al., 2020). By clearly hypothesizing the learning mechanism(s) that underlie teacher learning, researchers can design and test interventions that assess the validity of their theories and the efficacy of resulting interventions. For instance, if researchers posit that teachers gain instructional expertise by acquiring knowledge of content and how to teach it in ways that are responsive to students' emerging understandings, then they can attempt to define this knowledge, determine how to assess it, and determine how to structure teacher education interventions in ways that enable teachers to acquire such knowledge and test them empirically. By articulating theories of change, operationalizing them, and empirically testing them, researchers can develop a science of teacher learning.

Researchers also need valid measures of teacher outcomes that align with their theories of teacher learning—measures comprised of a common set of metrics that could be used across studies. These measures could address specific knowledge and instructional practices that would be unique to a content domain and those that might be common across content domains. For instance, if researchers believe that content knowledge for teaching undergirds instructional practice, they need to define that knowledge and develop valid ways to measure it. Tools for assessing content-specific approaches to instructional practices, such as use of reading comprehension strategies, would allow researchers to compare teacher intervention studies within a content domain. Metrics focused on more generic instructional practices (i.e., HLPs), such as the Recognizing Effective Special Education Teachers' Explicit Instruction Rubric (Johnson et al., 2022), could be employed to assess the degree to which teacher education interventions influence instructional practice across content domains. Such measures could be especially important in assessing the success of programmatic approaches to teacher change (i.e., initial teacher preparation and induction programs), as programmatic approaches seek to improve teachers working in a variety of content domains.

Our research on individual and contextual factors that influence teachers' implementation of EBPs and HLPs makes clear that teacher learning does not occur in a vacuum. If teachers' individual beliefs or motivation to learn play a role in their learning, then researchers need to attend to and assess these individual factors. Researchers, teacher educators, and school districts need to understand who is most likely to benefit from different types of teacher education innovations and under what conditions. Identifying key contextual factors that support teacher learning will be important for designing and implementing successful PD innovations. For instance, researchers need to examine how the structure and content of a curriculum support or hinder teachers' use of strategies targeted in teacher education interventions and programs. Or identify how collaboration among general and special education teachers, particularly as it relates to coordinating instruction and analyzing data, supports teachers' use of HLPs and EBPs acquired through teacher education interventions. An improved understanding of the implementation context is needed to support the system changes necessary for maximizing the efficacy of teacher education efforts across general and special education settings.

Need for Comprehensive Systems for Educating Teachers

Findings from our research, although not conclusive, combined with a substantive research base on implementation science, provide some evidence that individual teacher knowledge, the knowledge and skill of colleagues, access to focused, well-supported practice opportunities, time to collaborate with colleagues, and appropriate curriculum play a role in how teacher candidates and teachers apply what they are learning. Dingle et al. (2011), Benedict et al. (2020), and Brownell et al. (2017) also show that efforts to address the learning of special education teachers should simultaneously consider the learning of general education teachers. Effective instruction for students with SLD, provided within an RTI framework or via co-teaching, is enhanced by the collective knowledge of general and special education teachers and teachers' coordinated implementation of HLPs and EBPs. Taken together, findings from research on expertise, deliberate practice, and teacher education (Brownell et al., in press; Ericsson, 2014; Leko et al., 2024) implicate the need for a coherent system of teacher education that exposes general and special education teachers to a robust set of focused, collaborative, practice opportunities over time and supports teachers' efforts to apply what they are learning. This system should foster a clear vision for effective teaching for students with disabilities and support effective, ongoing learning opportunities and contextual supports to help teachers enact such a vision.

To establish a coherent system of teacher education, researchers argue that policies guiding teacher and student learning must focus and be aligned with teachers' opportunities to learn (e.g., Pak et al., 2020). Policies, such as teaching and program approval standards and those guiding initial induction, PD, and teacher evaluation systems, should be constructed to support the ongoing, effective, and collaborative practice opportunities that teachers need to develop expertise. Leko and colleagues (2024) assert that HLPs and selected EBPs (i.e., those with the strongest impact) provide a powerful lever for focusing the development of teacher standards and other policies that support teacher learning. Equally important are practice-based learning opportunities, defined by modeling, feedback, analysis, and reflection, that allow teacher candidates and teachers to learn about and refine the content knowledge and pedagogical skills they need to select and use HLPs and EBPs over time (Brownell et al., 2019). Well-constructed, focused, repeated, collaborative, practice-based learning opportunities that involve general and special education teachers should help teachers develop the needed expertise to educate students with SLD successfully.

Leadership at the school and district level is also important for ensuring that general and special education teachers have the ongoing collaborative learning opportunities needed and access to evidence-based curriculum that allows them to implement effective, coordinated instruction for students with disabilities (Billingsley et al., 2020; Brownell et al., in press). General and special education teachers' collaborative opportunities to learn about, enact, and analyze their implementation efforts can support the effective use of HLPs and EBPs (e.g., Benedit et al., 2024; Hill et al., 2020). Further, teachers need access to curricula that support their learning. Research suggests that curricula that support teachers' efforts to enact HLPs and EBPs in coordinated ways across general and special education will be important for supporting coherent, effective learning opportunities for teachers and students (Harn et al., 2015).

To help states, educator preparation programs, and local school districts establish systemic approaches to teacher learning, the Office of Special Education Programs has funded multiple national centers, including the Collaboration for Effective Educator, Development, Reform (CEEDAR) Center (*www.ceedar.org*), the Positive Behavioral and Interventions and Supports Center (*http://pbis.org*), the State Implementation and Scaling-Up of Evidence-Based Practices Center (*http://sisep.fpg.unc.edu*), and the National Center on Intensive Intervention (*http://intensiveintervention.org*). These centers work with states, universities, and local school districts to create the systemic conditions needed to develop (1) a system of focused, coherent practice-based learning opportunities, based on HLPs and EBPs, for general and special education teachers; (2) school and university capacity for supporting learning and enactment of HLPs and EBPs for students with disabilities; (3) state and district policies that support the ongoing preparation of teachers and leaders who can educate students with disabilities effectively; and (4) state and district policies that support the enactment of EBPs and HLPs and schooling for students with disabilities. Technical assistance from these centers can support states in creating conditions that promote effective teaching for students with disabilities and effective teacher education.

REFERENCES

Ball, D. L., Thames, M. H., & Phelps, G. (2008). Content knowledge for teaching: What makes it special. *Journal of Teacher Education, 59*(5), 389–407.

Benedict, A. E., Brownell, M., Bettini, E., & Sohn, H. (2021). Learning together: Teachers' evolving understanding of coordinated word study instruction within an RTI framework. *Teacher Education and Special Education, 44*(2), 134–159.

Benedict, A. E., Brownell, M. T., Griffin, C. C., Wang, J., & Myers, J. A. (2020). Leveraging professional development to prepare general and special education teachers to teach within response to intervention frameworks. In T. Petty, A. Good, & M. Putman (Eds.), *Accessibility and diversity in education: Breakthroughs in research and practice* (pp. 143–162). IGI Global.

Benedict, A. E., Brownell, M. T., Sohn, H., Williams, J., Kelcey, B., & Koziarski, G. (2024). Project Coordinate: Impact of content-focused lesson study on teacher knowledge, collaboration, and MTSS instruction. *Teacher Education and Special Education, 48*(1), 26–45.

Billingsley, B., Bettini, E., Mathews, H. M., & McLeskey, J. (2020). Improving working conditions to support special educators' effectiveness: A call for leadership. *Teacher Education and Special Education, 43*(1), 7–27.

Bishop, A. G., Brownell, M. T., Klingner, J. K., Leko, M. M., & Galman, S. A. (2010). Understanding differences in beginning special education teachers: The influence of personal attributes, preparation, and school environment on classroom reading practices. *Learning Disability Quarterly, 33*(2), 75–92.

Brock, M. E., Cannella-Malone, H. I., Seaman, R. L., Andzik, N. R., Schaefer, J. M., Page, E. J., et al. (2017). Findings across practitioner training studies in special education: A comprehensive review and meta-analysis. *Exceptional Children, 84*(1), 7–26.

Brock, M. E., & Carter, E. W. (2017). A meta-analysis of educator training to improve implementation of interventions for students with disabilities. *Remedial and Special Education, 38*(3), 131–144.

Brownell, M. T., Benedict, A. E., Leko, M. M., Peyton, D., Pua, D., & Richards-Tutor, C. (2019). A continuum of pedagogies for preparing teachers to use high-leverage practices (HLPs). *Remedial and Special Education, 6*(40), 338–355.

Brownell, M. T., Bishop, A. G., Gersten, R., Klingner, J. K., Penfield, R. D., Dimino, J., et al. (2009). The role of domain expertise in beginning special education teacher quality. *Exceptional Children, 75*(4), 391–411.

Brownell, M. T., Chard, D., Benedict, A., & Lignugaris/Kraft, B. (2018). Preparing general and special education teachers for response to intervention: A practice-based approach. In P. Pullen & M. Kennedy (Eds.), *Handbook of response to intervention and multi-tiered instruction* (pp. 121–145). Routledge.

Brownell, M. T., Haager, D., Bishop, A. G., Klingner, J. K., Menon, S., Penfield, R., & Dingle, M. (2007, April). *Teacher quality in special education: The role of knowledge, classroom practice, and school environment* [Paper presentation]. Annual Meeting for the American Education Research Association, Chicago, IL.

Brownell, M. T., Jones, N. D., Sohn, H., & Stark, K. (2020). Improving teaching quality for students with disabilities: Establishing a warrant for teacher education practice. *Teacher Education and Special Education, 43*(1), 28–44.

Brownell, M., Kiely, M. T., Haager, D., Boardman, A., Corbett, N., Algina, J., et al. (2017). Literacy learning cohorts: Content-focused approach to improving special education teachers' reading instruction. *Exceptional Children, 83*(2), 143–164.

Brownell, M. T., Lauterbach, A. A., Benedict, A. E., Bettini, E. A., & Murphy, K. (2012). Preparing teachers to effectively deliver reading instruction and behavioral supports in response to intervention frameworks. In B. G. Cook, M. Tankersley, & T. J. Landrum (Eds.), *Advances in learning and behavior disabilities* (pp. 247–277). Emerald Group.

Brownell, M. T., Lauterbach, A. A., Dingle, M. P., Boardman, A. G., Urbach, J. E., Leko, M. M., et al. (2014). Individual and contextual factors influencing special education teacher learning in literacy learning cohorts. *Learning Disability Quarterly, 37*(1), 31–44.

Brownell, M. T., & Leko, M. M. (2018). Advancing coherent theories of change in special education teacher education research: A response to the special issue on the science of teacher professional development. *Teacher Education and Special Education, 41*(2), 158–168.

Brownell, M. T., Leko, M. L., Sohn, H., & Williams, J. (in press). Facilitating professional learning across the career span: Securing the expert teachers we need to effectively educate students with disabilities. In M. Rock, B. Billingsley, L. Dieker, & M. Leko (Eds.), *Transforming the special education workforce: Research and complex systems perspectives.* American Educational Research Association.

Brownell, M. T., Ross, D. D., Colón, E. P., & McCallum, C. L. (2005). Critical features of special education teacher preparation: A comparison with general teacher education. *The Journal of Special Education, 38*(4), 242–252.

Brownell, M. T., Sindelar, P. T., Kiely, M. T., & Danielson, L. C. (2010). Special education teacher quality and preparation: Exposing foundations, constructing a new model. *Exceptional Children, 76*(3), 357–377.

Chernikova, O., Heitzmann, N., Stadler, M., Holzberger, D., Seidel, T., & Fischer, F. (2020). Simulation-based learning in higher education: A meta-analysis. *Review of Educational Research, 90*(4), 499–541.

Ciullo, S., Lembke, E. S., Carlisle, A., Thomas, C. N., Goodwin, M., & Judd, L. (2016) Implementation of evidence-based literacy practices in middle school response to intervention: An observation study. *Learning Disability Quarterly, 39*(1), 44–57.

Cohen, D. K., Raudenbush, S. W., & Ball, D. L. (2003). Resources, instruction, and research. *Educational Evaluation and Policy Analysis, 25*(2), 119–142.

Cook, B. G., & Odom, S. L. (2013). Evidence-based practices and implementation science in special education. *Exceptional Children, 79*(2), 135–144.

Cornelius, K. E., & Nagro, S. A. (2014). Evaluating the evidence base of performance feedback in preservice special education teacher training. *Teacher Education and Special Education, 37*(2), 133–146.

Council for Exceptional Children. (2014). *Council for Exceptional Children standards for evidence-based practices in special education. https://exceptionalchildren.org/sites/default/files/2021-04/EBP_FINAL.pdf*

Dall'Alba, G., & Sandberg, J. (2006). Unveiling professional development: A critical review of stage models. *Review of Educational Research, 76*(3), 383–412.

Desimone, L. M., & Hill, K. L. (2017). Inside the black box: Examining mediators and moderators of a middle school science intervention. *Educational Evaluation and Policy Analysis, 39*(3), 511–536.

Dingle, M., Brownell, M., Leko, M. M., Boardman, A., & Haager, D. (2011). Developing effective special education reading teachers: The influence of professional development, context, and individual qualities. *Learning Disability Quarterly, 34*(1), 87–103.

Ericsson, K. A. (2014). *The road to excellence: The acquisition of expert performance in the arts and sciences, sports, and games.* Psychology Press.

Fixsen, D. L., Naoom, S. F., Blase, K. A., Friedman, R. M., & Wallace, F. (2005). *Implementation research: A synthesis of the literature* (FMHI Publication #231). University of South Florida, Louis de la Parte Florida Mental Health Institute, National Implementation Research Network. *www.fpg.unc.edu/~nirn/resources/publications/Monograph/pdf/Monograph_full.pdf*

Fuchs, D., Fuchs, L., & Vaughn, S. (2014). What is intensive instruction and why is it important? *Teaching Exceptional Children, 46*(4), 13–18.

Gage, N. A., Scott, T., Hirn, R., & MacSuga-Gage, A. S. (2018). The relationship between teachers' implementation of classroom management practices and student behavior in elementary school. *Behavioral Disorders, 43*(2), 302–315.

Grossman, P. L., & McDonald, M. (2008). Back to the future: Directions for research in teaching and teacher education. *American Educational Research Journal, 45*(1), 184–205.

Harn, B., Basaraba, D., Chard, D., & Fritz, R. (2015). The impact of schoolwide prevention efforts: Lessons learned from implementing independent academic and behavior support systems. *Learning Disabilities: A Contemporary Journal, 13*(1), 3–20.

Harn, B. A., Chard, D. J., Biancarosa, G., & Kame'enui, E. J. (2011). Coordinating instructional supports to accelerate at-risk first-grade readers' performance: An essential mechanism for effective RTI. *The Elementary School Journal, 112*(2), 332–355.

Hiebert, J., Berk, D., & Miller, E. (2017). Relationships between mathematics teacher preparation and graduates' analyses of classroom teaching. *The Elementary School Journal, 117*(4), 687–707.

Hill, H. C., Lynch, K., Gonzaelz, K, & Pollard, C. (2020). Professional development that improves STEM outcomes: A meta-analysis attempts to discover what types of teacher learning are most likely to improve students' performance in STEM disciplines. *Phi Delta Kappan, 101*(5), 50–56.

Hill, H. C., & Papay, J. P. (2022). *Building better PL: How to strengthen teacher learning.* Research Partnership for Professional Learning. *https://annenberg.brown.edu/sites/default/files/rppl-building-better-pl.pdf*

Hudson, A. (2022). Upper elementary teachers' knowledge of reading comprehension, classroom practice, and student's performance in reading comprehension. *Reading Research Quarterly, 58*(3), 352–360.

Johnson, E., Zheng, Y., Crawford, A. R., & Moylan, L. A. (2021). The relationship of special education teacher performance on observation instruments with student outcomes. *Journal of Learning Disabilities, 54*(1), 54–65.

Johnson, E., Zheng, Y., Crawford, A. R., & Moylan, L. A. (2022). Evaluating an explicit instruction observation protocol through a validity argument approach. *The Journal of Experimental Education, 90*(2), 419–434.

Jordan, A., Glenn, C., & McGhie-Richmond, D. (2010). The supporting effective teaching (SET) project: The relationship of inclusive teaching practices to teachers' beliefs about disability and ability, and about their roles as teachers. *Teaching and Teacher Education: An International Journal of Research and Studies, 26*(2), 259–266.

Kennedy, M. M. (2016). How does professional development improve teaching? *Review of Educational Research, 86*(4), 945–980.

Klingner, J. K., Brownell, M. T., Mason, L. H., Sindelar, P. T., Benedict, A. E., Griffin, G. G., et al. (2016). Teaching students with special needs in the new millennium. In D. Gitomer & C. Bell (Eds.), *Handbook for research on teaching* (5th ed., pp. 639–717). American Educational Research Association.

Klingner, J. K., Urbach, J., Golos, D., Brownell, M. T., & Menon, S. (2010). Teaching reading in the 21st century: A glimpse at how special education teachers promote reading comprehension. *Learning Disability Quarterly, 33*(2), 59–75.

Kraft, M. A., Blazar, D., & Hogan, D. (2018). The effect of teacher coaching on instruction and achievement: A meta-analysis of the causal evidence. *Review of Educational Research, 88*(4), 547–588.

Lauterbach, A. A., Brownell, M. T., & Bettini, E. A. (2020). Expert secondary content-area teachers' pedagogical schemas for teaching literacy to students with learning disabilities. *Learning Disability Quarterly, 43*(4), 227–240.

Lefstein, A., Vedder-Weiss, D., & Segal, A. (2020). Relocating research on teacher learning: Toward pedagogically productive talk. *Educational Researcher, 49*(5), 360–368.

Leko, M. M., & Brownell, M. T. (2011). Special education preservice teachers' appropriation of pedagogical tools for teaching reading. *Exceptional Children, 77*(2), 229–251.

Leko, M. M., Brownell, M. T., O'Brien, K., & Nagro, S. A. (2024). Capitalizing on the potential of practice-based preparation in special education teacher preparation. In E. D. McCray, E. A. Bettini, P. T. Sindelar, J. McLeskey, & M. T. Brownell (Eds.), *Handbook of research on special education teacher preparation* (2nd ed., pp. 106–125). Routledge.

Leko, M. M., Kiely, M. T., Brownell, M. T., Osipova, A., Dingle, M., & Mundy, C. (2015). Understanding special educators' learning opportunities in collaborative groups: The role of discourse. *Teacher Education and Special Education, 38*(2), 138–157.

Leko, M. M., Kulkarni, S., Lin, M. C., & Smith, S. A. (2015). Delving deeper into the construct of preservice teacher beliefs about reading instruction for students with disabilities. *Teacher Education and Special Education, 38*(3), 186–206.

Leko, M. M., Roberts, C. A., & Pek, Y. (2015). A theory of secondary teachers' adaptations when implementing a reading intervention program. *The Journal of Special Education, 49*(3), 168–178.

Lemons, C. J., Vaughn, S., Wexler, J., Kearns, D., & Sinclair, A. C. (2018). Envisioning an improved continuum of special education services for students with learning disabilities: Considering intervention intensity. *Learning Disabilities Research and Practice, 33*(3), 131–143.

Lewis, C., & Perry, R. (2017). Lesson study to scale up research-based knowledge: A randomized, control trial of fractions learning. *Journal of Research in Mathematics Education, 48*(3), 261–299.

McDonald, M., Kazemi, E., & Kavanagh, S. S. (2013). Core practices and pedagogies of teacher education: A call for a common language and collective activity. *Journal of Teacher Education, 64*(5), 378–386.

McLeskey, J., Barringer, M. D., Billingsley, B., Brownell, M., Jackson, D., Kennedy, M., et al. (2017, January). *High leverage practices in special education.* Council for Exceptional Children and CEEDAR Center.

Nagro, S. A., & Cornelius, K. E. (2013). Evaluating the evidence base of video analysis: A special education teacher development tool. *Teacher Education and Special Education, 36*(4), 312–329.

Odom, S., Cox, A. E., & Brock, M. E. (2013). Implementation science, professional development, and Autism Spectrum Disorders. *Exceptional Children, 79*(3), 233–251.

Pak, K., Desimone, L. M., & Parsons, A. (2020). An integrative approach to professional development to support college- and career-readiness standards. *Education Policy Analysis Archives, 28*(111), 1–23.

Park, Y., Kiely, M. T., Brownell, M. T., & Benedict, A. (2019). Relationships among special education teachers' knowledge, instructional practice, and students' performance in reading fluency. *Learning Disabilities Research & Practice, 34*(2), 85–96.

Phelps, G., & Schilling, S. (2004). Developing measures of content knowledge for teaching reading. *Elementary School Journal, 105*, 31–48.

Pua, D., Peyton, D., Brownell, M. T., Contesse, V., & Jones, N. (2021). Preservice observation in special education: A validation study. *Journal of Learning Disabilities, 54*, 6–19.

Risko, V. J., Roller, C. M., Cummins, C., Bean, R. M., Block, C. C., Anders, P. L., & Flood, J. (2008). A critical analysis of research on reading teacher education. *Reading Research Quarterly, 43*(3), 252–288.

Rock, M. L., Gregg, M., Thead, B. K., Acker, S. E., Gable, R. A., & Zigmond, N. P. (2009). Can you hear me now? Evaluation of an online wireless technology to provide real-time feedback to special education teachers-in-training. *Teacher Education and Special Education, 32*(1), 64–82.

Scheeler, M. C., Budin, S., & Markelz, A. (2016). The role of teacher preparation in promoting evidence-based practices in schools. *Learning Disabilities: A Contemporary Journal, 14*(2), 171–187.

Sohn, H., Brownell, M. T., Huggins-Manley, C. A., Benedict, A. E., Williams, J., & Kelcey,

B. (2025). *Developing an observation protocol for tiered instruction: A validation study* [Manuscript submitted for publication].

Spear-Swerling, L., & Zibulsky, J. (2014). Making time for literacy: Teacher knowledge and time allocation in instructional planning. *Reading and Writing, 27*(8), 1353–1378.

Stanovich, P. J., & Jordan, A. (1998). Canadian teachers' and principals' beliefs about inclusive education as predictors of effective teaching in heterogeneous classrooms. *The Elementary School Journal, 98*(3), 221–238.

Stevens, E. A., Vaughn, S., Swanson, E., & Scammacca, N. (2020). Examining the effects of a Tier 2 reading comprehension intervention aligned to Tier 1 instruction for fourth grade struggling readers. *Exceptional Children, 86*(4), 430–448.

Stigler, J. W., & Hiebert, J. (1999). *The teaching gap: Best ideas from the world's teachers for improving in the classroom.* The Free Press.

Urbach, J., Moore, B. A., Klingner, J. K., Galman, S., Haager, D., Brownell, M. T., & Dingle, M. (2015). "That's my job" comparing the beliefs of more and less accomplished special educators related to their roles and responsibilities. *Teacher Education and Special Education, 38*(4), 323–336.

van Es, E. A., Tunney, J., Goldsmith, L. T., & Seago, N. (2014). A framework for the facilitation of teachers' analysis of video. *Journal of Teacher Education, 65*(4), 340–356.

Vaughn, S., Linan-Thompson, S., & Hickman, P. (2003). Response to instruction as a means of identifying students with reading/learning disabilities. *Exceptional Children, 69*(4), 391–409.

Wideen, M., Mayer-Smith, J., & Moon, B. (1998). A critical analysis of the research on learning to teach: Making the case for an ecological perspective on inquiry. *Review of Educational Research, 68*(2), 130–178.

Author Index

B

D

E

F

G

H

I

J

K

L

M

N

O

P

Q

R

S

T

U

V

W

Y

Z

Subject Index

Note. *f* or *t* following a page number indicates a figure or a table.

E

F

G

N

O

P

S

T

Z